Health Care Ethics
in Canada

Third Edition

Edited by

Françoise Baylis
Professor and Canada Research Chair
Dalhousie University

Barry Hoffmaster
Professor
University of Western Ontario

Susan Sherwin
University Research Professor, Emeritus
Dalhousie University

Kirstin Borgerson
Assistant Professor
Dalhousie University

NELSON

NELSON

Health Care Ethics in Canada
Third Edition

Edited by Françoise Baylis, Barry Hoffmaster
Susan Sherwin, and Kirstin Borgerson

Vice President, Editorial Higher Education:
Anne Williams

Acquisitions Editor:
Maya Castle

Senior Marketing Manager:
Amanda Henry

Senior Developmental Editor:
My Editor Inc.

Permissions Coordinator:
Natalie Russell

Content Production Manager:
Jennifer Hare

Production Service:
Integra

Copy Editor:
Erin Moore

Proofreader:
Integra

Production Coordinator:
Ferial Suleman

Design Director:
Ken Phipps

Managing Designer:
Franca Amore

Interior Design Revisions:
Dianna Little

Cover Design:
Martyn Schmoll

Cover Image:
© Diana Ong/SuperStock

Compositor:
Integra

**Library and Archives Canada
Cataloguing in Publication Data**

Health care ethics in Canada/
edited by Françoise Baylis…
[et al.].—3rd ed.

Includes bibliographical references.
ISBN 978-0-17-650464-9

1. Medical ethics—Canada.
I. Baylis, Françoise, 1961–

R724.H38 2011 174.20971
C2011-905303-9

ISBN-13: 978-0-17-650464-9
ISBN-10: 0-17-650464-8

Contents

Chapter 7: Clinical Research 301

Chapter 8: Reproduction 361

Preface

In 2004, when the second edition of *Health Care Ethics in Canada* was published, we noted with pride how in the time between the first and second editions, much had changed for the better in Canadian bioethics. That trend has continued such that both the quantity and quality of contemporary Canadian scholarship are very impressive. This has meant an even greater percentage of Canadian authors in the current edition, all of whom address issues of critical importance to the Canadian public. Indeed, with this third edition, Canadian content is at an all-time high at 70 percent. This is an important achievement as it means that students at Canadian institutions can now address ethical issues in a Canadian historical, political, social, and cultural context.

Students coming to ethics want to know what they will be studying, so they naturally seek a definition of "ethics." Despite the concerted efforts of philosophers, however, a comprehensive, rigorous, and plausible definition remains elusive. Yet the desire to know what ethics is cannot be evaded—particularly in a robustly practical area such as health care ethics, where "doing ethics" can have momentous impacts on people's lives and deaths. Instead of searching for a definition, another way to try to understand ethics in general, and health care ethics in particular, is by examining its methodology. Contemporary health care ethics began in a familiar, seemingly uncontroversial manner. It was taken to be an instance of "applied" ethics: the application of general moral theories and their associated rules or principles to the facts of particular cases to yield decisions about what ought to be done. A version of this "top-down" approach continues to dominate the practice and the pedagogy of health care ethics. In fact, a canonical set of principles for health care ethics has emerged: principles directed at preventing harm (non-maleficence), promoting good (beneficence), protecting freedom (respect for autonomy), and ensuring fairness (justice). These principles are routinely applied to problems that arise for patients and health care professionals, the kinds of problems that are widely regarded as constitutive of health care ethics because they implicate these principles.

As appealing as this methodological approach might be, it encounters serious difficulties. For a number of reasons, principles alone cannot always determine appropriate actions or justify decisions about how to resolve particular moral quandaries. Judgments have to be made about many crucial matters, including what features of a situation are morally salient; which principles are relevant to a situation; whether the specific features of a situation can be classified under the general terms of a principle; and which principle takes precedence when there is a conflict. Applying principles is by no means easy or straightforward, and the process requires resources beyond the principles themselves. That recognition has instigated considerable methodological development in health care ethics.

The first reaction to the difficulties inherent in a "top-down" approach to applied ethics was to shift from principles to particulars: to develop a "bottom-up" approach to health care ethics. Rather than beginning with principles and attempting to derive decisions from them, a "bottom-up" approach begins with cases and extrapolates decisions for new cases from decisions in previous cases. Its models are the operation of the doctrine of precedent in Anglo-American case law and the once influential tradition of moral casuistry. With this approach, a case with a clear resolution is identified, and then a decision for a related case is reached via an argument by analogy. Proponents of a "bottom-up" approach have more confidence in our ability to decide what is right and wrong for concrete, specific cases than our ability to justify decisions in terms of general principles. Nevertheless, it is hard to jettison principles from a "bottom-up" approach. Constructing a strong argument by analogy requires that relevant similarities and dissimilarities between cases be identified, and that the comparative significance of those similarities and dissimilarities be evaluated. Unguided by theoretical commitments of the sort embodied in principles, decisions about those matters can appear capricious.

The goal of "top-down" and "bottom-up" methodologies is to provide moral guidance and justification for moral decisions. In a "top-down" approach, the justification is a deductive argument; in a "bottom-up" approach the justification is an argument by analogy. The refractory problems with both approaches have prompted a more radical methodological move: the introduction of narrative ethics, which pursues the goal of understanding rather than justification. Narratives or stories connect events not in terms of temporal sequence, causation, or logical relationships, but in terms of meaning. Stories enable us to understand why a person or character perceived something in a certain way, felt and deliberated in a certain manner, and made a certain choice. They broaden our understanding of how other people live and what possibilities are open to us. It has even been proposed that we should regard our own lives as narratives and make decisions so as to create unified, coherent stories for ourselves. Narratives can convey the complexity, the quirkiness, and the messiness of life, can engage our emotions, and can reveal new sources of meaning. But how does the understanding they yield help us make moral decisions? How do we determine whether a story is true or whether one story is better than another? How does a story help us make a particular choice or adopt a way of life? Can concerns about justification simply be ignored?

The quest for understanding has also induced efforts to put moral issues in context. Principles are stated in spare and abstract terms, but the meanings those principles acquire and the moral problems on which they are brought to bear are dense and complicated. Those meanings are functions of the cultural, social, and historical backgrounds; the political, economic, and legal settings; the institutional and organizational structures; and the beliefs and values in which they are implicated. Real moral problems are complex, multi-layered, and ill-defined. Addressing them requires a perceptiveness that is formed by a variety of perspectives and that appreciates the realities that shape and constrain those problems. Feminist theories, for example, emphasize how the oppression of women (and other social groups) is located in and sustained by overlapping theoretical and practical contexts. The deeply contextual nature of moral problems makes moral progress a matter of social criticism and action, not just intellectual inquiry. But, again, concerns about justification are hard to ignore. What makes social criticism legitimate and telling? What vindicates movements for social reform? And what, ultimately, is the basis for determining that social change represents moral progress?

The methodological ferment in health care ethics is unlikely to abate. Providing accounts of what ethics is, and how ethics is done, remains a daunting theoretical and practical challenge. It is impossible to capture this challenge in a few readings, and Chapter 1 does not make that attempt. Rather, Chapter 1 offers a general orientation to ethics and health care ethics and presents conceptual terminology and tools that are helpful for identifying and addressing moral problems. It contains a selection of methodological perspectives illustrating the diverse approaches that are taken to specific topics in the readings that follow.

Topics addressed in the rest of the book raise important issues of health care ethics, and recognize the new directions and new guises these issues have assumed. Chapters 2 and 3 examine the Canadian health care system and the principled and practical challenges it faces. Chapter 2 focuses on the design, structure, and operation of our health care system with particular attention to underlying values. As we learn in this chapter, matters related to the just allocation of health care resources must be examined in the context of judicial decisions about the responsibilities of provincial governments to fund particular health care services. Chapter 3 then raises concerns about justice for more specific problems of resource allocation, recognizing that our publicly funded system is stretched to, and sometimes beyond, a point that both patients and providers find acceptable. Chapter 4 also examines issues of justice, but from a decidedly more communal perspective. The focus here is not on decision-making at the bedside (or in the research lab), but on policy choices from which all might benefit in terms of improved public health.

Chapter 5 is about the relationship between patients and providers. The relationship must be conceived in a way that fosters genuine trust, understands patient vulnerability, and promotes communication—communication that is more than just a professional dispensing intelligible information and a patient accurately recalling that information. Chapter 6, on autonomy and informed consent, addresses classic issues for contemporary North American bioethics where respect for patient autonomy is a predominant value. At the outset of this chapter there is an attempt to reframe this value in relational terms. Subsequent articles then consider the two key components of decision-making in health care: consent and competence. Chapter 7, on research involving humans, addresses a wide range of issues starting with an important debate on the meaning and scope of therapeutic misconception and its relevance for informed consent. An ethical assessment of research involving humans is no longer limited to protecting participants, but must also consider the just distribution of the benefits, not merely the burdens, of research. In addition, given the development of governmental and university partnerships with private companies, the manifold ways in which economic incentives can create conflicts of interest and corrupt research now require careful scrutiny as do conflicts of interest in multi-jurisdictional research.

Chapter 8 is devoted to topics in reproduction and includes articles on abortion, assisted human reproduction, and prenatal genetic testing. Chapter 9 is on end-of life care and it starts with a pointed discussion about the ever-challenging question: who decides who lives and who dies? There are articles on assisted suicide, euthanasia, and terminal sedation. The final chapter, Chapter 10, examines some of the challenges posed by scientific progress. Do we accept ourselves as we are, or embrace opportunities for enhancement be they surgical, chemical, or genetic enhancements? What about the prospect of human cloning? What is the proper response to stem cell research?

Each chapter includes a section on Useful Resources and most chapters also include brief summaries of relevant Canadian legal cases for discussion (along with questions to consider). This is not to suggest that the law and ethics are the same or even that they are always compatible. But legal decisions do shape the Canadian health care landscape and often involve moral reasoning. We think it important for an introductory textbook in Canadian bioethics to provide students with some background about "classic" Canadian cases.

With its expanded Canadian content, its new organization, and its new resources, the third edition provides a comprehensive introduction to health care ethics in Canada.

ACKNOWLEDGEMENTS

Sincere thanks are owed to Tom Wallwork for invaluable research assistance in the preparation of this book.

We also thank those instructors who provided comments and suggestions throughout the development of this third edition text:

Chris Kaposy, Memorial University of Newfoundland

Jeremy Snyder, Simon Fraser University

Jeff McLaughlin, Thompson Rivers University

Barbara Secker, University of Toronto

Ken Kirkwood, University of Western Ontario

Melany Banks, Wilfrid Laurier University

About the Editors

FRANÇOISE BAYLIS, Professor and Canada Research Chair in Bioethics and Philosophy at Dalhousie University, is one of Canada's public intellectuals. She is a frequent guest on CBC and Radio Canada and author of many news stories that give us a "behind the scenes" look at deep-seated ethical issues. Her interests are many and varied, and she has a love of thought-provoking questions. Stem cell research, research involving pregnant women, H1N1 vaccines, pharma funding of medical research and education, face transplantation—these are but a few of the issues on which she works. All of her research and policy consultation is informed by a strong commitment to the common good.

BARRY HOFFMASTER, Professor in the Department of Philosophy at the University of Western Ontario, teaches and writes about bioethics and philosophy of law. He was the Director of the Department's Ph.D. Program in Biomedical Ethics, and in preparing for that position over several years, he spent time in a diverse array of clinical settings. That experience changed his mind about the nature of morality; he learned that morality is a human endeavour, not a theory, and that people, not principles, are the centrepiece of morality. His participation in clinical settings continued while he served as the Director of the Westminster Institute for Ethics and Human Values and reaffirmed his conviction about the importance of empirical work in bioethics. He is a past President of the Canadian Bioethics Society and the first Canadian elected as a Fellow of The Hastings Center. With a former colleague, he is working on a book that recognizes the inevitability of judgment in bioethics, and everywhere else in life, and that provides an account of the rationality of judgment.

SUSAN SHERWIN, University Research Professor, Emeritus, Department of Philosophy at Dalhousie University is widely known in Canada and internationally for her theoretical contributions to bioethics and feminist ethics. Her books, *No Longer Patient* and *The Politics of Women's Health,* helped to launch the interdisciplinary field of feminist bioethics. She has served on national advisory committees dealing with reproductive and genetic technologies and public health ethics. Her influence in these areas has been recognized by her winning the Killam Prize in Humanities (2006) and the Lifetime Achievement Award of the Canadian Bioethics Society (2007).

KIRSTIN BORGERSON, Assistant Professor of Philosophy at Dalhousie University, is the newest member of the editorial team for *Health Care Ethics in Canada*. Kirstin researches and teaches in medical epistemology and medical ethics and spends quite a lot of time thinking about how health care professionals should answer the question, "What's your evidence for that?" She currently holds a CIHR Catalyst Grant in Ethics and is investigating whether medical researchers have an ethical obligation to adjust their methods or questions in order to conduct research on matters of greatest clinical importance. Kirstin's research and teaching is shaped by her upbringing in Saskatchewan and a deep commitment to the vision of public health care developed and defended by her parents, grandparents, and great-grandparents.

Chapter 1   THEORY AND METHOD

INTRODUCTION

Health care ethics (what many term "bioethics") encompasses questions regarding moral behaviour and policy in the realm of health. It is as vast and diverse as health practices themselves and includes different approaches to ethics as well as to health. Ethics includes both (1) questions of theory regarding such matters as the nature of right and wrong actions, good and bad character, valued and devalued outcomes, and justice and injustice, and (2) practical questions regarding the moral (ethical) acceptability of particular practices and policies. Those interested in the first set of questions seek to understand and properly apply central concepts such as right, good, and just along with their contraries. Those interested in the second set of questions want to know such things as whether we must always tell the truth, if it is ever morally permissible to end a human life deliberately, and how much information must be presented to ensure a research subject is giving informed consent. Neither set of questions can be answered satisfactorily without some engagement with the other set, but it is certainly possible to focus most of one's attention on one set over the other.

In health care ethics, attention is primarily focused on questions of the second sort, exploring practical decisions about specific types of behaviour and policies in the realm of health. Most discussions address questions that are in dispute—where reasonable people disagree about what morality requires in a particular realm. Hence, in this book, the articles deal with questions about health practices in Canada that are currently subject to debate. Although none of the articles address practices for which there is widespread agreement about the ethical demands of the situation, readers should not infer from this absence that there is no consensus on ethical matters. In fact, Canadians agree on the ethics of many familiar health practices, including the requirements that (barring exceptional circumstances) health care providers should seek to protect and promote the health and well-being of their patients, should not knowingly act in ways that will worsen their patients' health, should not mislead their patients, and should treat all patients fairly. Beyond the many areas of ethical agreement, there remain a large number of health practices that are contentious and the editors hope that the opportunity to explore on-going debates around some of these controversial topics will help readers learn valuable ways of identifying and engaging with these and other ethical topics in health care.

In most of the articles, the authors propose and defend normative (or prescriptive) positions regarding the morally correct behaviour or policy in the area they address; they propose that people *should* act in particular ways in certain types of circumstances (and *should not* act in contrary ways). The authors are well aware that some people hold different positions and so they provide reasoned arguments in defence of their own views, and, often, they offer reasons for rejecting some of the views with which they disagree. They argue that a certain type of action or policy is morally required, morally wrong, or morally permissible, explaining *why* they believe things should be done in a particular way in the domain they are addressing. In each case, readers will have to judge the quality of the reasons offered and consider carefully whether the author has provided a compelling case for the position proposed or whether there is something more to be said in defence of an alternative position. It is unlikely that any reader will agree with every author in this text, but it is hoped that each reader will be able to offer reasons in support of their own position— whether it is one of agreement or disagreement with the author of the target article.

In order to engage in the sort of ethical discussion represented by the authors of the various articles and encouraged of our readers, it is important to reflect on some of the first type of questions about ethics—namely those concerned with the nature of ethics and what makes particular actions, policies, or persons morally right or wrong. Theoretical ethics involves reflection on these sorts of questions, seeking guidance for determining what is morally expected of agents and also providing a basis for justifying moral positions that are articulated. There are many different approaches available for identifying and investigating questions in ethics and debate about these options occupies a great deal of the attention of philosophers who work in the realm of theoretical and normative ethics.

We offer a very brief summary of a few key theoretical positions within ethics that guide much of the discussion in practical moral debates, identifying the distinctions that characterize some of the central theoretical options. One common distinction has to do with the focus of ethics attention on either (1) persons or (2) actions (singly or collectively through policies). In the first category, virtue theories focus on the moral nature of persons and are concerned with determining and advising on questions of character (e.g., honesty, compassion, and fairness as well as moral failings such as greed, self-centredness, and rashness). This approach may discuss the goodness of persons overall or their moral goodness in particular roles (e.g., doctor, nurse, or spouse). Other approaches to the judgment of persons examine the role of individuals within relationships (personal, professional, and/or political).

The majority of ethical theorists situate themselves in the second category, in that they seek ways of determining whether actions are morally right, wrong, or neutral. Some argue that it is important to determine whether actions are required (or forbidden) as a matter of duty or as a response to someone's rights claim. Actions such as unjust killing, breaking promises, lying, stealing, and causing harm to others are prohibited unless there are overriding moral reasons for making an exception. Similarly, we have duties to care for those to whom we have particular obligations (e.g., our young children), to be compassionate, and to act fairly. Theorists who believe duty is at the heart of moral deliberation are called deontologists and the most famous of this group is the 18th century German philosopher Immanuel Kant. One of the rules he is best known for in bioethics commands us to treat other persons as ends and not merely as means—in other words, we must respect the independent judgment of persons and not use them for our own purposes without their voluntary consent.

Another way to make moral judgments about actions is to evaluate them according to the moral worth of their likely consequences. Those who adopt this strategy are known as consequentialists and they propose that we decide on the morally best actions (or practices or policies) by considering the available options, trying to predict the likely consequences or outcomes of each option, and then choosing the one that is most likely to produce the best outcome. In some circumstances, all options will produce undesirable outcomes and we must then choose the option likely to do the least amount of harm. There are many different versions of consequentialism since theorists disagree about what is morally important in judging the outcome of actions. Those known as utilitarians believe we should judge outcomes according to a single scale of positive and negative utility. A particularly influential utilitarian was the 19th century British philosopher John Stuart Mill who proposed happiness and unhappiness as the appropriate scale for measuring utility. He is credited with promoting the principle of utility, which says that actions are right in proportion to their tendency to promote happiness and wrong in proportion to their tendency to promote the reverse of happiness. (The principle is also summarized as saying we should act to promote the greatest overall happiness for the greatest number.) Like all utilitarians, Mill emphasized the importance of considering the consequences of actions on everyone likely to be affected and to weigh each person's interests equally with that of every other person. Many bioethics discussions involve some attention to likely consequences, though often in the context of a mixed approach that includes some commitments that cannot be altered by consequences (such as the rule against unjust killing).

Other theorists pursue other dimensions of ethics in their approach to moral dilemmas. Some attend to considerations of justice; others to principles of ideal social consensus (social contract theorists); still others to community cohesion (communitarians). And some theorists do not use the language of ethics explicitly at all. They offer descriptions of a situation that is framed by particular values such as fairness or a commitment to maximizing happiness and exploring ways in which the situation may be improved or worsened by a change in practice. They are doing ethics but their theoretical orientation is implicit rather than explicit. While many moral agents find their motivation for seeking to act morally in their religious beliefs, most find that they still need to interpret those beliefs in particular contexts. Many questions in bioethics involve new scientific knowledge and technologies (e.g., genetics, assisted reproduction, and life-supporting ventilation) that are not discussed in historical religious texts, requiring even the most devout agent to explore moral reasoning on these topics.

In this chapter, we offer articles that represent a few different kinds of positions that theorists adopt when wrestling with difficult moral questions without attempting to be either exhaustive or exclusive. These articles provide the reader with some vocabulary for identifying different types of moral theories and positions and strategies for applying them. It is important to reflect on the theoretical options authors take up, since each orientation directs readers' attention to specific types of concerns about the practice in question and also renders obscure some other features of the practice.

In the first article, Ruth Faden, Tom Beauchamp, and Nancy King outline an approach that has come to be known as principlism. Rather than endorse any particular foundational moral theory, they propose settling on some widely shared mid-level moral principles: respect for autonomy, beneficence, and justice. Together, these three principles can help to guide behaviour in health care contexts by supporting more specific moral rules such as seek patient consent. Principles may conflict in particular situations, requiring the agent to determine the appropriate balance among the three.

James Childress does not offer an alternative moral theory, per se, but discusses a key method widely used in bioethics: analogical and metaphorical thinking. Often, we can best understand a phenomenon by thinking of analogous cases on which we have clearer intuitions. Sometimes the process of appealing to analogy is made explicit, as, for example, when anti-abortion advocates claim that fetuses are similar to newborn children and should be accorded the same rights. Other times, the analogy is simply implied through the use of metaphors that suggest a way of thinking about a topic; for example, thinking of medicine as involved in a war against disease encourages certain attitudes, relationships, and practices that appear to be natural without further examination of the implicit metaphor.

Margaret Little and Joseph Kaufert remind us that bioethics is always situated in a particular historical, social, and political context and that, far too often, it reflects the interests and perspective of dominant political groups. Whatever ethical theory we might adopt, it is essential that we also attend to the distinct perspectives of voices that have historically been ignored or otherwise marginalized when thinking about issues in health care ethics. Little reviews some of the ways in which ethics and bioethics have tended to be male-centred and to appeal to gendered concepts. A feminist approach can help to reveal and counter the pervasive male bias within ethical thinking. Kaufert is interested in the ways in which bioethicists often appeal to case studies; he objects to their tendency to work with very thin case descriptions that are stripped of important details. In contrast, he provides a life narrative approach that is attentive to specific details of the life in question and shows its value for discussing the case of a person living with progressive disability who chooses to discontinue life support.

Readers of this volume are encouraged to try to identify the various ethical perspectives underlying specific articles and to consider how a different perspective might bring different dimensions of the situation to the fore. They should explore their own ideas about what is morally important on the various topics addressed. Ethics involves reflection and constructive debate on matters of moral concern and readers should see themselves as important participants in discussions of the matters addressed.

Foundations in Moral Theory

Ruth R. Faden, Tom L. Beauchamp, and Nancy M.P. King

PRINCIPLES, RULES, AND RIGHTS

Moral deliberation and justification rest on principles, rules, and rights, understood as abstract action-guides. These general guides and their relationships will be the focus of our attention in this section. However, before we turn directly to them, some background assumptions regarding the words "ethics," "morality," and "moral philosophy" deserve mention.

The Concept of Morality

The word "morality" has meanings that extend beyond philosophical contexts and professional codes of conduct. Morality is concerned with practices defining right and wrong that are usually transmitted within a culture or institution from generation to generation, together with other kinds of customs and rules. Morality denotes a social institution, composed of a set of standards pervasively acknowledged by the members of the culture. In this respect, it has an objective, ongoing status as a body of action guides. Like political constitutions and natural languages, morality exists prior to the acceptance (or rejection) of its rules and regulations by particular individuals. Its standards are usually abstract, uncodified, and applicable to behavior in many diverse circumstances.

The terms "ethical theory and "moral philosophy," by contrast, suggest *reflection* on the institution of morality. These terms refer to attempts to introduce clarity, substance, and precision of argument into the domain of morality. Moral philosophers seek to put moral beliefs and social practices of morality into a more unified and defensible package of action-guides by challenging presuppositions, assessing moral arguments, and suggesting modifications in existing beliefs. Their task often centers on "justification": Philosophers seek to justify a system of standards or some moral point of view on the basis of carefully analyzed and defended theories and principles, such as respect for autonomy, distributive justice, equal treatment, human rights, beneficence, nonmaleficence, and utility—some of the principles commonly employed in contemporary moral philosophy.

Despite these rough distinctions, we shall use the terms "moral" and "ethical" as synonymous, and "moral philosophy" and "ethical theory" will also be used interchangeably. "Morality," however, will be confined to social practice.

Reasoning by Principles

Philosophers try to exhibit how to avoid confusing a merely personal attitude or religious dogma with a reasoned and justified moral position.

Accordingly, moral philosophy offers principles for the development and evaluation of moral arguments. Rights, duties, obligations, and the like derive from these principles. ("Values" is a still more general term, and one we shall rarely employ.) Such principles—the choice and analysis of which are controversial—constitute the heart of modern ethical theory.... Most of these principles are already embedded in public morality and policies, but only in a vague and imprecise form. The job of ethical theory is to lend precision without oversimplification. It should always be remembered that moral debate about a particular course of action or controversy is often rooted not only in disagreement about the proper interpretation of applicable moral principles, but also in the interpretation of factual information and in divergent assessments of the proper scientific, metaphysical, or religious description of a situation.

Although it is neither possible nor necessary to outline a full ethical theory in this volume, three moral principles relevant to our subject matter need to be addressed and briefly analyzed: respect for autonomy, beneficence, and justice. These broad principles provide the basis for the more specific rules and requirements found in professional codes of medical and research ethics.... We shall not here debate whether these three principles jointly form a *complete* moral system nor whether other moral principles are distinct or derivative from these three principles....

Rights as Correlative to Duties

Only recently has Western society emphasized the importance of human rights, and only recently have rights come to play an important role in public policy discussions.... Rights are powerful assertions of claims that demand respect and status, and they occupy a prominent place in moral theory and political documents. If someone appeals to rights, a response is demanded. We must accept the person's claim as valid, discredit it by countervailing considerations, or acknowledge the right but show how it can be overridden by competing moral claims.

Legal rights are widely acknowledged and codified, but the status of moral rights is more puzzling. Some thinkers are skeptical of their validity; others find absurd the profusion of rights and the conflicts resulting from their various claims. Absurd or otherwise, rights language has been extended to many controversial arenas—rights to privacy, rights to health care, rights of children, rights of animals, rights of the elderly, rights to confidential information, rights to shelter, and so on. How, then, are we to understand the language and basis of rights in moral discourse, and what is the relationship between one person's rights and another's duties?

A plausible claim is that a right always entails the imposition of a duty on others either not to interfere or to provide something, both the duty and the right being justified by the same overarching principle. Thus, if as a matter of justice a state promises or otherwise incurs a duty to provide such goods as influenza shots or other medical care to needy citizens, then citizens can claim an entitlement or right to that care if they meet the relevant criteria. The right to die, the right to privacy, the right to be free to make a decision, and all other so-called negative rights, which are often grounded in respect for autonomy, may be treated as entailing someone else's duty to abstain from interference with one's intended course in life.

If our treatment of the "correlativity thesis" is correct, little is distinctive about rights as a moral category. As with duties, the moral basis for their assertion simply rests in moral principles. Although it remains controversial in contemporary ethical theory whether rights are based on duties, duties based on rights, or neither based on the other, we have tried to circumvent this controversy by holding that the principles in a moral system both impose duties and confer rights....

THREE PRINCIPLES

Respect for Autonomy

Respect for autonomy is... conceived as a principle rooted in the liberal Western tradition of the importance of individual freedom and choice, both for political life and for personal development. "Autonomy" and "respect for autonomy" are terms loosely associated with several ideas, such as privacy, voluntariness, self-mastery, choosing freely, the freedom to choose, choosing one's own moral position, and accepting responsibility for one's choices....

Historically, the word "autonomy" is a legacy from ancient Greece, where *autos* (self) and *nomos* (rule or law) were joined to refer to political self-governance in the city-state. In moral philosophy, personal autonomy has come to refer to personal self-governance: personal rule of the self by adequate understanding while remaining free from controlling interferences by others and from personal limitations that prevent choice. "Autonomy," so understood, has been loosely analyzed in terms of external non-constraint and the presence of critical internal capacities integral to self-governance.[1] But, again, major confusion can emerge over the precise analysis of autonomy if we move beyond the core idea that the autonomous person is not bound by controlling constraints and is in control of personal affairs.

Almost all existing analyses of autonomy focus on the autonomous *person*. Our central interest, however, is in autonomous *choice*—or, more generally, autonomous *action*. This distinction is between (1) persons who have the capacity to be independent and in control, and (2) the actions that reflect the exercise of those capacities. This distinction may be thought trivial because it might seem by definition that only autonomous persons act autonomously. However... the criteria of autonomous choices are not identical with the criteria of autonomous persons. Autonomous persons can and do make non-autonomous choices owing to temporary constraints such as ignorance or coercion....

It is one thing to be autonomous, and another to be *respected* as autonomous.... To respect an autonomous agent is to recognize with due appreciation that person's capacities and perspective, including his or her right to hold certain views, to make certain choices, and to take certain actions based on personal values and beliefs. Such respect has historically been connected to the idea that persons possess an intrinsic value independent of special circumstances that confer value. As expressed in Kantian philosophy, autonomous persons are ends in themselves, determining their own destiny, and are not to be treated merely as means to the ends of others.[2] Thus, the burden of moral justification rests on those who would restrict or prevent a person's exercise of autonomy.

The moral demand that we respect the autonomy of persons can be formulated as a *principle of respect for autonomy*: Persons should be free to choose and act without controlling constraints imposed by others. The principle provides the justificatory basis for the right to make autonomous decisions, which in turn takes the form of specific autonomy-related rights. For example, in the debate over whether autonomous, informed patients have the right to refuse self-regarding, life-sustaining medical interventions,[3] the principle of respect for autonomy suggests a morally appropriate response....

Beneficence

The welfare of the patient is the goal of health care and also of what is often called "therapeutic research." This welfare objective is medicine's context and justification: Clinical therapies are aimed at the promotion of health by cure or prevention of disease. This value of benefiting the person has long been treated as a foundational value—and sometimes as *the* foundational value—in medical ethics. For example, a celebrated principle in the history of medical codes of ethics is the maxim *primum non nocere*—"above all, do no harm"—commonly viewed as the fundamental maxim of the Hippocratic tradition in medicine. Recent scholarship has shown that in the Hippocratic writings the more precise formulation of the primary moral injunctions is "help, or at least do no harm,"[4] thus demanding the provision of benefit beyond mere avoidance of harm.

The principle of beneficence includes the following four elements, all linked through the common theme of promoting the welfare of others:[5] (1) one ought not to inflict evil or harm; (2) one ought to prevent evil or harm; (3) one ought to remove evil or harm; (4) one ought to do or promote good. Many philosophers have held that the fourth element may not, strictly speaking, be a duty; and some have claimed that these elements should be hierarchically arranged so that the first takes precedence over the second, the second over the third, and the third over the fourth.

There is a definite appeal to this hierarchical ordering internal to the principle of beneficence. In particular, good philosophical reasons exist for separating passive nonmaleficence (a so-called negative duty to avoid doing harm, as expressed in 1) and active beneficence (a so-called positive duty to afford assistance, as expressed in 2–4). Ordinary moral discourse and many philosophical systems suggest that negative duties not to injure others are more compelling than positive duties to benefit others.[6] For example, we do not consider it justifiable to kill a dying patient in order to use the patient's organs to save two others. Similarly, the duty not to injure a patient by abandonment seems to many stronger than the duty to prevent injury to a patient who has been abandoned by another (under the assumption that both are moral duties).

Despite the attractiveness of this hierarchical ordering rule, it is not firmly sanctioned by either morality or ethical theory. The duty expressed in (1) may not *always* outweigh those expressed in (2–4). For example, the harm inflicted in (1) may be negligible or trivial, while the harm to be prevented in (2) may be substantial. For instance, saving a person's life by a blood transfusion justifies the inflicted harms of venipuncture on the blood donor. One of the motivations for separating nonmaleficence from beneficence is that they themselves conflict when one must *either* avoid harm *or* bring aid. In such cases, one needs a decision rule to prefer one alternative to another. But if the weights of the two principles can vary, as they can, there can be no mechanical decision rule asserting that one principle must always outweigh the other.

In concrete cases, the conceptual distinctions between 1–4 begin to break down, at least in application. For example, if a physician pre-scribes morphine for a patient in extreme pain, is she providing a benefit (4) or removing a harm (3) or both? Similarly, when the state provides certain needed medical treatments to citizens, it can be argued that the state is not only providing a benefit (4), but also preventing and removing the harms of illness and death (2 and 3). To avoid running down a child playing in the street—that is, to refrain from doing harm (1)—requires positive steps of braking, turning, warning, and the like.[7]

Such problems lead us to unify the moral demands that we should benefit and not injure others under a single principle of beneficence, taking care to distinguish, as necessary, between strong and weak requirements of this principle. The strength of these requirements corresponds only in some cases to the ordering of 1–4. In its general form, then, the principle of beneficence requires us to abstain from intentionally injuring others, and to further the important and legitimate interests of others, largely by preventing or removing possible harms.

There are several problems with the principle, so understood. For example, to what extent does the principle require the benefactor to assume personal risk or to suffer harm? Although it is widely agreed that we are obligated to act beneficently only if we can do so with minimal personal risk or inconvenience,[8] are there no conditions—special circumstances or role relationships—in which we are obligated to act beneficently even in the face of significant personal risk? Are not parents morally bound to sacrifice time and financial resources for their children? But would a stranger to the child be so bound?

A related problem is determining in any given instance to whom duties of beneficence are owed. Whose interests count, and whose count the most? The principle of beneficence should not, as a *principle*, be restricted to single parties even in special contests such as the patient-physician or subject-researcher relationship. Thus, the principle itself leaves open the question as to whom one's beneficence should be directed. For example, in the soliciting of consent to therapeutic research, there may be duties of beneficence to numerous third parties (future patients, employers, the state, endangered parties, etc.), even if the patient-subject's interests are the primary reason for an action. But third parties may not always have interests that should count.

Another vexing problem in ethical theory concerns the extent to which the principle of beneficence generates moral *duties*. Any analysis of beneficence that includes element (4) potentially demands severe sacrifice and extreme generosity in the moral life—for example, giving a kidney for transplantation or donating bone marrow. As a result, some philosophers have argued that this form of beneficent action is virtuous and a moral *ideal*, but not a duty. From this perspective, the positive benefiting of others is based on personal ideals that are supererogatory rather than obligatory: We are not morally *required* to promote the good of persons, even if we are in a position to do so, and even if the action is morally *justified*. The underlying problem is that actions such as sacrificing bodily parts and loving one's enemies may be more costly to the agent than morality demands.

Several proposals have been offered in moral philosophy to resolve this problem by showing that beneficence *is* a principle of duty, but these theoretical ventures are extraneous to our concerns here.[9] The scope or range of acts required by the duty of beneficence is an undecided issue, and perhaps an undecidable one. Fortunately, our arguments do not depend on its resolution. That we are morally obligated on *some* occasions to assist others is hardly a matter of moral controversy. Beneficent acts are demanded by the roles involved in fiduciary relationships between health care professionals and patients, lawyers and clients, researchers and subjects (at least in therapeutic research), bankers and customers, and so on. For example, physicians on duty in an emergency room are obligated to attend to injured, delirious, uncooperative patients, sometimes at considerable risk both to themselves and to the patient.

We will treat the basic roles and concepts that give substance to the principle of beneficence in medicine as follows: The positive benefit the physician is obligated to seek is the alleviation of disease and injury, if there is a reasonable hope of cure. The harms to be prevented, removed, or minimized are the pain, suffering, and disability of injury and disease. In addition, the physician is of course enjoined from *doing* harm if interventions inflict unnecessary pain and suffering on patients. While these considerations are all included under beneficence, we view the idea of a lexical ordering of sub-principles as an expendable overgeneralization.

In therapeutic research, the benefits and harms presented to subjects parallel those in medicine—the cure, removal, or prevention of pain, suffering, disability, and disease. In nontherapeutic research, the subjects' interests are less at center stage, because the positive benefit sought by the scientist is new knowledge. Often (but not necessarily) this knowledge is desired because it is expected to contribute to the resolution of important medical or social problems. Therapeutic and nontherapeutic research thus differ in the kinds of benefits each hopes to achieve. Although in both there is an equally strong imperative to avoid harming the subject, therapeutic research may legitimately present increased potential for harms if they are balanced by a commensurate possibility of benefits to the subject.

Those engaged in both medical practice and research know that risks of harm presented by interventions must constantly be weighed against possible benefits for patients, subjects, or the public interest. The physician who professes to "do no harm" is not pledging never to cause harm but rather to strive to create a positive balance of goods over inflicted harms. This is recognized in the Nuremberg Code, which enjoins: "The degree of risk to be taken should never exceed that determined by the humanitarian importance of the problem to be solved by the experiment."[10] Such a balancing principle is essential to any sound moral system: Beneficence assumes an obligation to weigh and balance benefits against harms, benefits against alternative benefits, and harms against alternative harms.

Health care professionals and research investigators often disagree over how to balance the various factors, and there may be no objective evidence that dictates one course rather than another.[11] In clinical contexts, this balancing can also present situations in which health care professionals and patients differ in their assessments of the professional's obligations. In some cases, benefit to another is involved—as, for example, when a pregnant woman refuses a physician's recommendation of fetal surgery. In other cases the refusal may be exclusively self-regarding. Some health care professionals will accept a patient's refusal as valid, whereas others are inclined to ignore the fact that an informed consent to treatment has not been given, and so try to "benefit" the patient through a medical intervention.

This problem of whether to override the decisions of patients in order to benefit them or prevent harm to them is one dimension of the problem of medical paternalism, in which a parental-like decision by a professional overrides an autonomous decision of a patient....

In health care, professionals and patients alike see the authority for some decisions as properly the patient's and authority for other decisions as primarily the professional's. It is widely agreed, for example, that the choice of a birth control method is properly the patient's but that the decision to administer a sedative to a panicked patient in an emergency room is properly the physician's. However, many cases in medicine exhibit no clear consensus about legitimate decisionmaking authority—for instance, who should decide which aggressive therapy, if any, to administer to a cancer victim or whether to prolong the lives of severely handicapped newborns by medical interventions? Similar disputes appear in the research context—for example, as to whether the researcher has the authority to use persons without their knowledge as subjects in low-risk research.

Decisions regarding who ought to serve as the legitimate authority—patient, subject, or professional—can turn decisively on what will maximally promote the patient's or subject's welfare. Standing behind the position that authority should rest with the patients or subjects may be the goal of benefiting patients and subjects by enabling them to make the decision that best promotes their welfare. Promotion of the value of autonomous choice in medical decisionmaking by patients is often justified by arguments from beneficence to the effect that decisional autonomy by patients enables them to survive, heal, or otherwise improve their own health. These arguments range from the simple contention that making one's own decisions promote one's psychological well-being to the more controversial observation that patients generally know themselves well enough to be the best judges, ultimately, of what is most beneficial for them. Similar arguments are also used in research contexts where it is maintained that requiring the informed consent of subjects will serve as a curb on research risks. Here autonomous choice is valued extrinsically for the sake of health or welfare rather than intrinsically for its own sake.

Justice

Every civilized society is a cooperative venture structured by moral, legal, and cultural principles that define the terms of social cooperation. Beneficence and respect for autonomy are principles in this fabric of social order, but *justice* has been perhaps the subject of more treatises on the terms of social cooperation than any other principle. A person has been treated in accordance with the principle of justice if treated according to what is fair, due, or owed. For example, if equal political rights are due all citizens, then justice is done when those rights are accorded. Any denial of a good, service, or piece of information to which a person has a right or entitlement based in justice is an injustice. It is also an injustice to place an undue burden on the exercise of a right—for example, to make a piece of information owed to a person unreasonably difficult to obtain.

Many appeals to "justice" present a confused picture because they are not appeals to a *distinctive principle* of justice that is independent of other principles such as beneficence or respect for autonomy. These appeals to "what is just" use the term "just" in a broad and nonspecific sense to refer to that which is generally *justified*, or in the circumstances morally *right*. Claims of justice tend to emerge in literature on informed consent when it is believed that someone's legal or moral rights have been violated, and sometimes these claims also confuse justice with justification. For example, articles on psychological research involving deception often denounce the research as *unjustly* denying subjects information to which they are entitled. Yet, as the argument develops, it often turns out that the controlling moral principle in such a judgment is less one of justice per se than respect for autonomy. (The argument could, of course, involve appeal to both principles.) Similarly, proponents of a physician's obligation to withhold potentially harmful information from patients for therapeutic reasons sometimes argue that it would be *unjust* for the physician to provide less than the best possible medical treatment. Here the moral concern is one of beneficence rather than justice. Many complaints of "injustice" in the informed consent literature can be linked in this way to alleged violations of the principle of respect for autonomy or of the principle of beneficence.

However, not all issues of justice in biomedical ethics can be entirely accounted for by appeal to other principles. How to allocate scarce medical resources and the validity of claims to possess a right to health care are staple examples of justice-based problems. Although more difficult to isolate, various problems that plague the literature on informed consent also seem justice-based. For example, much of the controversy surrounding the use of prisoners as subjects in research centers less on whether prisoners can give valid informed consent in the coercive environment of incarceration than on whether justice permits creation of a ready pool of human volunteers out of the class of those incarcerated by the state, especially when the same pool of persons might be repeatedly used. This question turns on the just distribution of the burden of the risks of research participation in society and thus is *centrally* a problem about justice rather than beneficence or respect

for autonomy. The issue is whether this burden could be warranted even if the public welfare is enhanced by the practice (a consideration of beneficence in the form of public utility) and even if the prisoners are capable of giving, and *do* give, a voluntary informed consent (a consideration of autonomy). The point of many analyses of research involving frequently used and vulnerable subjects is whether autonomous consent is sufficient to *override reservations based on justice* about approaching such persons to be research subjects in the first place.

It has also been argued that rules of informed consent can be motivated less by a concern to promote autonomous choice than by a concern to promote justice. Charles Lidz and his associates maintain that some who have argued for rules governing informed consent in psychiatry, including rules promoting increased disclosure in such areas as consent to electroconvulsive treatment (ECT), have been motivated by a concern over the *fairness* of subjecting patients to a potentially harmful treatment because of administrative convenience. They note that the advocates of strict disclosure "sought to use informed consent as a technique to minimize the use of ECT by using premises of equity and justice." However, as so often occurs, the persons Lidz has in mind were probably motivated by a *mixture* of moral concerns of respect for autonomy, beneficence, *and* justice. Lidz and others describe their *own* concerns in studying multiple problems of informed consent as motivated by the question whether a "more equal and mutual participatory relationship" can be established between health professionals and patients. They too seem motivated by a mixture of considerations of respect for autonomy, justice, *and* beneficence.[12]...

BALANCING MORAL PRINCIPLES AND RIGHTS

Controversial problems about abstract moral principles such as "respect for autonomy" and "beneficence" inevitably arise over how much these principles demand and over how to handle situations of conflict with other moral principles, such as justice. Whatever the prominence of these principles, we must acknowledge that if they conflict—as they do on occasion—a serious weighting or priority problem is created. Successful novels and dramas often depict these moral principles in their baldest forms of conflict: A person steals in order to preserve a life, lies in order to protect a sworn secret, or breaks a duty to keep confidentiality in order to protect a person endangered by its maintenance. Under such conditions it must be decided which (if either) moral consideration has priority—a problem known in ethical theory as how to "weigh and balance moral principles."…

The philosopher W. D. Ross is celebrated for his attempt to handle this problem of conflict.[13] Ross provides a list of several valid moral principles, including principles similar to the three we have had under examination. According to him, we must find "the greatest duty" in any circumstance of conflict by finding "the greatest balance" of right over wrong in that particular context. This metaphor of weights moving up and down on a balance scale is vivid, but crude and potentially misleading. Ross sought to give as much precision as possible to his ideas through a fundamental distinction between *prima facie* duties and *actual* duties: "Prima facie duty" refers to a duty always to be acted upon unless it conflicts on a particular occasion with an equal or stronger duty. A prima facie duty is always right and binding, all other things being equal. Although a firm duty, it is nonetheless conditional on not being overridden or outweighed by competing moral demands. One's actual duty, then, is determined by the balance of the respective weights of the competing prima facie duties.

Consider the following example:[14] A seventy-three-year-old man was mortally ill in a hospital and required a mechanical respirator. Although he had been judged competent, his request to have the respirator disconnected was refused. He then disconnected it himself, only to have the hospital staff reconnect it. The matter wound up in court. The patient contended that the hospital and his physicians had an obligation to allow

him to make his own choices, even though his choice entailed his death. His physicians and legal representatives of the state of Florida argued that they had a duty to preserve life and to prevent suicide. Here the duty to preserve life is in direct conflict with the duty to respect the autonomous decisions of another person. Both are prima facie duties. A Florida court then had to fix the *actual* duty of the hospital and physicians. In a complicated balancing of the conflicting obligations, the court concluded that the patient's choice should be overriding because considerations of autonomy were *here* (though not *everywhere*) weightier. The court reasoned that "the cost to the individual" of refusing to recognize his choice in a circumstance of terminal illness could not be overridden by the duty to preserve life.

Partially as a result of Ross's arguments, moral philosophers have generally come to regard both duties and rights not as absolute trumps but, rather, as strong prima facie moral demands that may be validly overridden in circumstances where stringent opposing demands are presented by a competing moral principle. To call lying prima facie wrong means that if an act involves lying it *is* wrong, *unless* some more weighty moral consideration prevails in the circumstances. Moral principles and statements of rights thus have far greater moral importance than mere rules of thumbs, which do not have the same force of standing obligations.

As Ross admits, neither he nor any moral philosopher has yet been able to present a system of rules free of conflicts and exceptions. He argues that the nature of the moral life simply makes an exception-free hierarchy of rules and principles impossible. Contemporary moral philosophy has proved incapable of providing a solution to this problem of weighing and balancing that improves on Ross's approach. The metaphor of "weight" has not proved amenable to precise analysis, and no one has claimed to be able to arrange all moral principles in a hierarchical order that avoids conflicts.

Ross's thesis also applies to circumstances in which a single principle directs us to two equally attractive alternatives, only one of which can be pursued. For example, the principle of beneficence, when applied to problems of disclosing information to patients, could require both disclosure *and* nondisclosure; both options could lead to equally *beneficial*, albeit *different*, outcomes. Whether the conflict is of this sort or between two different principles, there may not be a *single* right action in some circumstances, because two or more morally acceptable actions may be unavoidably in conflict and prove to be of equal weight in the circumstances.

We assume... that respect for autonomy is but a prima facie principle, and that it therefore has the same *but only the same* prima facie claim to override as other valid moral principles of comparable significance, such as beneficence or justice. Neither respect for autonomy nor any moral principle has an absolute standing that allows it on every occasion to override conflicting moral claims. Our analysis presupposes, as an inherent feature of the moral life, a pluralism of moral principles equally weighted in abstraction from particular circumstances. (Ross does not entirely accept this thesis of "equal weight.") Therefore, we hold that the moral principles of beneficence and justice—as well as more particular role responsibilities such as providing the best professional care—can have sufficient weight under *some* conditions to override respect for autonomy.

The moral view underlying this claim is not meant to diminish the standing of autonomy. Autonomy gives us respect, moral entitlement, and protection against invasions by others. Few matters of morals could be more important. But we should step back and ask, as Daniel Callahan has put it, "what it would be like to live in a community for which autonomy was the central value... [and] sole goal."[15] There is an historical and cultural oddity about giving a standing of overriding importance to the autonomous individual. Moral communities—indeed morality itself—was founded at least as much on the other principles we have mentioned, and usually in a context of strong commitment to the public welfare.

Callahan has argued that making autonomy *the* moral value rather than *a* moral value, weighting it to trump every other moral value, buys the luxury of autonomy at too high a price, and we would agree. However, we would be well advised not to depress the value of autonomy relative to the other principles in our framework. Autonomy is almost certainly the most important value "discovered" in medical and research ethics in the last two decades.... The pertinent point is that autonomy not be either overvalued or undervalued....

This analysis of plural prima facie *duties* applies to *rights* as well. It has often been assumed, owing perhaps to political statements about fundamental human rights, that certain rights are absolute trumps. However, decisive counterexamples can be mounted against this thesis. For example, it is sometimes proclaimed that the right to life is absolute, irrespective of competing claims or social conditions. The dubious validity of this thesis is evidenced by common moral judgments about capital punishment, international agreements about killing in war, and beliefs about the justifiability of killing in self-defense. Most writers in ethics now agree that we have an *exercisable right* not to have our life taken only if there is not a *sufficient moral justification* to override the right. The right to life—like the right to make an autonomous decision, the right to give an informed consent, or a parent's right to decide for a child—is legitimately exercisable and creates actual duties on others if and only if the right has an overriding status in the situation. Rights such as a right to an informed consent, a right to die, and a right to lifesaving medical technology thus must compete with other rights in many situations, producing protracted controversy and a need to balance with great discretion the competing rights' claims.

Numerous authors in biomedical and research ethics believe that if a person is acting autonomously and is the bearer of an autonomy right, then his or her choices morally ought *never* to be overridden by considerations of beneficence or proper care. This is not our assumption. Although the burden of moral proof will generally be on those who seek to intervene in another's choice, as the need to protect persons from harm becomes more compelling, thereby increasing the "weight" of moral considerations of beneficence in the circumstances, it becomes more likely that these considerations will validly override demands to respect autonomy. Similarly, because some autonomy rights are less significant than others, the demands to protect those rights are less weighty in the face of conflicting demands....

CONCLUSION

...Philosophy can provide a reasoned and systematic approach to moral problems, but it does not supply mechanical solutions or definitive procedures for decisionmaking. Practical wisdom and sound judgment are its indispensible allies in applied contexts. However, this lack of finality is no reason for skepticism. Moral philosophy can still yield well-constructed arguments and criticisms that advance our understanding. Moral dilemmas require a balancing of competing claims in untidy circumstances, and moral philosophy can make a significant if not decisive contribution. In these respects philosophy is neither surpassed by nor superior to legal reasoning and legal solutions....

Notes

1. See Isaiah Berlin, *Four Essays on Liberty* (London: Oxford University Press, 1969), 130.
2. For some reflections on what Kant's views do and do not show, see Arthur Flemming, "Using a Man as a Means," *Ethics* 88 (1978): 283–98.
3. See, for example, President's Commission for the Study of Ethical Problems in Medicine and Biomedical and Behavioral Research, *Deciding to Forego Life-Sustaining Treatment* (Washington, D.C.: U.S. Government Printing Office, 1983), 244ff; and, for the theoretical grounding of this claim in autonomy, *Making Health Care Decisions* (Washington, D.C.: U.S. Government Printing Office, 1982), Vol. 1, 44ff, esp. 47.
4. See Ludwig Edelstein, "The Hippocratic Oath: Text, Translation, and Interpretation," *Supplements to the Bulletin of the History of Medicine* 30,

Supplement 1 (Baltimore: The Johns Hopkins University Press, 1943); reprinted in Owsei Temkin and C. Lilian Temkin, eds., *Ancient Medicine: Selected Papers of Ludwig Edelstein* (Baltimore: The Johns Hopkins Press, 1967). The translation provided here of the benefit injunction is from *Epidemics*, 1:11, in W.H.S. Jones, trans., *Hippocrates*, 4 vols. (Cambridge, MA: Harvard University Press, 1923), 1: 165.
5. See William K. Frankena, *Ethics*, 2nd ed. (Englewood Cliffs, N.J.: Prentice-Hall, Inc., 1973), esp. 47.
6. Perhaps the most important philosophical statement of this position is found in W.D. Ross, *The Right and the Good* (Oxford: Clarendon Press, 1930), 21.
7. For a discussion of such problems, see Joel Feinberg, *Harm to Others: The Moral Limits of the Criminal Law* (New York: Oxford University Press, 1984), 136–41; Richard Trammell, "Saving Life and Taking Life," *Journal of Philosophy* 72 (1975): 131–37, and "Tooley's Moral Symmetry Principle," *Philosophy and Public Affairs* 5 (1976): 305ff.
8. A widely held view is that one has a duty of beneficence only if one can prevent harm to others at minimal risk to oneself and if one's action promises to be of substantial benefit to the other person. This analysis of beneficence can be more tightly formulated as follows: X has a *duty* of beneficence toward Y only if each of the following conditions is satisfied: (1) Y is at risk of significant loss or damage, (2) X's action is needed to prevent this loss or damage, (3) X's action would probably prevent this loss or damage, and (4) the benefit that Y will probably gain outweighs any harms that X is likely to suffer and does not present significant risk to X. This formulation is indebted to Eric D'Arcy, *Human Acts: An Essay in Their Moral Evaluation* (Oxford: Clarendon Press, 1963), 56–57.
   Provision of benefit beyond these conditions would be to act generously but beyond the call of duty. Our formulation is only one plausible construal of the general duty of beneficence, but we believe it suffices for our purposes in this volume. For contrasting views, see Earl Shelp, "To Benefit and Respect Persons: A Challenge for Beneficence in Health Care," Allen Buchanan, "Philosophical Foundations of Beneficence," and Natalie Abrams, "Scope of Beneficence in Health Care," all in Earl Shelp, ed., *Beneficence and Health Care* (Dordrecht, Holland: D. Reidel Publishing Co., 1982).
9. See, for example, Frankena, *Ethics*, 47; Peter Singer, "Famine, Affluence, and Morality,"

Philosophy and Public Affairs 1 (1972): 229–43, and *Practical Ethics* (Cambridge: Cambridge University Press, 1979), 168ff; Marcus G. Singer, *Generalization in Ethics* (New York: Alfred A. Knopf, Inc., 1961), 180–89; and Michael A. Slote, "The Morality of Wealth," in William Aiken and Hugh LaFollette, eds., *World Hunger and Moral Obligation* (Englewood Cliffs, N.J.: Prentice-Hall, Inc., 1977), 125–47.

10. Nuremberg Code, Principle 6, from *Trials of War Criminals Before the Nuremberg Military Tribunals Under Control Council Law No. 10* (Military Tribunal I, 1947; Washington, D.C.: U.S. Government Printing Office, 1948–49).

11. A comprehensive treatment of this problem in the context of research is found in Robert J. Levine, *Ethics and Regulation of Clinical Research* (Baltimore: Urban & Schwarzenberg, 1981), chapter 3.

12. Charles W. Lidz, et al., *Informed Consent: A Study of Decisionmaking in Psychiatry* (New York: The Guilford Press, 1984), 7–8.

13. Ross, The Right and the Good, 19–42.

14. *Satz v. Perlmutter*, 362 S.2d 160 (Florida District Court of Appeals, 1978).

15. Daniel Callahan, "Autonomy: A Moral Good, Not a Moral Obsession," *The Hastings Center Report* 14 (October 1984): 40–42.

Metaphor and Analogy in Bioethics

James F. Childress

Many of our practices and much of our discourse in health care hinge on metaphors and analogies, whose significance is sometimes overlooked because they are considered merely decorative or escape notice altogether. Despite their relative neglect, they significantly shape our interpretations of what is going on as well as what should go on. In recent years they have received increasing attention, particularly from critics of principles-oriented approaches to bioethics who stress the role of imagination, emotion, and the like in morality and ethical reflection. I will examine metaphors before considering analogies, particularly in analogical reasoning, noting their overlap where appropriate....

METAPHORS IN BIOETHICS

The nature and function of metaphors. Perhaps because medicine and health care involve fundamental matters of life and death for practically everyone, frequently in mysterious ways, they are often described in metaphors. For instance, physicians may be viewed as playing God, or acting as parents, and nurses may be seen as advocates for patients; medicine itself may be interpreted as warfare against disease. Metaphors involve imagining something as something else, for example, viewing human beings as wolves or life as a journey. "The essence of a metaphor," according to Lakoff and Johnson, "is understanding and experiencing one thing through another."[1] More precisely, metaphors are figurative expressions that interpret one thing in terms of something else.[2]

In the large recent philosophical literature on metaphor, critics have challenged some traditional conceptions, contending that metaphors are more than merely ornamental or affective ways to state what could be stated in a more literal or comparative way and they can be and often are cognitively significant.[3] According to the traditional substitution view, a metaphorical expression is merely a substitute for some equivalent literal expression. For example, the metaphorical

James F. Childress, *Practical Reasoning in Bioethics* (Bloomington, IN: Indiana University Press, 1997), 3–24. Reprinted with permission. Much of the material appeared earlier in "Metaphor and Analogy" in *Encyclopedia of Bioethics*, 2nd. ed., ed. Warren T. Reich (New York: Simon & Schuster Macmillan, 1995), vol 3, pp. 1765–73.

expression "John is a fox" substitutes for the literal expression "John is sly and cunning." One common version of the substitution view, what Max Black calls a comparison view (elements of which can be found in Aristotle), construes metaphor as the presentation of an underlying analogy or similarity. Hence, metaphor is a "condensed or elliptical simile,"[4] or it is a "comparison statement with parts left out."[5] "John is a fox," for example, indicates that "John is like a fox in that he is sly and cunning." According to such views, metaphors are dispensable ways to express what could be expressed differently, but they often appeal to the emotions more effectively than their equivalent literal expressions or comparisons would do.

By contrast many recent theories of metaphor stress its cognitive significance. For instance, in an early and very influential essay, philosopher Max Black defended an interaction view of metaphor, in which two juxtaposed thoughts interact to produce new meanings through the metaphor's "system of associated commonplaces" or "associated implications."[6] The metaphor—for instance, "wolf" in "man is a wolf"—serves as a "filter" for a set of associated implications that are transferred from the secondary subject ("wolf") to the principal subject ("man") in the sentence. (In a full interaction or interanimation view of metaphor, the transfer of meaning occurs both ways, not merely from the secondary subject to the principal subject.)[7]

Metaphors highlight and hide features of the principal subject, such as the physician who is viewed as a parent or as a friend, by their systematically related implications.[8] When argument is conceived as warfare, for example, the metaphor highlights the conflict involved in argument while it hides the cooperation and collaboration, involving shared rules, that are also indispensable to argument. Our metaphors thus shape how we think, what we experience, and what we do by what they highlight and hide. They use us, just as we use them.

Metaphors are often associated with models. For instance, we have both metaphors and models of the doctor–patient relationship. The physician may be viewed through the metaphor of father and the patient through the metaphor of child, and their relationship may be interpreted through the model of paternalism. Models, for our purposes, state the network of associated commonplaces and implications in more systematic and comprehensive ways—according to Max Black, "every metaphor is the tip of a submerged model."[9]

Metaphors and models may be good or bad, living or dead. Both metaphors and models can be assessed by how well they illuminate what is going on and what should go on. We can distinguish descriptive and normative uses of metaphors and models without admitting a sharp separation between fact and value. For instance, the metaphor of physician as father (or parent), and the model of paternalism (or parentalism), may accurately describe some relationships in medicine, or they may suggest ideal relationships in the light of some important principles and values.

Medicine as war, business, etc. The metaphor of warfare illuminates much of our conception of what is, and should be, done in health care. Consider the way this metaphor emerges in the day-to-day language of medicine: The physician as the captain leads the battle against disease; orders a battery of tests; develops a plan of attack; calls on the armamentarium or arsenal of medicine; directs allied health personnel; treats aggressively; and expects compliance. Good patients are those who fight vigorously and refuse to give up. Victory is sought; defeat is feared. Sometimes there is even hope for a "magic bullet" or a "silver bullet." Only professionals who stand on the firing line or in the trenches can really appreciate the moral problems of medicine. And they frequently have "war stories" to relate. Medical organization, particularly in the hospital, resembles military hierarchy, and medical training, particularly with its long, sleepless shifts in residencies, approximates military training more than any other professional education in our society.10

As medicine wages war against germs that invade the body and threaten its defenses, so the society itself may also declare war on cancer, or on AIDS, under the leadership of its chief medical officer, who in the United States is the Surgeon General. Articles and books even herald the "Medical-Industrial Complex: Our National

Defense." As Susan Sontag notes, "Where once it was the physician who waged *bellum contra morbum,* the war against disease, now it's the whole society."[11]

The military metaphor first became prominent in the 1880s when bacteria were identified as agents of disease that threaten the body and its defenses. It both illuminates and distorts health care. Its positive implications are widely recognized—for instance, in supporting a patient's courageous and hopeful struggle against disease and in galvanizing societal support to fight against disease. But the metaphor is also problematic. Susan Sontag, who was diagnosed with cancer in the late 1970s, reports that her suffering was intensified by the dominance of the metaphor of warfare against cancer. Cancer cells do not just multiply; they are "invasive." They "colonize." The body's "defenses" are rarely strong enough. But since the body is under attack ("invasion"), by "alien" invaders, counterattack is justified. Treatments are also often described in military language:

> Radiotherapy uses the metaphors of aerial warfare; patients are "bombarded" with toxic rays. And chemotherapy is chemical warfare, using poisons. Treatment aims to "kill" cancer cells (without, it is hoped, killing the patient). Unpleasant side effects of treatment are advertised, indeed overadvertised. ("The agony of chemotherapy" is a standard phrase.) It is impossible to avoid damaging or destroying healthy cells (indeed, some methods used to treat cancer can cause cancer), but it is thought that nearly any damage to the body is justified if it saves the patient's life. Often, of course, it doesn't work. (As in: "We had to destroy Ben Suc in order to save it.") There is everything but the body count.[12]

Such "military metaphors," Sontag suggests, "contribute to the stigmatizing of certain illnesses and, by extension, of those who are ill." Other ill individuals have found the military metaphor unsatisfactory for other reasons. For instance, as a teenager, Lawrence Pray originally tried to conquer his diabetes, but his struggles and battles were futile and even counterproductive. Then over time he came to view his diabetes not as an "enemy" to be "conquered" but as a "teacher." Only then did he find a personally satisfactory way of living.[13]

Still others with illness, by contrast, have found the military metaphor empowering and enabling. In her wide-ranging study of pathographies, that is, autobiographical descriptions of personal experiences of illness, treatment, and dying, Anne Hunsaker Hawkins identifies several "metaphorical paradigms" that offer themes of "an archetypal, mythic nature."[14] In addition to illness as a battle, she concentrates on illness as a game or sport (a subset of the military metaphor), illness as a journey into a distant country, illness as rebirth or regeneration, and, on a somewhat different level, healthy-mindedness as an alternative to contemporary medicine. While pathographies are individualized statements, they provide "an immensely rich reservoir of the metaphors and models that surround illness in contemporary culture." These various metaphorical paradigms structure individuals' interpretations of their experiences of illness. Patterns emerge in individuals' selection of metaphors. They vary in part according to the illness involved—for example, the military metaphor is more common in descriptions of experiences with cancer and AIDS, while the rebirth metaphor is more common in descriptions of a critical life-threatening event, such as a heart attack. Furthermore, the military metaphor is generally more prevalent than the journey metaphor because it better fits the experience of modern medicine—for instance, it is easier to construe a physician as a "general" in a war than as a "guide" on a journey. Nevertheless, these various metaphors are often mixed and complementary. And they can be evaluated, Hawkins suggests, according to their capacity to enable and empower ill persons, for instance, by restoring a sense of personal dignity and worth. While expressing larger sociocultural patterns, the individual's choice of a particular metaphor is a creative act of assigning meaning to his or her illness.

The metaphor of warfare has been further challenged in modern medicine because of its apparent support for overtreatment, particularly of terminally ill patients, where death is the ultimate enemy and trauma, disease, or illness the immediate enemy. Physicians and families under the spell of this metaphor frequently find it difficult to let patients die. "Heroic" actions, with the best available weapons, befit the military effort that must always be undertaken against the ultimate enemy. Death signals defeat and forgoing treatment signals surrender. Some clinicians even feel more comfortable withholding (i.e., not starting) a treatment for cancer, for instance, than they do withdrawing (i.e., stopping) the same treatment, in part because withdrawing treatment implies retreat....

According to its critics, our invocation of the military metaphor often fails to recognize moral constraints on waging war. "Modern medicine," William F. May writes, "has tended to interpret itself not only through the prism of war but through the medium of its modern practice, that is, unlimited, unconditional war," in contrast to the just-war tradition.[15] In the spirit of modern total war, "hospitals and the physician-fighter wage unconditional battle against death." One result is that many patients seek assisted suicide or active euthanasia in order to escape from this warfare's terrorist bombardment. Traditional moral limits in the conduct of war include the principle of discrimination, which authorizes direct attacks on combatants but not on non-combatants. In medical care, the opposing combatant is the disease or death, not the patient. However, the patient is regularly the battleground and sometimes even becomes the enemy. This transformation into the enemy may occur if the patient betrays the military effort by not fighting hard enough or even by surrendering before the war ends. Finally, in accord with the just-war tradition's requirement of reasonable prospect of success and proportionality, the treatment should offer the patient a reasonable chance of success, and his or her suffering and other burdens must be balanced against the probable benefits of prolongation of life.[16]

Other problematic or ambiguous implications of the military metaphor appear in the allocation of resources for and within health care. It is not surprising that the two major terms for allocation and distribution of health care under conditions of scarcity emerged from, or were decisively shaped by, military experiences. These are triage and rationing. As Richard Rettig and Kathleen Lohr note,

> Earlier, policymakers spoke of the general problem of allocating scarce medical resources, a formulation that implied hard but generally manageable choices of a largely pragmatic nature. Now the discussion increasingly is of rationing scarce medical resources, a harsher term that connotes emergency—even war-time—circumstances requiring some societal triage mechanism.[17]

...I will only sketch some of the implications of the military metaphor for allocation, particularly macroallocation.

First, under the military metaphor, society's health care budget tends to be converted into a defense budget to prepare for and conduct war against disease, trauma, and death. As a consequence, the society may put more resources into health care in relation to other goods than it could justify, especially under a different metaphor, such as nursing or business (see below). Indeed, the society may overutilize health care, especially because technological care may contribute less to the national defense of health itself, through the reduction of morbidity and premature mortality, than other factors, such as the reduction of poverty.

Second, within the health care budget, the military metaphor tends to assign priority to critical care over preventive and chronic care. It tends to concentrate on critical interventions to cure disease, perhaps in part because it tends to view health as the absence of disease rather than as a positive state. It tends to neglect care when cure is impossible.

A third point is closely connected: In setting priorities for research and treatment, the military metaphor tends to assign priority to killer diseases, such as cancer and AIDS, over chronic diseases. Franz Ingelfinger once suggested that if we concentrated our research and treatment more on disabling diseases, such as arthritis, than on killer diseases, then national health expenditures would reflect the same values that individuals affirm: "It is more important to live a certain way than to die a certain way."[18] Anne R. Sommers has suggested that stroke is "a metaphor for the most difficult problems and challenges of geriatric medicine."[19] Although strokes are not limited to the elderly, they are more common among the elderly. Each year in the United States there are between 500,000 and 600,000 victims of stroke, 80 to 90 percent of them surviving their initial catastrophe, often with paralysis and aphasia, which have a terrible impact on both victims of stroke and their families. Approximately 2.5 million victims of stroke are alive today, 90 percent of them with varying degrees of incapacity and misery. Even though it has been called the single most costly disease in the United States, stroke received in 1979 only $18 million in research expenditures, in contrast to cancer, which received $937 million, and heart disease, which received $340 million. A major reason for this pattern of allocation is that, after the first acute phase, the stroke victim does not fit into the prevalent model of medical care, which emphasizes the specialist, who uses various technological weapons to fight specific problems. Hence this pattern continues.

Fourth, medicine as war concentrates on technological interventions over against non-technological modes of care and, within technologies, it tends to concentrate on more dramatic technologies, such as intensive care units and organ transplants, rather than less dramatic technologies, such as prostheses.

In short, the military metaphor has some negative or ambiguous implications for a moral approach to health care decisions: It tends to assign priority to health care (especially medical care) over other goods and, within health care, to critical interventions over chronic care, killer over disabling diseases, technological interventions over caring, and heroic treatment of dying patients rather than allowing them to die in peace.[20]

Some of the negative or ambiguous implications of the war metaphor for health care can be avoided if, as noted earlier, the metaphor is interpreted in accord with the limits set by the just-war tradition. However, the war metaphor may require supplementation as well as limitation. It is not the only prominent metaphor for health care, and since the early 1980s its dominance has been threatened by the language of economics and business, as reflected in the language of a health care industry: Providers deliver care to consumers, seek or are forced to seek productivity in light of cost-effectiveness or cost-benefit analyses, and may be concerned with "resource management, managed care systems, and market strategies."[21]

The business metaphor also highlights and hides various features of contemporary health care. Many critics of this metaphor worry that the language of efficiency will replace the language of care and compassion for the sick and equity in distribution of health care. Nevertheless, this metaphor has become more and more pervasive and persuasive as the structure of medicine and health care has changed and concerns about costs have become more central in societal discussions. Patients now often fear undertreatment as hospitals and professionals seek to reduce costs, in contrast to their fears of overtreatment under the war metaphor.

Both military and economic metaphors illuminate contemporary health care, but they may not be adequate, even together, to guide and direct health care. Whether any particular metaphor is adequate or not will depend in part on the principles and values it highlights and hides. Others have proposed nursing, a subset of health care, as a supplementary metaphor for the whole of health care, because of its attention to caring more than curing and to hands-on rather than technological care. Even though this metaphor of nursing—in contemporary discourse it is often more than a synecdoche—is also inadequate by itself, it could direct the society to alternative priorities in the allocation of resources for and within health care, particularly for chronic care....

Relationships between health care professionals and recipients of care. Relationships between physicians and other health care professionals, on the one hand, and patients, on the other, have been described and directed by a wide variety of metaphors and models.[22] For example, May has identified images of the physician as fighter, technician, parent, covenanter, and teacher, and Robert M. Veatch has identified several major competing models of physician-patient relationships: engineering, priestly (which includes the paternalistic model), collegial, and contractual models.[23] Other metaphors such as friend and captain of the ship have also been used.[24]

Some critics contend that such models are "whimsical gestalts," that many other arbitrary models could be invented—for example, bus driver or back-seat driver—and that moral points can and should be made more directly.[25] Such criticisms overlook how metaphors and models function in the interpretation and evaluation of interactions between physicians and patients. They miss the role of imagination, which can be defined as "reasoning in metaphors."[26] For example, opponents of paternalistic medical relationships usually do not eschew all use of metaphor; instead they offer alternative metaphors, such as partnership or contracts. And these various metaphors may be more or less adequate to describe what occurs and to direct what should occur in health care.

Metaphors and models highlight and hide features of the roles of physicians and other health care professionals by their various associated implications. For example, viewing the physician as a parent, or specifically as a father, based on the nineteenth-century model of the family, highlights some features of medical relationships, such as care and control, while hiding others, such as the payment of fees. The use of such metaphors to describe, interpret, and explain relationships is subject to criticism if they distort more than they illuminate. And when they are offered to guide relationships and actions, they

are subject to criticism if they highlight only one moral consideration, such as the physician's duty to benefit the patient or to respect patient autonomy, while hiding or obscuring other relevant moral considerations. It is also appropriate to consider the feasibility of various ideal relationships in light of significant personal, professional, and institutional constraints.

Several metaphors may be necessary to interpret health care as it is currently structured and to guide and direct actions, practices, and policies in health care. Some metaphors may fit some relationships better than others; for example, relations in clinical research, family practice, and surgery may be illuminated respectively by the metaphors of partner, teacher–student, and technician–consumer. Furthermore, not all of these metaphors conflict with each other; some may even be mutually supportive as well as compatible, for example, contractor and technician. However, conflicts can be expected if a physician interprets and directs relationships paternalistically, while his or her patient interprets and directs the interaction through metaphors of negotiation and accommodation....

Nursing as advocacy. Major changes in the conception of nursing correlate with alterations in its primary metaphors. Whether situated within the military effort against disease or viewed as physicians' handmaidens and servants, nurses have traditionally been expected to cultivate passive virtues, such as loyalty and obedience. Their moral responsibility was primarily directed toward physicians and institutions, such as hospitals, and only secondarily toward patients. This interpretation of responsibility was shaped in part by nursing's military origins in the nineteenth century as well as by societal conceptions of gender.[27] Then in the 1970s, nursing was reconceived through the metaphor of advocacy. Nurses became advocates for "clients" and "consumers" (the term "patient" was often rejected as too passive). This legal metaphor, drawn from the advocate as one who pleads another's cause, especially before a tribunal of justice, highlights active virtues, such as courage, persistence, perseverance, and courage, and views the nurse as primarily responsible to the patient or client. This metaphor is explicit or implicit in formal nursing codes, and it is also featured in a large number of nurses' stories of advocacy and conflict in health care.[28]

Critics, such as Ellen Bernal, note that the metaphor of advocacy reduces the range of services traditionally offered by nurses; it is thus insufficiently comprehensive. In addition to distorting the human experience of illness, it distorts nursing by focusing almost exclusively on patients' or clients' rights, construed mainly in terms of autonomy, and it neglects positive social relationships in health care.[29] It highlights conflict among health care professionals because it implies that some of them do not adequately protect the rights of patients. Thus, the metaphor frequently supports a call for increased nursing autonomy as a way to protect patient autonomy. Because of its adversarial nature, many question whether the metaphor of advocacy can adequately guide relationships among health care professionals in the long run, even if it is useful in the short run. The metaphor may also assume that the nurse's responsibility to the patient/client is always clear-cut and overriding, even though nurses may face serious conflicts of responsibility involving patients, other individuals, associates, and institutions.[30] At the very least, sympathetic commentators call for further clarification of the metaphor of advocacy, while critics seek alternative metaphors and models, such as covenant, partnership, teamwork, or collegiality, which appear to offer more inclusive, cooperative ideals.

Playing God and other metaphors of limits.
"Playing God" has been a common metaphor for both describing and (re)directing the activities of scientists, physicians, and other health care professionals. They have been criticized for usurping God's power—for instance, the power over life and death—by letting patients die or by using new reproductive technologies,

There are theological warrants for playing God in the Jewish and Christian traditions, which affirm the creation of human beings in God's image and likeness. Philosopher David Heyd builds on this idea of the image of God: "If indeed the capacity to invest the world with value *is* God's image, it elevates human beings to a unique (godly) status, which is not shared by any other creature in the world. This is playing God in a creative, 'human-specific' way."[31] And Paul Ramsey calls on those who allocate health care to play God in a fitting way: "Men should then 'play God' in the correct way: he makes his sun rise upon the good and the evil and sends rain upon the just and the unjust alike." We should emulate God's indiscriminate care by distributing scarce lifesaving medical technologies randomly or by a lottery rather than on the basis of judgments of social worth.[32] …

Despite a few such positive uses of the metaphor of "playing God," the metaphor is generally used to identify two aspects of divine activity that should not be imitated by humans: God's unlimited power to decide and unlimited power to act. On the one hand, users of this metaphor demand scientific and medical accountability over against unilateral decision making, for example, regarding life and death. On the other hand, they call for respect for substantive limits, for example, not creating new forms of life in violation of divinely ordained natural limits.[33] Critics frequently focus on human arrogance and rebellion in daring to "play God." In a more typical statement (in contrast to his positive use of the metaphor cited earlier), Ramsey writes: "Men ought not to play God before they learn to be men, and after they have learned to be men they will not play God."[34] Thus, critics of "playing God" usually demand scientific and medical accountability along with respect for substantive limits, such as not creating new forms of life. Objectors to negative uses of the metaphor of "playing God" often challenge the rationale for holding that a particular course of action, such as human genetic engineering, is wrong.

Edmund L. Erde contends that statements such as "doctors should not play God" are so unclear that they cannot function as commands and do not articulate a principle; thus, they cannot be followed because agents do not know how to conform their actions to them. Nor do they explain why certain actions should not be undertaken. Such phrases are, Erde argues, "metaphoric in that they tuck powerful feelings and images into descriptive language that cannot be understood literally." Any activity, such as mercy killing, that is "labeled 'playing god' carries the implication that it is clearly wrong." These phrases are used for situations in which agents face choices but one option is considered immoral and is rejected as arrogantly and presumptuously playing God. The background of intelligibility of this metaphor, according to Erde, is found in the Western idea of the great chain of being, which identifies appropriate responsibilities at each level and opposes the usurpation of power and the failure to respect limits.[35]

Other important and widespread metaphors of limits include the thin edge of the wedge and the slippery slope, both of which warn against undertaking certain actions because other unacceptable actions will inevitably follow. Examples regularly appear in debates about euthanasia. Such arguments about limits may take at least two different forms: (1) conceptual, and (2) psychological–sociological. The first focuses on the logic of moral reasoning, the hammer back of the wedge, and the other on what the wedge is driven into. Or, to shift to the slippery slope metaphor, the slope may be slippery for two different reasons. According to the first reason, the slope is slippery because the concepts and distinctions are vague, inadequately drawn, or ultimately indefensible. This first version derives its power from the principle of universalizability (discussed below), which commits us to treating relevantly similar cases in a similar way. Because of this principle of universalizability, Paul Ramsey argues, ethical (and legal) mistakes tend to replicate themselves: "It is quite clear that at the point of medical, legal, and ethical intersections at the edges of life... the so-called wedge argument is an excellent one. This is true because legal principles and precedents are systematically designed to apply to other cases as well. This is the way the law

'works,' and... also the way moral reasoning works from case to similar case."[36]

By contrast, the second version, which is more plausible in arguments against the legalization of physician-assisted suicide and euthanasia, considers the personal, social, institutional, and cultural context in order to determine the possible impact of changing rules or making exceptions. Even if certain distinctions between various acts are, in principle, clear and defensible, agents may not be able over time to draw them and act on them because of various psychological, social, institutional, and cultural forces, such as racisms, sexism, or ageism.[37]

Even though such metaphors of limits are often misused, they are appropriate in some contexts. In each use of these metaphor of limits, important moral questions require attention—the evaluation of the first action and subsequent actions—and important conceptual and empirical questions must be addressed in order to determine whether the putatively bad consequences will inevitably follow what might be innocuous first steps. (Similar points hold for analogies invoking moral limits.)...

Metaphors for bioethics and bioethicists. The role and function of the bioethicist have often been construed in metaphorical terms. The common langage of "applied ethics" invokes the metaphor of engineering as an application of basic science that does not contribute to basic science. The expertise of applied ethicists resides in their ability to apply general theories and principles to specific arenas of human activity. The metaphor of application has been widely challenged on the grounds that it is too narrow and distorts much that is important in bioethics. The term "applied" suggests that ethicists are problem solvers rather than problem setters, that they solve puzzles rather than provide perspectives, that they answer rather than raise questions, and that they begin from theory rather than from lived experience. It implies a limited technical or mechanical model of ethics.

The term "applied" distorts the numerous theoretical controversies in bioethics and neglects the way bioethics may help to resolve or recast some theoretical controversies. At the very least, the metaphor of application needs to be supplemented by various other metaphors for the task of practical ethics and the role of the practical ethicist: "Theoretician, diagnostician, educator, coach, conceptual policeman, and skeptic are also supplemental or alternative roles to that of the technician."[38] Some other metaphors are drawn from ancient religious roles, such as prophet or scribe. Yet another metaphor is "conversation," which is prominent in approaches to bioethics that emphasize interpretation, hermeneutics, and narrative. And the "stranger" has been proposed as the best metaphor for the ethicist in professional education because his or her outside perspective can challenge ordinary assumptions.[39]

No doubt several such metaphors are needed to interpret and direct the activities of ethicists. Which ones appear to fit best will depend in part on our operative conception of ethics and, in particular, on its breadth and richness....

Generative metaphors. Suggestions emerge at various times to retire all metaphors, not merely some metaphors, in some realm of discourse—for instance, Susan Sontag proposes retiring all metaphors for illness.[40] However, it is not possible to strip our discourse in science, medicine, and health care, or in biomedical ethics, of all metaphors. Instead, we must use metaphors with care and carefully assess their adequacy in their descriptive and normative functions.

For each use of metaphor, we have to ask whether, through highlighting and hiding features of subjects, it generates insights about what is or about what ought to be. A simple example of what Donald Schoen calls a generative metaphor, that is, one that generates insights, occurred when researchers were trying to improve the performance of a new paintbrush made with synthetic bristles. The new brush applied the paint to the surface in a "gloppy way." Nothing the researchers tried made the artificial bristles work as well as natural bristles. Then one day someone observed, " You know, a paintbrush is a kind of pump!" That was a generative metaphor: Pressing a paintbrush against a surface forces paint through the spaces or "channels" between the bristles, and painters sometimes even vibrate brushes to increase the flow. Once the researchers began to view the paintbrush as a kind of pump, they were able to improve the brush with synthetic bristles.[41] That is the kind of insight, both descriptive and directive, that we seek. Rarely, however, will it be so dramatic. In most issues confronted in biomedical ethics, the tests of adequacy of particular metaphors will be more complex and subtle. At the very least, tests of metaphors that function normatively to guide being and doing need to incorporate general moral considerations.

ANALOGIES IN BIOETHICS

Analogies and analogical reasoning. Often metaphors and analogies are presented in ways that indicate their substantial overlap. Indeed, in the comparison view of metaphor, there is little difference between them, because metaphors are compressed analogies. Some recent theories of metaphor have stressed, by contrast, that metaphors create similarities rather than merely expressing previously established and recognized similarities or analogies. According to Max Black, comparison views of metaphor fail because they reduce the ground for shifts of meaning (from the secondary subject to the primary subject) to similarity or analogy.[42] Nevertheless, there is a strong consensus that metaphorical statements presuppose some resemblance, even when they also create resemblance.[43] Black himself later conceded that metaphors "mediate an analogy or structural correspondence." Metaphor is, roughly speaking, "an instrument for drawing implications grounded in perceived analogies of structure between two subjects belonging to different domains."[44] And yet metaphor does not merely compare two things that are similar, but rather enables us to see similarities in what would be regarded as dissimilar.

Metaphors and analogies are thus closely related, with metaphors both expressing and creating similarities. In general, good metaphors function cognitively to generate new meaning and insight by providing new perspectives, while good analogies extend our knowledge by moving from the familiar to the unfamiliar, the established to the novel. In stretching language, concepts, and so forth for new situations, analogy does not involve the imaginative strain often evident in the use of metaphors.[45] Nevertheless, the differences in function between metaphors and analogies should not be exaggerated.

The term analogy derives from the Greek *analogia*, which referred to mathematical proportion. "An analogy in its original root meaning," Dorothy Emmet observes, "is a proportion, and primarily a mathematical ratio, e.g., 2:4::4:X." In such a ratio, given knowledge of three terms, and the nature of the proportionate relation, the value of the fourth term can be determined. Thus analogy is the repetition of the same fundamental pattern in two different contexts.[46]

Analogical reasoning thus proceeds inductively, moving from the known to the unknown. It appears prominently in problem solving and thus is featured in research in cognitive science and artificial intelligence.[47] For instance, computer problem-solving programs must search for analogous problems that have been successfully solved to generate solutions to new problems whether in highly structured domains such as law or in less structured domains.

Analogical reasoning has an important place in moral discourse, not only because of its importance in problem solving, but also because of the widely recognized moral requirement to treat similar cases in a similar way. Often stated as a principle of universalizability or of formal justice or formal equality, and dating back at least to Aristotle, the requirement to treat similar cases in a similar way also appears on the common law's doctrine of precedent. The basic idea is that one does not make an acceptable moral or legal judgment—perhaps not even a moral or legal judgment at all—if one judges that X is wrong but that a similar X is right, without adducing any relevant moral or legal difference between them. In general, analogical reasoning illuminates features of morally or legally problematic cases by

appealing to relevantly similar cases that reflect a moral or legal consensus (precedent). Of course, much of the moral (or legal) debate hinges on determining which similarities and differences are both relevant and significant....

Analogy and casuistry. Over the last decade or so analogical reasoning has received renewed attention from philosophers and theologians focusing on case-oriented or casuistical judgments in bioethics and elsewhere, particularly in the wake of perplexities often associated with new technologies that appear, at least at first glance, to create or occasion unprecedented problems. In *The Abuse of Casuistry*, Albert R. Jonsen and Stephen Toulmin identify "the first feature of the casuistic method" in its classical formulations as "the ordering of cases under a principle by paradigm and analogy."[48] For instance, the rule prohibiting killing is set out in "paradigm cases" that illustrate its most manifest breaches according to its most obvious meaning. Moving from simple and clear cases to complex and uncertain ones, casuists examine various alternative circumstances and motives to determine whether those other cases violate the rule against killing. They seek analogies that permit the comparison of "problematic new cases and circumstances with earlier exemplary ones," that is, the similar type cases that constitute presumptions.[49]

Despite the claims of some modern casuists, it is not clear that analogical reasoning distinguishes casuistical from principlist approaches. For instance, in analyzing the novel microallocation problems of modern medicine, Ramsey, a strongly rule-oriented ethicist, appealed to the analogous "lifeboat" cases—when some passengers have to be thrown overboard to prevent the lifeboat from sinking—as a way to interpret the requirements of the principle of equality of opportunity in distributing such scarce lifesaving medical technologies as kidney dialysis.[50] Because principles and rules are indeterminate and because they sometimes conflict, analogical reasoning can be expected in case judgments— mere application cannot be sufficient in ethical frameworks that appeal to principles and rules....

Analogies are often divided into two main types, analogies of attribution and analogies of proportion.[51] The analogy of attribution involves a comparison of two terms or analogates, both of which have a common property, the analogon, that appears primarily in one and secondarily in the other. As Thomas Aquinas noted, "healthy" is used primarily for a person in a state of health (a "healthy" person) and secondarily for those medicines and practices that help to maintain or restore health (e.g., a "healthy" diet) or specimens that provide evidence of the body's health (e.g., "healthy" blood). By contrast, in the analogy of proportion, the analogates lack a direct relationship, but each of them involves a relationship that can be compared to a relationship in the other.[52] This second type is most common in analogical reasoning in biomedical ethics, as is evident in debates about maternal–fetal relations and abortion, where analogies of attribution also appear, particularly with reference to the fetus.

Analogical reasoning in debates about maternal–fetal relations. Debates about maternal–fetal relations, including pregnant women's decisions to abort and to decline caesarean sections, illustrate the pervasiveness and importance of analogical reasoning. Traditionally, abortion has been construed as directly killing the fetus, an innocent human being, in violation of the duty of nonmaleficence. Hence, in traditional Roman Catholic moral theology, direct abortions are tantamount to homicide. Sometimes the analogy of the "unjust aggressor" appears in situations where the pregnancy threatens the pregnant woman's life or health, but it has not been accepted in official Catholic thought the same way the similar analogy of the "pursuer" has been accepted in some Jewish thought to justify abortions when the pregnant woman's life or health is threatened.

Some feminists and others have attempted to recast the debate about abortion to focus on the basis and extent of the pregnant woman's obligation to provide bodily life support to the fetus. Often accepting, at least for purposes of argument, the premise that the fetus is a human being from the moment of conception (or at some time during the pregnancy), they argue that this premise does not entail that the pregnant woman always had a duty to sustain the fetus's life, regardless of the circumstances of pregnancy, the risks and inconveniences to the pregnant woman, and so forth. Their arguments often proceed through analogies to other hypothetical or real practices or cases, on the assumption that a judgment about those practices or cases will entail a similar judgement about abortion.

The fantastic abortion analogies introduced by Judith Jarvis Thomson have been particularly influential and controversial.[53] In one of her artificial cases, an individual with a rare blood type is kidnapped by the Society of Music Lovers and attached to a famous violinist who needs to purify his system because of his renal failure. Part of the debate is whether relevant analogies can be found in such fantastic, artificial cases, in contrast to actual real cases. For example, over against Thomson, John Noonan opposes abortion in part by appeal to a U.S. tort law case, in which the court held liable the hosts who had invited a guest for dinner but then put him out of the house into the cold night even though he had become sick and fainted and requested permission to stay.[54]

Some feminists and others contend that other analogous real-life legal and moral cases support the pregnant woman's free decision to continue or to discontinue her pregnancy. For many the relevant analogous cases concern living organ and tissue donation. Such donations are conceived as voluntary, altruistic acts that should not be forced by others even to save the potential recipient's life. They are "gifts of life." Requiring a pregnant woman to continue the pregnancy until birth imposes on her a heavier burden than others are expected to bear in analogous circumstances, such as a parent who could save a child's life by donating a kidney. Thus, the provision of bodily life support, whether through donating an organ or allowing the fetus to use the uterus, has been conceived as a gift of life that should not be legally enforced.[55]

According to Lisa Sowle Cahill, much analogical reasoning about pregnancy overlooks what is unique about maternal–fetal relations and thus obscures the morally relevant features of pregnancy or makes some relevant features more significant than they are. Many analogies problematically narrow our moral perspective on abortion by portraying the inception of pregnancy as accidental and the fetus as strange, alien, and even hostile. Furthermore, they often rely on the connotative meanings of their terms, particularly as embedded in a story, such as Thomson's case of kidnapping the unconscious violinist. Examples also appear in the rhetoric of abortion opponents who, for instance, speak of the fetus as a "child" and thereby distort the unique dependence of the fetus on the pregnant woman. Finally, Cahill contends, justifications of abortion based on analogy often rest on liberal convictions that special responsibilities derive only from free choice.[56]

For all these reasons, Cahill holds that analogical reasoning needs supplementation through direct examination of the unique features of maternal–fetal relations, particularly total fetal dependence, and of the ways these unique features qualify maternal, professional, and societal obligations. She argues that, as a category or class of moral relations, pregnancy "is unique among human relations at least because in it one individual is totally and exclusively dependent on a particular other within a relation which represents in its physical and social aspects what is *prima facie* to be valued positively."[57] Hence, she argues, most analogies hide what is distinctive and unique about pregnancy, even though they identify some morally relevant features of maternal–fetal relations.

With the emergence of other maternal–fetal conflicts, particularly regarding caesarean sections to benefit the fetus, similar debates have emerged about the appropriateness of the analogy with living organ and tissue donation. For instance, in the case of *In re A.C.* (No. 87–609, District of Columbia Court of Appeals, April 26, 1990), the majority of the court held that just as courts do not compel people to "donate" organs or tissue to benefit others, so they should not compel caesarean sections against the will of pregnant women to benefit potentially viable fetuses. The dissenting opinion rejected the analogy with organ and tissue donation, insisting that the pregnant woman "has undertaken to bear another human being, and has carried an unborn child to viability," that the "unborn child's" dependence upon the mother is unique and singular, and that the "viable unborn child is literally captive within the mother's body."

Even though analogies with organ and tissue donation are now widely invoked to oppose state control of pregnant women's decisions regarding both abortion and caesarean sections, there are important differences between these two sorts of issues in maternal–fetal relations. In the abortion debate, pregnancy is viewed as the provision of bodily life support and is itself analogous to the donated organ. In the debate about caesarean sections, the surgical procedure is analogous to organ donation—the potentially viable fetus is removed for its own benefit rather than to benefit some other party as in organ or tissue donation. In the abortion debate, the pregnancy is viewed as invasive; in the debate about caesarean sections, the surgical procedure is invasive. However, the central issue is whether state coercion to benefit the fetus is morally and legally acceptable in these cases, and the debate hinges in part on the appropriateness of living organ and tissue donation as an analogy. Even the critics of the analogy engage in analogical reasoning, but they deny that the similarities are more morally or legally relevant and significant than the dissimilarities. Defenders of governmental coercion could also hold that the moral or legal precedent is mistaken and that organs and tissues should sometimes be conscripted or expropriated from living persons.

Similar disputes appear in other areas of contemporary bioethics, for instance, in debates about whether mandatory testing or screening for antibodies to the human immunodeficiency virus, which causes AIDS, can be justified by analogy to accepted practices of mandatory testing or screening (and what precedents it would create for additional testing and screening, for example, for various genetic conditions), and in debates about whether transplantation experiments using human fetal tissue, following deliberate abortions, are analogous to the complicitous use of materials or data from the morally heinous Nazi experiments. In these cases, as in many others, the debates focus to a great extent on the relevance and significance of the proposed analogies....

CONCLUSIONS

Debates in biomedical ethics are often debates about which metaphors and analogies illuminate more than they distort. Far from being merely decorative or affective, metaphors and analogies are central to both discourse and practice, for framing our problems as well as for shaping our responses to them. They cannot be evaluated in general but rather must be evaluated specifically according to how well they function to describe and/or direct actions, relationships, and the like. Even though in recent bioethics they have sometimes been offered as ways to circumvent or transcend principles and rules, particularly through attention to cases, narratives, and aesthetic dimensions of experience, they are not necessarily incompatible with principles and rules. For instance, analogical reasoning is important within frameworks of principles and rules, as well as in casuistry, and metaphors and models often succeed or fail depending on how well they express the full range of relevant moral considerations....

Notes

1. George Lakoff and Mark Johnson, *Metaphors We Live By* (Chicago: University of Chicago Press, 1980), p. 5.
2. Janet Martin Soskice, *Metaphor and Religious Language* (Oxford: Clarendon Press, 1985).
3. See, for instance, Max Black, "Metaphor," in *Models and Metaphors: Studies in Language and Philosophy* (Ithaca: Cornell University Press, 1962), pp. 25–47; Paul Ricoeur, *The Rule of Metaphor,* trans. Robert Czerny (Toronto: University of Toronto Press, 1977); and Soskice, *Metaphor and Religious Language.*
4. Black, "Metaphor."
5. George Miller, "Images and Models, Similes and Metaphors," in *Metaphor and Thought*, ed. Andrew Ortony (Cambridge: Cambridge University Press, 1979), pp. 202–50.
6. Black, "Metaphor," and Black, "More about Metaphor," in *Metaphor and Thought*, ed. Ortony, pp. 19–43.
7. Soskice, *Metaphor and Religious Language.*
8. Black, "Metaphor," and Lakoff and Johnson, *Metaphors We Live By.*
9. Black, "More about Metaphor," p. 31.
10. Childress, *Who Should Decide?* chap. 1. See also Childress, *War as Reality and War as Metaphor: Some Moral Reflections,* The Joseph A. Reich, Sr., Distinguished Lecture, November 18, 1992 (Colorado Springs: U.S. Air Force Academy, 1993). For other discussions of military metaphors in health care, in addition to the ones that appear in these notes, see Virginia Warren, "A Powerful Metaphor: Medicine as War" (unpublished paper), and Samuel Vaisrub, *Medicine's Metaphors: Messages and Menaces* (Oradell, NJ: Medical Economics Company, 1977).
11. Susan Sontag, *Illness as Metaphor* and *AIDS and Its Metaphors* (New York: Doubleday Anchor Books, 1990), p. 72. Her essay "Illness as Metaphor" was first published separately in the *New York Review of Books* in 1978 and later that year by Farrar, Straus and Giroux, which also published the essay *AIDS and Its Metaphors* separately in 1989 before the combined edition appeared.
12. Ibid., p. 68.
13. Lawrence Pray, *Journey of a Diabetic* (New York: Simon and Schuster, 1983), and "How Diabetes Became My Teacher," *Washington Post*, July 31, 1983.
14. Anne Hunsaker Hawkins, *Reconstructing Illness: Studies in Pathography* (West Lafayette: Purdue University Press, 1993).
15. William F. May, *The Physician's Covenant* (Philadelphia: Westminster Press, 1983), p. 66.
16. For an explication of the just-war tradition, see James F. Childress, *Moral Responsibility in Conflicts* (Baton Rouge: Louisiana State University Press, 1982), esp. chap. 3 on "Just-War Criteria."
17. Richard Rettig and Kathleen Rohr, "Ethical Dimensions of Allocating Scarce Resources in Medicine: A Cross-National Study of End-Stage Renal Disease," unpublished manuscript (1981).
18. Franz Ingelfinger, Editorial, *New England Journal of Medicine* 287 (December 7, 1982): 1198–99.

19. Anne R. Somers, "The 'Geriatric Imperative' and Growing Economic Constraints," *Journal of Medical Education* 55 (February 1980): 89–90, which is also the source of the figures in the remainder of this paragraph.

20. For these points, see James F. Childress, "Ensuring Care, Respect, and Fairness for the Elderly," *Hastings Center Report* 14 (October 1984): 27–31.

21. Howard F. Stein, *American Medicine as Culture* (Boulder: Westview Press, 1990).

22. James F. Childress and Mark Siegler, "Metaphors and Models of Doctor-Patient Relationships: Their Implications for Autonomy," *Theoretical Medicine* 5 (1984): 17–30, which is reprinted below as chapter 3. See also Mark Siegler, "The Physician-Patient Accommodation: A Central Event in Clinical Medicine," *Archives of Internal Medicine* 142 (1982): 1899–1902.

23. May, *Physician's Covenant,* and Robert V. Veatch, "Models for Ethics in Medicine in a Revolutionary Age," *Hastings Center Report* 2 (June 1972): 5–7. See also May, "Code, Covenant, Contract, or Philanthropy," *Hastings Center Report* 5 (December 1975): 29–38.

24. Nancy M. P. King, Larry R. Churchill, and Alan W. Cross, eds., *The Physician as Captain of the Ship* (Dordrecht: D. Reidel, 1988).

25. K. Danner Clouser, "Veatch, May, and Models: A Critical Review and a New View," in *The Critical Encounter,* ed. Earl E. Shelp (Dordrecht: D. Reidel, 1983), pp. 89–103.

26. David Eerdman, "Coleridge as Editorial Writer," in *Power and Consciousness*, ed. Conor Cruise O'Brien and William Dean Vanech (New York: New York University Press, 1969), p. 197.

27. Gerald Winslow, "From Loyalty to Advocacy: A New Metaphor for Nursing," *Hastings Center Report* 14 (June 1984): 32–40; Ellen W. Bernal, "The Nurse as Patient Advocate," *Hastings Center Report* 22 (July/August 1992): 18–23.

28. Winslow, "From Loyalty to Advocacy," and Bernal, "Nurse as Patient Advocate."

29. Bernal, "Nurse as Patient Advocate."

30. Winslow, "From Loyalty to Advocacy."

31. David Heyd, *Genethics: Moral Issues in the Creation of People* (Berkeley: University of California Press, 1992), p. 4 (emphasis in original).

32. Paul Ramsey, *The Patient as Person* (New Haven: Yale University Press, 1970), chap. 7, esp. pp. 256 and 259. Ramsey waffles, sometimes holding that human beings should not play God, at other times (as in this context) suggesting that there are proper ways to play (and not to play) God.

33. See the discussion in the President's Commission for the Study of Ethical Problems in Medicine and Biomedical and Behavioral Research, *Splicing Life* (Washington, D.C.: U.S. Government Printing Office, 1983).

34. Paul Ramsey, *Fabricated Man: The Ethics of Genetic Control* (New Haven: Yale University Press, 1970), p. 138.

35. Edmund L. Erde, "Studies in the Explanation of Issues in Biomedical Ethics: (II) On 'On Playing God', Etc., *Journal of Medicine and Philosophy* 14 (1989): 593–615.

36. Paul Ramsey, *Ethics at the Edges of Life* (New Haven: Yale University Press, 1978), pp. 306–307.

37. For fuller analyses and assessments of wedge and slippery slope arguments, from which some of these points have been drawn, see Tom L. Beauchamp and James F. Childress, *Principles of Biomedical Ethics,* 4th ed. (New York: Oxford University Press, 1994), pp. 228–31.

38. Arthur L. Caplan, "Ethical Engineers Need Not Apply: The State of Applied Ethics Today," *Science, Technology and Human Values* 6 (1980): 30.

39. Larry Churchill, "The Ethicist in Professional Education," *Hastings Center Report* 8 (December 1978): 13–15.

40. Sontag, *Illness as Metaphor* and *AIDS and Its Metaphors.*

41. Donald Schoen, "Generative Metaphor: A Perspective on Problem-Setting in Social Policy," in *Metaphor and Thought*, ed. Ortony.

42. Black, "Metaphor."

43. Ricoeur, *The Rule of Metaphor.*

44. Black, "More about Metaphor."

45. Soskice, *Metaphor and Religious Language.*

46. Dorothy Emmet, *The Nature of Metaphysical Thinking* (New York: St. Martin's Press, 1945), p. 6

47. See David H. Helman, ed., *Analogical Reasoning: Perspectives of Artificial Intelligence, Cognitive Science, and Philosophy* (Dordecht: Kluwer, 1988); and Mark T. Keane, *Analogical Problem Solving* (Chichester: Ellis Norwood, 1988).

48. Albert R. Jonsen and Stephen Toulmin, *The Abuse of Casuistry: A History of Moral Reasoning* (Berkeley: University of California Press, 1988), p. 252.

49. Ibid., p. 316.

50. Ramsey, *Patient as Person*, chap. 7.

51. Lisa Sowle Cahill, "Abortion and Argument by Analogy," *Horizons* 9 (1982): 271–87.

52. Ibid.

53. Judith Jarvis Thomson, "A Defense of Abortion," *Philosophy and Public Affairs* 1 (1972): 47–66.

54. John T. Noonan, "How to Argue about Abortion," (New York: The Ad Hoc Committee in Defense of Life, 1974).

55. See Susan Mattingly, "Viewing Abortion from the Perspective of Transplantation: The Ethics of the Gift of Life," *Soundings* 67 (1984): 399–410; and Patricia Beattie Jung, "Abortion and Organ Donation: Christian Reflections on Bodily Life Support," *Journal of Religious Ethics* 16 (1988): 273–305.

56. Cahill, "Abortion and Argument by Analogy."

57. Ibid., p. 283.

Why a Feminist Approach to Bioethics?

Margaret Olivia Little

Those who work in feminist bioethics are all too familiar with the question, "Why think that feminism offers a distinctive contribution to bioethics?" When asked respectfully, I take it to be a fair question. After all, even if we were to stipulate that the tenets of feminism are profound and wise, it would not guarantee that they offer substantial illumination in every subject matter. However, while it is a good question to ask, it also has a good answer. In this essay, I outline why it is, and how it is, that feminist insights provide such a valuable theoretical aid to the study of bioethics.

First, however, certain misunderstandings need to be addressed. Some individuals seem to understand feminist bioethics to be talk about women's issues in bioethics or, again, to be women talking about bioethics. But while the subject bears some relation to each, it is equivalent to neither. Feminist bioethics is the examination of all sorts of bioethical issues from the perspective of feminist *theory*. The question of feminism's contribution to bioethics can be understood, then, as a question about how and why bioethics might benefit from excursions into this sort of theory. And here the potential for dialogue is too often stunted by a tendency, on the part of those who pose the question, to measure feminism's contribution solely in terms of any distinctive policy recommendations its advocates might give to familiar bioethical controversies. This tendency is often joined by frustration among those who have encountered the diversity within feminist thought, as they wonder how feminism's contribution to specific bioethical topics can be assessed until feminists resolve which camp—liberal, cultural, or radical, say—is correct. But this policy-oriented view of feminism, and of what would count as a "distinctive contribution," sets the stage for far too flat a conception of how feminist theory can enrich bioethics.

At its most general, feminist theory can be thought of as an attempt to uncover the ways in which conceptions of gender distort people's view of the world and to articulate the ways in which these distortions, which are hurtful to all, are particularly constraining to women. These efforts involve *theory*—and not merely benign protestations of women's value or equality—because the assumptions at issue are often so subtle or so familiar as to be invisible, and, crucially, because the assumptions about gender have shaped not only the ways in which we think about men and women, but also the contours of certain fundamental concepts—from "motherhood" to "rationality"—that constitute the working tools of theoretical analyses. According to feminist theory, that is, distorted and harmful conceptions of gender have come to affect the very ways in which we frame our vision of the world, affecting what we notice, what we value, and how we conceptualize what does come to attention.

Little, Margaret. "Why a Feminist Approach to Bioethics?". *Kennedy Institute of Ethics Journal* 6:1 (1996), 1–18.

If these claims are correct, then feminist theory will be useful to disciplines whose subject-matter or methods are appreciably affected by such distortions—and it will be useful in ways that far outstrip the particular policy recommendations that feminists might give to some standard checklist of topics. For one thing, feminist reflection may change the checklist—altering what questions people think to ask, what topics they regard as important, what strikes them as a puzzle in need of resolution. Or again, such reflection may change the analyses underlying policy recommendations—altering which assumptions are given uncontested status, which moves feel persuasive, what elements stand in need of explanation, and how substantive concepts are understood and deployed. If such reflections sometimes yield policies similar to those offered by nonfeminists, the differences in approach can still matter, and matter greatly, by influencing what precedent one takes oneself to have set, what dangers one is alerted to watch for, what would later count as reason to abandon or re-think the policy. And if such reflections are sometimes followed by diverse policy recommendations, we should not be surprised, much less frustrated; for the diagnostic work that forms the core enterprise of feminist theory leads to policy recommendations only in combination with commitments on a variety of other fronts, from economic theory to the empirical facts of the case, about which feminists will understandably disagree.

This, however, is so far rather abstract. To give a more concrete sense of how feminist theory might contribute to bioethics, we need to dip into the theory itself. Accordingly, I want to outline two central themes common to virtually all feminist reflection and use them to illustrate two quite different ways in which attention to feminist insight offers illumination in health care ethics.

ANDROCENTRISM

One of the central themes of feminist theory is that human society, to put it broadly, tends to be androcentric, or male-centered. Under androcentrism, man is treated as the tacit standard for

human: he is the measuring stick, the unstated point of reference, for what is paradigmatic of or normal for humans. To start with an obvious example, man is used as the supposedly generic representative of humanity. That is, when we want to refer to humans independently of gender, it is man that is cast for the job: in language ("Man does not live by bread alone"), in examples (such as the classic illustration of syllogistic reasoning, "All men are mortal, Socrates is a man, therefore Socrates is mortal"); in pictorial representations (according to the familiar depiction of evolution—still used in current biology texts—the indeterminate primate, gradually rising to bipedalism, is inevitably revealed in the last frame to be a man).

This depiction of "human" arguably places man in an unfairly privileged position, since he is not only a constituent, but the representative, of all humanity. But much deeper problems than this are at issue, for these supposedly neutral uses of man are not actually neutral. They are *false generics*, as revealed in our tendency to drop the so-called gender-neutral "he" in favor of "she" when speaking of professions (such as nanny) that are held mostly by women, or again by our difficulty in imagining the logic professor saying, "All men are mortal, Sally is a man (woman?), therefore Sally is mortal."

The first problem resulting from this hidden bias is that androcentrism has a disturbing cumulative effect on our understanding of "human": over time, our substantive conception of what is normal for humans has come to be filled in by what is normal for men (excellent discussions of this general theme can be found in Bem 1993, especially Chapters 3 and 6; Minow 1990; and MacKinnon 1987, Part I). Certain features of men—their experiences, their bodies, their values—have subconsciously come to be regarded as constituting the human norm. His psychology, for instance, tends to define the human mind. In a famous study (Broverman et al. 1970), when psychologists were canvassed and asked to describe the "healthy" man, the "healthy" woman, and the "healthy" human, the list for men and humans turned out to be virtually identical, the list for women divergent. His body tends to define the human body. A clear, if depressing, example can be found in the Supreme Court decision in *General Electric Co. v. Gilbert* (429 U.S. 125, 1976). In a decision finally superseded legislatively by the Pregnancy Discrimination Act, the Court decided that businesses could permissibly exclude pregnancy disabilities from general insurance coverage. Their reasoning was that "pregnancy-related disabilities constitute an additional risk, unique to women, and the failure to compensate them for this risk does not destroy the presumed parity of the benefits that accrue to both men and women," even though (as the Court was aware) the list of traditionally protected benefits included all manner of medical procedures that were unique to men, such as prostate operations and circumcisions. As Sandra Bem (1993, p. 76) puts it:

> The Court is androcentrically defining the male body as the standard human body; hence it sees nothing unusual or inappropriate about giving that standard human body full insurance coverage for each and every condition that might befall it. Consistent with this androcentric perspective, the Court is also defining equal protection as the granting to women of every conceivable benefit that this standard human body might require—which, of course, does not include disability coverage for pregnancy.

In addition, man's biography tends to define norms of practice in the work place. We need go no further than the academic tenure system for an example. Presumably, the idea of evaluating faculty for tenure after their first seven years of employment is premised on the supposition that job performance during those seven years provides some rough indication of performance over the remainder of academic life. But, while this may be true for men, the same cannot be said for women. Factoring in the average time spent at graduate school, those seven years precisely correspond to likely childbearing years for women

faculty—years most likely to involve pregnancy, birth, and breast-feeding, and hence most likely to involve severe sleep deprivation and time pressure. Of all the years of her academic career, these will be the ones *least* likely to represent her overall potential.

Second, treating man as the human norm affects, in subtle but deep ways, our concept of "woman." Males and females obviously differ from one another in various ways. "Different from" is a relation, of course, and a symmetrical one at that: if x is different from y, it is just as true that y is different from x. Under androcentrism, however, we tend to anchor man as the reference point and view woman's nature as a departure from his. A subtle but powerful message is communicated when we always anchor one side of what is logically a symmetrical relation as the fixed point of reference: the anchored point gains the status of the center; the other receives the status of the margin. Because man has been fixed as the reference point for so long, part of our very conception of woman has become the conception of "other"—she is, as Simone de Beauvoir (1952) put it, the *second* sex. Instead of thinking that men differ from women who differ from men, a subtle conceptual shift occurs, and we begin to think of women as simply "different"—as though "different" were an intrinsic property that adheres to them, instead of a relational property men also instantiate (see Minow 1990, pp. 53–56). In the end, it is a short step to regarding aspects of woman's distinct nature as vaguely *deviant*.

Further, woman becomes closely defined by the *content* of her departure from man. The fundamental ways in which women and men differ are, of course, in certain biological features. But when man's body is regarded as the neutral "human" body, woman's biological sex becomes highlighted in such a way that, in the end, awareness of woman very often is awareness of her sex. The phenomenon is akin to one that occurs with race. In white-dominated societies, being white gets anchored as the tacit reference point; over time, the fact that whites have a race tends to fade from consciousness, while people of color are seen as somehow more intrinsically raced (think of how many Americans use the phrase "ethnic restaurants" to refer to non-European cuisine, as though Europeans had no ethnicity, or of how Western history books use the phrase "Ethnic Hoards" to refer, say, to the Mongolian invaders of Europe, but not, say, to the United States' invasion of Okinawa). In a similar way, woman's sex comes to be seen as more essential to her nature than man's sex is to his. We are more likely to see woman as ruled by the whims of her reproductive system than man is by his; more subtly, if no less dangerously, we are simply more likely to think of and be concerned with reproductive issues when thinking of women than of men.[1]

Finally, under androcentrism, woman is more easily viewed in instrumental terms—in terms, that is, of her relation to others and the functions she can serve them. We tend, for instance, to specify a woman's identity in relation to the identity of some man (think of how traditional titles of respect for women indicate her marital status while those for men do not). Or again, the norms of a good woman, unlike those of a good man, tend to value her function for others: an excellent man is one who is self-directive and creative; an excellent woman is one who is nurturing of others and beautiful for them to behold. More concretely, women's legal status often reflects an instrumentalist interpretation of her being. In certain countries, indeed, the interpretation is still as stark as it was in early English common law's doctrine of coverture, which declared, as the legalist William Blackstone ([1765–1769] 1979, Vol. 1, p. 430) wrote:

> By marriage, the husband and wife are one person in law: that is, the very being or legal existence of the woman is suspended during the marriage, or at least incorporated and consolidated into that of the husband; under whose wing, protection, and cover, she performs everything.

Awareness of these general androcentric themes will give new food for thought on any number of topics in bioethics. The medicalization of childbirth, for instance—too often packaged as a tiresome debate between those generically loyal to and those generically suspicious of technology—takes on more suggestive tones when we consider it in light of the historical tendency to regard women as "other" or deviant and hence in need of control (see, e.g., Rothman 1982). Certain patterns of research on women and AIDS emerge with greater clarity when viewed against our proclivity to view women instrumentally: until very recently such research focused almost entirely on women as transmitters of the disease to their fetuses, rather than on how the disease manifests itself, and might be treated, in the women themselves (Faden, Kass, and McGraw, in press). Let me develop in slightly more detail, though, an example that brings to bear the full range of androcentric themes outlined above.

Many people were taken by surprise when a 1990 U.S. Government Accounting Office report (GAO 1990) indicated that women seemed to be underrepresented in clinical trials. To give a few now-famous examples, the Physicians Health Study, which concluded in 1988 that an aspirin a day may help decrease the risk of heart disease, studied 22,000 men and no women; the Baltimore Longitudinal Study, one of the largest projects ever to study the natural processes of aging, included no women at its inception in 1958 and still had no data on women by 1984, although women constitute 60 percent of the population over age 65 in the United States (see Laurence and Weinhouse 1994, p. 61). It is difficult to be precise about women's overall representation in medical research because information on participants' sex often is not gathered; but there does seem to be legitimate cause for concern. For one thing, U.S. Food and Drug Administration (FDA) guidelines from 1977 to 1993 barred all women of childbearing potential from early clinical trials, which seems to have discouraged their representation in later stages of drug research (Merton 1994). More broadly, a review of medical studies published in JAMA in 1990 and 1992 revealed that, in studies on non-gender-specific diseases, women were underrepresented in 2.7 times as many studies than were men (Bird 1994; see also Laurence and Weinhouse 1994, pp. 64–67).

The possibility of significant underrepresentation has raised concerns that women are being denied equal opportunity to participate in something they may regard as valuable and that women may face compromised safety or efficacy in the drugs and procedures they receive (for instance, the difference in the average weights of women and men raises questions about the effects on women of drugs that are highly dosage-sensitive). Now, determining what policy we should advocate with respect to women's inclusion in medical research is a complicated matter—if only because adding sex as a variable in research protocols can significantly increase the cost of research.[2] What is clear, though, is that awareness of various androcentric motifs can highlight important issues that might otherwise remain hidden or camouflaged. Without the perspective of feminist theory, that is, certain concerns are likely not even to make it to the table to be factored in when policy questions arise (for a related discussion, see DeBruin 1994). Let me give some examples.

One argument against the inclusion of women commonly offered by those running clinical trials is that women's hormones represent a "complication": the cyclicity of women's hormonal patterns introduces a variable that can make it harder to discern the effects of the drug or procedure being studied. Now this is an interesting argument, for acknowledging the causal power of women's hormonal cyclicity might also suggest the very reason that it might be important to include women in studies, namely, the possibility that the cyclicity affects the underlying action of the drug or procedure. Medicine has only begun to consider and study this possibility in earnest (see Cotton 1990; Hamilton and Parry 1983). Early results include preliminary evidence that surgical treatment for breast cancer is more effective if done in the second, rather than the first, half of a woman's menstrual cycle, and that the effectiveness of antidepressants varies across a woman's menstrual cycle, suggesting that women currently receive too much

for one half of the month and too little for the other (see Laurence and Weinhouse 1994, p. 71). Trust in all-male studies seems to reflect a broad confidence in the neutrality of treating the male body as the human norm and a familiar tendency to regard that which is distinct to woman as a distortion—in this case, by regarding women's hormonal pattern as merely distorting the evidence concerning the true effect of a drug or procedure, and hence as something that is best ignored, rather than regarding it as an important factor in its own right, one influencing the actual effect of the object studied.

Another reason often given for the underrepresentation of women by those running clinical trials is that women are harder to find and to keep in studies. There is an important element of truth here: questionnaires reveal that women report greater problems navigating the logistics of participating in drug trials—they find it more difficult, for instance, to arrange for transportation and child care (Cotton 1993; Laurence and Weinhouse 1994, pp. 70–71). But if it is currently harder for women to participate than for men, it is not because of some natural or neutral ordering of things; it is in large part because drug trials are currently organized to accommodate the logistical structure and hassles of men's lives. Organizers routinely locate trials where men are, such as the military, for instance, and to organize activities around work schedules in the public economy. Again, there is a tendency to anchor what is normal for "participants" to features that are more typical of men. If women's distinctive needs show up on the radar screen at all, they appear as needs that would require "special" accommodation—and hence accommodation one may decline to make—as though accommodations for men have not already been made.

A different concern lay behind the now-defunct FDA guidelines barring women of childbearing potential from early clinical trials. Here the explicit rationale was fetal protection: the drugs women would be exposed to might harm fetuses they knowingly or unknowingly carried. A closer look, however, once again reveals the subtle presence of androcentrism: granting society's interest in fetal health, protective measures are applied quite differently to men and women. The guidelines in essence barred all fertile women from early trials—including single women not planning to have intercourse, women using reliable birth control, and women whose partners had had vasectomies (Merton 1994). In contrast, when trials were conducted on drugs suspected of increasing birth defects by affecting men's sperm (a possibility often forgotten), fertile men were simply required to sign a form promising to wear condoms during the trial (Laurence and Weinhouse 1994, pp. 72–73). The regulation was able to think of men under guises separate from their reproductive capacities, but, as Vanessa Merton (1994, p. 66) says, it "envisions all women as constantly poised for reproductive activity." Further, and again granting that fetal protection is important, one might argue that respect for parental autonomy argues in favor of allowing the individual to decide whether participation is worth the risk. But when respect for parental autonomy conflicts with protection for fetuses or children, society is much more willing to intrude on the autonomy if it belongs to a woman than to a man. Courts, for instance, have forced women to undergo cesarean sections in attempts to gain slight increases in a fetus's chance for survival, while they routinely deny requests to force fathers to donate organs—or even blood—to save the life of their children (see Daniels 1993).

GENDERED CONCEPTS

A second core theme of feminist theory maintains that assumptions about gender have, in subtle but important ways, distorted some of the broad conceptual tools that philosophers use. Certain key philosophical concepts, such as reason and emotion or mind and body, seem in part to be *gendered* concepts—that is, concepts whose interpretations have been substantively shaped by their rich historical associations with certain narrow conceptions of male and female.

One such distortion stems from the fact that, historically, that which is tightly and consistently associated with woman tends to become devalued. Throughout history, woman has been regarded as a deficient human: as a group, at least, she does not measure up to the standard set by man. (Indeed, it would be surprising if there were not some such evaluation lurking behind the scenes of androcentrism, for it would otherwise be puzzling why it is man who is ubiquitously cast as the human norm.) Aristotle *defined* woman as "a mutilated male," placing her just above slaves in the natural hierarchy (*Generation of Animals*, Books I and II; *Politics*, Book I). In post-Darwinian Victorian society, when a theory emerged according to which "lower forms" of human remained closer to embryonic type, a flurry of studies claimed to demonstrate the child-like aspects of woman's anatomy. She was, as one chapter heading called her, "Undeveloped Man"; in the words of James Allan, a famous and particularly succinct anthropologist, "Physically, mentally, and morally, woman is a kind of adult child… Man is the head of creation" (both cited in Russett 1989, pp. 74, 55). Against this background, those things associated with woman can gradually inherit a depreciated status. "Womanly" attributes, or aspects of the world regarded as somehow "feminine," become devalued (which, of course, only serves to reinforce the poor judgment of women, as they are now associated with things of little value). To give just one illustration, think of the associations we carry about voice types and authority. A resonant baritone carries a psychological authority missing in a high squeaky voice. This is often cited as a reason women have trouble being viewed as authority figures; but it is also worth asking why authority came to be associated with a baritone rather than a soprano in the first place. Clearly, the association both reflects a prior conception of man as naturally more authoritative and reinforces that commitment, as women's voices then stand in the way of their meeting the "neutral" standard of authority.

Another common distortion stems from the fact that pairs of concepts whose members are associated with man and woman, respectively, tend to become interpreted in particularly dualistic ways. For much of Western history, but especially since the Scientific Revolution, men and women have been understood as having different appropriate spheres of function (see, e.g., Gatens 1991, Pateman 1989, Bordo 1986, Lloyd 1983, Okin 1979).[3] Man's central role was in the public sphere—economics, politics, religion, culture; woman's central role was in the private sphere—the domestic realm of care taking for the most natural, embodied, and personal aspects of humans. This separation of spheres was understood to constitute a complementary system in which each contributed something of value that, when combined, made an ideal whole—the marriage unit. Of course, given the devaluation of that which is associated with woman, it is not surprising that woman's sphere was regarded as less intrinsically valuable: it is man, and what is accomplished in the public sphere, that represents the human ideal (a view reflected in history books, which are histories of wars and political upheavals, not of hearth and home). In any event, because the division was understood as grounded in the natures of man and woman, the separation was a rigid one; the idea that either side of the division could offer something useful to the other's realm would simply not emerge as a possibility. This dualistic picture of the nature and function of women and men, with its subtle devaluing of women, can bleed over to concepts that have been tightly associated with the sexes. When abstract concepts, such as, say, mind and body, come to be paired with the concepts of male and female consistently enough, their substantive interpretations often become tainted with the dualism that characterizes the understanding of those latter concepts. The nature of each comes to be understood largely in opposition to the other, and, while the pair is understood as forming a complementary whole, the functions of the components are regarded as rigidly separated, and the one that is regarded as "male"—here, mind—is held in higher philosophical esteem.

These themes are mirrored in the interpretation of certain central philosophical concepts. An important instance is the traditional conception of reason and emotion, which plays a large role in moral philosophy. For all the hotly disputed debates in the history of ideas, one theme that emerges with remarkable consistency is an association of women

with emotion and men with reason (see Tuana 1992, Chapters 2–4; Lloyd 1984). According to Aristotle (*Politics*, 1260a15), women have rationality "but without authority"; Rousseau (1979, p. 386) gives Sophie a different education from Emile because "the search for abstract and speculative truths, principles and axioms in the sciences, for everything that tends to general ideas, is not within the competence of women"; and according to Kant (1960, p. 79), "women's philosophy is not to reason but to sense." Science has contributed its support—for example, tracing woman's supposedly greater proclivity towards volatile emotions to disorders of the womb (hence "uterus" as the root of "hysteria") and her restricted intellect to the "hormonal hurricanes" of her menstrual cycle (see Smith-Rosenberg 1972; Russett 1989, especially Chapter 4; and Fausto-Sterling 1992, Chapter 4). As James Allan wrote, "In intellectual labor, man has surpassed, does now, and always will surpass woman for the obvious reason that nature does not periodically interrupt his thought in application" (cited in Russett 1989, p. 30). (Apparently Allan suffered no concern that man's rather more constant hormonal activity might be rather more constantly interrupting his thought!)

The conception of reason and emotion found in much of traditional ethical theory bears the mark of these entrenched associations (see Jaggar 1989, Lloyd 1983). There is a tendency to regard reason and emotion as having completely separate functions and to regard emotion, at best, as irrelevant to the moral enterprise and, at worst, as something that infects, renders impure, and constantly threatens to disrupt moral efforts. Emotion is conceptualized as something more to do with the body we have as animals than the mind we have as humans; it is viewed as a faculty of blind urges, akin to pains and tickles, rather than as responses that reflect evaluations of the world, and that hence can be "tutored" or developed into mature stances.

Thus, most traditional moral epistemology stresses that the stance appropriate to moral wisdom is a dispassionate one. To make considered, sound moral judgments, we are told to abstract from our emotions, feelings, and sentiments. Emotions are not part of the equipment needed to discern moral answers; indeed, only trouble can come of their intrusion into deliberations about what to do, for they "cloud" our judgment and "bias" our reasoning. To be objective is to be detached; to be clear-sighted is to achieve distance; to be careful in deliberation is to be cool and calm. Further, the tradition tends to discount the idea that experiencing appropriate emotion is an integral part of being moral. Moral theory tends to focus exclusively on questions about what actions are obligated or prohibited, or perhaps on what intention or motive one should have in acting, not on what emotional stance a moral agent should be feeling. Indeed, much of traditional moral theory has a positive suspicion of emotion as a basis for moral action. Emotions such as love or indignation, as opposed to some cerebral "respect for duty," are deemed fickle and unreliable (metaphors, of course, for the female); they "incite" and "provoke" us, rather than moving us by way of their reasonability. Finally, traditional moral theory vastly underplays the importance of the "emotional work" of life—of nurturing children, offering sympathetic support to colleagues, or displaying felt concern for patients. To the extent that the value of such work is recognized at all—as, for example, in treatises on "mother love"—it is often accorded a lesser status, regarded as reflective of instinct rather than skill, and hence not qualifying as moral work at all, or as relevant only in limited spheres of life, such as nursing or parenting, that are accorded lower value than other more impersonal enterprises.

Feminists argue that these presuppositions may not survive their gendered origins. Possession of appropriate emotion, for instance, arguably forms an indispensable component of a wise person's epistemic repertoire (see Little 1995). While our passions and inclinations can mislead us and distort our perceptions, they can also guide them. To give just one example, if one is deprived of felt concern for a patient, it is unlikely that one will be attuned to the subtle and unique nuances of his situation. Instead of discerning the contours of his particular needs, one is likely to see his case as an instance of one's current favorite generality. Distance, that is, does not always clarify. Sometimes truth is better revealed, the landscape most clearly seen, from a position that has been called "loving perception" or "sympathetic thinking" (Lugones 1987, Jaggar 1989, Walker 1992b). And again, emotion arguably forms an integral part of being moral. Simply to perform a required action—while certainly better than nothing—is often not enough. Being moral frequently involves feeling appropriate emotions, including anger, indignation, and especially caring. The friend who only ever helps one out of a sense of duty rather than a feeling of generous reciprocity is not in the end a good friend; the citizen who gives money to the poor, but is devoid of any empathy, is not as moral as the one whose help flows from felt concern. This is not to say that we owe personal love to all who walk the earth—proper caring comes in different forms for different relationships. Nor is proper caring to be conflated with self-abnegation. Suspicions about the moral imperative to care often tacitly rely on self-sacrificial models of care, in which the boundary between self and other is overly blurred. From a feminist perspective, it is not surprising that this is the model of care we have inherited, for caring has usually been regarded as women's work, and traditional norms for women have stressed a denial of self. Feminist reflection, acutely aware of the limitations of these norms, precisely invites us to develop a healthier and more robust conception of proper caring (for further discussion, see Carse and Nelson 1996).

In another important instance, that which is associated with the private or domestic sphere is given short shrift in moral theory. Relations in the private sphere, such as parent-child relations, are marked by intimacies and dependencies, appropriate kinds of partiality, and positive but unchosen obligations that cannot be modelled as "contracts between equals." Furthermore, few would imagine that deliberations about how to handle such relations could be settled by some list of codified rules—wisdom here requires skills of discernment and judgment, not the internalization of set principles. But traditional moral theory tends to concentrate on moral questions that adjudicate relations between equal and self-sufficient strangers, to stress impartiality, to acknowledge obligations beyond duties of noninterference only when they are incurred by voluntary contract, and to emphasize a search for algorithmic moral principles or "policies" that one could apply to any situation to derive right action (Walker 1992a, Baier 1987).

This tendency to subsume all moral questions under a public "juridical" model tends, for one thing, to restrict the issues that will be acknowledged as important to those cast in terms of rights. "The" moral question about abortion, for instance, is often automatically cast as a battle between maternal and fetal rights, to the exclusion of, say, difficult and nuanced questions about whether and what distinctly maternal responsibilities might accompany pregnancy. And it often does violence to our considered sensibilities about the morality of relations involving dependencies and involuntary positive obligations. For instance, in considering what it is to respect patient autonomy, many seem to feel forced into a narrow consumer–provider model of the issue, in which the alternative to simply informing and then carrying out the patient's wishes must be regarded as paternalism. While such a model may be appropriate to, say, business relations between self-sufficient equals, it seems highly impoverished as a model for relations marked by the unequal vulnerabilities inherent in physician–patient relations. In these sorts of relations, all of the rich moral possibilities lie in between the two poles of merely providing information, on the one hand, and wresting the decision from the patient, on the other. For example, a proper moral stance might involve proactively helping a patient to sift through options, or proactively fostering the patient's independence by, say, discussing sensitive questions outside the presence of overly interfering family members.

Finally, when ethical approaches more characteristic of the private sphere do make it onto the radar screen, there is still a tendency to segregate these approaches from those we take to the public sphere. That is, in stark contrast to the tendency to subsume the morality of intimates into the morality of strangers, rarely do we ask how the moral lessons garnered from reflecting on private relations might shed light on moral issues that arise outside of the purely domestic context. To give just one example, patients often feel a deep sense of abandonment when their surgeons do not personally display a caring attitude toward them: the caring they may receive from other health care professionals, welcome as it may be, seems unable to compensate for this loss. This phenomenon will seem less puzzling if, borrowing a concept from the private realm, we realize that surgery involves a special kind of *intimacy*, as the surgeon dips into the patient's body. Seen under this guise, the patient's need becomes more understandable—and the surgeon's nontransferable duty to care clearer—for reflection on more familiar, domestic intimacies, such as those involved in sexual interactions, reminds us that intimacy followed by a vacuum of care can constitute a kind of abandonment.

In summary, then, reflection in feminist theory is important to bioethics in at least two distinct ways. First, it can reveal androcentric reasoning present in analyses of substantive bioethical issues—reasoning that can bias not only which policies are adopted, but what gets counted as an important question or persuasive argument. Second, it can help bioethicists to rethink the very conceptual tools used in bioethics—specifically, helping to identify where assumptions about gender have distorted the concepts commonly invoked in moral theory and, in doing so, clearing the way for the development of what might best be called "feminist-inspired" moral theory.

Notes

1. For excellent discussions of this theme in the history of science, see Russett (1989), Fausto-Sterling (1992, Chapter 4), and Rosenberg (1976, Chapter 2).
2. For extensive analysis of issues relating to public policy, see the essays in Institute of Medicine (1994, vol. 1).

3. Portions of this and the next few paragraphs are taken from my article, "Seeing and Caring: The Role of Affect in Feminist Moral Epistemology" (Little 1995).

References

Baier, Annette. 1987. The Need for More than Justice. In *Science, Morality and Feminist Theory*, ed. Marsha Hanen and Kai Nielsen, pp. 41–56. Calgary: University of Calgary Press.

Beauvoir, Simone de. 1952. *The Second Sex.* New York: Alfred A. Knopf.

Bem, Sandra L. 1993. *The Lenses of Gender.* New Haven and London: Yale University Press.

Bird, Chloe E. 1994. Women's Representation as Subjects in Clinical Studies: A Pilot Study of Research Published in JAMA in 1990 and 1992. In *Women and Health Research: Ethical and Legal Issues of Including Women in Clinical Studies,* vol. 2, Institute of Medicine, pp. 151–173. Washington, DC: National Academy Press.

Blackstone, William. [1765–1769] 1979. *Commentaries on the Laws of England.* Chicago: University of Chicago Press.

Bordo, Susan. 1986. The Cartesian Masculinization of Thought. *Signs* 11: 439–56.

Broverman, Inge K., Broverman, Donald M., Clarkson, Frank E., et al. 1970. Sex-Role Stereotypes and Clinical Judgments of Mental Health. *Journal of Consulting and Clinical Psychology* 34 (1): 1–7.

Carse, Alisa L., and Nelson, Hilde Lindemann. 1996. Rehabilitating Care. *Kennedy Institute of Ethics Journal* 6: 19–35.

Cotton, Paul. 1990. Examples Abound of Gaps in Medical Knowledge Because of Groups Excluded from Scientific Study. *Journal of the American Medical Association* 263: 1051, 1055.

———. 1993. FDA Lifts Ban on Women in Early Drug Tests. *Journal of the American Medical Association* 269: 2067.

Daniels, Cynthia. 1993. *At Women's Expense: State Power and the Politics of Fetal Rights.* Cambridge and London: Harvard University Press.

DeBruin, Debra A. 1994. Justice and the Inclusion of Women in Clinical Studies: An Argument for Further Reform. *Kennedy Institute of Ethics Journal* 4: 117–46.

Faden, Ruth; Kass, N.; and McGraw, D. In press. Women as Vessels and Vectors: Lessons from the HIV Epidemic. In *Feminism and Bioethics: Beyond Reproduction,* ed. Susan Wolf. New York: Oxford University Press.

Fausto-Sterling, Anne. 1992. *Myths of Gender: Biological Theories About Women and Men.* New York: HarperCollins.

GAO. U.S. General Accounting Office. 1990. *National Institutes of Health: Problems in Instituting Policy on Women in Study Populations.*

Gatens, Moira. 1991. *Feminism and Philosophy.* Bloomington: Indiana University Press.

Hamilton, Jean, and Parry, Barbara. 1983. Sex-Related Differences in Clinical Drug Response: Implications for Women's Health. *JAMWA* 38(5): 126–32.

Institute of Medicine: Committee on the Ethical and Legal Issues Relating to the Inclusion of Women in Clinical Trials. 1994. *Women and Health Research,* vols. 1 and 2. Washington, DC: National Academy Press.

Jaggar, Alison. 1989. Love and Knowledge: Emotion in Feminist Epistemology. In *Women, Knowledge, and Reality,* ed. Ann Garry and Marilyn Pearsall, pp. 129–55. Boston: Unwin Hyman.

Kant, Immanuel. 1960. *Observations on the Feeling of the Beautiful and Sublime,* Section Three (Of the Distinction of the Beautiful and Sublime in the Interrelations of the Two Sexes). Berkeley: University of California Press.

Laurence, Leslie, and Weinhouse, Beth. 1994. *Outrageous Practices: The Alarming Truth about how Medicine Mistreats Women.* New York: Fawcett Columbine.

Little, Margaret Olivia. 1995. Seeing and Caring: The Role of Affect in Feminist Moral Epistemology. *Hypatia* 10(3): 117–137.

Lloyd, Genevieve. 1983. Reason, Gender, and Morality in the History of Philosophy. *Social Research* 50: 490–513.

———. 1984. *The Man of Reason: Male and Female in Western Philosophy.* London: Methuem.

Lugones, Maria. 1987. Playfulness, World-Traveling, and Loving Perception. *Hypatia* 2(2): 3–19.

MacKinnon, Catharine A. 1987. *Feminism Unmodified: Discourses on Life and Law.* Cambridge and London: Harvard University Press.

Merton, Vanessa. 1994. Impact of Current Federal Regulations on the Inclusion of Female Subjects in Clinical Studies. In *Women and Health Research: Ethical and Legal Issues of Including Women in Clinical Studies,* vol. 2, Institute of Medicine, pp. 65–83. Washington, DC: National Academy Press.

Minow, Martha. 1990. *Making All the Difference: Inclusion, Exclusion, and American Law.* Ithaca and London: Cornell University Press.

Okin, Susan Miller. 1979. *Women in Western Political Thought.* Princeton: Princeton University Press.

Pateman, Carole. 1989. *The Disorder of Women.* Stanford: Stanford University Press.

Rosenberg, Charles. 1976. *No Other Gods: On Science and American Social Thought.* Baltimore: Johns Hopkins University Press.

Rothman, Barbara Katz. 1982. *In Labor: Women and Power in the Birthplace.* New York: Norton.

Rousseau, Emile. 1979. *Emile, or On Education.* New York: Basic Books.

Russett, Cynthia E. 1989. *Sexual Science: The Victorian Construction of Womanhood.* Cambridge and London: Harvard University Press.

Smith-Rosenberg, Caroll. 1972. The Hysterical Woman: Sex Roles in 19th Century America. *Social Research* 39: 652–78.

Tuana, Nancy. 1992. *Woman and the History of Philosophy.* New York: Paragon House.

Walker, Margaret Urban. 1992a. Feminism, Ethics, and the Question of Theory. *Hypatia* 7(3): 23–38.

———. 1992b. Moral Understandings: Alternative Epistemology for a Feminist Ethics. In *Explorations in Feminist Ethics,* ed. Eve Browning Cole and Susan Coultrap-McQuinn, pp. 165–75. Bloomington: Indiana University Press.

The Cultural Context of Ethicists' Case Examples and Consumer Narratives of Decisions About Life Supporting Technology

Joseph M. Kaufert

INTRODUCTION

This paper applies the perspective of anthropology to interpretation of constructed case studies and narrative approaches to decision-making involving mechanical ventilation. It contrasts clinical ethicists' case studies, illustrating the application of principles in initiating or discontinuing life support, with ventilator users' accounts of their own decisions about mechanical ventilation. It explores the cultural, structural and methodological context of case examples constructed by ethicists and life narratives of ventilator users describing the complexity of their own decisions. One case example of end of life decision-making constructed by ethicists is contrasted with a consumer's complex and contextualized life narrative using the approaches of "thick description" and narrative reconstruction.

I will focus on cultural construction of case examples describing decisions involving mechanical ventilation technology in clinical ethics and use of consumer narratives in the emerging literature in disability studies. I will draw on more culturally contextualized narratives of people living with disability which are utilized extensively within the field of disability studies. Anthropological approaches emphasize need for development of case studies based on life narratives emphasizing cultural context and rich descriptive narratives of the decision-makers. I will examine anthropological approaches to developing more culturally contextualized case studies in the field of ethics through the use of "thick" description and narrative reconstruction.

Ethicists and clinical decision-makers commonly use constructed case studies to illustrate moral, legal, and cultural dimensions of end of life decision-making. Authoritative interpretation is often sustained by reference to precedent cases and principles of moral philosophy. Ethicists, for example, have documented and then constructed case studies centered

From *Disability Studies Quarterly* 21(3), pp. 76–91. Copyright 2001. Reprinted by permission of the author.

on discontinuation of life support by persons living with disabilities. Widely disseminated case studies, including popular films such as "Whose Life is It Anyway," depict situations involving acceptance, rejection or discontinuation of life supporting technologies.

Implicit in ethicists' perspective in building case studies is a series of medico-legal narratives that support their assumptions about the quality of life of persons living with disability who need mechanical ventilation. This perspective is reflected in constructed examples where descriptions sustain values about life quality prevalent among physicians, ethicists and members of the general public. Ethicists deal with the whole medical legal spectrum of clinical practice and often are asked to advise on both clinical and resource allocation decisions. The clinical ethicist is rewarded for giving pragmatic advice based on [principles] and widely held values. They may also be called upon to communicate approaches to decision making through case examples.

Because ethicists and clinicians frequently interpret and construct cases from a professional perspective emphasizing medical data and an ethical aesthetic, their case studies may represent the "quality of life" and prospects for independent living in ways that contrast dramatically with personal narratives of persons living with disabilities. In an attempt to reconstruct the broad sequence of medical decision making, many ethicists' case examples typically omit biographical and contextual information to present a clearer moral analysis of the decision. Decisions described in such constructions thus are seldom anchored in the decision-makers' life history. In addition, formal case studies rarely acknowledge the past experience of the technology user, the care-provider, or the relationship they share. Nor is recognition typically given to the institutional context in which such decisions are made or to structural barriers, which from the person with a disability's perspective may critically influence decisions. The importance of these factors in understanding the principles and issues which constructed studies

profess to illustrate is the central focus of this paper.

BIOGRAPHICAL CONTEXT

As a medical anthropologist my awareness of the contrasting approaches to case studies of ethical decision evolved as I became more committed to research and advocacy activities within the independent living movement. My involvement shifted from more epidemiological studies of disability prevalence to doing qualitative research on consumer narratives describing their experiences in accessing and using enabling technologies and the independent living movement. I worked with members of post-polio support groups to record life narratives describing technology access experience and involvement with the independent living movement. Their life narratives provided critical and policy relevant insights about the ethics of access to life supporting technology and consumer perspectives on autonomy in end of life decision-making. My identification with the disability movement has been reinforced by personal experience with the consumer movement, cardiovascular disability, bypass surgery and encounters with the rehabilitation system.

Case Examples

In this paper I contrast a single reconstructed, decontextualized case presented by ethicists at a disability studies conference with a long term ventilator user's account of decisions to use mechanical ventilation.[1] The conference was convened by The World Institute on Disability, Rehabilitation International and the World Rehabilitation Fund. It was held simultaneously with the Society for Disability Studies. The conference was attended by disability studies researchers, ethicists and representatives of consumer organizations. The ethicists' case study describes one person's decision to discontinue life support designed to illustrate moral, legal, and cultural dimensions of end of life decision-making. The consumer narrative is one of ten life histories I collected among people who used mechanical ventilation after sustaining respiratory impairment in the 1952–53 polio epidemics. They described their experiences with successive generations of mechanical ventilation technology.[2] Participants had been using mechanical ventilators for more than 35 years. In the context of an integrated biographical narrative, they described repeated experiences of respiratory insufficiency, equipment failure, and anxieties related to future crises. In this paper I will compare consumer narratives describing crisis events involving respiratory failure with more recent experience in deciding whether to use more effective, but more invasive life support technology. More particularly, several informants expressed concerns over how their voice—documented in advance directives—would be represented in end of life decisions.

The Ethicists' Case Example

The distance between the formal case studies and the histories of consumers with personal experience was highlighted at this national conference on ethical decision making and disability. Meeting participants included social scientists, ethicists, and clinicians. In addition, more than half the participating membership was composed of persons with disabilities. At the final session of the two-day meeting, a case involving end of life decision making was presented by two physician ethicists from a rehabilitation hospital. Neither had attended the rest of the conference.

The speakers opened with a 40 minute long videotaped reconstruction of the case-history of a 50 year old man with progressive impairment resulting from Amyotrophic Lateral Sclerosis (A.L.S.). Its focus was his decision to discontinue his life support. Made six months after the man's death, the tape showed the clinical ethicist and another attending physician discussing the sequence of events leading up to the final decision to disconnect the patient's respirator. One speaker described the course of the person's illness, the progressive impairment of his respiratory system, and the initial decision to perform

a tracheotomy and support breathing using a portable ventilator.

The ethicist then described other events occurring in the man's life, particularly his profound depression following the sudden death of his wife. The speakers emphasized that the death of his primary family caregiver made it extremely unlikely that the man would be able to return home. The two clinicians then described their efforts to help him explore alternative ways of enhancing his life quality. Rather than pursuing other options, the man requested that his ventilator be turned off, saying that he found the current quality of life and his prospects for future suffering unbearable.

The videotape then described a sequence of repeated consultations with the patient, psychiatrists and representatives of the hospital's Institutional Review Committee. These culminated in an agreement that the man was fully informed, understood the limited prospects for the future quality of his life, and was making a valid and consistent request for discontinuation of life support. The presentation concluded with a description by physicians of their role in disconnecting the ventilator and providing him with palliative care.

Reaction

The two speakers then turned to the audience. Expecting to lead the usual academic discussion, they faced instead a series of critical, often angry, comments and questions. While none of the commentators questioned the man's right to decide that life support should be discontinued or the validity of this experience of suffering, the constructed case study was criticized for what it did not discuss or portray. Further, as one discussant noted, the tape revealed an attitude prevalent within the medical rehabilitation community and shared by many members of general public. This perspective was characterized by devaluation and emphasis on quality and resource implications of technology use.[3] Several discussants with personal experience using life support focused on the man's isolation and dependence on the two clinicians for information about the options available to him. He had not been encouraged to meet with people living at home with life supportive technology or to speak with other users of mechanical ventilators, for example. Others criticized the clinician's decision not to involve people with high-level quadriplegia as consultants. Other discussants decried the lack of effort made to help the man to fully explore the various alternative services that might have enabled the man to live at home.

Criticism was not limited to audience members with long term ventilator experience. One ethicist commented on the compressed time frame of the case study's reportage, noting that no account seemed to have been taken of the length of the usual period of depression following the death of a spouse. Another stated that, from her perspective as an ethicist and as a woman with a disability, the presentation reflected both the hazards of oversimplification and the lack of consumer input she had experienced during her participation in a state ethics commission. Her primary criticism was that the "rehabilitation personnel in charge had not offered the man a vision of a good life in spite of his disability."[4]

A spokesperson for consumer perspectives commented on the way in which the clinician's account served to decontextualize the man's decision.[5] Structural barriers, such as the limitations of state and federal benefits, the shortage of community living options, the lack of respiratory home care, while perhaps critical to decision making were ignored in their case presentation. The final discussant noted that the tape revealed an attitude, prevalent within the medical rehabilitation community (and among the general public), that life with a disability was a devalued life and one perhaps not worth living.[6]

The outraged reaction surprised the presenters who clearly thought they had presented a sympathetic account of their role in helping a patient accomplish his own decision. For its part, the audience saw the video as a demonstration of the powerlessness of an individual totally dependent on health care providers for information, and without full knowledge of potential living options.

The audience's reaction to the case example presented at the disability studies conference may reflect criticism of ethicists' construction of key medical legal cases involving discontinuation of life support or active euthanasia. The audience emphasized that the case presented by the ethicist did not acknowledge the full impact of resource constraints or decision maker's isolation from peer advice from other ventilator users.

We need to recognize that these conflicting approaches to case study development reflects not just a conflict between interpretations emphasized by ethicists and accounts of consumers. The consumer reaction may also reflect a more global critique of ethicists' and physicians' approaches to defining quality of life. It may reflect more general concerns about the power of professionals in proxy decision-making where the person's "best interest" is externally defined.

The ethicists' lack of awareness of culture and ethical context of the field of disability studies meant that they did not expect to have their case analysis contested. Their inability to anticipate the consumer response reflected their own cultural orientation as benevolent and pragmatic clinical and ethical decision-makers.

Anthropological interpretations may contribute to understanding of both consumer's perspective on end of life decision-making and the cultural context of clinical ethics. Professional and clinical cultures inculcate and reinforce the importance of physicians and clinical ethicists' roles in helping to interpret the availability and quality of life achievable using alternative life supporting technologies.[7]

Description and Authenticity in Case Studies

The clinicians' account of the decision to discontinue life support differed in many critical respects from the narratives that my colleagues and I documented in interviews with long term ventilator users. Their account was reconstructed after the man's death from the perspective of the attending physician and the consulting clinical ethicist. It did not use thick description to convey either a sense of the patient's own voice or a detailed description of the context of his decision. Their case was strategically constructed to sustain an analysis emphasizing autonomy and beneficence.

Part of the technology users' criticism of the case was that, although it was based on a real experience, it did not contain the detailed descriptions or narrative quotes which adequately conveyed his perspective on his own decision. Several members of the audience emphasized that the clinicians' account of actual decision-making failed to convey a sense of authenticity and voice.

Thick Description and the Perspective of the Narrator

Chambers has described the limitations of teaching cases like this one which are constructed to illustrate a particular principle or theory.[8] As an alternative to constructed case studies to illustrate principles, Davis draws on the perspectives of anthropologists like Clifford Gertz in emphasizing that detailed descriptions of "real" experiences keep the ethicist "honest" and invite varying interpretations.[9] Davis has proposed the use of "thick description" to develop "rich cases" describing in detail the context of ethical decision-making and sense of meaning as an alternative approach.

In the ethnographic tradition rich case descriptions can either be drawn from actual incidents, from cases that are documented in the media or from fictional accounts. Davis asserts the benefits of using rich cases to develop a more detailed moral response. At the same time she has also recognized the dilemmas of using "thick descriptions" of actual cases because of the need to protect the confidentiality of the decision-makers in the actual case while at the same time conveying detail. Despite these constraints, Davis asserts that thick descriptions of real experiences allow ethicists to draw conclusions while also allowing readers to make their own independent moral and social analysis. Davis concludes: "We need thick descriptions to allow cases to remain open to different interpretations over time and also to enable cases to ground an ethics of care."[10]

The other dimension of the consumer critique of the ethicists' representation of the man's decision to discontinue mechanical ventilation centered on the question: whose point of view was represented in the case narrative? Chambers analysis of the literary dimension of ethicists' cases concluded that they can be constructed from multiple perspectives and that the ethicists' relationship to the participants is often unclear.[11] In many case studies the narrator will adopt the position of an unseen or non-participant observer. They also frequently adopt the perspective and voice of the clinician.

In recent case studies in narrative ethics, the perspective of the person with a disability has been featured. Despite this growing recognition that the cases can be constructed from multiple perspectives, Chambers concludes: "narrative continues to be used by most ethicists in a somewhat naive way, as if it simply reproduced reality without also interpreting the world in a manner that colors the reader's perspective."[12]

The remainder of this paper will examine the impact of reconstructing descriptions of decisions about mechanical ventilation from the perspective of the technology user, recognizing that this narrative may not fully represent the perspective of either the clinician or ethicist.

Chambers asserts that "all representations must adopt a particular point of view and that point of view will always carry with it a partial and limited understanding of the world."[13] I examine the process of narrative construction to understand consumers' accounts of life threatening events and decisions about treatment and non-treatment.

Narrative Reconstruction of Threatening Events

In contrast to ethicists' formal case examples, the life historical accounts of key decisions made by long term ventilator users include both thick description, a sense of personal voice and detailed information about the context in which the decision was made. The process of integrating consumer accounts of illness and treatment/non-treatment decisions into life narrative is explained by Williams' sociological approach to the concept of narrative reconstruction.[14] In William's approach, narratives explain: "How and why people see their illness originating in a certain way, and how people account for the disruption that disablement has wrought in their lives."[15] His approach to reconstruction emphasizes that individual narratives reconstruct causal connections between disease and antecedent factors. They also explain the context of illness by providing "narrative reference points between the individual and society in an unfolding process which has become profoundly disrupted."[16] Williams' initial research involved life narratives of persons with disabilities associated with rheumatoid arthritis. He conducted life historical interviews with thirty individuals who had been diagnosed with rheumatoid arthritis for at least five years. His qualitative interviews focused on the experience of living with arthritis including explanations of the origins and genesis. Examples of reconstructed narratives among Williams' informants explained causation in terms of political or environmental determinants, social or psychological explanations, such as stress and narratives describing overcoming the impact of disability through personal faith.

Williams' interpretation of the process of narrative reconstruction to understanding the persons' perspective on the genesis of chronic illness is also applicable to interpreting the technology user's accounts of key decisions. We will apply it in key treatment/non-treatment decisions within the context of long term ventilator users' life narratives. These life narratives provide reconstructed accounts that contain thick description and a sense of the person's voice.

Life Narratives of Ventilator Users

In my life historical interviews discussion of treatment and discontinuation occurred within the context of an integrated biographical narrative. Living for from 30 to 40 years "on and with" life support technology had given them many opportunities to define life priorities in terms of both personal values and their rights as consumers. Their descriptions of these decisions were characterized by: a sense of biographical integration and temporality; an awareness of the complex patterns of social interaction between the machine (e.g. the technology itself), the user, (professional) care givers and…members of [the] family; a recognition of the impact of structural barriers limiting options for independent living and empowerment.

This is precisely the type of data omitted in the case study of the ALS patient. The biographical connections and critical awareness which characterize long term ventilator users' narratives of past crisis events also appear to have influenced the technology users' approach to negotiating advance directives and do-not-resuscitate orders. Clearly, the approach of ventilator users to defining the criteria for discontinuing treatment or giving consent to alternative forms of life support was very different to the reasoning process emphasized in ethicists' case examples.

Several informants' life narratives described near death situations in which treatment/non-treatment decisions were interpreted in the context of past biographical and social experience. These narratives were used, in William's words, to "reaffirm the impression that the self has a purpose or telos."[17] Ventilator users also applied their long term biographical experience in defining the terms of advance directives. In these statements they frequently referenced crisis situations associated with respiratory insufficiency which had resulted in the adoption of more efficient, but more invasive and less easily controlled technology.

A Narrative Example

It is useful to focus on a single ventilator user's interpretation of decisions about adoption or discontinuation of life support technology. One of the persons from our interview series, a 45 year old man, had used a range of different mechanical ventilation systems over a thirty five year period following the onset of respiratory paralysis associated with poliomyelitis. His approach to decision-making is characterized by biographical integration, engagement of the complexity of technology choices, an understanding of the dynamics of social interaction in decision-making, and an awareness of structural barriers to consumer choice. In his narrative he described his experience as an adult, living independently in the community and working as a senior hospital administrator and civil servant. Despite use of a rocking bed and a single cycle respirator at night, when in his mid 40s the narrator started to experience increasing respiratory difficulty. He then asked his physician if he could explore more efficient forms of mechanical ventilation using a mask or mouth tube. The initial response of the physician was to limit discussion of treatment options to continuous positive ventilation requiring a tracheotomy and permanent rather than periodic respirator dependence. In his narrative, the man described his interaction with his physician's argument for a more invasive, but more effective mechanical ventilation than the patient wanted.

> It's not bad enough yet, you are still functioning, carry on with your rocking bed but you are probably going to have to have a tracheotomy or tracheostomy. (I never could understand which is which, but anyway it is a hole in the neck.)

> At the same time Dr.___ was having discreet chats with me saying, "Have you thought about the tracheotomy sort of thing?" So that is how things were left at that time. I continued on the rocking bed and things were getting worse and worse and I was trying to struggle to keep working. I remember at the end of those days just crawling home and getting into bed. I was absolutely, totally exhausted, completely drained. So that I was sort of beginning to realize I was coming to the end of the line. I should be checking out what my pension was going to be and if there was something that I could do to continue.

As his breathing problems increased, his medical caregivers remained committed to the single invasive treatment the narrator hoped to avoid. His physician advised him that less efficient technology would result in respiratory failure. In describing these events, and his efforts to negotiate

an alternative form of life support, the man discussed what he thought was his physician's interpretation of the biographical experience of people with polio related respiratory impairment.

> I believe Dr.___ has a theory that all us post-polios have this recollection of the acute stages of people having trachs, you know—they come in the middle of the night and rush you down the hall and they stick this tube in your neck—that this is supposed to be a kind of subconscious phobia or fear of tracheotomies—it seems to be a pretty strong tendency to go ahead and give a tracheotomy and if you don't want it, well maybe there is some mental block there that is preventing you from seeing the light and getting this done.

In describing his rejection of his physician's advice, he asserted the validity of his resistance to being tracheostomized.

> I don't really feel I have to defend or explain why I don't want somebody to punch a hole in my neck. It seems to me that if I can find some way of shoving air through some orifice that is already there, that to me has a certain ring of logic to it. I really don't think I have to be psycho-analyzed for making that decision.

Complexity and Social Interaction in Consumer Narratives

The complexity of the narrator's interpretation—including his understanding of the physician's perceptions—provides a more grounded and personally owned account of the choices available to him, one which may be difficult for clinicians and others to perceive. As Linn et al. put it in terms of cancer decision making:

> The person without cancer can afford to be more dogmatic about cancers and likely to think in stereotypes. The closer he comes to dealing with the disease, the less clear cut and more complex the explanation becomes.[18]

Discussing the negotiation of options, this man described his search for alternatives. He compared his preference for adopting some form of nasal ventilation over his physician's decision to "push" for a tracheotomy as a more familiar and less ambiguous treatment option:

> I think that with nasal ventilation, it seems to me that there is a lot more patience required, a lot more innovation in playing around with it. It is not something which is a black and white sort of thing, there are a lot of grays and you have got to gradually play around and get the hue up to the right level. It is much more of a personal thing. I think that is probably the hardest part for the professionals to deal with... and I guess that is my concern; getting the professional help you need to get it working.

The complexity of treatment options and the need for innovative, long term co-participation is not usually captured in ethical case studies which tend to focus on acute situations and decisions involving tracheotomy and short term ventilation of patients in emergency room settings.

In his search for an alternative, the narrator discussed his situation and concerns with other ventilator users, care givers, and leaders of the consumer movement he met at an international post-polio meeting. There he also learned about an alternative means of connecting his ventilator.

> And then I was able to make the trip to St. Louis and that gave me—if I was thinking of giving up on this type of ventilation—the trip to St. Louis convinced me that I wasn't playing with something that was sort of pie in the sky; which I think it was viewed as by some of the doctors. You could see the vision from the outside that there were more alternatives.

Following the conference, he then found a respiratory therapist with recent experience using nasal masks, one willing to work with him to develop efficient, alternative means of life support that would be less invasive than that recommended by the physician:

> I kind of lucked into [name of Respiratory Therapy Technician] who helped me set up alternative therapy... that she was trying to make a point and wasn't about to let me slip out, to let the thing fail.

The man recognized the active role that he played in the decision process and in researching his own treatment options:

> Obviously not everybody is going to have the luck or the resources to follow the kind of approach that I took (e.g. going to consumer conferences and finding alternative care providers and technology options). The person on the street is not going to be able to go somewhere else and have this kind of access. They don't have the capability to do the research and keep looking for other solutions.

Structural Barriers and Empowerment Strategies in Consumer Narratives

Case examples used in teaching ethics typically adopt a microanalytic perspective, one de-emphasizing the impact of structural barriers and the limited access to alternative modalities of life support or options for independent living. These include barriers to assessing information about treatment and technology options, economic constraints and inadequate or inaccessible services. Structural barriers practically diminish the option of living independently with disabilities.

In the first case, for example, the ethicist's presumption that the person with ALS had the information and resources to make an informed choice was criticized by long term users of ventilation for ignoring the myriad ways of using technology and services to live with autonomy and dignity. As Koch et al. have noted, the failure to assure logistical, informational and peer support resources present structural barriers that impede access to interesting and active continuance.[19] In cases where persons who depend on technology do not have access to resources to sustain quality of life the only option presented may be "death with dignity."[20]

The effect of structural barriers is also considered in medical and ethical summaries of two well-known Canadian Supreme Court decisions. Nancy B. requested discontinuation of mechanical ventilation.[21] Susan Rodriguez's requested euthanasia.[22] Consumer reaction to both decisions emphasized that Nancy B. had very limited information about the availability of independent living options, such as home respiratory care programs in Quebec. Disability organizations also emphasized that Sue Rodriguez may not have been informed about home hospice care options in British Columbia.

In contrast to the reconstructed case of the ALS patient, the narratives of long time users of life support technology often incorporated structural critiques emphasizing their experience in overcoming barriers to accessing alternative treatment or their strategies for empowerment and advocacy. Their experience was consistent with that of arthritis patients interviewed by Williams whose narratives explained the impact of disability in terms of structural or political determinants such as occupational risks, barriers to service access, and the impact of social inequality on prospects for independent living.[23]

Thus for this narrator, and for other narrators in our group, issues of treatment choice may be dependent on barriers to information, travel, and knowledge access. More generally long term technology users may...more accurately identify structural barriers to alternative treatment and living options, describing experiences of empowerment and advocacy in which they were able to overcome systemic barriers.

Proxy Decision-Making

A final theme in consumer narratives describing decision to accept or discontinue the use of life support technology centers on the need for the person to maintain control of the definition of the quality of their own life. Some of the initial reaction to the clinical ethicist's case presentation of a man's decision to discontinue mechanical ventilation centered on the perception that the physicians acted inappropriately as proxy decision-makers. Among the ten long term ventilator users, half commented on the hazards of allowing clinicians to interpret present or prospects for future quality of their lives related to their present or future respiratory function. A psychologist and ventilator user, Audrey King, at another conference, captured their perceptions.

She stated: "No one can prejudge or project 'quality of life' issues for those who are ventilator dependent. Neither can an individual facing ventilator dependency express a valid opinion until he/she is well into the experience."[24] King then described consumer concerns about professionals' control within institutional settings:

> Support structures [that] enable him/her to live within their communities have provided greater opportunities to become empowered, regain autonomy and consequently enjoy a better quality of life. However, this autonomy is increasingly threatened as well meaning health care providers impose institutional models within the community and encroach on individual rights and freedoms in doing so."[25]

Her statement emphasizes the importance of the consumer's long term experience with technology. It also clearly focuses on the questions of whether the autonomy of the technology dependent person may be restricted by resource constraints and the range of treatment and living options made available. King's analysis recognizes the interaction of resource availability, self-advocacy, social network and quality of life.[26]

The majority of the ventilator users I interviewed described the problems of proxy decision-making when they were asked to develop advance directives and do not resuscitate orders. Several voiced their reservations about orders which would place the power of final decision-making in the hands of a clinician who was not aware of their long term life experience and previous decisions about continuation or discontinuation of life support. They also voiced concerns over the dual roles of clinicians' proxy decision-makers and as gatekeepers with control over allocation of resources for community living.

CONCLUSION

In the context of interviews with an anthropologist, long term ventilator users contextualized their current and future decisions about continuing mechanical ventilator accepting alternative form of technology or negotiating advance directives within the structure of their life historical narratives. In contrast, ethicists' clinical case description of ventilator users' life historical narratives are intended to enable their caregivers and family to understand contemporary decisions and future choices within the context of multiple crisis situations, evolving definitions of quality of life, and the consumer's long term experience with uncertain technology.

Long term users of life support technology describe a life time experience characterized by crisis events and continuing vulnerability that they draw on when making choices about their future. From their perspective, a series of issues bear upon their decisions regarding continuation or removal of life support. These are relational involving familial and professional caregivers and structural barriers to service access, knowledge and prospects for empowerment. This multi-layered, grounded portrait is in sharp contrast with the decontextualized and principle centered account dominating the ethicist's case study. Consumer narratives also reveal the importance of knowing the nature of the structural barriers that must be overcome in achieving control over their lives. The biographical connections and critical awareness which characterize narratives describing past crisis events also influence the technology user's approach to negotiating advance directives and do-not-resuscitate orders.

An anthropological presentation of the thick description emphasizing the richness of consumer narratives provides a balance to the assumptions of ethicists and clinicians who, with the best intentions, may counsel patients without understanding the complex personal or social realities of the person. It is one thing to

promise patient autonomy, another to assure that the support systems are available to make the appearance of individual choice a reality. As a result, anthropological approaches to narratives reconstructing personal experience teach the medical decision-maker about the socially constructed options they often do not perceive. They also provide a sense of the life context of the decision-maker and an indication of the structural constraints which influence choice. Like all case-based presentations, neither clinical cases constructed by ethicists nor life narratives reconstructed at the request of an anthropologist by people who depend on technology, can fully represent either an individual nor represent the perspective of all decision-makers or claim general applicability. As complementary modalities, together they can inform us about both general theory in ethical decisions and its relationship to the lived reality of complex decisions that draw on individuals' experience over the life course.

Acknowledgements

The author would like to acknowledge the significant editorial assistance in the development of this manuscript by Tom Koch, Devva Kasnitz, and Patricia Leyland Kaufert. I would also like to thank Jackie Pantel for her assistance in data management and manuscript preparation.

Notes

1. David Locker and Joseph Kaufert, "The Breath of Life: Medical Technology and the Careers of People with Post- Respiratory Poliomyelitis," *Sociology of Health and Illness* 10 (1988): 24–40.
2. Joseph Kaufert and David Locker, "Rehabilitation Ideology and Respiratory Support Technology," *Social Science and Medicine* 30, no. 8 (1990): 867–877.
3. Barbara Duncan, "Conference Overview," in *Ethical Issues in Disability and Rehabilitation*, ed. B. Duncan and D. Woods, World Institute on Disability, Rehabilitation International, World Rehabilitation Fund, New York (1989) 7: 12.
4. See note 3 Duncan (1989): 12.

5. See note 3 Duncan (1989): 7.

6. See note 3 Duncan (1989): 8.

7. See note 2 Kaufert and Locker (1990): 868.

8. Ted Chambers, "From the Ethicist's Point of View: The Literary Nature of Ethical Inquiry," *Hastings Center Report* (January-February 1996): 25–32.

9. Dena S. Davis, "Rich Cases: The Ethics of Thick Description," *Hastings Center Report* (July-August 1991): 12–16.

10. See note 9 Davis (1991): 15.

11. See note 8 Chambers (1996).

12. See note 8 Chambers (1996): 31.

13. See note 8 Chambers (1996): 32.

14. Gareth Williams, "The Genesis of Chronic Illness: Narrative Re-construction," *Sociology of Health and Illness* 6, no. 2 (1984): 175–200, 179.

15. See note 14 Williams (1984): 177.

16. See note 14 Williams (1984): 175.

17. See note 14 Williams (1984): 176.

18. M. Linn, B. Linn and S. Stein, "Beliefs about Causes of Cancer in Cancer Patients," *Social Science and Medicine* 16 (1982): 836.

19. Thomas Koch, K. Braun and J. Pietsch, "Social Necessity, Individual Rights, and the Needs of the Fragile: Euthanasia in the Context of End-of-Life Decision-Making," *Journal of Ethics, Law and Aging* 5, no. 1 (1999): 17–27.

20. Thomas Koch, "Living versus Dying with Dignity—A New Perspective on the Euthanasia Debate," *Cambridge Quarterly on Healthcare Ethics* 5 (1996): 50–60.

21. *Nancy B. v. Hotel-Dieu de Quebec*, (1992) 86 D.L.R. (4th) 385 (Que. Sup. Ct.).

22. *Rodriguez v. Attorney General of Canada* (1993) 3 S.C.R. 519.

23. See note 14 Williams (1984): 175.

24. Audrey King, "Autonomy, Empowerment and Perception: Issues in Achieving Quality of Life for Ventilator Dependent Individuals." Paper presented at *National Symposium: The Ventilator: Muscular Dystrophy, A.L.S., Emphysema, and Other Diseases.* April 26–28, 1990. Foundation of Thanatology, New York: 1.

25. See note 24 King (1990): 1.

26. See note 24 King (1990): 1.

Useful Resources

ONLINE

American Society for Bioethics and Humanities (ASBH), Resource Links

ASBH has an extensive list of links divided into groups such as academic centres, organizations and networks, and government offices for science and technology.

Bioethics.net

This website provides links to various journals and current news stories under various headings.

BioethicsWeb

Wellcome Library, BioethicsWeb offers free access to a searchable catalogue of Internet sites and resources covering biomedical ethics.

Canadian Bioethics Society (CBS)

CBS has a number of useful links to Canadian bioethics resources.

Canadian Institutes of Health Research (CIHR), Ethics Useful Links

The CIHR website's ethics section provides links divided into four categories: Guidelines for Health Research, Relevant Agencies and Organizations, Academic Bioethics and Health Law Centres/ Institutes, and Bioethics Information Resources on the Web.

EthicShare

EthicShare is a research and collaboration website. The site includes a comprehensive collection of "ethics resources including searchable research materials, group discussions, current news articles, and upcoming events."

MedlinePlus

This is a Web-based service of the U.S. National Library of Medicine and the National Institutes of Health that provides links to resources about ethics.

Nuffield Council on Bioethics

The Nuffield Council on Bioethics is an independent body in the United Kingdom that "examines and reports on ethical issues raised in biological and medical research." It was established by the trustees of the Nuffield Foundation in 1991.

PubMed

PubMed is a useful search engine that now includes Bioethicsline.

United Nations Educational, Scientific and Cultural Organization (UNESCO), Bioethics

"Since the 1970s, UNESCO's involvement in the field of bioethics has reflected the international dimensions of this debate. Founded on the belief that there can be no peace without the intellectual and moral solidarity of humankind, UNESCO tries to involve all countries in this international and transcultural discussion."

U.S. National Institutes of Health (NIH), Bioethics Resources on the Web

The brief annotations in this directory are divided into five categories: Bioethics at NIH, General Resources, Organizations, Federal Bioethics Resources, and Specific Topics (Research Ethics, Genetics, and Medicine and Health Care).

U.S. National Reference Center for Bioethics Literature, Bioethics Resources on the Web (Scope Note 38)

This page offers links to databases, electronic journals, full-text documents, news, and teaching resources in bioethics.

World Health Organization (WHO), Links to Bioethics Resources on the Web

The WHO website's ethics section provides links divided into five categories: Collaborating Centres in Bioethics, United Nations Organizations, International Organizations, Regional and National Organizations, and Related Health Topics.

ENCYCLOPEDIAS

Chadwick, R. (Ed.) (2012). *Encyclopedia of applied ethics* (Vols. 1–4) 2nd Edition. New York, NY: Academic Press.

Cooper, D. (Ed.) (2003). *Nature encyclopaedia of the human genome* (Vols. 1–5). Hampshire, England: Nature Publishing Group, Macmillan.

Clark, A. et al. (2010). *Encyclopedia of life sciences* (Vols. 1–32). London, UK: John Wiley & Sons, Ltd. Available from http://www.els.net/default.asp

Heggenhougen, K. (Ed.). (2008). *International encyclopedia of public health* (Vols. 1–6). Amsterdam: Elsevier; Oxford, UK: Academic Press.

Lafollette, H. (Ed). (forthcoming 2013). *International encyclopedia of ethics*. (Vols. 1–12+). London, UK: Wiley-Blackwell.

Mitcham, C. (Ed). (2005). *Encyclopedia of science, technology and ethics* (Vols. 1–4). Toronto, ON: Macmillan.

Post, S. G. (Ed.). (2003). *Encyclopedia of bioethics* (Vols. 1–5). New York, NY: Macmillan Reference USA. Online version 2004.

Zalta, E. N. (Ed). *The Stanford encyclopedia of philosophy*. Available from http://plato.stanford.edu/

HEALTH LAW

Downie, J., Caulfield, T., & Flood, C. (Eds). (2011). *Canadian health law and policy*, 4th ed. Toronto: Butterworths.

Downie, J. & Gibson, E. (Eds). (2007). *Health law at the Supreme Court of Canada.* Toronto: Irwin Law.

Picard, E. & Robertson, G. (Eds). (2007). *Legal liability of doctors and hospitals in Canada*, 4th ed. Toronto: Carswell.

Judgments of the Supreme Court of Canada

This collection includes the decisions rendered by the Supreme Court of Canada since 1948. While the database is not comprehensive for previous years, many decisions before 1948 are available, including all decisions originating from Ontario and British Columbia back to 1876.

Chapter 2 CANADIAN HEALTH CARE

INTRODUCTION

The structure and operation of a health care system are an historical and political amalgamation of evolving conceptual understandings, social values, scientific and technological advances, professional responsibilities and influences, legal regulation, and economic circumstances. Conceptual understandings and social values provide the ethical framework of the system. What does "health" mean? Are people healthy simply when they do not have a disease or illness, or is there more to being healthy and staying healthy? What factors contribute to good health, and to what extent should a health care system promote them? How much should a health care system focus on prevention and treatment? On physical health and mental health? On acute care and chronic care? How are priorities among services to be established, and how can access to services be made equitable? These questions require policy choices. The foundational choices establish budgets that fund and circumscribe the resources of the system. Federal and provincial governments decide how much money to allocate to health care compared to national defence, education, and transportation, for example. Administrators of provincial health care systems then allocate the money they receive. How much will go to hospitals and how much to public health, for example? Hospital administrators in turn allocate their funding across programs such as obstetrics, cardiology, surgery, and intensive care. At the bottom of this decision-making hierarchy, health care providers decide which patients receive which services and in what order.

The first article by Pat Armstrong and Hugh Armstrong provides a comprehensive, critical analysis of the fundamental understandings and assumptions that shape our health care system. Most basic are a definition of health and a recognition of the five determinants of health: social environments, physical environments, psychological environments, productivity and wealth, and health care. Armstrong and Armstrong then identify and challenge the assumptions integral to the prevailing structure of health care: health as primarily biological; the engineering model of the body; medicine as cure; medicine as scientific; and the authority and expertise of doctors. Appreciating the weaknesses and limitations of these powerful assumptions, and the alternatives to them, is crucial to informed criticism and productive reform of the health care system.

In the second article Kai Nielsen provides a philosophical examination of the core values of a health care system. Nielsen argues that, contrary to the standard liberal view, the values of autonomy and equality do not have to conflict because "autonomy cannot be widespread or secure in a society which is not egalitarian." He then asks what kind of health care system a moderately abundant, autonomy-respecting egalitarian society would have. His answer is that this kind of society would have a health care system that does not just meet health care needs, but also meets such basic needs as the need to be healthy and the need to ameliorate conditions that cause suffering, impede functioning well, or adversely affect well-being. Moreover, Nielsen believes that this kind of system could exist only if medicine were entirely removed from the private sector.

How limited resources should be allocated across a diverse, expansive, and dynamic health care system is a challenging and controversial issue. In the next article Christine Overall replies to a familiar criticism of the current allocation of health care resources: that too much money is spent on caring for people in their last years of life and on the health problems of old age. This criticism, Overall points out, assumes that health care needs, or at least the cost of health care needs, should be the same at all stages of life. The costs of care for elderly people can be regarded as unduly burdensome, if not "wildly disproportionate" as one journalist charges, only if elderly people are getting more than their fair share of health care and if "fair" means approximately equal. But there are real differences between the health care one needs at age 80 and age 40, just as there are real differences between the health care one needs at age 40 and age 4. Overall proposes a "life-course approach" to recognizing health care needs that would support "a strong public policy of affirmative prolongevitism." But, similar to Nielsen, she believes such a policy would require "a social-democratic approach to human well-being, not an approach based only on what can be provided by market forces, for which cost containment and the maximization of profit are the ruling values."

The final article by Colleen Flood and Bryan Thomas provides the background to and the information about the Canadian health care system that are needed to make informed, critical moral assessments of the role of private funding in the system. If the resources of our health care system are inadequate because public funding is limited, why not, contrary to the views of Nielsen and Overall, allow private sector companies to provide health care services and allow patients to pay for health care services privately? In other words, why not have a "two-tiered" health care system? Private entrepreneurship has long operated in Canadian health care, and the pressure to expand private funding of health care services continues to intensify. Can sweeping private funding be fairly blended with public funding? Flood and Thomas present an insightful history and analysis of the blurring of the public and private sectors in health care. After reviewing the basic features of the public/private mix in Canadian health care, they discuss the decision of the Supreme Court of Canada in *Chaoulli v. Québec*, which involved a challenge to the province's legislative ban on private health insurance for services covered by its public insurance plan. (This case is summarized at the end of the chapter.) The Supreme Court held, in a 4–3 decision, that given long waiting lists, the ban violates the right to personal security guaranteed in Québec's provincial *Charter of Human Rights and Freedoms*. As Flood and Thomas put it, this important decision "has let the genie out of [the] bottle in terms of legitimizing privatization as a policy option" for Canadian health care.

From Cuts and Chemicals to Carrots and Condoms: The Development of Canadian Health Care

Pat Armstrong and Hugh Armstrong

Health is about much more than health care services. Indeed, as various provincial and federal government reports make clear, health is not primarily determined by health care. What happens outside health care institutions and services is much more important for the overall health of the population than what happens within them. Recognizing that health is about much more than cuts and chemicals, these reports question the need for additional or even continued government investment in health care. Indeed, they recommend less care and more prevention, defined more in terms of carrots and condoms than secure employment and guaranteed incomes. Although the reports suggest a variety of ways the delivery system could be improved, the main concern is saving money by providing less of the same. They do little to challenge the medical model on which the system is based or to apply research on health determinants to health care delivery.

In this chapter, we do just that. We argue that the set of assumptions which together constitute the medical model needs to be questioned if health care is to be reformed in a way that takes the established determinants of health into account. We do not argue that the system should be dismantled or that the assumptions should be simply discarded and replaced by their opposites. Rather, we reject the notion of simple choices between such alternatives as prevention and cure; promotion and intervention. We argue for the necessity of recognizing the fundamental contradictions between such assumptions as the doctor as expert and the patient as empowered. At issue is not which side to choose, but how to retain and manage the tension between the two. There is no single or simple solution to reforming the health care system. Health is determined by social, physical, and psychological environments, by work and income.

DEFINING HEALTH

In 1947, the World Health Organization (WHO) defined health as 'a state of complete physical, mental, and social well-being and not merely the absence of disease and infirmity'. This definition was repeated again in the *Ottawa Charter for Health Promotion* in 1986, suggesting that ideas about what constitutes health changed little in the intervening years.[1] Although the definition was criticized for being too broad, too much about a condition rather than about a process and impossible to achieve,[2] it nevertheless became a standard way of defining health. The WHO's claim that an individual's

state of health was influenced by much more than biology and personal practices also became widely accepted.

Variations on this definition of health have been adopted by all the Canadian ministries responsible for health. And there is a broad consensus on what determines a state of physical, social, and mental well-being. As the Ontario Ministry of Health explains in *Goals and Strategic Priorities,* 'Our health is much more than the traditional health care system. Our health is profoundly affected by the social and physical environments, by access to education, adequate housing, by a sense of control and the ability to contribute in meaningful ways in the workplace, by individual choices and responses, and by the wealth and productivity of society—the determinants of health.'[3]

DETERMINING HEALTH

These determinants are critical to the positions taken in various government reports and in the strategies for change. Indeed, they provide the shared framework that justifies a wide range of reform. An Ontario report, *Nurturing Health: A Framework on the Determinants of Health,* provides details on the research and theory behind the consensus on what determines health.[4] According to this report, health is determined by five factors: social environments, physical environments, psychological environments, productivity and wealth and, finally, health care. Because they are central to the new health strategies, how these factors are presented is worth examining more closely.

1. Social Environments

As the Ontario report points out, study after study has demonstrated that social relations and social support are critical to health. Interpersonal contacts and recognition as a person count in health terms. According to the Ontario report, 'People with more social contacts and friends tend to live longer than those with fewer.'[5]

What the report fails to discuss, however, is the considerable research indicating that social support is even more important to those who are ill or disabled. Comfort and support provided to people undergoing treatment can not only speed recovery but can also make a difference in whether or not recovery happens at all.[6] Social interaction based on knowledge of the person and the particular problems is also essential to the health of the disabled. Providing such comfort to the sick is not simply a reflection of caring for someone, something women do naturally, or an additional frill offered by those with the time. Rather it is a skill long recognized in nursing as central to what constitutes health care and is increasingly being acknowledged in other areas as well.[7]

...

Such caring is not a separate activity but one which is integral to all health care work, whether it be administering drugs or giving a bath. And it is critical to helping a patient 'attain or maintain health, or die a peaceful death'.[8]

Moreover, the kinds of social support people want and need varies with their cultural origins. Cultural sensitivity is particularly important in providing care, given that familiar practices are especially supportive in stressful situations.[9]

Social support, then, is a critical component in a variety of environments. And an important ingredient in that support and these environments is a sense of security. Indeed, security in social relations is important to health, and in work relations as well.

As Ontario's *Nurturing Health* points out, a secure paid job is a significant determinant of health. 'Statistics Canada's 1989 General Social Survey found that the unemployed and those in insecure full-time employment reported lower health and life satisfaction than those employed in secure jobs.... Unemployment, especially among poorer people, is associated with deteriorating physical and mental health.'[10]

It is not only employment security that is important, however. The nature of the work is also critical to health. According to the Ontario report, 'The lifespan and the health of an individual is linked to his or her location in the job hierarchy and to associated factors such as degree of authority, freedom to make decisions and level of social support in the workplace.' As well, workplace 'social supports, as measured by the number and quality of interactions with co-workers, also have an effect on health.' And health is 'affected by the stress related demands of the job'.[11]

...

2. Physical Environments

It has long been recognized that the physical conditions under which people work and live are fundamental to health. In fact, these were the major concern of the public health movement that first appeared in the last century.[12] Nutritional food, clean water, and clean hands are essential to good health. And it is difficult to remain healthy if homes and workplaces are dirty, crowded, noisy, lack facilities, or are poorly ventilated. Clean air is also vital. As *Nurturing Health* makes clear, 'Indoor air pollution, especially secondhand smoke, is a major health hazard.'[13] But healthy physical environments are even more critical to those who are ill because their immune systems are weaker, a fact that the report fails to point out. It also fails to consider the part played by food, crowding, noise, and ventilation in health care.

...

3. Psychological Environments

Nurturing Health draws attention to the importance of mental states in remaining healthy. According to the report, 'There is growing evidence that mental health influences physical well-being although the exact pathways and the biological mechanisms are not yet clear.... Psychoneuroimmunology, an emerging and still controversial field of knowledge, may go a long way to explaining a biological pathway linking social and environmental factors with the performance of the immune system and hence the health status of individuals.'[14]

As is the case with the discussion of social and physical environments, however, the report fails to consider that mental states are even more important when the immune system is weakened by surgery or disease. And by classifying the issue as one of individual response, the report ignores the importance of social, physical, and psychological environments in creating these responses.

4. Productivity and Wealth

It is not only secure employment but also secure income that is important to health. As *Nurturing Health* makes clear, the economy establishes the context for health. 'National prosperity is important for health and the narrower the gap between the rich and the poor in a prosperous nation, the better the overall national health.'[15] 'Greater wealth (socio-economic status) is associated with greater health; poorer and middle income people appear to be more vulnerable than wealthy people to a variety of ailments. The type of ailments that disproportionately affect poor people change over time.'[16] Social policy also plays a role. 'There is a strong relationship between socio-economic status and health status. The evidence indicates that when socio-economic differences are narrowed, population health status improves.'[17] The young are particularly at risk. 'The harmful effects of poverty on the physical and mental health of children can be partially offset by public programs. Intervention can reduce the number of Low Birth Weight babies, who are prone to suffer major health problems.'[18]

If prosperity and equity are important to maintaining the health of the overall population, they must also be important to health services. In fact, although differences related to sex, race, and class remain,[19] governments have successfully reduced inequality in access to care through the collective provision of a wide range of services and supports. However, the various government reports that outline the determinants of health explicitly call for cost reductions in health care. Indeed, they use the determinants of health as an argument for cost reductions. Reform is taking place within a context of restraint, with cost reduction all too often the top or even the sole priority. But, as we shall see, cutbacks are bound to increase inequality in access and thus contribute to reducing the possibilities for health.

5. Health Care

'Since the traditional medical care system concentrates on the treatment of ill health and disability, it can only make a limited contribution to the prevention of illness by nurturing overall good health,' says the Ontario report.[20] In keeping with other reports, it maintains that 'Research suggests there may be an optimal ceiling for spending on the formal health care system—past a certain point such spending could be a drag on the nation's economy and hence on its health.'[21]

Few would contest the report's claim that 'there is limited scope for effective medical intervention with many of the leading causes of death' or its contention that there must be a limit on health care spending.[22] However, the critique is mostly about health care based on a medical model and its failure to cure biologically defined ills. There is little discussion of how the services could be designed to improve health in ways that apply the knowledge about the determinants of health to the system itself. Moreover, the critique is for the most part based on overall population trends, not on the individuals who have been helped by the system. Whatever has caused our illness or disability, we want to have access to good health care when we are ill or disabled. Too often, the individuals who need care disappear in the emphasis on health determinants.

The Ontario report, like similar ones in other provinces, treats health care as one factor determining health. It does little to explore the links among the other determinants and with the health care system. Instead, the reports focus primarily on reducing the government's contribution to the health care system because health care is defined as only one determinant of health. Rather than link health care to the determinants of health, the reports see care as competing with these determinants.

GOVERNMENT RESPONSIBILITIES

The WHO definition of health makes clear that ensuring health is a government responsibility. It does not see health as simply an individual problem. According to WHO, governments must provide adequate health and social measures not only because citizens have a right to health but also because the promotion of health is critical to the attainment of peace and security. In addition, all governments have an interest in promoting health measures throughout the world, because poor health in one country could be a threat to all. AIDS has clearly demonstrated the reason for collective concern and government involvement.

The recent Canadian government commissions and reports certainly do not deny the need for government intervention. According to these reports, governments must play a leadership role in health but this role must be fundamentally changed. The British Columbia report, *Closer to Home,* makes it clear that the 'traditional focus of our health care system is the curing of illness and not the prevention of disease.... It is time to change this focus. Increased spending on hospitals, equipment or health care will not necessarily improve health status. More money should be spent on prevention of illness or injury and on protecting health. The least amount of money possible should be spent on providing the necessary, high quality curative services.'[23] All the reports and commissions echo this claim. The emphasis in government action is to shift from treatments and cures to prevention and health promotion.

Governments have for a long time taken responsibility for some aspects of health determinants. They have provided clean water and education, regulated housing and waste, offered inoculations and lunch programs, and provided some protection against unemployment and health hazards at work. Public health services devoted to prevention have been in place since the last century. Yet, although cutbacks are being carried out in health care in the name of new research demonstrating that these are the determinants of health, governments are at the same time removing the regulations designed to protect health, privatizing those services that promoted health, and reducing the supports available to the unemployed and those without homes. At the same time, they are laying off health care workers and threatening the security of those that remain.

Although all the provincial reports stress the need to 'review the efficiency, effectiveness and suitability of our health system',[24] there is little indication that we need to challenge the assumptions on which 'the high quality, curative services' are based. Effectiveness, efficiency, and suitability are mainly defined in terms of the traditional assumptions of the system and of the 'free' market. They are not considered in relation to how health is determined within the system. Rather, we are to have less of the same provided by the public system and more provided in the private sphere.

With prevention as the focus, we will have fewer cuts and chemicals, not a new approach to care. For example, the report of the Saskatchewan Commission, *Future Directions for Health Care in Saskatchewan,*[25] is concerned that 'Despite sophisticated delivery systems and advanced technology and specialization, there will always be those in society for whom complete treatment and recovery is not possible.' While the report goes on to say that those who cannot be treated and cured should be cared for with 'compassion and understanding', the implication is that the same concerns do not apply when dealing with those who can be treated and cured. The determinants of health are listed as an addition to, rather than a fundamental critique of, current practices in the curative system.

. . .

In order to understand how reforms can serve to emphasize some of the worst aspects of the system while ignoring the determinants of health, let us now examine what is meant by the medical model and the assumptions about health that are part of that model.

THE BASIC ASSUMPTIONS OF CANADIAN HEALTH CARE DELIVERY

The Canadian health care system is centred around, and dominated by, allopathic medicine. Although we have come to think of this approach to health care as the only approach, a system focused on penetration of the body 'physically by surgery and chemically by drugs'[26] is just one of many ways to deal with illness or disability. There are other ways of addressing health problems and of constructing a health care system. Chiropractic, for example, is based on 'locating, correcting and adjusting the interference with nerve transmission and expression in the spinal column and other articulations without the use of drugs or surgery'.[27] Unlike allopathic approaches, chiropractic treatment does not require hospitalization or very expensive technology. Nor usually does acupuncture. 'Acupuncture and acupressure both stress how the work of their therapies is to release blockages in the flow and balance of the body after which the body will heal itself.'[28] A system based on acupuncture would also create health care structures different from those found in Canada today.

Allopathic, or what we often think of as regular or orthodox medicine, is based on a particular set of assumptions. These assumptions are reflected in both the structure and the relations of the health care system. Yet many of these assumptions are quite different from those identified by the various reports as the determinants of health; they are also different from those found in what we usually call alternative therapies. For our analytical purposes, these assumptions are set out explicitly, simply, and separately in the following section....

Assumption 1. The Determinants of Illness Are Primarily Biological

As Shorter points out in *Bedside Manners,* diagnosis in modern allopathic medicine stems from 'linking changes observed in the tissues after death to the patient's signs and symptoms during life' and from the 'new science of microbiology' that made it possible to see how germs produce disease.[29] To a large extent, mind and body are defined as separate, with diagnosis of illness or disability focused on discovering a specific injury, germ, or cancerous cell that causes the problem. While psychological problems are recognized, they are often treated in the same way as biological ones, with drugs or surgery, and usually treated as separate from other biological complaints. Little attention is paid to the interaction between mind and body, because it is assumed that there are largely different causes for problems in each.

Directly related to the assumption of a biological base for health problems is the use of tests designed to identify the cause of symptoms. Given that illness is assumed to be identifiable in tissues, blood, organs, or bones, tests that allow us to 'see' the specific cause are a central part of diagnosis. If test results are negative, problems are often attributed to mental rather than physical causes and the two kinds of cause are usually considered distinct. All too often, if a physical cause cannot be readily identified, the complaint will be dismissed as 'all in the head'. This is especially the case for women.

This assumption of biological causes also has an impact on doctor-patient relationships. With identifiable biological causes in mind, doctors need only spend a very limited time with patients to determine the specific problem. A prescription can be offered immediately or tests can be ordered and solutions provided over the phone. Walk-in clinics, where patients are served quickly by a stranger trained in the diagnosis of these biological ills, become possible when it is assumed that there is a readily identifiable cause that requires little knowledge about the person as an individual. Moreover, patients are usually seen individually in the doctor's office, without the involvement of family or friends, because it is assumed that physiological problems need not be situated within a social context. The assumption means people are treated as isolated individuals.

Assumption 2. The Engineering Model of the Body

To a large extent, modern medicine assumes that the body works much like any other machine. It is made up of a series of parts that can be fixed. Once the part and the problem are identified, there are recognized procedures to follow and specific locations for treatment.

It is this model that allows for specialization in allopathic medicine. Because the body is conceived of as a collection of components, these parts can be separated for the purposes of diagnosis and treatment by experts in particular parts. Sections of hospitals or even whole hospitals can be structured to deal with particular component parts. So, for example, Sunnybrook Medical Centre in Toronto can specialize in what the then President called 'six major "product lines": trauma, cancer, aging, heart and circulation, mental health, and rehabilitation'.[30] Like the hospitals, patients can be classified according to the part with the problem.

This engineering model of the body, combined with the assumption of specific cause, also makes possible a fee-for-service system to determine doctors' pay. Fee-for-service is very similar to piece-work payments in factories, where workers are paid for each component made. In our health care system, most doctors' fees are based on the specific part treated or task done, rather than on the basis of the number of people treated. In addition, this model allows hospitals and other institutions to calculate the amount of work time required from other workers on the basis of the specific part being fixed. With an approach that assumes parts to be fixed, work for and with a patient can be divided into discrete tasks that are measured and counted.

Assumption 3. Health Care Is Primarily About Curing Illness or Disability

Central to modern medicine is the notion of intervention to bring about cure. The assumption is that most physical and mental health problems are subject to treatment and cure. Furthermore, it is often assumed that it is better to intervene if intervention is possible. Drugs and surgery are used to cure the diagnosed illness or injury. The purpose is to return patients to 'normal'.

This curative approach, combined with the engineering model of the body, provides a basis for constructing acute care hospitals that focus primarily on fixing a specific part as quickly as possible. On the assumption that a cure is primarily about applying a particular technique, hospitals can put a great deal of energy into shortening patient stays to cover only the minimum period required for the particular treatment. Surgery can be done on an out-patient basis, with people arriving at and leaving from the hospital within hours of surgery or other treatment, because the major concern is getting the procedure done. Psychological support before and after treatment, feeding, bathing, and talking with the patient are defined as non-medical tasks. Increasingly, jobs related to food, cleaning, and laundry are called 'hotel services', reflecting the assumption that these have nothing to do with cure or even health. Similarly, management techniques developed in industry are transferred to health care on the assumption that fixing a care part is not much different from fixing a car part. The care process, like making cars, can be assessed in value-added terms.[31] Anyone who does not fit into the category of quickly cured is assigned to another kind of institution, such as chronic care hospitals, group homes, or nursing homes.

Assumption 4. Medicine Is Scientific

Allopathic medicine is scientific medicine. 'Scientific medicine taught that each disease had a single well-defined cause, and that the control of the disease could best be achieved by attacking the causative organism or by correcting the function of the diseased part of the body.'[32] Science determines cause, effect, and cure. It is assumed that the effectiveness of tests, drugs, surgery, and other techniques used in treatment has been scientifically established and agreed upon. This is taken to mean that all procedures have been rigorously examined, following strict, value-free procedures that take all relevant factors into account. It is assumed not only that such research has been done, but also that it can be done and that everyone agrees on what constitutes scientific evidence. At the same time, it is assumed that any treatment that cannot be examined or explained by such procedures is not effective or useful.

When both physiological cause and scientific 'proof' are taken for granted, it is possible to define medicine as the application of standard techniques. It is assumed that all patients with the same problem will display very similar symptoms, will follow basically the same pattern of disease development, and will take very similar times for treatment and recovery. It is therefore possible to develop formulas to determine the times for patient cures and discharge. It is also possible to divide up the tasks into separate parts, many of which can be done by people quickly trained to apply the specific, proven technique.

Assumption 5. The Doctor as Authority and Expert

Throughout most of this century, doctors' training and position have both reflected and reinforced these assumptions. Doctors' education has stressed the biological and physical sciences upon which drug therapy and surgery are based. This lengthy training in the scientifically established procedures that are to be applied to largely physiologically determined problems was assumed to make doctors the objective experts who name the appropriate diagnosis and treatment and apply the necessary cure.

Doctors' authority over both patients and other health care workers is justified in terms of these assumptions. Because only doctors have the training in the scientific evidence and correct procedures, they need to determine what patients do and what is done to them. It is assumed that patients lack the necessary knowledge and often the necessary will to follow appropriate procedures. Similarly, it is assumed that doctors' superior knowledge means only they can know what procedures can be safely delegated to others who work in the system. Doctors' power

over both patients and the system is necessary and desirable because health care is about fixing body parts based on expert knowledge of scientifically established procedures, and only doctors have this knowledge. And it is often assumed that most of the improvements in health care over the century can be attributed to the curative powers of doctors.

CHALLENGING THE ASSUMPTIONS

These assumptions are so integral to our health care system and have been around for so long that they seem just common sense. To a large extent, within the system alternatives have become unthinkable. But the health care system came to be based on these assumptions not simply or even primarily because they were demonstrated to be the most effective means of improving the health of the population. Doctors became dominant mainly as a result of a power struggle, although they have retained much of their strength because many of their techniques have proved effective in restoring health.

Challenge 1. Doctors' Authority and Expertise

Indeed, allopathic doctors' authority did not begin with their knowledge of scientific evidence. Rather, it preceded the development of the kinds of scientific techniques on which today's medicine is based. As early as the eighteenth century, a group of medical practitioners tried to gain dominance by pressuring the state to give them the exclusive right to practise medicine."[33] Although the struggle between 'regular' and 'irregular' healers lasted for many years, the dominance of allopaths was eventually established.

Their demands for a monopoly, however, were not based on the demonstrated efficacy of their treatments or on biomedical science. And their demands were met largely because of their class, race, and sex rather than because of their treatments and cures. By the mid-nineteenth century, before most discoveries based on biomedical science were made, Colleges of Physicians and Surgeons were incorporated in many jurisdictions to ensure that these practitioners had the right to control who practised and to eliminate other alternatives such as the Thomsonian herbalists, the homeopaths, and the eclectics who 'rejected certain of the theories and practices of the mainstream profession'.[34] As Naylor makes clear in *Private Practice: Public Payment,* the 'emergence of rival schools such as homeopathy and eclecticism can be taken as evidence that there was no firm scientific consensus concerning most aspects of practice.'[35] One group was successful in using their political connections to win state support and exclude competition. Moreover, in restricting entry to those who attended particular university programs, they ensured dominance by men of particular classes and races.

But they were not as successful in convincing the population that their treatments were better than those of the many others offering their services. Although one group of doctors was legitimated by the state, alternative approaches did not disappear. As Bilson points out in his study of cholera, the brutal, often irrelevant, or even dangerous treatment provided by the licensed doctors encouraged many people 'to abandon the regular medical men and turn to those offering less daunting regimes'.[36]

This was particularly the case with midwifery. In 1865, organized medical men in Ontario were successful in getting the state to grant them the exclusive right to attend childbirths.[37] Because there was a surplus of graduates from medical school, they wanted not only to eliminate competition from the unorganized women who served as midwives but also to use childbirth as a way of becoming family practitioners.[38] But this monopoly was not based on evidence that these allopathic practitioners were safer and more effective in attending birth. In fact, a Saskatchewan medical officer reported in 1919 that 'maternal mortality was much higher in the 50 per cent of confinements attended by medical men.' Although the higher death rate may have partially reflected the more risky cases covered by doctors, the officer went on to explain that 'a very large number of women were

confined without either nurse or doctor in attendance, and in these cases, maternal mortality was much lower'. When the officer presented his report to the practitioners with the monopoly, he 'was very strongly taken to task by some of the members for even compiling the figures'.[39]

Not surprisingly, some women continued to resist the medical control over childbirth. A Prairie woman interviewed for *A Harvest Yet to Reap* explained that she first called a doctor to attend her child's birth when she was told she had to have a doctor in attendance. 'So we sent for one and they was three hours late and I had everything done, had the baby dressed and myself washed and the afterbirth taken out and put in the heater. And then he came and felt my pulse and said, "Well you're just as nature led you. That's forty-five dollars please."'[40] That was the last time she called the doctor when she was ready to give birth. Indeed, midwifery never entirely disappeared, in spite of doctors' state-backed power, precisely because many women resisted doctors' claims and fees.

However, with the discovery of germs and the gradual acceptance of germ theory among practitioners, intervention by the licensed practitioners became less risky for patients. With the development of chloroform, surgery became less painful. With practice and with some new knowledge about anatomy and microbiology, allopaths developed more effective and less dangerous techniques. With better sanitation, nutrition, and housing, health improved as well and medicine claimed much of the credit. These developments contributed to doctors' power and legitimacy, but were not the only factors in establishing their authority. Allopaths used their political connections and their collective strength to establish not only their monopoly on treatment but also the dominance of their assumptions throughout the health care system.

. . .

The assumption, then, that doctors' authority is based simply on their knowledge and expertise is incorrect. Their right to a monopoly, to self-government, and to direct the system preceded much of the scientific knowledge on which the claim is based. State support was critical to the establishment and continuation of medical authority, although a number of medical breakthroughs helped considerably in gaining popular acceptance of doctors' claims. Certainly doctors continue to be challenged by patients, by alternative therapists, and by other health care workers. And attempts to reduce state expenditures and the dramatic changes taking place within the system are placing some limits on doctors' power. But even though various reports suggest more team work or that the physician is no longer 'the only person qualified to decide what treatment or studies are appropriate for a patient',[41] governments have resisted directly taking on the question of doctors' authority or the [hierarchical] structure of most health care. Doctors remain both the gatekeepers for other doctors and patients and the most powerful group within the system. Doctors are still in charge of treatment and cure. Indeed, many cutbacks have meant an increasing focus on quick treatment and cure, thus ensuring that doctors are at the centre of acute care.

This is not to argue that doctors should be stripped of all their powers over patients, other doctors, and other workers in health care. Nor is it to argue that doctors have no expertise based on scientific evidence. In many circumstances, doctors' knowledge is critical, as is their right to direct a team quickly and to insist a patient follow treatment. But it is to argue that this is not inevitably or self-evidently the case. Instead of assuming either that doctors must be in control or that they should not have any independent power, we need to retain the tension between scepticism about doctors' power and knowledge and recognition of an expertise in particular fields that requires considerable independence. We need to do so without firmly rejecting or embracing either doctors' authority or their subjugation to others.

...

Challenge 2. Medicine Is Scientific

There are also questions to be raised about the science on which the doctors' authority and expertise are assumed to be based. There is considerable evidence to suggest that not all drugs, devices, and procedures have been rigorously and systematically tested to ensure that they are safe and effective. And there is also a great deal of evidence to suggest that doctors do not always know or properly apply the information that is available.

In Canada, the testing of drugs for safety and effectiveness is largely left to those developing and manufacturing them for profit. Although the federal government's Health Protection Branch does examine a summary of the company's test data before issuing the notice of compliance which allows drugs to be marketed in Canada, it does no independent testing of its own. There are two approval stages in this federal process. The first requires testing done on tissue cultures or on small animals to see if the drug has any therapeutic value, to see how it is processed, and to see whether it has any major negative impact on the rest of the body. Tests must be done on at least two mammalian species, one of which is not a rodent, to determine the dosage range.[42] Once the Health Protection Branch has examined the reports on these tests, it can approve the drug for three kinds of clinical testing on humans. Healthy volunteers are given the drug to see if there are significant side effects. Then small pilot studies and larger clinical trials on ill people, some of whom are given the drug and others who are given a non-drug, are done. A notice of compliance is given after the company submits reports on these trials. Once approved, drugs do not have to undergo regular reviews, although companies are required to report side effects that have been established by additional research. The government also accepts voluntary reports on side effects from other sources, although this is not a very systematic process.

The testing of medical devices is also left to the manufacturers. Only those devices that are to be implanted for thirty days or more and menstrual tampons, long-term contact lenses, and test kits for aids need a notice of compliance from the government. And these controls were introduced only after considerable protest and evidence gathering by those who used the devices.... The testing of medical procedures is not really covered by formal regulation. This helps explain why it is estimated that only 15 to 20 per cent of medical procedures have ever been subjected to any clear, scientific examination and why there are no systematic data on how the others have been developed and tested.[43] ...

There are a number of reasons why the apparently thorough processes to assess drugs and devices do not always ensure that those on the market are safe and effective. First, drugs introduced before this procedure was established in the early 1960s were not subject to these requirements, and many of them remain on the market today. Many devices have never been tested. In *Safety Last,* Regush maintains that 'only 5 per cent of medical devices are assessed for safety by federal reviewers.'[44] The Health Protection Branch found that 450 of the 7,000 prescription drugs on the market before the new rules were introduced were worthless or lacked medical benefit.[45] Non-prescription drugs were not reviewed and many remain on the counters today. The United States Food and Drug Administration concluded that 40 per cent of the drugs they studied that were introduced before 1962 had 'no effective indication'.[46]

Second, companies produce test reports in ways that stress the benefits but downplay the risks. As a result, many drugs are approved that, at best, have little or no effect or, at worst, may cause serious damage. In 1977, the World Health Organization reported that only 230 of the many thousands of drugs on the market were 'indispensable for health'.[47] In the United States, where regulations for approving drugs are at least as rigorous as those in Canada, a Senate inquiry found that 'of the 348 new drugs introduced by US manufacturers between 1981 and 1988, 292 made "little or no" contribution to therapy and only 12 (3.5 per cent) were rated as providing an important therapeutic gain.' In Canada, the 1990 Pharmaceutical Inquiry found there were a large number of 'suboptimally effective drugs' paid for in the Ontario Drug Benefit Plan.[48] Some of these drugs and devices are not simply useless. The Dalkon Shield is only the most famous of similar contraceptive devices that had to be removed from the market after a public outcry about the 'alarmingly high rate of pelvic inflammatory disease'.[49] In this case, such problems had been reported from the time similar devices were first introduced in 1909.[50]

In addition to the problem of how the reports are structured, there is also the problem of how the tests are carried out. There is no guarantee that the tests have been conducted as described. Perhaps the best known example of this is the case of a Canadian doctor who has been found guilty of falsifying research data on breast cancer patients.[51] The Meme silicone breast implant provides another example. It was never subjected to pre-market approval. But some Canadian scientists suspected problems with the implants and many concerns were raised about it even within the federal Department of Health and Welfare. Eventually, the Department commissioned a surgeon who had been using the Meme to summarize the research. Her report, written in a month, concluded the implant was safe. Two years later, the American Food and Drug Administration found low traces of suspected cancer-causing agents. The Meme was voluntarily removed from the market by the manufacturer at about the same time.[52]

Third, although the requirements may seem quite rigorous, many side effects cannot be assessed through such a short and limited process. More in-depth research done long after a drug is on the market can reveal serious consequences. For example, a study published in *The New England Journal of Medicine* found that the drug Indomethacin, used for 20 years to prevent premature labour, could seriously harm very premature infants.[53] Manitoba researchers have found that several commonly used antihistamines promoted the growth of cancer in mice.[54] A seven-year study at six Canadian hospitals indicated that the drug ritodrine, prescribed to prevent premature birth, did little to reduce the length of pregnancy but did cause chest pain, irregular heart beat and fluid-filled lungs.[55] However, there is no organized means of ensuring such research on long-term effects is done. Moreover, when individual doctors or specific hospitals happen to notice patterns in side effects, there is no systematic way of collecting these data. Canada often depends on the United States for such data. For example, sales of silicone breast implants were suspended only after many individuals reported complaints to the Federal Drug Administration in the United States. A member of Parliament, herself an implant recipient, claimed that 'We have been after the federal government for well over a year to do some proper research into safety. The minister said he was not interested in anecdotal evidence and was waiting to see what the FDA would do.'[56]

...

We do not simply get the drugs or devices scientific surveys say we need, either. The selection of drugs and devices available is more a reflection of where profits are to be made than of where drugs or devices are needed.[57] Much of what companies produce are 'me-too' drugs that simply reproduce drugs already on the market. In the period 1988 to 1990, less than 5 per cent of new drugs introduced in Canada were a substantial improvement on those already available.[58] As one executive sympathetic to the industry put it, 'No manufacturer can afford to restrict his production to genuinely significant pharmaceutical innovations.'[59] Sometimes research on drugs that could be quite useful is abandoned or not undertaken because the potential profits are low. So, for example, the therapeutic possibilities of garlic are not explored by the drug companies because it is much too accessible to the general population. And some products are developed to treat problems that do not call for

intervention. While, for example, the best treatment for diarrhoea is fluid intake and 'specific drugs are neither available or required', pharmaceutical companies produce a wide range of products to treat diarrhoea.[60]

And these unnecessary treatments produced by the drug companies are frequently prescribed by doctors who rely on the same companies for much of their information. As Lexchin makes clear in his survey of the research, the 'more doctors rely on commercial sources for their information, the less rational they are as prescribers: they are more likely to prescribe the wrong drug in the wrong formulation for the wrong reason in an incorrect dosage for an inappropriate length of time.'[61] A comprehensive review of the literature on drug utilization concluded that there continue to be problems in physicians' prescribing practices that relate 'both to over-prescribing of drugs for which there is no evidence of efficacy, as well as under-prescribing of preventative medications like vaccines for immunization of children and adults'.

...

Inappropriate prescribing does not simply reflect the training of doctors and the education they receive from drug companies. It also reflects doctors' values and specific interests. Women and the elderly, a majority of whom are also women, receive more prescriptions for mood-modifiers than do men in part because doctors define women as more emotional and are more likely to see women's problems as 'all in their heads'.[62] It is also much easier for doctors to prescribe pills than to discuss the social conditions that may give rise to the problem treated with mood modifiers. The values of doctors and the interests of the drug companies often combine to create treatments that do not conform to the scientific application of scientifically demonstrated cures.

It is not only the assumption that drugs and devices have been thoroughly tested and proven effective that needs to be challenged. It is also the assumption that such research can always be done in traditional scientific ways. For example, a doctor who has been prescribing histamines to patients has been challenged by the College of Physicians and Surgeons of Ontario because there is no scientific evidence to support his treatment, although no patient has complained and most maintain that they have been helped significantly by this approach.[63] It was not study of tissues or reactions of laboratory animals that has led to a Canadian hospital to use cuddling to a human breast as a treatment for premature babies. Instead, it was experience in a Bogata hospital, where incubators were scarce. In both examples, the treatment appears effective but scientific trials may not be able to establish the connection.

Even drugs and devices that have been examined according to the protocols, following all the rules, are still only best guesses in terms of their effectiveness. Decisions about approving and using drugs are always based on a weighing of risks, not on sure bets. The best science in health care is about probabilities, both because each individual is unique and because treatments interact with a complex, thinking, human being.

It is simply not possible to test all the combinations of drugs or combinations of individual circumstances and conditions that may influence the impact of any treatment. Individual variations in patients and practitioners help explain why a recent Ontario study found significant geographical variations in surgery rates and why simple formulas for procedures based on 'science' would limit the possibilities for taking such factors into account.[64]

As we shall see in the next sections, scientific procedure in medicine excludes the social context and social values that may be at least as important as what happens in the particular tissue that is the focus of concern. And it often excludes the complex interrelationships within the human body and mind. Moreover, a focus on science that stresses overall patterns tends to ignore the fact that each of us is an individual who responds in a different way. Although there are rules to follow, both research and the practice of medicine are arts as well as sciences and much of medical practice cannot be largely transformed into measurable procedures that follow the same rules each time. The techniques used in medicine 'share the features of all human activity in that they are a combination of serendipity, painstaking accumulation of knowledge and inspired guesswork'.[65] They also reflect human values and structural constraints. The devotion to science can be at the expense of the 'inspired hunch' which is the most common means of medical advance.[66] It also may be at the expense of the individual patient and practitioner. While we do need better science, we also need to remain sceptical of all science and to remember that no two human beings are the same.

Although a variety of studies have indicated problems with how drugs and devices are both approved and used, the federal state has been reducing the time taken for testing and the number of people available to do the testing. Regush reports that there are only 'sixty or so' scientists to evaluate manufacturers' reports on thousands of medical devices.[67] The number available to assess reports on tests of new drugs has not increased in two decades, even though the workload has grown rapidly.[68] The process for granting a notice of compliance has been sped up, some drugs are allowed to fast-track, and some assessment work has been contracted out.[69] Managers, rather than scientists, have more power in the assessment. No systematic procedures have been introduced to collect and review information from individual doctors. Little has been done to ensure that doctors are trained in how to monitor and report on complications created by drugs and devices, or in how to create alternative sources of information on drugs. Although there are now guidelines for relationships between doctors and drugs companies, drugs companies are playing an even greater role in doctors' education, a role that is encouraged by state cutbacks in education funding.[70] Moreover, the guidelines remain silent on drug company advertising in medical journals, even though research indicates that such advertisements are often misleading.[71] All these changes make it less rather than more likely that rigorous, scientific procedures will be followed in those areas where they could be the most useful.

...

This is not to argue that there is no place for science, that scientific procedures are either useless or ignored, or that no research has contributed to the development of new means of treatment and cure. Certainly we are far better to have rigorous procedures and every effort should be made to ensure systematic, long-term research is carried out by independent researchers who do not depend on the companies making the drugs or devices for support. It is to argue, however, that here too we should retain the scepticism about whether the research has been or can be done while supporting efforts to promote the safety of procedures through the support of a variety of research methods. Quantitative, experimental, and survey techniques cannot easily examine ethical and legal questions, many of the social and psychological issues, or even many of the problems with more recognizable biological roots. At issue is not whether to use a scientific approach but rather the recognition that science is limited and cannot produce simple objective truth. Also at issue is the question of control, of who decides what research is done, how it is done, what information is provided, and how products are disseminated. These decisions are now more likely to be made with profits, rather than health, in mind.

Challenge 3. Medicine as Cure

The assumption that medicine provides treatment and cure rests on the assumption that science has determined cause and cure. Yet, as the previous section makes clear, there are many treatments that have not been scientifically established and many that cannot be established through traditional scientific means. Many are irrelevant or dangerous.

This is partly the reason why allopathic cures are not the main reason for the improved health and increasing longevity of the Canadian population. In recent years, some drugs have been credited with preventing heart disease, although heart problems are still a major killer in Canada and improvements may be at least as much the result of changes in diet as they are of changes in cures....

Although surgery and drugs certainly make some people better, most of those who pass through the health care system are not cured in the process. Many of those treated in the health care system have one of two problems that cannot be fixed by current medical means. Some have chronic diseases or disabilities that are not subject to cure through currently available drugs or surgery. Those with chronic diseases may have their pain relieved by drugs or surgery and may improve through physical therapy, but they are seldom cured.... Many others seeking help have viruses or other diseases that cannot be effectively treated by medical means. Antibiotics, for example, are not infrequently prescribed for viral infections, which they do not effectively treat. Even though little of what is done in the health care system results in cure, the system is structured around the assumption that this is mainly what happens. People can certainly be helped by caring professionals but the stress on cure makes it less likely that those who cannot easily be cured will get the assistance they need, assistance based on a different view of what determines health.

...

While the focus on cure means that some people get treatment that they do not need, it also means that others do not receive the help that could provide long-term benefit because they cannot easily be cured. As Eakin puts it in her study of stroke patients, they fall outside the central focus on 'doing something'.[72] When stroke patients are admitted to acute care hospitals, they initially do receive intensive care but are often neglected after that. The reason for the neglect, Eakin maintains, can be found in the focus on 'immediate and intensive treatment'. Staff assumed 'nothing could be done', even though there was much that could be done; 'physical, emotional and social support and rehabilitation were clearly not "nothing".[73]

For a number of reasons, this problem is not easily solved simply by dividing the curables from the incurables and sending each group to different institutions. First, it is often not possible to determine whether or not people can be restored to their former state of health. Second, the treatments cannot and should not be separated. The 'physical, emotional and social support' Eakin discusses, or the 'compassion and understanding' the Saskatchewan report says are necessary for those who cannot be cured, are critical whatever the diagnosis and treatment. They should not be the last resort when 'nothing can be done'. Third, all the health care institutions are based, to a large extent, on the same assumptions, so merely dividing up the problems does little to address them, although it may make care cheaper. Too often those defined as incurable receive only the minimum care required. Indeed, the care is often defined as custodial, as if the care is simply about maintenance.

For similar reasons, the problems inherent to the curative approach cannot be solved simply by focusing more on prevention and promotion, defined as a way of maintaining health outside the curative system. As is the case with curables and incurables, the line between prevention and cure is not so easily drawn. Diabetes can be treated but not cured. Although we are very unsure about ways to prevent it, we do know that diet may reduce the possibilities of additional complications. The diet, exercise, security, housing, cleanliness, and support that are the central features of prevention are also central features of cure. And more stress on advanced technology and specialization, as the Saskatchewan report suggests, begs the question of why we have so much ineffective technology and so few cures.

Yet the solutions offered in most government reports involve a new emphasis on prevention outside the curative system and an allocation of patients both to different institutions and to different practitioners, depending on their curability. More of doctors' work that is not specifically curative would be done by nurses and more of those who cannot be cured would be placed in special facilities or sent home to be maintained. Within the curative system, there is to be greater emphasis not on prevention but on cure measured in terms of outcomes. These outcomes are defined primarily in terms of length of patient stays. Such an approach could only be based on the assumption that patients can be quickly and accurately diagnosed and cured. Yet it is clear that many who enter the curative system do not emerge from it cured, that cure cannot be easily separated from prevention and care, and that the curables cannot be easily separated from the incurables. Nor can health care work be neatly packaged into those tasks that contribute to treatment and those that do not. For example, even though cleaning in hospitals is often classified as housekeeping, it bears little relation to the kinds of cleaning women do in the home. What is cleaned and how it must be cleaned are very different in both places.

This is not to argue that there are no cures, that treatment is irrelevant, or that everyone should be served by the same type of hospital and by a doctor. There can be no question that the curative system saves many lives and improves many others, and that some specialization in terms of facilities and caregivers is appropriate. Rather, it is to argue that cure and prevention should not be treated as alternative approaches but rather as combined approaches, albeit ones that remain in considerable tension.

...

Challenge 4. The Engineering Model

Similar questions need to be raised about the engineering model of the body. It is even more difficult to separate body parts from each other to determine treatment and cure than it is to separate the curables from the incurables. Chest pain may indicate gall bladder problems and antibiotics for ear infections can encourage yeast infections in the vagina.

This interconnectedness of body parts is one of the reasons there is such a high rate of iatrogenic illnesses, those caused by medical treatment. Treatment for one body part often conflicts with treatment for another part or affects other body parts....

...

The engineering model, especially when combined with the curative approach, contributes to the over-prescribing patterns of doctors. A study of prescribing patterns among New Brunswick doctors treating patients over age 65 found that the busiest doctors were the ones prescribing the most drugs.[74] The greater use of drugs was linked to very short visits with the doctor. Such short visits can be explained only by a focus on parts to be fixed by specific cures, with little concern for the links among parts or for the whole person. Walk-in clinics are more likely to be focused on parts, given that it is assumed that service can be easily provided to the stranger who brings in the parts.

The fee-for-service system, which attaches a price to treatment of particular body parts, also contributes to these short visits and the tendency to prescribe more than one drug. A researcher in the New Brunswick study said of the fee-for-service system: 'It's not rewarding the physician who sits down and talks to the patients. It rewards the physician who sits there with his hand cocked like a trigger, ready to write a prescription as soon as you have a complaint out of your mouth.'[75] ... The body parts approach not only affects doctors; it also affects the entire organization of work in health care. With this assumption, it is possible to assign the responsibility for different parts to different people and to divide up the work of individual health care workers into tiny, interchangeable parts. So, for example, a nurse long employed by an organization providing home care has had her full-time job transformed into a part-time one. Although she now works at least as many hours as she did previously, she is no longer assigned to follow particular patients through their illnesses. Instead, she is constantly moved around among patients to ensure, as much as possible, that every minute of her time is devoted to treatment. She is therefore unable to help the same patient over a period of time adjust to such problems as a diagnosis of diabetes or cancer. This fragmentation is even more obvious in hospitals. As one hospital worker interviewed for 'Voices from the Ward' put it: 'We process people just ... like in a chocolate factory.'[76]

Specialization is also based on the assumption of parts to be fixed and it, too, can be questioned. While clearly there are advantages in having practitioners develop expertise in particular areas, there are also problems with this approach. In treating the part, one specialist may provide treatment that conflicts with, or masks, problems created in another. A dermatologist, for example, may prescribe cream for a skin ailment but the rash may be the result of blood pressure pills prescribed by the heart doctor. Moreover, specialization means patients must travel from doctor to doctor, none of whom is likely to have a full view of the entire patient.

There is considerable evidence that fee-for-service payment promotes quick-fix treatments that may be useless or harmful. There is also plenty of evidence to indicate that the body is a complex, interconnected organism that cannot easily be carved up for service. However, while the various government reports talk about '*people* being the focus of the health system',[77] they do little to challenge the engineering model of the body. Instead, in many ways they encourage specialization in services and the allocation of specific parts to different health care workers. The separation of aging from mental health, for example, is integral to the current restructuring programs. With new monitoring systems care of the patient will be fragmented further, as each patient is classified according to the part to be fixed and each function measured as if it were the same as an oil change on the car. As much as possible, the part to be fixed will be quickly treated in the doctor's office, the out-patient clinic, or the day-surgery, with little time for consideration of other, connected body parts, let alone for social and psychological support.

This is not to argue that expertise should be abandoned or that all institutions should respond to all needs. But it is to argue that health care should begin with the assumption that people are the focus and that systems must be designed to make whole people, rather than body parts, the central concern. The tension between specialization and integration must be recognized and maintained, not resolved by simply choosing one alternative.

Challenge 5. Health as Mainly Biological

The challenge to the assumption that illness and disability are primarily the result of readily identifiable biological causes is directly linked to the fact that people are not simply or even mainly collections of parts to be fixed.

...

The determinants of health identified in the government reports and set out in the earlier sections of this chapter clearly show that the social context is critical to maintaining health. What is much less clear in these reports is that the same factors are critical in both diagnosis and cure. There is a recognition that 'social and physical environments ... have a major impact on people's health.'[78] But these environments are not discussed in relation to the provision of care, even though the assumptions of allopathic medicine largely ignore them. And although there is a recognition that psychological factors are critical to the body's immune system and the capacity to both resist and recover from disease,[79] there is also no discussion of how this conflicts with the current assumptions of health care.

The determinants of health as set out in these reports directly challenge some basic assumptions of allopathic medicine. Biological causes cannot be separated from social contexts, minds cannot be separated from bodies, and body

parts cannot be separated from each other. The recognition that bodies must be understood and problems with them be diagnosed in their social contexts necessarily leads to the conclusion that each individual is unique, given that the social influences on bodies and minds vary from individual to individual.

This is not to argue that no tests should be done, that no research focused on biological factors should be conducted, or that no doctor should see a patient alone. However, it is to argue that it is necessary to recognize the contradiction between establishing the importance of social and physical environments outside the health care system while restructuring health care to focus more exclusively on biological causes and the fixing of body parts. We need to integrate this knowledge into the restructuring of care to ensure that care delivery links body part and body part, mind and body, body and social context.

...

Notes

1. World Health Organization, *Ottawa Charter for Health Promotion*. Ottawa: Canadian Public Health Association, 1986.
2. Irving Rootman and John Raeburn, 'The Concept of Health'. Pp. 56–71 in Ann Pederson, Michel O'Neill, and Irving Rootman (eds) *Health Promotion in Canada*. Toronto: W.B. Saunders, 1994.
3. Ontario Ministry of Health, *Working Document: Goals and Strategic Priorities*. Toronto: Ontario Ministry of Health, 19 January 1992, p. 1. Also see Sharmila L. Mhatre and Raisa B. Deber, 'From Equal Access to Health Care to Equitable Access to Health: A Review of Canadian Provincial Health Commissions and Reports', *International Journal of Health Services* 22, 4 (1992): 656.
4. Ontario Premier's Council on Health Strategy, *Nurturing Health: A Framework on the Determinants of Health*. Toronto: Author, 1991.
5. Ibid., p. 8.
6. James House, Karl Landis, and Debra Umberson, 'Social Relationships and Health'. Pp. 85–94 in *The Sociology of Health and Illness: Critical Perspectives*. New-York: St Martin's Press, 1990.

7. See Carol Baines, Patricia Evans and Sheila Neysmith (eds), *Women's Caring.* Toronto: McClelland and Stewart, 1991.

8. Kathleen MacPherson, 'Looking at Caring and Nursing Through a Feminist Lens' in *Caring and Nursing,* 1991, p. 26.

9. Nancy Waxler-Morrison, Joan Anderson, and Elizabeth Morrison (eds), *Cross-Cultural Caring.* Vancouver: U.B.C. Press, 1990, and M. Judith Lynam, 'Towards the Goal of Providing Culturally Sensitive Care: Principles upon Which to Build Nursing Curricula', *Journal of Advanced Nursing* 17 (1992): 149–57.

10. *Nurturing Health,* p. 8. See also Robert L. Jin, Chandrakant P. Shah, and Tomislav J. Svoboda, 'The Impact of Unemployment on Health: A Review of the Evidence', *Canadian Medical Association Journal* 153, 5 (1 Sept. 1995): 529–40.

11. Ibid., p. 7.

12. See, for example, Heather MacDougall, *Activists and Advocates.* Toronto: Dundurn Press, 1990.

13. *Nurturing Health,* p. 11.

14. Ibid., p. 12.

15. Ibid., p. 17.

16. Ibid., p. 14.

17. Ibid., p. 15.

18. Ibid., p. 9.

19. B. Singh Bolaria and Rosemary Bolaria (eds), *Racial Minorities in Medicine and Health.* Halifax: Fernwood, 1994.

20. *Nurturing Health,* p. 6.

21. Ibid., p. 17.

22. Ibid., p. 6.

23. British Columbia, Royal Commission on Health Care and Costs, *Closer to Home.* Victoria: Author, 1991, pp. 12–13.

24. The Premier's Commission on Future Health Care for Albertans, *The Rainbow Report: Our Vision for Health.* Edmonton: Author, 1989, p. 38.

25. Saskatchewan Commission on Directions in Health Care, *Future Directions For Health Care in Saskatchewan.* Regina: Author, 1990, p. 19.

26. Evan Willis, *Medical Dominance.* Sydney: George Allen and Unwin, 1983, p. 2.

27. Quoted in Bernard Blishen, *Doctors in Canada.* Toronto: University of Toronto Press, 1991, p. 113.

28. Rosalind Coward, *The Whole Truth: The Myth of Alternative Therapies.* London: Faber and Faber, 1989, p. 49.

29. Edward Shorter, *Bedside Manners: A Troubled History of Doctors and Patients.* New York: Simon and Shuster, 1985, pp. 75–6.

30. Daniel Stoffman, 'Losing Patience. Are Hospital Costs Killing the Taxpayer?', *Canadian Business,* November 1988, p. 72.

31. Sara Dimers, 'Total Quality Management—A Strategy for Success', *Housecall.* Women's College Hospital, 1992, pp. 10–11.

32. Joel Lexchin, *The Real Pushers: A Critical Analysis of the Canadian Drug Industry.* Vancouver: New Star, 1984, pp. 209–10.

33. Blishen, *Doctors in Canada,* p. 9; and C. David Naylor, *Private Practice: Public Payment.* Montreal: McGill-Queen's University Press, 1986, pp. 16–17.

34. Naylor, p. 18.

35. Ibid.

36. Geoffrey Bilson, 'Canadian Doctors and the Cholera' in *Medicine in Canadian Society,* S.E.D. Shorn (ed.), Montreal: McGill-Queen's Press, 1981, p. 118.

37. David Cayley, *Doctoring the Family.* Montreal: CBC, 1985, p. 7.

38. Quoted in Cayley, p. 15.

39. Cayley, p. 44.

40. Linda Rasmussen, Lorna Rasmussen, Candace Savage, and Anne Wheeler, *A Harvest Yet to Reap.* Toronto: Women's Press, 1976, p. 76.

41. British Columbia Royal Commission on Health Care and Costs, *Closer to Home: A Summary Report.* Victoria: Author, 1991, p. 8.

42. Nicholas Regush, *Safety Last; The Failure of the Consumer Health Protection System in Canada.* Toronto: Key Porter Books, 1993, p. 12. See also James McRae and Francis Tapon, 'Prices, Patents, and R&D Location in the Canadian Pharmaceutical Industry' in *Limits To Care,* Ake Blomqvist and David M. Brown (eds). Montreal: C.D. Howe Institute, 1994, p. 380.

43. Philip Hassen, *Rx for Hospitals: New Hope for Medicare in the Nineties.* Toronto: Stoddart, 1993, p. 80.

44. Regush, p. 36.

45. In Regush, p. 16.

46. In Andrew Chetley, *A Healthy Business: World Health and the Pharmaceutical Industry.* London: Zed Books, 1990, p. 48.

47. In Lexchin, 1984, p. 83.

48. Report of the Pharmaceutical Inquiry of Ontario, *Rx: Prescriptions for Health.* Toronto: Ontario Ministry of Health, 1990.

49. Ann Pappert, 'The Rise and Fall of the IUD' in *Adverse Effects. Women and the Pharmaceutical*

Industry, Kathleen McDonnell (ed.). Toronto: Women's Press, p. 168.

50. Pappert, p. 167.

51. Canadian Press and Reuters, 'Breast Cancer Researcher Falsified Data in Major Study', *Globe and Mail* (14 March 1994): A2.

52. Gord McIntosh, 'Ottawa Overlooked Implant Concerns, Documents Indicate', *Globe and Mail* (18 June 1992): A9.

53. Reuters News Agency, 'Drug That Delays Labour May Harm Fetus, Study Finds', *Globe and Mail* (25 November 1993) p. A4.

54. The Medical Tribune News Service, 'Allergy Drugs Cancer Suspects', *The Toronto Star* (18 May 1994): A18.

55. Lisa Priest, 'Labour-Halting Drug called Ineffective and Risk to Health', *Toronto Star* (31 July 1992): C1.

56. Quoted in Paul Taylor and Rod Mickleburgh 'Breast Implant Sales Suspended', *Globe and Mail* (8 January 1992): A4.

57. See Lexchin, *The Real Pushers;* and Donald Drake and Marian Uhlman, *Making Medicine, Making Money.* Kansas City: Andrews and McMeel, 1993.

58. Joel Lexchin, 'Profits First: The Pharmaceutical Industry in Canada' in *Health, Illness and Health Care in Canada,* 2nd edn, B. Singh Bolaria and Harley Dickinson (eds). Toronto: Harcourt, Brace and Company, 1994, p. 708.

59. Quoted in Lexchin, 1994, p. 708.

60. Quoted in Chetley, p. 45.

61. Lexchin, 1994, p. 710.

62. See Jim Harding, 1986; Dorothy Smith, and Sara David (eds), *Women Look at Psychiatry.* Vancouver: Press Gang Publishers, 1975; and Deborah Findlay and Leslie Miller, 'Through Medical Eyes: The Medicalization of Women's Bodies and Women's Lives' in B. Singh Bolaria and Harley Dickinson, *Health, Illness and Health Care in Canada.* Toronto: Harcourt Brace and Company, 1994, pp. 276–306.

63. Joan Breckenridge 'Unorthodox … or Incompetent?', *Globe and Mail* (2 July 1994): A4.

64. C. David Naylor, Geoffrey M. Anderson, and Vivek Goel (eds), *Patterns of Health Care in Ontario,* vol. 1. Toronto: The Institute for Clinical Evaluative Sciences in Ontario, 1994.

65. Grant Gillett, *Reasonable Care.* Bristol: Bristol Press, p. 12.

66. Ibid., p. 13.

67. Regush, p. 37.

68. Regush, p. 15.

69. Regush, Ch. 2.

70. Art Chamberlain, 'Doctor, Drug Firm Ties Coming into Question', *Toronto Star* (10 May 1994): C1, C4.

71. Warren McIsaac, C, David Naylor, Geoffrey M. Anderson, and Bernie J.O'Brien, 'Reflections on a Month in the Life of the Ontario Drug Benefit Plan', *Canadian Medical Association Journal* 150, 4 (1994): 476.

72. Joan M. Eakin, 'Stroke Patients in a Canadian Hospital' in Coburn et al., (eds), p. 535.

73. Eakin, p. 535.

74. In Paul Taylor, 'Busiest MDs Prescribe the Most Drugs', *Globe and Mail* (15 March 1994): A1.

75. In Taylor: A2.

76. Pat Armstrong, Jaqueline Choinière, Gina Feldberg, and Jerry White, 'Voices from the Ward' in Pat and Hugh Armstrong, Jacqueline Choinière, Gina Feldberg, and Jerry White, *Take Care: Warning Signals for Canada's Health System.* Toronto: Garamond, 1994, p. 57.

77. Premier's Commission on Future Health Care for Albertans, *The Rainbow Report: Our Vision for Health,* vol. II. Edmonton: Author, 1990, p. 43.

78. Ontario Premier's Council on Health Strategy, *Nurturing Health.* Toronto: Author, 1991, unpaginated.

79. Ontario Premier's Council on Health Strategy, *A Vision of Health: Health Goals For Ontario.* Toronto: Author, 1991, unpaginated.

Autonomy, Equality and a Just Health Care System

Kai Nielsen

I

Autonomy and equality are both fundamental values in our firmament of values, and they are frequently thought to be in conflict. Indeed the standard liberal view is that we must make difficult and often morally ambiguous trade-offs between them.[1] I shall argue that this common view is mistaken and that autonomy cannot be widespread or secure in a society which is not egalitarian: where, that is, equality is not also a very fundamental value which has an operative role within the society.[2] I shall further argue that, given human needs and a commitment to an autonomy respecting egalitarianism, a very different health care system would come into being than that which exists at present in the United States.

I shall first turn to a discussion of autonomy and equality and then, in terms of those conceptions, to a conception of justice. In modernizing societies of Western Europe, a perfectly just society will be a society of equals and in such societies there will be a belief held across the political spectrum in what has been called *moral equality*. That is to say, when viewed with the impartiality required by morality, the life of everyone matters and matters equally.[3] Individuals will, of course, and rightly so, have their local attachments but they will acknowledge that justice requires that the social institutions of the society should be such that they work on the premiss that the life of everyone matters and matters equally. Some privileged elite or other group cannot be given special treatment simply because they are that group. Moreover, for there to be a society of equals there must be a rough equality of condition in the society. Power must be sufficiently equally shared for it to be securely the case that no group or class or gender can dominate others through the social structures either by means of their frequently thoroughly unacknowledged latent functions or more explicitly and manifestly by institutional arrangements sanctioned by law or custom. Roughly equal material resources or power are not things which are desirable in themselves, but they are essential instrumentalities for the very possibility of equal well-being and for as many people as possible having as thorough and as complete a control over their own lives as is compatible with this being true for everyone alike. Liberty cannot flourish without something approaching this equality of condition, and people without autonomous lives will surely live impoverished lives. These are mere commonplaces. In fine, a commitment to achieving equality of condition, far from undermining liberty and autonomy, is essential for their extensive flourishing.

If we genuinely believe in moral equality, we will want to see come into existence a world in which all people capable of self-direction have, and have as nearly as is feasible equally, control over their own lives and can, as far as the institutional arrangements for it obtaining are concerned, all live flourishing lives where their needs and desires as individuals are met as fully as possible and as fully and extensively as is compatible with that possibility being open to everyone alike. The thing is to provide institutional arrangements that are conducive to that.

People, we need to remind ourselves, plainly have different capacities and sensibilities. However,

---

Nielsen, K. (1989) "Autonomy, Equality and a Just Health Care System." *International Journal of Applied Philosophy* 4(3): pp. 39–44. Reprinted by permission.

even in the extreme case of people for whom little in the way of human flourishing is possible, their needs and desires, as far as possible, should still also be satisfied in the way I have just described. Everyone in this respect at least has equal moral standing. No preference or pride of place should be given to those capable, in varying degrees, of rational self-direction. The more rational, or, for that matter, the more loveable, among us should not be given preference. No one should. Our needs should determine what is to be done.

People committed to achieving and sustaining a society of equals will seek to bring into stable existence conditions such that it would be possible for everyone, if they were personally capable of it, to enjoy an equally worthwhile and satisfying life or at least a life in which, for all of them, their needs, starting with and giving priority to their more urgent needs, were met and met as equally and as fully as possible, even where their needs are not entirely the same needs. This, at least, is the heuristic, though we might, to gain something more nearly feasible, have to scale down talk of meeting needs to providing conditions propitious for the equal satisfaction for everyone of their *basic* needs. Believers in equality want to see a world in which everyone, as far as this is possible, have equal whole life prospects. This requires an equal consideration of their needs and interests and a refusal to just override anyone's interests: to just regard anyone's interests as something which comes to naught, which can simply be set aside as expendable. Minimally, an egalitarian must believe that taking the moral point of view requires that each person's good is afforded equal consideration. Moreover, this is not just a bit of egalitarian ideology but is a deeply embedded considered judgment in modern Western culture capable of being put into wide reflective equilibrium.[4]

II

What is a need, how do we identify needs and what are our really basic needs, needs that are presumptively universal? Do these basic needs in most circumstances at least trump our other needs and our reflective considered preferences?

Let us start this examination by asking if we can come up with a list of universal needs correctly ascribable to all human beings in all cultures. In doing this we should, as David Braybrooke has, distinguish *adventitious* and *course-of-life* needs.[5] Moreover, it is the latter that it is essential to focus on. Adventitious needs, like the need for a really good fly rod or computer, come and go with particular projects. Course-of-life needs, such as the need for exercise, sleep or food, are such that every human being may be expected to have them all at least at some stage of life.

Still, we need to step back a bit and ask: how do we determine what is a need, course-of-life need or otherwise? We need a relational formula to spot needs. We say, where we are speaking of needs, B needs x in order to y, as in Janet needs milk or some other form of calcium in order to protect her bone structure. With course-of-life needs the relation comes out platitudinously as in 'People need food and water in order to live' or 'People need exercise in order to function normally or well'. This, in the very identification of the need, refers to human flourishing or to human well-being, thereby giving to understand that they are basic needs. Perhaps it is better to say instead that this is to specify in part what it is for something to be a basic need. Be that as it may, there are these basic needs we *must* have to live well. If this is really so, then, where they are things we as individuals can have without jeopardy to others, no further question arises, or can arise, about the desirability of satisfying them. They are just things that in such circumstances ought to be met in our lives if they can. The satisfying of such needs is an unequivocally good thing. The questions 'Does Janet need to live?' and 'Does Sven need to function well?' are at best otiose.

In this context David Braybrooke has quite properly remarked that being "essential to living or to functioning normally may be taken as a criterion for being a basic need. Questions about whether needs are genuine, or well-founded, come to an end of the line when the needs have been connected with life or health."[6] Certainly to flourish we must have these things and in some instances they must be met at least to a certain extent even to survive. This being so, we can quite properly call them basic needs. Where these needs do not clash or the satisfying them by one person does not conflict with the satisfying of the equally basic needs of another no question about justifying the meeting of them arises.

By linking the identification of needs with what we must have to function well and linking course-of-life and basic needs with what all people, or at least almost all people, must have to function well, a list of basic needs can readily be set out. I shall give such a list, though surely the list is incomplete. However, what will be added is the same sort of thing similarly identified. First there are needs connected closely to our physical functioning, namely the need for food and water, the need for excretion, for exercise, for rest (including sleep), for a life supporting relation to the environment, and the need for whatever is indispensable to preserve the body intact. Similarly there are basic needs connected with our function as social beings. We have needs for companionship, education, social acceptance and recognition, for sexual activity, freedom from harassment, freedom from domination, for some meaningful work, for recreation and relaxation and the like.[7]

The list, as I remarked initially, is surely incomplete. But it does catch many of the basic things which are in fact necessary for us to live or to function well. Now an autonomy respecting egalitarian society with an interest in the well-being of its citizens—something moral beings could hardly be without—would (trivially) be a society of equals, and as a society of equals it would be committed to (a) *moral* equality and (b) an equality of *condition* which would, under conditions of moderate abundance, in turn expect the equality of condition to be rough and to be principally understood (cashed in) in terms of providing the conditions (as far as that is possible) for meeting the needs (including most centrally the basic needs) of everyone and

meeting them equally, as far as either of these things is feasible.

III

What kind of health care system would such an autonomy respecting egalitarian society have under conditions of moderate abundance such as we find in Canada and the United States?

The following are health care needs which are also basic needs: being healthy and having conditions treated which impede one's functioning well or which adversely affect one's well-being or cause suffering. These are plainly things we need. Where societies have the economic and technical capacity to do so, as these societies plainly do, without undermining other equally urgent or more urgent needs, these health needs, as basic needs, must be met, and the right to have such medical care is a right for everyone in the society regardless of her capacity to pay. This just follows from a commitment to *moral* equality and to an equality of condition. Where we have the belief, a belief which is very basic in non-fascistic modernizing societies, that each person's good is to be given equal consideration, it is hard not to go in that way, given a plausible conception of needs and reasonable list of needs based on that conception.[8] If there is the need for some particular regime of care and the society has the resources to meet that need, without undermining structures protecting other at least equally urgent needs, then, *ceteris paribus,* the society, if it is a decent society, must do so. The commitment to more equality—the commitment to the belief that the life of each person matters and matters equally—entails, given a few plausible empirical premises, that each person's health needs will be the object of an equal regard. Each has an equal claim, *prima facie,* to have her needs satisfied where this is possible. That does not, of course, mean that people should all be treated alike in the sense of their all getting the same thing. Not everyone needs flu shots, braces, a dialysis machine, a psychiatrist, or a triple bypass. What should be equal is that each person's health needs should be the object of equal societal concern since each person's good should be given equal consideration.[9] This does not mean that equal energy should be directed to Hans's rash as to Frank's cancer. Here one person's need for a cure is much greater than the other, and the greater need clearly takes precedence. Both should be met where possible, but where they both cannot then the greater need has pride of place. But what should not count in the treatment of Hans and Frank is that Hans is wealthy or prestigious or creative and Frank is not. Everyone should have their health needs met where possible. Moreover, where the need is the same, they should have (where possible), and where other at least equally urgent needs are not thereby undermined, the same quality treatment. No differentiation should be made between them on the basis of their ability to pay or on the basis of their being (one more so than the other) important people. There should, in short, where this is possible, be open and free medical treatment of the same quality and extent available to everyone in the society. And no two- or three-tier system should be allowed to obtain, and treatment should only vary (subject to the above qualification) on the basis of variable needs and unavoidable differences in different places in supply and personnel, e.g., differences between town and country. Furthermore, these latter differences should be remedied where technically and economically feasible. The underlying aim should be to meet the health care needs of everyone and meet them, in the sense explicated, equally: everybody's needs here should be met as fully as possible; different treatment is only justified where the need is different or where both needs cannot be met. Special treatment for one person rather than another is only justified where, as I remarked, both needs cannot be met or cannot as adequately be met. Constrained by ought implies can; where these circumstances obtain, priority should be given to the greater need that can feasibly be met. A moral system or a social policy, plainly, cannot be reasonably asked to do the impossible. But my account does not ask that.

To have such a health care system would, I think, involve taking medicine out of the private sector altogether including, of course, out of private entrepreneurship where the governing rationale has to be profit and where supply and demand rules the roost. Instead there must be a health care system firmly in the public sector (publicly owned and controlled) where the rationale of the system is to meet as efficiently and as fully as possible the health care needs of everyone in the society in question. The health care system should not be viewed as a business anymore than a university should be viewed as a business—compare a university and a large hospital—but as a set of institutions and practices designed to meet urgent human needs.

I do not mean that we should ignore costs or efficiency. The state-run railroad system in Switzerland, to argue by analogy, is very efficient. The state cannot, of course, ignore costs in running it. But the aim is not to make a profit. The aim is to produce the most rapid, safe, efficient and comfortable service meeting travellers's needs within the parameters of the overall socio-economic priorities of the state and the society. Moreover, since the state in question is a democracy, if its citizens do not like the policies of the government here (or elsewhere) they can replace it with a government with different priorities and policies. Indeed the option is there (probably never to be exercised) to shift the railroad into the private sector.

Governments, understandably, worry with aging populations about mounting health care costs. This is slightly ludicrous in the United States, given its military and space exploration budgets, but is also a reality in Canada and even in Iceland where there is no military or space budget at all. There should, of course, be concern about containing health costs, but this can be done effectively with a state-run system. Modern societies need systems of socialized medicine, something that obtains in almost all civilized modernizing societies. The United States and South Africa are, I believe, the only exceptions. But, as is evident from my own country (Canada), socialized health care systems often need altering, and their costs need monitoring.

As a cost-cutting and as an efficiency measure that would at the same time improve health care, doctors, like university professors and government bureaucrats, should be put on salaries and they should work in medical units. They should, I hasten to add, have good salaries but salaries all the same; the last vestiges of petty entrepreneurship should be taken from the medical profession. This measure would save the state-run health care system a considerable amount of money, would improve the quality of medical care with greater cooperation and consultation resulting from economies of scale and a more extensive division of labor with larger and better equipped medical units. (There would also be less duplication of equipment.) The overall quality of care would also improve with a better balance between health care in the country and in the large cities, with doctors being systematically and rationally deployed throughout the society. In such a system doctors, no more than university professors or state bureaucrats, could not just set up a practice anywhere. They would no more be free to do this than university professors or state bureaucrats. In the altered system there would be no cultural space for it. Placing doctors on salary, though not at a piece work rate, would also result in its being the case that the financial need to see as many patients as possible as quickly as possible would be removed. This would plainly enhance the quality of medical care. It would also be the case that a different sort of person would go into the medical profession. People would go into it more frequently because they were actually interested in medicine and less frequently because this is a rather good way (though hardly the best way) of building a stock portfolio.

There should also be a rethinking of the respective roles of nurses (in all their variety), paramedics and doctors. Much more of the routine work done in medicine—taking the trout fly out of my ear for example—can be done by nurses or paramedics. Doctors, with their more extensive training, could be freed up for other more demanding tasks worthy of their expertise. This would require somewhat different training

for all of these different medical personnel and a rethinking of the authority structure in the health care system. But doing this in a reasonable way would improve the teamwork in hospitals, make morale all around a lot better, improve medical treatment and save a very considerable amount of money. (It is no secret that the relations between doctors and nurses are not good.) Finally, a far greater emphasis should be placed on preventative medicine than is done now. This, if really extensively done, utilizing the considerable educational and fiscal powers of the state, would result in very considerable health care savings and a very much healthier and perhaps even happier population. (Whether with the states we actually have we are likely to get anything like that is—to understate it—questionable. I wouldn't hold my breath in the United States. Still, Finland and Sweden are very different places from the United States and South Africa.)

IV

It is moves of this *general* sort that an egalitarian and autonomy loving society under conditions of moderate scarcity should implement. (I say 'general sort' for I am more likely to be wrong about some of the specifics than about the general thrust of my argument.) It would, if in place, limit the freedom of some people, including some doctors and some patients, to do what they want to do. That is obvious enough. But any society, any society at all, as long as it had norms (legal and otherwise) will limit freedom in some way.[10] There is no living in society without some limitation on the freedom to do some things. Indeed a society without norms and thus without any limitation on freedom is a contradiction in terms. Such a mass of people wouldn't be a society. They, without norms, would just be a mass of people. (If these are 'grammatical remarks,' make the most of them.) In our societies I am not free to go for a spin in your car without your permission, to practice law or medicine without a license, to marry your wife while she is still your wife and the like. Many restrictions on our liberties, because they are so common, so widely accepted and thought by most of us to be so reasonable, hardly *seem* like restrictions on our liberty. But they are all the same. No doubt some members of the medical profession would feel quite reined in if the measures I propose were adopted. (These measures are not part of conventional wisdom.) But the restrictions on the freedom of the medical profession and on patients I am proposing would make for both a greater liberty all around, everything considered, and, as well, for greater well-being in the society. Sometimes we have to restrict certain liberties in order to enhance the overall system of liberty. Not speaking out of turn in parliamentary debate is a familiar example. Many people who now have a rather limited access to medical treatment would come to have it and have it in a more adequate way with such a socialized system in place. Often we have to choose between a greater or lesser liberty in a society, and, at least under conditions of abundance, the answer almost always should be 'Choose the greater liberty'. If we really prize human autonomy, if, that is, we want a world in which as many people as possible have as full as is possible control over their own lives, then we will be egalitarians. Our very egalitarianism will commit us to something like the health care system I described, but so will the realization that, without reasonable health on the part of the population, autonomy can hardly flourish or be very extensive. Without the kind of equitability and increased coverage in health care that goes with a properly administered socialized medicine, the number of healthy people will be far less than could otherwise feasibly be the case. With that being the case, autonomy and well-being as well with be neither as extensive nor so thorough as it could otherwise be. Autonomy, like everything else, has its material conditions. And to will the end is to will the necessary means to the end.

To take—to sum up—what since the Enlightenment has come to be seen as the moral point of view, and to take morality seriously, is to take it as axiomatic that each person's good be given equal consideration.[11] I have argued that (a) where that is accepted, and (b) where we are tolerably clear about the facts (including facts about human needs), and (c) where we live under conditions of moderate abundance, a health care system bearing at least a family resemblance to the one I have gestured at will be put in place. It is a health care system befitting an autonomy respecting democracy committed to the democratic and egalitarian belief that the life of everyone matters and matters equally.

Notes

1. Isaiah Berlin, "On the Pursuit of the Ideal," *The New York Review of Books* XXXV (March 1987), pp. 11–18. See also his "Equality" in his *Concepts and Categories* (Oxford, England: Oxford University Press, 1980), pp. 81–102. I have criticized that latter paper in my "Formulating Egalitarianism: Animadversions on Berlin," *Philosophia* 13:3–4 (October 1983), pp. 299–315.

2. For three defenses of such a view see Kai Nielsen, *Equality and Liberty* (Totowa, New Jersey: Rowman and Allanheld, 1985), Richard Norman, *Free and Equal* (Oxford, England: Oxford University Press, 1987), and John Baker, *Arguing for Equality* (London: Verso Press, 1987).

3. Will Kymlicka, "Rawls on Teleology and Deontology," *Philosophy and Public Affairs* 17:3 (Summer 1988), pp. 173–190 and John Rawls, "The Priority of Right and Ideas of the Good," *Philosophy and Public Affairs* 17:4 (Fall 1988), pp. 251–276.

4. Kai Nielsen, "Searching for an Emancipatory Perspective: Wide Reflective Equilibrium and the Hermeneutical Circle" in Evan Simpson (ed.), *Anti-Foundationalism and Practical Reasoning* (Edmonton, Alberta: Academic Printing and Publishing, 1987), pp. 143–164 and Kai Nielsen, "In Defense of Wide Reflective Equilibrium" in Douglas Odegard (ed.) *Ethics and Justification* (Edmonton, Alberta: Academic Printing and Publishing, 1988), pp. 19–37.

5. David Braybrooke, *Meeting Needs* (Princeton, New Jersey: Princeton University Press, 1987), p. 29.

6. *Ibid.*, p. 31.

7. *Ibid.*, p. 37.

8. Will Kymlicka, *op cit.*, p. 190.

9. *Ibid.*

10. Ralf Dahrendorf, Essays *in the Theory of Society* (Stanford, California: Stanford University Press, 1968), pp. 151–78 and G.A. Cohen, "The Structure of Proletarian Unfreedom," *Philosophy and Public Affairs* 12 (1983), pp. 2–33.

11. Will Kymlicka, *op cit*, p. 190.

Adopting a Life-Course Approach

Christine Overall

Jeffrey Simpson (2000, A17) writes "A wildly disproportionate amount of [Canada's] health-care budget is spent caring for people in their last year of life and dealing with the inevitable health problems associated with old age. For those worried about the costs of health care, here are the knotty issues such as cutting off treatment for the incurable." The crucial question, however, is whether those health-care costs should be described as "wildly disproportionate." They would be genuinely disproportionate only if we made an a priori assumption that every decade, or even every year, of human life should receive approximately the same share of health-care resources. But such an assumption takes for granted precisely the point that is at issue, namely, whether people at different ages legitimately need and should be able to access different kinds and amounts of health-care resources.

Elderly people are the heaviest users of out-patient and inpatient services (Hanson 1995, 3). In the United States, the average annual expenditures for health care per person from 1985 to 1997 ranged from $425 for those under twenty five to $2,900 for those aged sixty-five to seventy-four. But the statistics do not suggest that those who are elderly receive all the benefits to the utter neglect of the young. The average annual health-care costs of those who were aged twenty-five to thirty-four were more than twice those of the under-twenty-fives, at $1,236. And the average annual health-care costs of persons seventy-five years of age or older were, at $2,799, lower than the costs of the next younger group (U.S. Bureau of the Census 1999). Nonetheless, even if the goal of compressing morbidity into the last years or months of life is achieved, so that the most concentrated use of medical care is required only at the very end of life, we should still expect that, over the course of their aging elderly people will have different health-care needs than younger ones and hence that it is appropriate, in both practical and moral terms, to allocate resources differentially to that stage of life.

The implicit error of politicians, journalists, ethicists, and policy analysts who engage in hand wringing about the costs of caring for elderly people is their assumption that health-care needs should be the same, or at least cost the same, at all stages of life. Interpreting elderly people as a "burden" relies, I suggest, on this key assumption. The costs of sustaining elderly people's lives and health can be understood as burdensome only if it is assumed that such people are demanding more than their fair share and if "fair" is implicity construed as meaning "approximately equal." But there are real differences between being forty years old and being eighty years old, just as there are real differences between being forty years old and being four years old. If we would not expect the four-year-old's health-care needs to be the same

Overall, C. (2003) "Adopting a Life-Course Approach." In Overall, C. *Aging, Death, and Human Longevity: A Philosophical Inquiry* (pp. 205–217). Berkeley, CA: University of California Press. Reprinted by permission of University of California Press.

and cost the same as those of the forty-year-old, so also we should not expect the eighty-year-old's health-care needs to be the same and cost the same as those of the forty-year-old.

It is simply ageism to suppose that the eighty-year-old must be like the forty-year-old in order for his needs to be considered legitimate or that the typical (if there is one) forty-year-old—or thirty-year-old or twenty-year-old—provides the standard by which health-care expectations, needs, and demands should be evaluated. We should not play into stereotypes that depict the old as adversaries or competitors of the young; nor should we condone a situation in which old people must fear the bitterness of younger people who are "forced" to support them. We cannot continue to sustain or even tolerate what Jean-Nesmy calls our culture's "lopsided glorification of youth." Human life is valuable to its possessors because it affords the ongoing opportunity for activities and experiences, and, in the absence of debilitating pain or total loss of consciousness, that opportunity exists at every age. Hence, as Jean-Nesmy (1991, 148–149) points out, there is a contradiction between extending human lives, "which means *ex hypothesi* additional years during the last third of life, and the belief that only the first third is worth living." Of course the last third is worth living, and those in the first third and second third must recognize that fact.

Many commentators have registered their anxiety that, because of demographic unevenness, a smaller proportion of people will be in the workforce by 2010 than are working now. Callahan (1999, 191), for example, is worried about "an excessive tax burden on the young to pay for the health care of the elderly." And Simpson (2000, A17) writes, "If we think the costs of health care are large today, just wait for 10 or 15 years, unless there are miracle cures around the corner for such diseases as cancer. The ratio of those working to those over 65 could fall as low as 2 to 1, compared with more than 3 to 1 today."

But the prospect is highly exaggerated. First, the technologies (including "better treatment of hip fractures, degenerative joints, osteoporosis,

circulatory diseases, cataracts and other visual disorders, and diabetes") that enable people to live longer lives also permit them to remain in a healthy condition, with reduced incidence of disability, for a longer period (Posner 1995, 46). It is ironic, as Susan McDaniel points out, that growing successes in promoting healthy aging and extending people's lives are taken to challenge the health-care system and are used by so-called reformers to justify the reduction of funds for health care. In this fashion, the very successes of modern health care are claimed to undermine the viability of modern health care. Yet without good health care in a fair and supportive society, people are likely to be sicker, more vulnerable, more dependent, and in need of even more health care (McDaniel 2000, 144).

Second, the dependency ratio—that is, the ratio of nonworkers to workers—has fallen steeply since the mid-1960s in the United States, mostly because women have entered the labor force in greater numbers than before. The dependency ratio is predicted to rise after 2005 but not return to the level of the mid-sixties (Posner 1995, 40). In Canada, current projections indicate that even when the members of the baby boom are old, the dependency ratio will not be as high as it was when the members of the babyboom were children—that is, Canada has already experienced a high dependency ratio, handled it successfully, and is not likely to return to it (Gee 2000, 11).[1] In addition, the baby-boom generation will not all hit old age simultaneously. There is at least a fifteen-year difference between the youngest and the oldest boomers, so although the generation is large, its size does not pose the unmanageable challenge predicted by apocalyptic demographers. Moreover, although the children of the boomers, the so-called echo boomers, do not constitute as large a cohort as their parents do, nonetheless they are a substantial group and they will still be in the labor force when the boomers are elderly.

Third, we should not assume that old people, most of whom have already worked and paid taxes all their adult lives,[2] do not want to and will not continue to work and pay taxes. When postretirement employment is included, and comparisons are made with the recent past, the labor-force participation of old people is growing rather than declining (Posner 1995, 41). Even though the average age of retirement is falling, 25 percent of workers take up part-time or full-time jobs, after their retirement (Posner 1995, 44). Posner suggests also that the average age of retirement may not continue to fall and may even rise, partly because of the future demographic decline in the number of young workers and the resulting costs to employers of replacing older with younger workers and partly because, with the prospect of living a longer life, workers will choose to retire later in order to maximize their retirement income (Posner 1995, 48–49). In addition, as workers stay healthy for longer, their productivity will decline more slowly, and mid-life career changes will become more frequent (Posner 1995, 56).

Perls and Silver (1999, 215) cite examples of corporations in which employees over seventy make significant contributions. According to the U.S. Bureau of the Census (1999), in 1998 2,200,000 men and 1,600,000 women over the age of sixty-five were in the labor force. That number may increase. The Bureau predicts that in 2006, the numbers will be 2,600,000 men and 1,700,000 women. In Canada, 10.6 percent of men sixty-five and over and 3.4 percent of women sixty-five and over are in the labor force. In Japan, which has the world's highest life expectancy, the figures are much higher: 35.9 percent of elderly men and 15.2 percent of elderly women participate in the workforce (Statistics Canada 1998). Perls and Silver (1999, 215–216) describe policies in place in Japan that encourage the hiring and retention of older workers and the retraining and reemployment of workers nearing retirement age.

In addition there is a huge national value, less easily calculated, of unpaid labor contributed by older people (Posner 1995, 45; Gee 2000, 11–12), both formally to organizations that employ them as volunteers and informally, especially in the case of old women, through domestic work such as childcare, care of those who are sick or disabled, and care of other aging relatives in the homes of their families.[3] For example, in the 1996 Canadian census, 18.7 percent of men and 22.8 percent of women sixty-five and over reported engaging in fifteen to twenty-nine hours of housework per week (Statistics Canada 1996). Moreover, in 1998, 23 percent of Canadians over sixty-five participated in formal volunteer activities (Statistics Canada 1999). By assuming that old people are not working and not willing or able to work, apologists make a direct inference that such people are a burden. On the contrary, the U.S. Bureau of the Census (1999) estimates that the "mortality cost" (financial loss) to the nation of each death of a person sixty-five or older in 1996 was $38,153, calculated on the basis of individuals' age, sex, life expectancy at time of death, labor-force participation, annual earnings, and homemaking services. The total mortality cost of the deaths of these persons was $29,836,000. We can anticipate that as medical research enables people to live longer in a healthy state, the economic value of the lives of elderly people, as producers and consumers, will increase.

Still, many elderly people do not engage in paid or unpaid labor because they choose not to do so or are unable to do so. Although, on the one hand, we should appreciate the real work that elderly people contribute, on the other hand, we ought not to expect that all elderly people can, will, or must work, and it is illegitimate and unfair to draw conclusions about the moral entitlements of those who do not. As I argued in Chapter 4, their not working does not make them undeserving of longer life. Most elderly people have already contributed two-thirds of a lifetime or more of labor to the well-being of their families and their employers. A life-course approach to aging acknowledges that people are not all alike and are different at different stages of their lives. Social policy and medical services must take into account the varying health-care and other needs that people in old age have regardless of whether they are currently working.

So I argue both that the costs of supporting elderly people are not likely to be as great as the hand wringers suppose and that younger people—by which I mean those under the age of sixty-five—should be prepared to support old people, those over sixty-five, simply because it is in the nature of human life, at least as we have lived it so far, that different stages involve different contributions and different needs. Contributing toward the collective support of elderly people reduces the demands on individuals to carry the sole responsibility for their elderly relatives. Aging is a human fate that most of us will share; hence, it is fair to expect younger people to contribute to the support of those in a group that they will one day join, just as they were supported when they were very young. When resources are not needed for the relatively healthy stages of life, they can and should be devoted to the support of the more vulnerable stages, both at the beginning and at the end of life. In taking account of human needs, societies must recognize the full spectrum of the human condition from prenatal development to death and understand that every individual will go through these stages in one way or another. Hence, there can be no genuine conflict between young and old, healthy and ill, because the young become the old and the healthy do get sick.

So far my view is not much different from that of Battin, who, drawing on the work of Norman Daniels, suggests that "the elderly should be viewed as the same persons at a later stage of their lives….[Distributive problems] are more correctly understood as problems of allocating resources throughout the duration of lives" (1987, 322). In her life-course approach, however, Battin argues that a Rawlsian "veil-of-ignorance" approach would induce people to direct health-care funding to stages early in life, but, as we saw in Chapter 3, "not to underwrite treatment which would prolong life

beyond its normal span. By freeing resources which might otherwise have been devoted to prolonging the lives of the elderly for use instead in the treatment of diseases which cause death or opportunity-restricting disability earlier in life, such a policy would maximize one's chances of getting a reasonable amount of life within the normal species-typical, age-relative opportunity range"(322).[4]

There are several problems with Battin's interpretation of the life-course approach to health-care funding. First, as I argued in Chapter 3 in criticizing the claim that there is a duty to die, the deliberate and substantial reallotment of social support from old people to young people generates serious problems. Most relevant to the current discussion is the fact that the first cohort of midlife and elderly people would literally sacrifice a portion of their lives for the sake of this reallotment, without profiting personally from it. The members of this cohort would be too old to have benefited from the redistribution of savings to younger people and so would not have received improved care in their youth and middle age. Then, they would be expected to give up their lives prematurely for the sake of those who would receive both better health care earlier in life and improved life expectancy as a result.

A second problem in Battin's interpretation of the life-course approach is that self-interest ordinarily has a wider purview than merely one's own survival. As social beings, we have interests in the survival of our parents, grandparents, siblings, friends, and co-workers. Hence, even from a Rawlsian veil-of-ignorance perspective, it would be unreasonable to assume that there are no elderly people or potential elderly people who might play key roles in our life. Even in a culture that countenances a duty to die, social engineering is unlikely to induce us to look on the deaths of elderly loved ones and colleagues with equanimity. So when choosing the allocation of health-care funds, we have a strong motivation not to deprive elderly people, our relatives, friends, and co-workers, of crucial treatments and services.

My third criticism of Battin's life-course approach is more general. Although I agree that resources should be devoted to the treatment of serious diseases in early life and that, over the long run, persons at all life stages will thereby benefit, the arguments in this book have demonstrated that seeking to prolong one's life is justified and that policies devoted to the extension of life expectancy are warranted. If the prolongevist perspective defended here is correct, then persons behind the Rawlsian veil of ignorance would have objective reasons for wanting to live longer. Hence, they would not rationally choose to reject resources for and methods of prolonging human life, at least provided that that life could be lived in an acceptable minimum state of health.

Battin's sights are lower. She refers only to a goal of promoting "a reasonable amount of life within the *normal* species-typical, age-relative opportunity range" (1987, 322, my emphasis). Similarly, Daniels says that in the context of distributive justice the function of health care is "the maintenance or restoration of species-typical *normal* functioning." He believes that the normal opportunity range for an individual is relative to his or her stage of life and that the health-care budget must be allocated across all stages of life (1996, 211, my emphasis). His idea is that people would opt for a distribution that favors good health care at the beginning of life to set the stage for a longer life and then a lower allocation of resources for later stages. But the arguments in this book call into question the unexamined concepts of normality that underlie most discussions of human longevity. It is not evident that we must settle for the maintenance or restoration of what is currently considered "normal" functioning in old age. At the very least, the concept of typical species functioning in elderly people should be up for discussion. Given the enormous extensions, in the previous two centuries, in average life expectancy, the improved health of the North American population, the growing achievements of elderly people in education[5] and their increasing participation in physical activities,[6] and the improvements in health-care treatments and support for persons with disabilities, it is at least premature to suppose that what is "normal" now for some statistical average old person should constitute the norm for determining the allocation of health-care resources.

Suppose, for example, as Jecker suggests, that a means could be found that is both inexpensive and virtually unlimited to sustain memory functioning in extreme old age.

> On Daniels' analysis, such treatment is not important, because normal species functioning in extreme old age does not include clear and vivid recall. Moreover, memory loss does not diminish the age-relative normal opportunities of someone who is, say, ninety years old, since the opportunities a sound memory affords are not normally available to the very old. Consequently, government would not be under a strict obligation to make such treatment available to the elderly, for example, by reimbursing it under Medicaid and Medicare programs. This is so, even if the treatment in question were extremely cheap and abundant. (Jecker 1989, 667–668)

As Jecker (1989, 668) points out, such an approach seems unjustified "because normal functioning can be sorely inadequate," and hence altering what is currently considered to be normal species functioning could be a requirement of justice. Societies already accept this principle when they devote research time and money to developing improved hearing aids and eyeglasses, as well as surgical alterations of the eyes and ears, all of which mitigate the "normal" age-related decline in hearing and sight (672). Because existing social practices reflect skepticism about the normative force of species-typical functioning and have the power to alter it, we ought not to settle for unexamined definitions of the acceptable and "normal" capacities in elderly people.

Thus, the life-course approach suggests not that there must be a distributive competition among the different age groups—a competition that young people would win and old people would lose—but rather that adequate funds should be allocated for the last stages of life. When younger people become old, they too, in their turn, will be supported. This perspective acknowledges that it is in one's interest to support elderly people and not regard them as a "burden" because one will likely some day be elderly and in need of support oneself. So, even from a self-absorbed perspective, it is irrational to regard old people as nothing but "burdens" who have a "duty to die." Younger people should not see elderly people as some "other" group whose interests are contrary to their own but as a concrete presentation of their own future. From the perspective of younger people, elderly people are also their own parents, aunts and uncles, grandparents, friends, and co-workers. The question then is, What kind of relationships with old people do young people want? And what sort of future do they want for themselves:

Undeniably, the availability of social resources, including health care, social security, and family support, can be a constraint on achieving the goal of enabling people to live longer. Thus, Gillon (1996, 200) argues that even when life-prolonging technologies (LPTs) "can he expected to produce net benefit for the patient, and the patient or proper proxy desire[s] the LPT, justice in the allocation of scarce resources may require rationing of the available LPTs and some patients may thus morally justifiably (though regrettably) be denied LPTs." But the scarcity or availability of resources is not a fixed, divinely ordained feature of human societies. Collectively we do have choices about where to put our money, our educational efforts, and our research. Collectively we can also choose whether to foster life-enhancing attitudes such as the willingness to donate blood or the commitment to make one's body parts available after death for donation and transplantation. This book is, in part, a plea for

a reconsideration of how social resources are allocated and is an attempt to call into question the knee-jerk impugnment of elderly and disabled people who refuse to accept death with meek acquiescence.

A strong public policy of affirmative prolongevitism requires a social-democratic approach to human well-being, not an approach based only on what can be provided by market forces, for which cost containment and the maximization of profit are the ruling values. A social-democratic perspective rejects the assumption that good health care and abundant social resources are only for the wealthy. Gillon (1996, 205) claims that "respect for the autonomy of those who provide the resources for health care"—that is, taxpayers—could override the provision of life-prolonging technologies for those who need them. He believes that if taxpayers collectively do not want their money to support longer life for aging persons, then it ought not to be used in that way. But many elderly people, including those who now need or may eventually need life-prolonging technologies, are also taxpayers, and, as such, they may well want some resources to be directed toward measures to prolong their lives. Taxpayers do not speak with one voice.

But even if they did, it would be both dangerous and immoral in the extreme to allow the fiat of taxpayers to determine directly who lives and who dies, for such a fiat would provide no protection for members of disadvantaged groups. They are the ones without the means to purchase alternative care and services. What role would ignorance, lack of foresight, or failure to identify with elderly people, especially those from minority populations, play in such decisions? How might some taxpayer attitudes play out in deciding the fate of vulnerable populations—native people, ex-inmates, single mothers, and those who are poor? A social-democratic perspective does not support the health of the wealthy at the expense of that of the poor. Instead, it commits us to support all members of society, whether or not they have the wherewithal to pay for medical care and social support at the ends of their lives.

In addition, a social-democratic perspective is skeptical of unthinking consumption and the elevation of spending and acquiring as ultimate social values, skeptical of the idea that having money means one should be able to purchase whatever one wants and that buying things is the main source of happiness.[7] The alternative for which I've argued here is a life—whatever kind of self, career or seriatim, one is or chooses to be—that is built primarily on experiences and relationships and not so much on the acquisition of material things. The justification for this alternative is that such a life is likely to be healthier and more fulfilling, both individually and collectively, than a life that requires the consumption of indefinitely large amounts of resources. Granted, a life that is founded on experiences rather than on the acquisition of things can also be costly and can deplete natural and social assets in ways that are morally unjustified. To take one example, a skier who insists on being transported in comfort into back-country, difficult-to-access ski areas and on being provided there with every luxury while he indulges in his sport might contribute to the degradation of the environment and the exhaustion of resources almost as much as someone who owns a couple of cars and replaces them every year or two. Obviously the mere substitution of experiences for things is not an inevitable source of greater health and satisfaction; it does not automatically reduce resource depletion and environmental contamination. But it can, depending on the experiences sought. Backpacking into a wilderness area is preferable to going in by helicopter, plane, or car; taking the kids to the playground is preferable to buying them yet another set of expensive toys; living in solar-powered, well-insulated houses of modest size is preferable to choosing "monster homes" that require huge amounts of nonrenewable energy to heat and light.

Choices can be made, and some choices may involve the accumulation of things— a beautiful sweater, a useful kitchen tool, a hockey stick, a clarinet. I do not propose that there is just one way of having a meaningful life, although I do think that some are better than others, and I believe that some life activities can be shown to have more value and meaning than others. But, in general, if we choose to manufacture and to buy things based on their capacity to provide positive and interesting experiences at low cost, we are less likely to be pursuing a life-style that is incompatible with a social policy of affirmative prolongevitism. Such a policy requires genuine concern for truly long-range planning and the stewardship of resources so that there is a sustainable environment for future people (as well as nonhuman animals). As my suggestions indicate, the genuine application of prolongevitism requires a rethinking of the kind of society that the Western world created and tolerated over the previous century. A prolongevist social policy requires, I believe, a deep commitment to social change, change that would probably have to be fundamental. If the vast majority of people can count on living a long life, and if thereby they experience their grandchildren and other people's grandchildren growing to maturity and having children of their own, they will come to have an increased awareness of the connections among different age cohorts and of the implications of actions in the present for the well-being of members of future generations.

Notes

1. Some evidence suggests that in Canada eliminating all aggressive treatments, hospice care, and advance directives for persons sixty-five and over would save only 1 percent of total national health-care costs (Gee 2000, 20).

2. Posner (1995, 295) argues not only that elderly people receiving social security payments have already contributed to social security throughout their lifetimes but also that they "paid in the form of school taxes for a large part of the taxpaying generation's human capital that in turn generates the tax revenues that defray the cost of social security retirement benefits.

3. For example, my grandmother, Hazel Irene Bayes, cared for both my grandfather and my mentally disabled uncle in their home right up until she had a stroke at the age of eighty-six. At that point, my grandfather was ninety-one and my uncle fifty-nine.

4. In a real-world context, the impetus to direct health-care funding to the first parts of life might be exacerbated if, as I suggested in Chapter 6, people underwent transformations throughout their lives. The self that I am now might fail to anticipate the needs and aspirations of the self that I will be in old age. As Posner (1995, 266–267) remarks, " To allow the young to make life and death decisions for the old is to give one person, the younger self, undue control over a resource (a body) shared with another, the individual's older self.… The young self may scant his future self's interest in extending life not because the voting self is short-sighted or lacks self-control but simply because it has different preferences." If so, there will be urgent reasons for young selves to develop a better awareness of the moral entitlements both of their own future old selves and of present-day old selves.

5. According to the U.S. Bureau of the Census (1999), whereas, in 1980, 8,200,000 persons over sixty-five had one to three years of college, and 8,600,000 had four or more years of college, by 1998 the comparable figures were 17,200,000 and 14,800,000.

6. Statistics from the U.S. Bureau of the Census (1999) indicate that elderly people are more active than many who are younger. To take just a few examples, while 24.3 percent of males eighteen to twenty-nine years old participate in regular sustained activity (defined as any activity that occurs five times or more per week and lasts for thirty minutes or more per occasion), 25.5 percent of males sixty-five to seventy-four participate in such activity. And whereas 10.8 percent of females aged eighteen to twenty-nine participate in regular vigorous activity (defined as rhythmic contraction of the large muscle groups performed at 50 percent or more of estimated age-and sex-specific maximum cardiorespiratory capacity three times per week or more for at least twenty minutes per occasion), 15.4 percent of women aged sixty-five to seventy-four participate in such activities.

7. If, as Malcolm Cowley suggests (1980, 37), elderly people are less avid consumers than young people because their wants are fewer, then elderly people are thereby contributing, at least indirectly, to the betterment of society. I'm grateful to Carlos Prado for giving me Cowley's book.

References

Battin, Margaret Pabst, 1987. "Age Rationing and the Just Distribution of Health Care: Is There a Duty to Die?" *Ethics* 97 (January): 317–340.

Callahan, Daniel.1999. "Age, Sex, and Resource Allocation." In *Mother Time: Women, Aging, and Ethics,* edited by Margaret Urban Walker. Lanham, Md.: Rowman & Littlefield, pp. 189–199.

Cowley, Malcolm. 1980. *The View from 80.* New York: Penguin Books.

Daniels, Norman. 1996. "On Permitting Death in Order to Conserve Resources." In *Intending Death: The Ethics of Assisted Suicide and Euthanasia,* edited by Tom L. Beauchamp. Upper Saddle River, N.J.: Prentice-Hall, pp. 208–216.

Gee, Ellen M. 2000. "Population and Politics; Voodoo Demography, Population Aging, and Canadian Social Policy." In *The Overselling of Population Aging: Apocalyptic Demography, Intergenerational Challenges, and Social Policy*, edited by Ellen M. Gee and Gloria M. Gutman, Toronto: Oxford University Press, pp. 5–25.

Gillon, Raanan. 1996. "Intending or Permitting Death in Order to Conserve Resources." In *Intending Death: The Ethics of Assisted Suicide and Euthanasia,* edited by Tom L. Beauchamp. Upper Saddle River, N.J.: Prentice-Hall, pp 199–207.

Hanson, Mark J. 1995. "How We Care for the Elderly." In *A World Growing Old: The Coming Health Care Challenges,* edited by Daniel Callahan, Ruud H.J. ter Meulen, and Eva Topinková. Washington, D.C.: Georgetown University Press, pp. 1–8.

Jean-Nesmy, Claude. 1991. "The Perspective of Senescence and Death: An Opportunity for Man to Mature." In *Life Span Extension: Consequences and Open Questions,* edited by Frédéric C. Ludwig. New York: Springer, pp 146–153.

Jecker, Nancy S. 1989. "Towards a Theory of Age-Group Justice." *Journal of Medicine and Philosophy* 14: 655–676.

McDaniel, Susan A. 2000. "What Did You Ever Do for Me? Intergenerational Linkages in a Restructuring Canada." In *The Overselling of Population Aging: Apocalyptic Demography, Intergenerational Challenges, and Social Policy,* edited by Ellen M. Gee and Gloria M. Gutman. Toronto: Oxford University Press, pp. 129–152.

Perls, Thomas T., and Margery Hutter Silver. 1999. *Living to 100: Lessons in Living to Your Maximum Potential at Any Age.* New York: Basic Books.

Posner, Richard A. 1995. *Aging and Old Age.* Chicago: University of Chicago Press.

Simpson, Jeffrey. 2000. "Touting 'Wellness' Is Laudable, but Not Enough." *Globe and Mail* (Toronto), 5 April, A17.

Statistics Canada. 1996. *Population 15 Years and Over by Sex, Age Groups, and Hours of Unpaid Housework, for Canada, Provinces, Territories and Census Metropolitan Areas, 1996 Census.* Ottawa: Government of Canada.

———. 1998. "Participation Rates and Unemployment Rates by Age and Sex, Canada and Selected Countries." Retrieved January 11, 2001, from http://www.statcan.ca/english/Pgdb/People/Labour/labour23a.htm.

———. 1999. *The Daily* (October 1). Retrieved January 31, 2001, from http://www.statcan.ca/Daily/English/991001/d991001a.htm.

U.S Bureau of the Census. 1999. *Statistical Abstract of the United States: 1999.* 119th ed. No. 127: Expectation of Life at Birth, 1970 to 1997, and Projections, 1995 to 2010; no. 154: Deaths—Life Years Lost and Mortality Costs, by Age, Sex, and Cause: 1996; no. 184: Average Annual Expenditure per Consumer Unit for Health Care: 1985 to 1997; no. 222: Days of Disability, by Type and Selected Characteristics: 1980 to 1996; no. 248: Percentage of Adults Engaging in Leisure-Time Physical Activity: 1996; no. 650: Civilian Labor Force and Participation Rates, with Projections: 1970–2006; no. 1421, Expectation of Life at Birth by Race and Sex: 1900 to 1997. Washington, D.C.

Blurring of the Public/Private Divide: The Canadian Chapter

Colleen M. Flood and Bryan Thomas

...

2. CONTEXT OF THE CANADIAN SYSTEM—BASIC FEATURES OF THE PUBLIC/PRIVATE MIX

The Canadian health care system is generally characterized as a "single payer" system, implying that the government, through taxation revenues, pays for all health care spending. This term is misleading, for in Canada, as in all countries, there is a mixture of public and private financing for health care goods and services; indeed the share of private financing proportional to public financing is high in Canada relative to other countries.[1] Moreover, the private share of total health care spending in Canada has been steadily increasing over time and is now 29.8 per cent, while the public share of health care spending in Canada is 70.2 per cent.[2] What distinguishes Canada is that the importance of private financing varies significantly depending on the particular health service or good under discussion, with, for example, private financing of retail prescription drugs accounting for 61.5 per cent of the total spent thereon.[3] Thus, even within Canada's "single payer" system, private financing plays a large and important role and its importance varies drastically depending on the sector in question. The total effect of this approach is that a massive 65% of the Canadian population holds private health insurance and it accounts for 11.4% of total spending.[4] This context is important as proposals in Canada to expand the role for private health insurance

Flood, C. and Thomas, B., "Blurring of the Public/Private Divide: The Canadian Chapter", *European Journal of Health Law* (173). © 2010 Mantinjus Nijhoff Publishers.

are often aired without considering the fact that a significant proportion of the population presently hold private health insurance (generally employer-subsidized). The impact of significantly broadening the scope of what may be privately insured could thus be very different than in other countries which start with much lower per capita rates of private health insurance.

In terms of delivery, the Canadian system is often generically described as publicly funded yet privately delivered.[5] Many are surprised to learn that there is nothing in the *Canada Health Act* preventing the supply of health services by private firms, even if they are for-profit organizations; for example, diagnostic clinics are usually owned by for-profit companies, pharmacies are owned by for-profit entities, etc. Canadians describe their hospitals as "public" but they are in fact private non-for-profit entities, heavily regulated by government.... Canadian physicians, both general practitioners and specialists, are generally private for-profit contractors (albeit not incorporated into firms) and independent contractors. They contract with provincial governments through their provincial medical associations to supply publicly funded health services to Canadians.[6] Generally, medical associations negotiate overall increases to the total amount of government funding for physician services, and the medical associations determine how to allocate this increase between different physician services.[7] Physicians are still largely reimbursed by fee-for-service payment, although there have been shifts to paying family physicians on mixed models of payment (e.g., blended capitation, fee-for-service, etc.).

Canada's particular approach to public/private in its health care system is sourced in law. The courts have interpreted the constitution so that the ten provincial governments have primary jurisdiction over health care management and delivery within their respective provincial boundaries. Consequently, in order to achieve national standards the federal gov-

ernment uses its taxation and spending powers to try to entice provincial governments to meet certain standards of access. The federal government's legislative vehicle is the *Canada Health Act* (CHA).[8] The CHA sets out five criteria that each provincial insurance plan must comply with in order to obtain a federal funding contribution for "insured health services;" namely, comprehensiveness, accessibility, universality, portability, and public administration. The CHA also expressly prohibits user charges and extra-billing for "insured health services." "Insured health services" are defined in the Act to include all "medically necessary" hospital services, "medically required" physician services, and surgical-dental services that need to be performed in a hospital. The five criteria and the prohibitions against user charges and extra-billing *do not* apply to other services and treatments, e.g. home care, long-term care, medical devices and prescription drugs used outside hospital walls.

It is important to reiterate that the CHA does not protect many important health services which are becoming of even greater prominence in the system due to technological shifts; for example, pharmaceuticals and medical equipment consumed or used outside of hospitals, ambulance services, or home care services. There is no federal commitment to ensuring universal access to these goods and services and there are no impediments to patients being charged directly for their provision or for coverage through private health insurance.

Although not required to do so by the CHA, provinces do provide some coverage for prescription drugs, home care, etc., but coverage varies significantly from province to province.[9] With respect to pharmaceuticals most provinces emulate the US model of insurance (as of 2009) and provide the poor and elderly and with some catastrophic coverage—leaving the bulk of Canadians to obtain insurance for prescriptions drugs from private insurers through their employer (hence why some 65% of Canadians have private health insurance compared, for example, to just 2.5% of the Swedish population where prescription drugs are part of the core benefits of the universal plan).[10] Similar to the US, Canadian employers are allowed to deduct what they pay on behalf of employees for private insurance premiums from their income tax, and individuals who pay directly for health insurance premiums may be able to claim this cost as a deduction from their income tax.[11] As in the US this approach to financing is regressive and leaves a portion of the population uninsured—about 10 per cent of Canadians have no drug insurance (although for catastrophic costs this proportion falls to about 3 per cent), and a further 10 per cent are under-insured (pay 35 per cent or more of their costs out of pocket).[12]

...

5. CHAOULLI DECISION

Private financing already plays a very significant role in the Canadian health care system ..., however, its role is pronounced in certain areas (pharmaceuticals, etc.) and what distinguishes Canada internationally is that hospital and physician services attract close to 100% public financing in order to comply with the CHA. The Canadian system has long valued the concept of equity at least with respect to "medically necessary" physician and hospital services and has resisted the concept of allowing those with private financing and/or private health insurance to buy their way ahead of queues existing in the public system—the assumption being that such queues reflect prioritization of need for health care services. Nonetheless some question whether or not overturning the particular Canadian model of financing for hospital and physician services would result in greater efficiency and, in particular, shorter waiting times.[13] Certain stakeholders are, unsurprisingly, in favour of this because of the ability to increase their own revenues. Few, however, directly confront the fact that what is at issue is a commitment to redistribute resources to ensure timely access for all; advocates for privatization think

that they as individuals should be able to pay for timely treatment but not that they should contribute more resources so that all individuals can achieve timely access.

In compliance with the prohibitions against user charges and extra-billing for medically necessary care in the CHA, the provinces have each enacted multiple layers of regulation.[14] Some provinces ban private health insurance for medically necessary care, all provinces require physicians who wish to work for private payment vis-à-vis "medically necessary" services (i.e. those that are publicly insured) to opt out of the public health care system, some provinces regulate the prices that can be charged privately to match those which are paid publicly, and all provinces explicitly ban extra-billing and/or user charges. This complicated array of regulations is usually over-simplified in public discourse and scholarly writing to a blanket statement that, in Canada, private health insurance and/or private health care is "illegal". Indeed that is far from the case—as already explained close to 30% of the system is privately financed, there are flourishing and largely unregulated private sectors, for example, for IVF treatments, cosmetic surgery, etc., and increasingly for what appear to be medically necessary diagnostic services, as entrepreneurs exploit loop-holes in or failure to enforce provincial legislation.

The Canadian public health care system contains its own internal seeds of erosion, for at its core it protects hospitals and physician services and yet increasingly the locus of care is shifting outside of hospital walls and delivered by a wide range of health professionals. Technological advancements have altered the kinds of care needed and provided, expanding the role of sectors that are not protected, resulting in passive privatization.[15] A more direct assault to the particular Canadian model of financing health care came in the form of the case of *Chaoulli*.[16] As it attacks a Canadian icon—it is said that Canadians are but Americans with good health care!—one commentator writes that *Chaoulli* "may be the most controversial Supreme Court of Canada decision to date."[17] The 2005 case involved a challenge to Québec's legislative ban on private health insurance for services covered under the province's public insurance plan. The goal of this legislative ban is to avoid a 'two-tiered' healthcare system, wherein physicians have a financial incentive to prioritize privately-insured patients over those in the public system.[18] The problem arises when patients—such as Mr. Zeliotis, the co-claimant in *Chaoulli*—endure pain and suffering, and even endangerment to their lives, as they wait for care in the public system. In *Chaoulli*, a 4:3 majority of the Supreme Court agreed that a ban on private insurance, given long wait lists for certain health services, violates the right to personal security, guaranteed in Québec's provincial *Charter of Human Rights and Freedoms*.[19] The decision came as a surprise to many, as the court had previously taken a deferential approach to legislative acts of health care regulation.[20] In *Chaoulli*, by contrast, the majority considered social science evidence on foreign health care systems, and concluded that a ban on private insurance was not necessary for the preservation of the public system. The court pointed to the fact that other countries, such as England, maintain a viable public health system without a ban on private insurance.

The court's grasp of comparative evidence of health care system performance was subsequently roundly criticized—it did not, for example, consider the different roles that private health insurance plays across different health care systems, nor did it closely examine the extent of wait times in countries that allow parallel private health insurance. It simply concluded that many systems allowing private health insurance have "superior" health systems to that of Canada.[21] Having reached this astonishing conclusion—it being far from clear what parameters were assessed to determine "superiority" or that a sufficient evidentiary base had been canvassed to reach such a judgment—the majority then concludes that allowing private

health insurance would not harm Canadian Medicare.

As the decision was handed down, its broader implications for Canadian health care were unclear, for a variety of reasons. To begin, the *Chaoulli* ruling was decided under Québec's provincial *Charter;* only a minority of the court was prepared to conclude that the ban also violated the federal *Charter of Rights and Freedoms* (thus having application across all Canadian provinces and not just the province of Québec). The decision's narrowness on this score left it an open question how similar challenges might fare if advanced, under the analogous provisions in the federal *Charter,* in other provinces where private insurance is banned. Moreover, the relevant section of the federal *Charter* contains a limitations clause:

> 7. Everyone has the right to life, liberty and security of the person and the right not to be deprived thereof *except in accordance with the principles of fundamental justice.* [emphasis added]

As the court noted in *Chaoulli,* the analogous provision in the Québec *Charter* contains no limitations clause, making it "potentially broader."[22] Those advancing claims in other provinces, under the federal *Charter,* will bear the additional burden of proving that the legislation they are challenging is arbitrary. It remains to be seen how much of an added burden that will be.[23]

It has always been unclear what precisely the *Chaoulli* decision requires by way of a response from the Québec government—a fact that further complicates efforts to surmise the decision's broader implications for Canadian health care and the public/private mix.... Crucially, it is the pain, suffering and risk of death arising from unreasonable wait times that grounds the court's finding of a rights infringement; a ban on private insurance is permissible, so long as wait times in the public system are reasonable.[24] The dissent in *Chaoulli,* however, expressed grave concern that courts would now be responsible for monitoring the 'reasonableness' of wait times.[25]

6. QUÉBEC'S RESPONSE

In responding to the decision, the Québec government has played upon this open-endedness, lifting the ban on private insurance for those procedures highlighted in Chaoulli as having unreasonable wait times: hip and knee replacement surgery, and cataract surgery.[26] The government simultaneously introduced wait time guarantees for these same procedures, pledging that they will be delivered within six months, and that where delays exceed nine months, the service will be procured from a private clinic, or out of province, at public expense.[27] Bearing in mind as well that patients with pre-existing conditions in these areas will be refused coverage by private insurers, the predictable effect of these policy manoeuvres is that very few Quebeckers to date appear willing to exercise their newly-won freedom to purchase private insurance.[28] On the supply side, it is unclear as well to what extent private health insurers will be interested in entering the narrow market space opened by Chaoulli. On this last point, though, it bears noting that private insurers already have an established presence in Québec, for things not covered by the public plan—pharmaceuticals and dental care, for example. Private insurers in Canada appear to be beginning to press into markets. For example, some companies offer so-called "wait list insurance." According to the website of one of such companies, an insured person will have access to expedited diagnostic procedures and/or treatments in the U.S. or through Canadian private clinics when he/she is placed on a medical wait list that will be longer than 45 days. The scheme is supposedly legal because it "supplements" the public health insurance coverage.[29] Another insurance product presently available in Canada is the "critical illness insurance." In most cases, an insurer will pay a lump sum to an insured person if he/she is diagnosed with a covered critical illness and survives 30 days thereafter. This lump sum can be used by the insured in any way that he/she chooses, including accessing medical treatment privately in Canada or elsewhere. In fact, one company has billed such insurance as a way to "bypass hospital line-ups and receive immediate treatment." It further claims that having such insurance "is like having your own private health care program."[30]

Although ominous, the present uptake of private health insurance appears still small and thus it can be said that the Chaoulli decision has not, over the last five years at least, completely revolutionized the financing of health care in Québec, let alone across Canada. And, indeed, arguably it can be said to have had a positive effect in Québec, at least in the short term, in that the government response was to introduce wait time guarantees for hip, knee and cataract surgeries *within* the public health care system. . . .

But whatever the real impact of Chaoulli to date in terms of policy reforms, it has let the genie out of bottle in terms of legitimizing privatization as a policy option.[31] Prior to Chaoulli, advocates of privatization were discounted as either ideologues or as speaking from the perspective of their own vested interests—for example, private clinics that would reap financial gains from further privatization of Canadian Medicare. Now, the pro-privatization position has the normative imprimatur of legitimacy from no lesser body than the Supreme Court of Canada; it now does seem more like a matter of "when" Canada will move formally from its position of one-tier medicine rather than "if".[32] What is at stake here is both the level of Canada' commitment to redistribution and its ability to manage a coherent system. With a move towards a greater role for private finance, the Canadian system will take a step back from the goal of ensuring reasonable and needs-based access for all its citizens and will instead implicitly condone the concept of a mediocre public system and preferential and better treatment of those with more resources and/or private insurance.[33] Wealthier Canadians will then be able to pay for and have access to timely treatment, but not be expected or required to contribute to ensure the same level of access and timeliness for all Canadians. Apart from issues of access and fairness, a two-tier system will make overall management of the system even more difficult than it presently is. Challenges here involve the organization of health care delivery and the supply, regulation and remuneration of health care practitioners, and the appropriate locus for governance and managerial decisions. Such challenges are arguably exacerbated with a greater role for private financing.

...

Notes

1. Canadian Institute for Health Information. 2009. *National Health Expenditure Trends, 1975–2009* (Ottawa: CIHR 2009) at 63.
2. *Ibid.*, at 9.
3. *Ibid.*, at 19.
4. F. Colombo, N. Tapay. 2004. "Private Health Insurance in OECD Countries: The Benefits and Costs for Individuals and Health Systems." OECD Health Working Papers no. 15, p. 11. Retrieved www.oecd.org/dataoecd/34/56/33698043.pdf.
5. See generally R.B. Deber, "Delivering Health Care: Public, Not-for-Profit, or Private?" in: G.P. Marchildon, T. McIntosh and P.G. Forest (eds), *The Fiscal Sustainability of Health Care in Canada* (Toronto, University of Toronto Press, 2004).
6. Provincial medical associations are generally charged with representing physicians and promoting their professional interest. A separate body in each province, the College of Physicians and Surgeons, is charged with regulating the profession in order to protect and serve the public interest, and has powers to discipline individuals who fall short of professional standards.
7. C. Tuohy, *Accidental Logics: The Dynamics of Change in the Hoealth Care Arena in the United States, Britain, and Canada* (New York: Oxford University Press, 1999) at 244 writes that:

   it is important to note than in almost all provinces (the notable exception being Québec...) what was negotiated was the overall rate of increase to the schedule: the determination of the relative value of particular services was accomplished entirely through the committee structures of the provincial medical associations.
8. *Canada Health Act* (R.S., 1985, c. C-6).
9. Virginie Demers et al., "Comparison of provincial prescription drug plans and the impact on patients'

   annual drug expenditures", 178(4) *Canadian Medical Association Journal* (2008) 405–409; V. Kapur, K. Basu, "Drug coverage in Canada: who is at risk", 71(2) Health Policy (2005) 181–193.
10. F. Colombo, N. Tapay. 2004. "Private Health Insurance in OECD Countries: The Benefits and Costs for Individuals and Health Systems." OECD Health Working Papers no. 15, p. 11. Retrieved www.oecd.org/dataoecd/34/56/33698043.pdf.
11. For deductions by employers, see Income Tax Act, R.S.C. 1985, c. 1 (5th Supp.), s. 18(l)(a). For deductions by individuals for medical expenses, see Income Tax Act, s. 118.2, as am.
12. See Applied Management. 2000. "Canadians' Access to Insurance for Prescription Medicines: Executive Summary", A Report Submitted to Health Canada, March 2000 at 6. Retrieved March 10, 2010 www.frasergroup.com/downloads/execsum_eng.pdf. This is a measure of a "first dollar index" being defined as the proportion of the first $1,000 of annual drug expenses covered by the plan. Full coverage is defined as 100 per cent; underinsured is where 64 per cent or less is covered; and uninsured is zero coverage.
13. See for example N. Esmail, M. Hazel, Waiting Your Turn: Hospital *Waiting Lists in Canada, 2008 Report* (18th Edition) (Vancouver, B.C.: Eraser Institute) pp. 13–16 (arguing that 'non-price rationing' is inefficient). In U.S. debates, proponents of free market solutions have pointed to Canadian wait times as evidence of the perils of 'socialized' health care. See for example, D. Gratzer, *The Cure: How Capitalism Can Save American Health Care* (New York: Encounter Books, 2006).
14. For a discussion, see C.M. Flood, T. Archibald, "The Illegality of Private Health Care in Canada", 164(6) *Canadian Medical Association Journal* (2001) 825–830.
15. R. Deber, "Thinking Before Rethinking: Some Thoughts about Babies and Bathwater", 1(3) *Health-care Papers*, (2000) 25–31.
16. *Chaoulli v. Québec* [2005] 1 S.C.R. 791.
17. J. King, "Constitutional Rights and Social Welfare: A Comment on the Canadian *Chaoulli* Health Care Decision", 69(4) *Modern Law Review* (2006) 631–643.
18. *Chaoulli* v. Québec [2005] 1 S.C.R. 791 at para. 49.
19. *Charter of Human Rights and Freedoms*, R.S.Q. c. C-12.

20. See *Auton (Guardian ad litem of) v British Columbia (Attorney General)*, 2004 SCC 78, [2004] 3 SCR 657. An unsuccessful Charter challenge to the B.C. government's decision to deny public funding for Lovaas-type Intensive Behavioral Autism Treatment for children. *Cameron v. Nova Scotia (Attorney General)* (1999), 172 N.S.R. (2d) 227. (N.S. C.A. Sep 14, 1999) Leave to appeal refused by: *Cameron v Nova Scotia (Attorney General)*, [2000] 1 S.C.R. viii, 190 N.S.R. (2d) 198 (note), [*Cameron*]. A Charter claim brought by an infertile couple seeking reimbursement for having to pay out of pocket for a specialized in vitro treatment.

21. C.M. Flood, Kent Roach and Lorne Sossin (eds.), Access to Care, Access to Justice, (Toronto: University of Toronto Press, 2005).

22. *Chaoulli* at para. 30. (per Deschamps)

23. It bears noting though that three members of the court, in their decision concurring with the majority, did indeed find the ban on private insurance to be arbitrary. See *Chaoulli* at paras. 134–143. For a critique of this finding, see C.M. Flood, '*Chaoulli's* Legacy for the Future of Canadian Health Care Policy", 44(22) *Osgoode Hall Law Journal* (2006), 273–310 at 279–293.

24. *Chaoulli* at paras. 14 and 34 (per Deschamps J.).

25. *Chaoulli* at para. 163 (per Binnie and Lebel J.J.).

26. An Act to Amend the Act respecting health services and social services and other legislative provisions, R.S.Q., ch.43 (2006).

27. Québec, Ministère de la Samé et des Services sociaux, *Guaranteeing access: meeting the challenges of equity, efficiency and quality* (consultation document) (Québec: Direction des communications du ministère de la Santé et des Services Sociaux, 2006). Retrieved March 10, 2010 publications.msss.gouv. qc.ca/acrobat/f/documentation/2005/05–721–01A.pdf. The proposals set out in this consultation document were largely carried into law. See *An Act to Amend the Act respecting health services and social services and other legislative provisions*, R.S.Q., ch. 43 (2006).

28. Phillipe Couillard, "The *Chaoulli* Ruling and the Government Response: 4 Years Later", (Paper presented to the CIHR Health Law, Ethics and Policy Seminar Series, Faculty of Law, University of Toronto, January 14, 2010) [unpublished]. C.f. Marie-Claude Prémont who argues that it is conceivable, however, that some Quebeckers may wish to purchase insurance in order to avoid the 6–9 month waiting periods permitted under the guarantee. Marie-Claude Prémont, "Wait-time Guarantees for Health Services: An Analysis of Québec's Reaction to the *Chaoulli* Supreme Court Decision", 15 *Health Law Journal* (2007) p. 43 at 56.

29. See http://ww.acurehealth.com/.

30. See http://www.cheaplifeinsurnace.ca/Critical_Illness_Insurance.htm.

31. C.M. Flood, "*Chaoulli*'s Legacy for the Future of Canadian Health Care Policy", 44(22) *Osgoode Hall Law Journal* (2006), 273–310.

32. Even the CBC played a documentary called "Medicare; Schmedicare" on Thursday, 8 December 2005. It is reported to have been filmed in private clinics in Montreal, Toronto and Vancouver and compares the waiting times for those who use the private services to those who use the public system; online: CBC News—The Passionate Eye <http://www.cbc.ca/passionateeye/medicare.html>.

33. Proponents of two-tier health care will spin a golden story that it is win-win and that the wealthy will no longer be a drain on public resources; conveniently overlooking the fact that public resources (manpower) will be diverted from attending to the needs of those in the public health care system to those who are able to pay.

CASES

Chaoulli v Québec (Attorney General), 2005 SCC 35, [2005] 1 SCR 791

Summary prepared by Leah Hutt

Over many years, George Zeliotis sought health care services in Québec's public system for a variety of health problems. Hip problems and other medical issues had rendered him unable to work and in pain. Mr. Zeliotis spoke out publicly, denouncing the lengthy wait times he experienced in the public health care system. Dr. Jacques Chaoulli wanted to establish a private medical practice. Together, he and Mr. Zeliotis challenged the validity of the part of Québec's health care insurance legislation that prohibited citizens from buying insurance for health care services in the private sector if these services were available under the public system. The goal of the prohibition was to preserve the integrity of the public health care system. Mr. Zeliotis and Dr. Chaoulli argued that the delays resulting from waiting lists unjustifiably violated their right to personal inviolability (specifically to life, liberty and security of the person under the *Canadian Charter of Rights and Freedoms*). They argued the legislative prohibition deprived them of access to health care services that are available without delays.

Discussion Questions

1. Should provincial governments prevent citizens from spending their own money to purchase health care insurance? Are there justifications for restricting access to private health care services where the services are offered in the public system?
2. Is the enforcement of a "single-tier" health care plan justifiable? Is the allowance of a "two-tier" system justifiable?
3. What mechanisms are appropriate for managing costs in a publicly funded health care system? What considerations other than costs are important?

Reprinted by permission of the author.

Reference re Assisted Human Reproduction Act, 2010 SCC 61, [2010] 3 SCR 457

Summary prepared by Matthew Herder

The *Assisted Human Reproduction Act* was enacted by Parliament in 2004. The *Act* encompasses a set of "prohibited activities" (which, if practiced within Canada, carry criminal penalties), as well as a number of "controlled activities" that are permitted if practised in accordance with the regulations and a license granted by the regulatory body Assisted Human Reproduction Canada.

Reprinted by permission of the author.

According to the Attorney General of Québec, many of the *Act*'s provisions aim to regulate medical practice and research related to assisted human reproduction, which, under the *Constitution Act 1867*, are typically matters of provincial jurisdiction. Therefore, a reference to determine the constitutionality of those provisions was sent to the Québec Court of Appeal. In June 2008, the Court of Appeal ruled that various sections of the *Act* (including two prohibited activities, but mostly sections pertaining to controlled activities) were beyond the federal government's legislative competence and thus invalid.

In turn, the Attorney General of Canada appealed to the Supreme Court of Canada asserting that the *Act* was a valid exercise of the federal government's criminal law power. To decide whether the provisions in question were within Parliament's powers under the *Constitution Act 1867*, the Supreme Court of Canada had to determine what the "pith and substance" of the legislation as a whole was, and whether its parts—most notably, the controlled activities—usurped provincial authority. That is, the Supreme Court had to decide whether the purpose and effects of the legislation were to regulate and promote the benefits of medical practice and research related to assisted human reproduction (as Québec argued), or to protect morality, safety, and public health (as the federal government argued).

Discussion Questions

1. Should health be a provincial or a federal responsibility? In other words, do you think that it is best for Canadians to have multiple provincial health care systems, or should there be one health care system with the same rules and benefits for all Canadians?

2. Do you think that the federal or provincial governments should regulate research involving human embryos? Should this be done with guidelines or legislation?

Useful Resources

ONLINE

Canadian Policy Research Networks (CPRN)

Contains numerous research reports on a variety of topics such as healthy public policy, patient-centred health care, and delivering services to vulnerable populations.

Canadian Policy Research Networks and The Change Foundation

Nuala Kenny, "What's Fair? Ethical Decision-making in an Aging Society" (May 2004), Research Report F/44: Canadian Policy Research Networks Inc. and The Change Foundation.
Proposes an ethical framework for analyzing intergenerational connections and dependencies and for promoting intergenerational equity.

A New Perspective on the Health of Canadians: A Working Document

A Report released by Marc Lalonde (Minister of Health and Welfare for Canada) in 1974. It is one of the founding documents on health promotion and is highly regarded both nationally and internationally for challenging traditional thinking about health.

Ottawa Charter for Health Promotion

Drafted at the first international conference on health promotion, held in Ottawa in 1986. An important document in the World Health Organization's campaign "to achieve Health for All by the year 2000."

The Royal Commission on the Future of Health Care in Canada

Also known as the Romanow Report, this committee study led by Roy Romanow and published in 2002 makes 47 recommendations for reform of the Canadian health care system that address issues such as primary health care and prevention, prescription drugs, home care, aboriginal health, health care in rural and remote communities, and the globalization of health care.

What Determines Health?

Discussion of the 12 key determinants of health according to current Canadian analysis; this report is available on the website of the Public Health Agency of Canada.

Chapter 3 CHALLENGES FOR CANADIAN HEALTH CARE

INTRODUCTION

Resources are limited. No government can do everything it should for everybody, and given recent economic developments, every government now does less than it used to do for everybody. The resources of publicly funded health care systems are stretched to, and sometimes beyond, a point that both patients and providers find acceptable. The two most important health care resources are the people who provide services and the time those people can devote to patients. A shortage of personnel or time can mean that jobs are not done properly. A hospital room might not get cleaned and disinfected as thoroughly as it should, for example. As a result, an infection could spread to critically ill patients and to hospital employees. Less portentously, hospital admissions could get backed up, as a result of which patients could be stranded in an emergency room or a hall, while health care providers scramble to solve a problem that interferes with their responsibilities for patient care.

Shortages of labour affect not only the care that patients receive but the people who provide the care. The adverse impact on health care providers is particularly dramatic and dismaying in nursing. In a health care "crunch," patients do not receive the nursing care they used to receive, both in hospitals and in their homes. For example, hospital nurses no longer have time to listen to, comfort, and support patients who are anxious and fearful, and public health nurses no longer visit new mothers in their homes to check on them and their babies. More generally, nursing care has declined because there are fewer nurses overall, as well as fewer nurses with advanced training. Nurses well know what they should do for their patients, but all too often they are unable to do their jobs professionally and ethically. This causes them to suffer "moral distress," which is sometimes so severe that it drives nurses to leave the profession. In the first article, Colleen Varcoe and Patricia Rodney provide a highly contextualized analysis of the phenomenon of moral distress and the ways in which nurses respond to it. They embed moral distress in a culture of health care that is shaped by a powerful corporate ideology. They outline how nurses who provide direct patient care are regarded as disposable and how the well-being of patients, families, and communities is overlooked, and then describe the tactics nurses use to engage in moral resistance.

Funding constraints mean that potentially beneficial health care resources and services cannot be provided to every patient who has a legitimate need, or cannot be provided as expeditiously as they should be. Expensive medical devices and technologies often count as scarce resources. Consider, for example, implantable cardioverter defibrillators (ICDs) used to protect patients from sudden cardiac death. Suppose 300 patients customarily receive ICDs from a hospital each year, but for financial reasons, the administration decides the hospital can afford only 250 this year. How should those fewer ICDs be rationed? Should this be on the basis of first-come, first-served? Most urgent need? Or, greatest potential benefit? And, what happens if the allocated number of ICDs is exhausted before year-end? A different scarce resource might be operating rooms in a hospital, or nurses to properly staff the operating rooms. In each of these instances, priorities have to be set—criteria for eligibility have to be developed, and waiting lists have to be established and managed.

In the second article Benjamin Freedman, James Gilbert, and Lois Kaltsounakis present the even more complicated example of whether a patient should be removed from an air-support bed that prevents pressure sores and helps them to heal so that it can be used by a patient who could benefit more. The hospital has only one air-support bed, and there always is a queue for it. How can the hospital develop a rational policy for ethically allocating this limited resource?

A particularly troublesome aspect of determining eligibility for a scarce treatment is whether patients may be assigned lower priority because they are regarded as personally responsible for their medical problem. In the third article, Walter Glannon examines whether personal responsibility is a relevant consideration in the fair treatment of individuals who need a liver transplant because they have alcohol-related, end-stage liver disease. In what ways and to what extent are the factors that cause this disease within the control of patients? Assuming these factors are controllable, should patients be held morally responsible for failing to exercise that control and for this reason assigned a lower priority for a liver transplant?

Restrictions on what services are available in a health care system and how readily they are accessible raise questions about whether, and if so, how, patients should be able to acquire information about services and access to services outside the public health care system. The last four articles address this issue.

Although most Canadians obtain genetic services through the public health care system, they also can purchase them internationally, most easily by using the Internet. Bryn Williams-Jones and Michael Burgess use a case study of how the development of a commercial genetic susceptibility test for hereditary breast cancer by the U.S. biotechnology company Myriad Genetics (and the subsequent patenting of this test) have affected Canadians' access to the test. They endorse an approach designed to ensure "accountability for reasonableness" combined with public consultation as a just and rational way of making decisions about the provision of health care services. Durhane Wong-Rieger and Barbara Mintzes then debate whether direct-to-consumer advertising of prescription drugs should be legal in Canada, as it is in the United States and New Zealand. Wong-Rieger contends that such advertising fulfills an unmet patient need by providing information about prescription drugs, whereas Mintzes argues that this kind of advertising causes harm and that whatever benefits it might provide could be better achieved through public health campaigns.

In the final article, Gillian Crozier and Françoise Baylis review the nature and scope of international travel to obtain medical services. They describe the circumstances and considerations that prompt patients to travel abroad for medical care and explore what physicians can do to help patients who are thinking about or embarking on that journey.

Constrained Agency: The Social Structure of Nurses' Work[1]

Patricia Rodney and Colleen Varcoe

INTRODUCTION

Driven by neo-liberalism and corporatization as part of economic globalization, several decades of Canadian health care reform have worsened the conditions of nurses' work and thus the care nurses are able to provide.[2] Yet, nurses are not mere pawns at the mercy of change. They have the capacity to critically analyze and influence their conditions of work—in other words, they have agency, albeit constrained. In this chapter we outline key elements of the current sociopolitical context of health care, examine the consequences for nurses' work in the culture of health care characterized by a corporate ideology, and explore nurses' roles in shaping their work and work environments. We close by commenting on what we have learned about actions to improve the moral climate[3] of health care delivery.

We are particularly interested in how corporate ideology operates in the everyday work of nurses and other health care providers, and in particular how the ideology of scarcity (Varcoe, 1997; 2001)—the pervasive assumption that resources are too scarce to provide adequate care—works with management technology in the control of work. We will consider how nurses' work is organized within scarcity and how nurses participate in corporate ideology. Patterns of practice foster a certain kind of "efficiency" by limiting and devaluing the body care and emotional labour of nursing. Nurses then donate unpaid time to limit the moral distress[4] they experience while working under such conditions. At the same time, nurses take multiple actions to limit the impact of their work environments on themselves and

their patients, with some actions being more effective than others. In this chapter we consider both the moral distress and the health risks faced by nurses working in these conditions. We also examine the impact on nurses and other health care providers as well as patients, and possibilities for improving such conditions. This critical analysis of the culture of health care[5] is offered in the spirit of building on the strengths of the current system. Thus, we will conclude by exploring how individuals and groups might develop a critical awareness of the culture of health care and the social structure of work, and how a greater nursing "voice" in policy might benefit all.[6]

THE CORPORATE CONTEXT OF CONTEMPORARY HEALTH CARE

The Canadian health care system is increasingly shaped by globalization, in which capital flows around the world to serve the interests of an economically dominant elite (Coburn, 2010; Saul, 2005, 2008). While the espoused intent of the health care reforms occurring in Canada and other Western countries is to improve the quality and accessibility of health care, the implementation of the reforms is fuelled by a powerful corporate ideology (Hiraki, 1998; Myrick, 2004). Canadian health care reforms are being enacted in an era of escalating inequities in the distribution of human resources—and a corresponding acceptance that actions to save money in health care or other social services are inherently justifiable (Lynam et al., 2003; Moorhouse & Rodney, 2010; Rankin & Campbell, 2006; Stein, 2001; Storch, 2010).

Varcoe, C., Rodney, P. (2002) "Constrained Agency: The Social Structure of Nurses' Work." In Bolaria, B.S. & Dickenson, H. (eds.) *Health, Illness, and Health Care in Canada*, Third Edition (pp. 102–128). Scarborough, ON: Nelson Thomas Learning. Reprinted by permission of the authors.

This has resulted in a mechanistic, reductionist approach to health services that threatens the Canadian commitment to universal and equitable health care (Armstrong & Armstrong, 2003; Coburn, 2010; Commission on the Future of Health Care in Canada, 2002; Picard, 2000). Cost constraint has, to a significant extent, trumped the quality and accessibility of health care.

Economic trends in Canada, including budget deficits and restrictions in the role of the federal government in maintaining the principles of medicare, put tremendous pressure on provincial and territorial governments to economize on health spending (Armstrong & Armstrong, 2003; Storch, 2010). Consequently, over almost two decades Canada has experienced "a climate for change in the organization and management of health services that transcend[s] anything since the foundation for the current system was completed in 1968" (Storch & Meilicke, 1994, p. 32). This climate has generated extensive cost constraint measures within health care over a prolonged period of time.[7] In the 1990s, hospital units and entire hospitals were closed, community services shuffled, and health care staff moved around or dismissed at unprecedented rates.

Canadian research began to evaluate the impact of these changes in the early 1990s and some beginning progress was made in reversing some of the earlier damages. Unfortunately, as this revised chapter goes to press, we are witnessing yet another round of sweeping cost constraint measures (Pringle, 2009). In the meantime, disparities in access to care are increasingly apparent in rural and remote settings, home care, mental health care, palliative care, elder care, care of Aboriginal peoples, and acute care in large centres (Browne, Smye, Rodney et al., 2011; Health Council of Canada, 2008; Lynam et al., 2003; Penning & Votova, 2009; Stadjuhar, 2003). Overall, the research warns that as the conditions of nurses' work deteriorate through casualization of the workforce, increased workload, loss of clinical leadership, and shortages of skilled health care providers, morbidity and mortality rises, and patient satisfaction is reduced.

Nurse satisfaction is also reduced, and there are now serious problems with nurse illness, injury, and attrition as well as patient safety (Canadian Nurses Association and the Registered Nurses Association of Ontario, 2010; Storch, 2005).

The impact of corporatized health care reform has not been uniform across all people. Rather, because such reforms are occurring at the nexus of multiple ideologies that are raced, classed, and gendered, the impact is greatest on those who are least privileged. As cost savings in health care reform are achieved primarily through lower wages, poorer care, and a shift of costs and responsibility to patients and their families (Armstrong, 2001; Björnsdóttir, 2001), women, racialized people, those with debilitating conditions, those who are impoverished, and those who are homeless are most affected (Anderson, Rodney, Reimer-Kirkham et al., 2009; Anderson, 2004; Coburn, 2010; Frankish, Hwang, & Quantz, 2005; Lynam, 2005; Stephenson, 1999).

Why has a corporate ideology, with its aforementioned problems, taken such hold in Canada? An ideology is a set of ideas and images: "a shared set of fundamental beliefs, attitudes, and assumptions about the world that justify 'what is'" (Thomas, 1993, p. 8). Ideologies are usually taken for granted because they are unconscious—they are not in and of themselves good or bad, but they provide the conceptual machinery for questions, for the data gathered or ignored, and for the chosen interpretations (Thomas, 1993, p. 8). A corporate ideology takes direction from the operation of the marketplace and management and organizational theories (Hiraki, 1998, p. 117). And, as Coburn points out, a corporate ideology is used "to make citizens powerless in their own countries…[with the] doctrine of 'we have no choice'" making adherence to corporate interests seem inevitable (2001, p. 60; see also Coburn 2010). As a consequence of taking this ideology for granted, health policy and health care delivery are "based upon economic and political values rather than values reflecting the broader social responsibilities of individuals in community" (Storch, 1996, p. 25).

In this chapter we will therefore attempt to unmask what has been taken for granted. We will explore the consequences of corporate ideology for the everyday work of nurses and other health care providers, as well as for patients and their families. What has been taken for granted must be made visible if nurses and other health care providers are to work beyond constraints to their ability to provide good and ethical care (in other words, to work beyond constraints to their moral agency), and if the nation is to move toward the more equitable health care system that most Canadians desire and all deserve.

CORPORATISM AT THE LEVEL OF PATIENT CARE

Both the ideologies and the practices of the corporate culture of health care are played out at the level of direct patient care (Browne, 2001; Myrick, 2004; Rankin & Campbell, 2006; Rodney & Street, 2004; Rodney & Varcoe, 2001; Weiss et al., 2002). The research cited earlier indicates that each cost constraint measure has a direct impact on nursing practice, creating more work, more uncertainty, and less control over how nursing time is spent. Perhaps most importantly, "redesign" strategies, such as those aimed at reducing the length of hospital stay, have resulted in an increase in patient acuity and turnover, which in turn directly affect nursing workload. Nurses find themselves caring for more acute patients and processing more patients more quickly. Downsizing activities such as bed closures require nurses to organize those closures, move to new practice areas, and organize the reopening of beds and work areas. The consolidation of hospital boards and executive management, staff layoffs, and the elimination of levels of management (and often the managers) create a climate of instability and uncertainty. Further, with less contact between direct care providers and management, nurses generally have less impact on decision making. Moving nurses to unfamiliar patient care areas and replacing registered nurses with practical nurses and/or care aides dilutes levels of skill, placing heavier responsibilities on the remaining staff.

AN IDEOLOGY OF SCARCITY

Our research indicates that nurses adjust their work to this evolving corporate context and make sense of the changing conditions of work in various ways. Nurses participate in the corporate ideology and organize their work to maximize a certain kind of efficiency. One of the most profound ways that the ideas and images of corporatism are enacted at this level is through an ideology of scarcity (Varcoe, 2001). Ideas and images of resources as scarce and unattainable abound in the day-to-day world of nursing practice. And these ideas and images in turn drive practices that emphasize certain kinds of streamlining and efficiencies. So, for example, nurses might put diapers on competent adults because they do not have time to assist them to the toilet, justifying such practice as arising out of the necessity of scarce resources.

Corporate rhetoric and ideas dominate thinking both within the health care system and in the wider social context. Nurses receive messages about the state of the economy and health care from many sources, ranging from media messages, including local and health care specific media, to managers, coworkers and patients. In the settings we have studied, messages about scarcity predominate. Along with increasing concern about "wait lists" and "wait times", news media continue to emphasize budget constraints in health care. Managers, responsible for implementing such budgets, promote ideas that resonate with the ideas of efficiency in a time of scarcity. In the words of a hospital manager, "To do the best job with the resources that you have, that is what exemplary is." (Varcoe, 1997, p. 125)

In our research on nursing work in these settings, this ideology of scarcity was primarily expressed in talk about time and enacted in nurses' work in the form of certain "efficiencies." In our early studies, nurses' talk revealed an acceptance of scarcity as the driving force in health care and as the driving force that organizes nursing practice. One nurse said, "It's money, it's management, it's things I can't really argue with." (Varcoe, 1997, p. 124). Another said:

> You'd like more staff and you'd like more participation but in reality there isn't the money, you aren't going to get the staff, so don't spend the time whining and sniveling, it's not going to be there. Just do the best you can with what you have. (Varcoe, 1997, p. 124)

In our more recent work, *Ethics in Action*,[8] nurses continued to echo such sentiments, although to us the overall tone was at once both more defeated and angrier, with "frustration" being perhaps the most common descriptor of practice. One nurse said of her work:

> There are great people here and they're doing a great job under I think very stressful, high-pressure circumstances. I'm going to use a catch phrase: it's like its own war zone. (Staff Nurse Interview, *Ethics in Action*, 2005)

Another voiced other nurses' widespread concerns about not being able to practice according to their professional standards: "I don't feel like I have control over my practice and I'm not meeting [patient care] standards." (Staff Nurse Interview, *Ethics in Action*, 2005)

Despite the sense of acceptance of "fiscal realities," nurses' talk also conveyed a profound awareness of the discrepancies between the care they valued and the care they were able to provide. Much of this talk was couched in terms of time: time that nurses did not have to provide the care that their patients required. Time was described as "lacking," "inadequate," and "nonexistent," and the predominant impact of this scarcity was seen as inadequate attention to nonphysical care. In our more recent work, nurses' awareness of the influence of the wider context on their work seemed more acute, with expressions of frustration aimed not only at the impact on their work, but also at the immediate organizational conditions that gave rise to that impact—poor communication, lack of direction from managers, and unending change:

> Sometimes you get pulled like a piece of toffee. You know. People calling you names, the phones are ringing, you're having to put out a fire or you're having to start a fire under somebody, keep things moving, dealing with the administration, and that's the biggest problem is trying to get something going throughout the day so you can get your day done. (Staff Nurse Interview, *Ethics in Action*, 2005)

Nurses identified their attention to the non-physical needs of patients as the aspect of care that suffered most, both during the provision of routine care and when patients experienced significant emotional crises. Nurses talked about the ways they routinely curtailed their conversation and attention to the emotional needs of patients, and as researchers we observed nurses letting patients know that they were busy so that patients did not expect to engage in conversation. Nurses routinely mentioned that they did not have time for "the psychosocial," meaning attention to patients' nonphysical needs. One nurse said that when patients request extra attention, "you think 'just don't bother me anymore, I want to do my work and get out of there.'" (Staff Nurse Interview, *Ethics in Action*, 2005)

Even during devastating events, nurses felt they were unable to afford the time required for emotional care. Throughout all of our studies, most who were interviewed told at least one story that exemplified such situations. Each nurse told a story about a patient who had experienced a profound loss, such as the death of a child or partner, or a terminal diagnosis, in which he or she was unable to provide the support the patient needed:

It is really hard for a nurse to just sit there and do nothing at a bedside when she's got a gazillion things to do, but with some people that is almost what you need to do, just sit there for five minutes and not say anything, just be there and that builds the trust. Anyway that's a dream, we don't have the time to do that any more. (Varcoe, 1997, p. 165)

Note that this nurse refers to her emotional care as doing "nothing." It should also be noted that throughout all of our studies we have noted that nurses and other health care providers sometimes (unwittingly) embraced a corporate ideology by not questioning it.

Ideas of scarcity in health care are dominant in public spheres, at all levels of government, and among health care providers at various levels within the system and among patients. Nurses accepted these ideas to a large extent and shaped their practice to conform to corporate ideology and imperatives. Time, nurses' most valuable resource, was viewed as a scarce commodity and was often spent in the service of corporate goals rather than nursing or patient priorities. Thus, these ideas of scarcity supported cost constraint measures, and both the ideas and constraints structured nurses' work. As a result of corporate streamlining, nurses' work became structured as "efficient" practice (Rodney & Varcoe, 2001).

CORPORATE STREAMLINING AND "EFFICIENT" PRACTICES

In response to cost constraint measures and messages about the inevitability of scarcity in health care, and with at least a partial acceptance of those messages, nurses' work is organized to maximize their "efficiency." This efficiency is organized by what Smith (1990) calls "the relations of ruling"—structures, institutions, and regulations—that create understandings taken up by the nurses themselves (see also Stein, 2001). For example, in many organizations "patient care coordinators" have been re-labeled as "bed utilization managers"

creating new understanding regarding what is important. The relations of ruling between management and nurses are mediated by various management technologies that organize nurses' efforts to efficiently process patients. The introduction of management technology to manage nurses' labour shaped the relationship between fiscal restraint and nursing, and as a consequence much of the less visible skilled practice of nurses—especially the emotional support of patients and their families—becomes "indeterminate work" (Campbell, 1994; see also Rankin & Campbell, 2006).

Over the past several decades, then, staffing patterns have been adjusted by using various management technologies to the point that the indeterminate work of nursing and other health care providers has been squeezed almost out of existence. Because only certain practices are "counted," because physiological care and medical treatment are valued over other forms of care, and because scarcity has been accepted, patterns of practice have developed to accommodate these values. Thus, the form of "efficiency" that has evolved is one that provides physiological care and medical treatment as quickly and as cheaply as possible.

In the units we studied initially, the patterns of practice reflected this sort of "efficiency," patterns that persist in units we studied more recently. In the emergency units, the predominant practice pattern was one of "efficient processing." In this pattern of practice, patients were: a) "stripped down" (literally and figuratively), to b) identify a manageable problem (such as a chest pain, laceration, or fever), and c) processed according to this manageable problem in order, to d) empty the stretcher. Various strategies were used to keep patients "on track." Assessments were routinized and circumscribed, and patients were encouraged to give only the information needed to identify the problem. Such strategies began with opening questions at triage such as, "What brings you to emergency today?" and continued with checklists and flow sheets tailored to identify physiological problems. These strategies were facilitated by behaviours that let patients know how busy the staff were and discouraged them from making demands for attention beyond what nurses could meet.

Similarly, in the medical units, the actual running of departments was often seen to have priority over the needs of patients, including both physical and nonphysical needs. Patient needs often were subordinated to the needs of departments, so, for example, an unstable patient might be transported without adequate personnel and equipment (such as oxygen, a stretcher, and a nurse, rather than a wheelchair and a porter) in order to prevent delays in the X-ray department; home care patients with disabilities might be admitted to hospital and anesthetized repeatedly for small procedures because those procedures could not be coordinated.

One of the ways in which these "efficient"[9] practices were maintained by nurses was the use of workplace sanctions. Nurses let one another know what was expected, rewarded one another for maintaining "efficiency," and penalized each other for not maintaining expectations. Nurses expressed regard for those who were "efficient" in terms of providing physical care and "getting the tasks done," and expressed derision for those who were "slow," were "bleeding hearts," spent "too much time talking," and so on:

> here are a few [nurses] in particular who deal with the emotional aspect first, unless of course [patients] are bleeding out or whatever. They meet the wrath of some of the other staff members quite significantly. "She's not pulling her load, she's doing that PR crap." (Varcoe, 1997, p. 173)

However, although we continued to observe such sanctions in our current work, we also observed active defiance of both workplace requirements and sanctions by colleagues that interfered with what individuals saw as "good care." For example, in our *Ethics in Action* study, one of the nurses with whom we worked closely vehemently declared that "I am NOT going to have a 52 year old patient die in the

hall on my shift!" (Staff Nurse Interview, *Ethics in Action*, 2005) and defied rules to enact that declaration. We also witnessed the power of taking action collectively. For example, in the medical oncology unit, nurses banded together to block a policy of mixing men and women in the same rooms.

Paradoxically, accommodating the efficiencies of other health care providers and departments, and defying such constraints both sometimes threatened already thin nursing resources. The oncology nurses had to engage in multiple bed moves to prevent "co-ed" rooms, and the nurse with the critically ill patient had to add advocating for his care to her already impossible workload. Clearly, this is not the type of efficiency intended by a cost-benefit analysis that purportedly has health as the intended outcome.

Sanctions enacted by staff nurses were also evident at administrative levels. Administrators applied sanctions for "inefficiencies" such as an increased length of stay. A manager in an acute medical unit explained that her unit was held to a standard of a length of stay of seven days. That standard had been decreased from 11 days the year before, despite the fact that the population of patients that the unit served had changed to include more patients with complex health problems that required even more care.

She went on to explain how the failure to comply with corporate edicts resulted in consequences that in turn created more problems:

> [T]here's no money so we ended up closing. Summertime last year we closed twelve beds to try and reap in the money so the outcome was … nursing lay off... if you can't shut down any more beds, then what we're going to do is [use] aides, not nurses. (Rodney, 1997, p. 241)

Failure to meet corporate goals, such as in this case decreasing the increased length of stay, often carried the risk of sanctions for managers, units, and staff, including staff layoffs, and/or the replacement of registered nurses with less prepared staff.

CORPORATE CASUALTIES[10]

Thus far, we have argued that the corporate culture of health care is made manifest in an ideology of scarcity. We further argued that corporate streamlining and efficient processing shape direct patient care. But what is the impact on nurses as individuals and for nursing as a profession? What are the consequences for the patients, families, and communities that nurses serve? Overall, the social organization of "cost efficiency" exacts both a professional and personal toll when nurses are expected to accept responsibility for delivering a safe and sufficient level of care under conditions that become less and less capable of sustaining this work. The consequences are serious, not just because of the human costs to nurses, but because of the impact on the quality of care received by patients, families, and communities.

Disposable Nurses

Nurses providing direct care are treated as if they are disposable in at least four ways. Their intellectual labour, emotional labour, personal time, and well-being are too often sacrificed for the efficiency of the system. For example:

> [W]hen it gets busy, when it gets so busy you're so busy coping sometimes with just the actual immediate physical needs and their meds getting out and stuff like that that you often don't have the time to really think through the assessments...when I go home afterwards I think, "Wow, what about such and such?"...and you know, you hit yourself.... There's things that I forget too, like I go home and I think, "Now I wonder if..." (Rodney, 1997, p. 184).

First, let us look at the nurse's intellectual labour. This experienced medical nurse took pride in her ability to assess her patients and was acknowledged as a clinical resource by her colleagues. Yet in the interview cited above, she went on to tell a story of how she had missed picking up bladder distention on a

patient who was showing many of the classic signs. Indeed, this nurse was what Benner and her colleagues (1996) would have recognized as an expert at clinical judgment. She knew "the particular patient, his typical pattern of responses, his (sic) story and the way in which illness has constituted his story. [She knew this] through advanced clinical knowledge...gained from experience with many persons in similar situations" (Benner, Tanner, & Chesla, 1996, p. 1). Yet she had little opportunity to employ that judgment in her work. In this sense, her intellectual labour was not valued.

Second, being busy with "just the actual immediate physical needs" means that nurses' emotional labour—the labour of dealing with emotional needs—is compromised (Varcoe, 1997; Yyelland, 1994).[11] For example, a nurse working in an emergency department said:

> There was a young fellow...diagnosed with leukemia down there, first thing in the morning they wheeled him in and told him what he had and he didn't want me to leave. Of course you are torn because you've got a lot of other things to do and in many respects he is a priority but the way we worked down there is ABC, life-threatening, limb-threatening, and he is neither of those....I waited for awhile and then I said, "Do you want to be alone or do you still want me to stay until your family comes...or can I get you a Social Worker or something?" I'm trying everything to get another body in there so I can get out and that's wrong, but what do you do? (Varcoe, 1997, p. 128)

And, as noted, nurses sometimes demeaned one another for attending to patients' emotional needs.

Thus, both intellectual and emotional labour are devalued by the way work is organized and by nurses themselves. Nurses in our studies did not have time to "think through" their care. Nor did they have time to "talk about it." Such concerns about excessive workloads—workloads that get in the way of nurses meeting the professional standards of their practice—are by no means new. At least five decades of empirical work in diverse studies from various practice contexts echo this concern (Rodney & Starzomski, 1993; Rodney & Street, 2004). What is more recent is the escalation of workloads and the concomitant reduction of professional resources. Nurses in our studies conveyed their distress, frustration, anger, and sometimes resignation, about this. For example, in the *Ethics in Action* study, the nurses in emergency routinely would begin each shift with what we called their "mantra": "we're 5 [nurses] short, have 22 admits (admitted patients awaiting beds), one stretcher open, and the wait time [for patients] is over 4 hours." (Field Notes, *Ethics in Action*, 2004) We witnessed the consequences of this mantra almost every day that we did our observational fieldwork. Patients who were supposed to be admitted to hospital filled most of the emergency beds, patients were lined up in the halls in stretchers, and anxious (and often angry) patients and their family members spent long hours waiting to be seen. Nurses and other health care providers repeatedly expressed that they worried that they were going to "miss something."

Third, nurses' personal time was often treated as disposable. Not surprisingly, in order to complete their tasks, nurses routinely stayed past the end of their designated work shift but often did not claim overtime pay. In other words, they "donated" time to the health care system. Nurses' "donations" often jeopardized their personal time. This was particularly apparent for nurses who faced concurrent child care demands, who frequently had to incur extra child care costs or arrangements in order to finish their work.

Nurses' commitments to their patients and their own families, and their difficulty in meeting these commitments, exact significant personal costs. Therefore, the fourth "disposable" to be explored is nurses' well-being. Campbell (1994) noted that nurses working under excessive workloads suffer frustration, anxiety, and self-blame about the care they are able to give (p. 594). Nurses in our studies often experienced profound guilt and fatigue. One emergency nurse was embarrassed and apologetic about her work

environment. After several hours of dashing from patient to patient, providing only urgent care and using techniques to forestall patient demands, she turned to one researcher, nearly in tears. "I'm sorry," she said, gesturing back to the unit, which was crowded, noisy, and crawling with people pushing various pieces of equipment about. "You should see it the way it should be, not like this." (Varcoe, 1997, p. 124; see also Sanders at al., 2011)

Nurses from all practice settings spoke of how tired they felt at the end of most shifts. The physical demands of providing basic nursing care to elderly and/or dependent patients were substantial, and there was almost always a sense that nurses were racing against the clock to complete the required tasks. Confounding the physical demands was the fatigue generated both by shift work and by the "second shift" that many nurses experienced in caring for their families—fatigue that is receiving increasing attention as a serious threat to nurses' health and safe patient care (Aiken et al., 2002; Canadian Nurses Association and Registered Nurses Association of Ontario, 2010; O'Brien-Pallas et al., 2006).

As well as the guilt and fatigue that nurses in the studies experienced, there was an ever-present (but not often discussed) level of personal risk, both physical and psychological. The physical risk was multidimensional. As she spoke of the risks posed by the complexity of the patients on her unit, one nurse manager warned:

> The other thing that we've got going on now is a lot more infectious diseases. You know with the AIDS patients, they're coming in with chicken pox and stuff.... We're having a lot more dangerous [exposure to illnesses]... HIV, TB [tuberculosis], we've had a meningitis outbreak and... it's a personal threat to ourselves [as well as] violence by patients.... I think it contributes to the fatigue.... and threat of injury. (Rodney, 1997, p. 201).

During fieldwork in our studies we were told that a significant amount of "sick time" was taken by staff due to events such as back injuries, which had escalated with the increased acuteness and heavy care requirements of patients. In the emergency units, nurses told of often taking "mental health days" both informally and through stress leave programs. On the basis of our experiences in all of our research studies, and on the basis of the related research we have cited above, it is clear that nurses routinely practice in environments that are not conducive to their well-being. Nor are such environments conducive to the care of either patients, families, or communities.

Overlooked Patients

In the corporate culture of health care today, nurses all too often are treated as disposable, while the well-being of patients, families, and communities all too often is overlooked.[12] Throughout our studies we observed situations in which, for example, elderly patients did not receive the basic physical care they required, patients with substance use problems were not treated appropriately for their withdrawal, and family members of dying patients were not adequately supported. Such situations arose at least partly because nurses and other members of the health care team (including physicians) were working under almost impossible structural constraints. Some administrators with whom we spoke also felt powerless to challenge or reverse these constraints. One nurse manager whose unit chronically functioned at 110 percent of the workload index (itself a poor estimate that undermeasured nursing work) found that despite staff working "flat out," they were routinely unable to meet basic patient needs. Another manager noted that unless staff came to work with "100 percent energy, a clear mind, and an open heart," the demands of the workplace were impossible to meet.

In today's era of cost constraint, nurses and other health care providers often are unable to meet patients' complex health care needs. Indeed, even basic physical needs often are not adequately met, particularly for the elderly. The "body care" inherent in nursing work—the

work that addresses people's experiences of their embodied existence, especially when their bodies fail to function normally (Lawler, 1993, p. vi)—is overlooked. The nurse mentioned earlier elaborated on missing bladder distention:

> [A] lady…was in with neck pain, back pain and knee pain and they thought she possibly had some collagen disease, [she was] very stiff and all this kind of stuff. She had an IV [intravenous], she wanted to go on the [bed]pan constantly, she was on a slipper [small] pan because she couldn't get on a bigger one she was too stiff constantly [the urine] would back flow and get on the pad or she'd squirt over the front or something you know, and…I didn't really think about it, I just thought "It's the IV that's going," so the second night I capped [stopped] the IV, she was still going…something was going on in my mind you know, like she's not going [voiding] that much [quantity]… so I did an in and out catheter post void, eleven seventy-five [1,175 millilitres] I got, so it was all overflow [her bladder was full and overflowing]….But I didn't pick up on that the first night.… I was just trying to…get everything together you know and…we had a couple of [patient] transfers in, a couple of admissions and things like that so you don't always pick up on those things (Rodney, 1997, p. 188).

The woman had a serious and debilitating medical condition, yet it was extraordinarily difficult for the nurse who was an expert to assess even her basic physiological functions. Beside the immediate pain the woman might have experienced, a variety of complications, including infections might have arisen as a consequence. In another situation, an elderly woman immobilized with serious rheumatoid arthritis was to be discharged into the care of her daughter and son-in-law. The daughter was ill with cancer, and the son-in-law was in his sixties. Yet the body care involved in toileting the elderly woman, feeding her, washing her, and so on was not recognized or planned for in "the system." Nor was there the opportunity to devise a comprehensive inter-disciplinary plan to help her with her pain and mobility. And there was certainly not the time to help her adjust to her altered level of independence or to listen to the concerns she might have for her daughter. Further, the needs of her family were not taken into account. In fact, we observed patients being discharged and returning to the emergency department in full-blown crisis. In our *Ethics in Action* study, one of our research colleagues relayed an account of a patient with cancer who, having been discharged from hospital and refused readmission to hospital, walked to the hospital barefoot in the middle of the night in her nightdress. She and her husband had been unable to obtain support for her escalating physical problems, so she returned to hospital alone and without identification so that hospital staff would be unable to return her home (Hartrick-Doane & Varcoe, 2005, p. 251).

Although the intent of health care reform has been to limit the costs of *treatment*, it has been *care* that has been limited.[13] Although nurses in our studies rationed their most valuable resource, their time, primarily based on patient acuteness, social judgments based on age, class, ethnicity, substance use, and so on, also figured into their allocation of resources. For example, the nurse who militated against the threat of her patient dying in the hallway had witnessed many elderly patients in similar circumstances, but the age of the patient seemed to add weight, not only to the nurses' concern, but to the likelihood of others sharing that concern.

CONSTRAINED AGENCY

Clearly, the well-being of nurses, patients, families, and communities is threatened in the corporate culture of health care. In closing this portrait of the social structure of nurses' work, we consider some of the implications for nurses as moral agents. Moral agency can be understood as referring to how people, in this case nurses, fulfill their moral responsibility and accountability and deal with ethical problems (Rodney,

1997; Rodney, Brown, & Liaschenko, 2004). Traditional perspectives on moral agency reflect a notion of individuals engaging in self-determining or self-expressive choice (Sherwin, 1992; Taylor, 1992). In contrast to this traditional view, there are emerging perspectives that see moral agency as *relational;* that is, enacted through interconnected relationships in particular contexts (Baylis, Kenny & Sherwin, 2008; Rodney, 1997; Sherwin, 1998). It is this interconnectedness that is a source of both challenges and strengths for nurses.

Moral Distress

Nurses are often in situations which challenge their abilities to fulfill their moral responsibility and accountability, and they too often are overwhelmed by ethical problems; they experience a great **moral distress** because of this. The ethical problems they face are sometimes dramatic questions of life and death decision-making, for instance, how to help a family decide whether or not to initiate tube feeding for a person who has suffered a stroke. More often, however, the ethical problems that nurses face are everyday questions, such as whether to restrain or "tie down" a confused patient. These questions are ethical because they revolve around "the good" in practice (Rodney, 1997; Rodney, Brown, & Liaschenko, 2004).

Significantly, the ethical problems faced by nurses in our studies frequently emerged as a result of constraints and cutbacks in the workplace. For example, the need to physically restrain confused patients or to rapidly force-feed dependent elders was increased by inadequate staffing levels that precluded alternative approaches to care. Thus, the ethical problems with which nurses dealt were embedded in everyday practice in an era of health reform—problems that, as Liaschenko (1993) has warned, are frequently "discounted or trivialized or sentimentalized" in biomedical ethics (p. 9). Nurses felt badly about the abrogation of their professional responsibility and accountability, and about the difficulties they experienced in trying to deal with ethical problems in their practice.

An emergency nurse cited earlier in this chapter was frustrated and tearful when she said, "You should see the way it should be, not like this" (Varcoe, 1997, p. 124). Almost every nurse we have encountered during our fieldwork in our seven studies has expressed this kind of distress, distress that has been echoed by managers, physicians, physiotherapists, radiation therapists, social workers, patients, family members, and others involved (both directly and indirectly) in patient care.

The nurses' distress was not just fatigue. Their distress reflected the anguish and powerlessness inherent in moral distress. That is, nurses made moral choices, but situational constraints made it difficult to translate moral choices into moral actions (Austin, 2007; Hamric & Blackhall, 2007; Rodney, Brown, & Liaschenko, 2004). For example, we observed nurses working with social workers to set up support for a caregiver who had been physically abusive to an elderly parent, only to have the patient discharged (to make room for other patients) before those supports could be put in place. The moral distress that nurses experience is a reflection of their difficulty enacting their moral agency. As the enactment of moral agency is prerequisite to professional practice, the social structure of nurses' work (within current health care contexts dominated by corporatism and narrow definitions of efficiency) threatens the foundation of professional practice as well as the well-being of nurses.

Moral Resistance

Nurses in our studies did not passively acquiesce to the constraints inherent in the social structure of their work. They resisted in various overt and covert ways. Despite the constraints, nurses made efforts to "get to know" their patients, to work with others as a team, and to negotiate better care, particularly when they faced ethical problems. For example, in the *Ethics in Action* study, nurses in the acute medical oncology unit negotiated as a group with the hospital administration to prevent (or at least ameliorate) the implementation of co-ed rooms, which they thought would be contrary to dignity and choice

(values from the CNA Code of Ethics, 2008) for many of their patients. In the Emergency setting, nurses worked against a policy that would permit narcotic administration in the hallway advocating instead for strategies that would allow patients to receive more timely admission and pain management under conditions where the nurses could monitor the patients. In a recent survey conducted in our program of research (Varcoe, Pauly, Storch, in review), participants described undertaking considerable effort to effect change, calling into question the utility of defining moral distress as an 'inability to act due to institutional constraints' or a 'failure to pursue a right course of action'.

Nurses also attempted to enact their moral agency by bending the rules. In other words, they went outside of what was officially sanctioned in their attempts to provide good care. For instance, a nurse in a medical unit where there were no regular venues for communication with physicians (such as patient care rounds) explained how she requisitioned blood tests without waiting for a physician's order when worried about a patient's electrolyte status. She explained, "You always have to work a way around the system to make it work." (*Ethics in Action*, Field Notes, 2004) Similarly, nurses in emergency bent the rules, for example, by giving patients unordered pain medications to take home (see also Hutchinson, 1990). And in our recent survey (Varcoe, Pauly, Storch, in review), nurses continued to report practices to circumvent policies that impaired their abilities to address patient needs.

The nurses we observed were usually motivated by what they saw as the best interests of the patients for whom they were caring, and they were caught in conflicts between institutional and medical rules (e.g., to monitor electrolytes only on a physician's order) and their own beliefs about what patients needed (e.g., to have electrolytes monitored during replacement therapy). Importantly, at least some of this subversion was a result of trying to "make up for" workplace constraints (e.g., the lack of patient care rounds and workloads that limited communication with physicians and others).

However, such actions, dubbed "responsible subversion" by Hutchinson (1990), may have negative as well as positive consequences. Nurses who bend the rules may experience sanctions if they are "caught," and rules may become more rigid once this happens. Moreover, if rules are not applied consistently, patients and families may become concerned about inconsistent (and possibly unjust) treatment. Further, there are a number of ethical questions about such subversion. These include questions about the rightness or wrongness of nurses practicing according to their own rules, about the ethical principles that underlie nurses' actions when they bend or break rules, about what would happen if everybody broke rules, about whether rule-breaking is the only course of action available to the nurse, and so on (Munhall, 1990). Thus, although this subversion often helped nurses to mediate the constraints inherent in the social structure of their work, it also had the potential to jeopardize their role and their care of patients and families. Further, in our studies we observed that rule-bending became so entrenched that practice problems were hidden and remained unexamined. Paradoxically, then, such subversion has the potential to jeopardize the nurses' enactment of their moral agency. In a sense, "responsible subversion" may be a "guerrilla tactic" that has the potential to backfire.

CONCLUSION

At the same time as health care workers participate in corporatism, they engage in tactics that mitigate these dominant influences. However, most of these tactics are at the level of the individual and are not necessarily based on a critical awareness of the dominance of corporate ideologies and practices. Thus, efforts to preserve quality in the health care system must become increasingly conscious, deliberate, and organized. In particular, nurses' work must be restructured to align with goals of health and in defiance of corporatism as the exclusive driving force in health care. The warnings we cited at the outset of this chapter about the danger to health and health care

posed by corporatism must be heeded. Ideologies must be exposed and challenged, "efficiency" re-envisioned, and space for the intellectual, emotional, and body work of nursing must be carved out of the wasteland that corporatism has created in health care. Nurses must take active roles individually and collectively both in countering the erosion of health care and nursing practice, and in formulating policy. Collective action will require proactive work through professional nursing associations and unions. Through our *Ethics in Action* and other studies, we have learned that such collective action *must* systematically engage nurses at all levels especially those in direct care roles, who often feel particularly powerless and disenfranchised.

This chapter has attempted to make visible some of the ways in which corporate ideologies are enacted within health care, within nursing practice, and by nurses themselves. It is hoped that this will be revealing for nurses and that they will be able to operate with a greater critical awareness of the ways in which ideologies function to structure their work and of the ways in which they participate in undermining their own values. With this awareness, nurses might challenge the often taken for granted idea that "there is no more money," and recognize such ideas as tricks to hide the fact that money is simply being spent elsewhere (sometimes on expensive systems to keep track of their labour). Nurses might then refuse the corporate rhetoric and challenge corporate ideologies. They might also then decide that accepting such ideas and sanctioning one another to work in compliance with corporatism is unacceptable, that it is neither in their own interests nor in the interests of their patients. Collective refusal to comply with corporatism would necessarily put patient needs and health outcomes ahead of corporate imperatives, would foreground alternate ideologies (perhaps ideologies of health, social justice, and the common good), and would require rethinking "efficiency."

Of course, individual nurses cannot do this work alone. There must be sufficient critical awareness of the issues and operating ideologies to make resistance the norm rather than simply the maverick behaviour of an individual. Shifting away from an environment of sanction and compliance would require and contribute to the creation of environments where relationships and trust flourish. Collective action within units, and in collaboration with existing groups such as professional organizations and unions, is necessary to move beyond guerrilla tactics to a full-scale assault on corporatism as the only or prevailing value in health care. A key initiative here is to find a safe—and constructive—venue to open up conversations between nurses and other health care providers, administrators, and policy makers. For example, after two years of hosting focus groups and workshops to support interdisciplinary staff at the British Columbia Cancer Agency, we learned how the professional practice leaders on our research team could promote change by bringing our findings to the clinic staff, to regional managers, to provincial leaders, and to national cancer and ethics conferences (Serrano, Martin, & Rodney, 2011). The work is ongoing, but it has made possible a dialogue that focuses more explicitly on values than was possible before.

Years of "reform" have eroded the culture of health care to one based predominantly on corporate values. Within this culture, the emphasis on efficiency has eroded the foundation for professional nursing practice. In addition to "righting" staffing to levels that can sustain safe care, space needs to be created for nurses to provide the emotional labour patients require during illness and death experiences. Space needs to be created for nurses to provide reasoned care, based on evidence and research. Such space needs to be created for nurses who provide direct care, rather than allocating the thinking space only to those who practice in roles removed from direct care. This cannot be achieved simply by allocating reasonable staffing levels, but must also be supported by the continued development of clinical advanced nursing practice roles such as clinical nurse specialists, clinical practice leaders, clinical resource nurses, and clinical nurse researchers roles that can contribute to and support direct care. Intellectual and emotional work must also be supported by greater attention being given by ethicists as well as researchers and educators who are not in direct care to linking practice, especially body work and emotional and intellectual labour, to health care and health outcomes. Realistically capturing the indeterminate work of nursing and other health care providers will require voices from nurses and all other health care providers to be heard in policy development from the unit to organizational to social levels.

This chapter was titled "constrained agency" to draw attention to the ideological and structural constraints to agency within nursing. However, nurses are never completely without agency. Whether it is an individual nurse offering an alternative to corporate images (perhaps we could see mentally ill patients as casualties of deinstitutionalization rather than as "repeaters" or "users"), or a group lobbying for change or participating in public policy formulation, the structure of nurses' work can be shaped by nurses to the extent that they are willing to take action. Questioning that which has been taken for granted is the first step. In the three years of our engagement with nursing colleagues in *Ethics in Action*, and the subsequent three years with our nursing and interdisciplinary colleagues in *Building a Moral Community for Collaborative Practice in Ambulatory Oncology Care* we have learned that nurses in direct care roles are more than ready and capable of taking that step.

Acknowledgements

The authors gratefully acknowledge all the research participants and the team of researchers with whom we work, especially Dr. Jan Storch, Dr. Gweneth Hartrick Doane, Dr. Bernie Pauly, Dr. Lee Ann Martin, Ms. Elena Serrano, and Dr. Rosalie Starzomski.

Notes

1. This chapter is an adapted and updated version of Varcoe C., & Rodney P. (2009) Constrained agency: the social structure of nurses' work. In B.S. Bolaria & H.D. Dickinson (Eds.). *Health,*

illness, and health care in Canada. (4th ed; pp. 122–151). Toronto, ON: Nelson Education.

2. While our focus in this chapter is on nurses, it should be noted that the constrained agency we address applies to *all* health care providers, at all levels of leadership in the health care system. The constraints to agency for each individual and group may differ, but in our current interdisciplinary research we have found striking similarities in the experiences of diverse health care providers (Pauly, Storch, & Varcoe, 2010; Serrano, Martin, & Rodney, 2011).

3. By *moral climate* we mean the "implicit and explicit values that drive health-care delivery and shape the workplaces in which care is delivered" (Rodney, Doane, Storch & Varcoe, 2006, p. 24).

4. *Moral distress* occurs when nurses (or other moral agents) are unable to translate their moral choices into moral action. It can be understood as "incoherence between one's beliefs and one's actions, and possibly also outcomes" (Webster & Baylis, 2000, p. 218). The initial definition of moral distress by philosopher Andrew Jameton (1984) emphasized external constraints as causing moral distress, but further theorizing by Webster and Baylis and work done [by] our own research team indicates that the causes of moral distress are embedded in a complex network of internal and external moral relationships—moral agents (such as nurses) can internalize their own "constraints" and contribute to their own moral distress, and that of their health care colleagues (Rodney, Brown, & Liaschenko, 2004; Pauly, Varcoe, Storch, & Newton, 2009). The aftermath of moral distress can be cumulative and long term, including anger, frustration, guilt, and powerlessness as well as decisions to leave the nursing role or profession (Austin et al., 2005; Jameton, 1984; Hamric & Blackhall, 2007; Rodney, Brown, & Liaschenko, 2004; Webster & Baylis, 2000). A growing number of scholars are calling for more careful theoretical and empirical work on the concept of moral distress so as to delineate it from other forms of stress and to posit effective strategies to ameliorate it (McCarthy & Deady, 2006; Pauly, Varcoe, Storch, & Newton; Repenshek, 2009).

5. *Culture* is more than race or ethnicity. It includes the processes that occur between people as individuals and as groups within organizations and society, and that confer meaning and significance (Geertz, 2000; Rodney, Pauly, & Burgess, 2004; Stephenson, 1999). Those of us in health care tend to see culture as residing in patients/clients and families. We need to understand that the health care system that we operate in has its own culture(s) (Coward & Ratanakul, 1999).

6. This chapter builds on our individual and shared programs of research, which we have conducted over the past 14 years with colleagues in nursing and other disciplines (Hartrick Doane, Storch, & Pauly, 2009; Pauly, Varcoe, Storch, & Newton, 2009; Rodney, 1997; Rodney, Varcoe, Storch, McPherson, Mahoney, Brown et al., 2002; Rodney, Doane, Storch, & Varcoe, 2006; Serrano, Martin, & Rodney, 2011; Storch, Rodney, Pauly et al., 2009; Storch, Rodney, Varcoe et al., 2009; Varcoe, 1997; 2001; Varcoe, Doane, Pauly, Rodney, Storch, Mahoney et al. 2004; Varcoe, Pauly & Storch, in review).

7. These cost constraints measures include capping (setting a predetermined level or number of activities to be done within a specific program, e.g., limiting the number of specific surgeries to be done over a year); downsizing (bed closures, staff layoffs, and redesign of the remaining activities, e.g., reducing the length of hospital stay); and consolidation of activities (e.g., merging hospital boards and executive management, which often includes a downgrading of the status and role of medicine and nursing in the new organizational structure). The measures further include restructuring and work redesign strategies such as reducing the levels of management, "cross training techniques" that allow staff to be moved between patient care areas, and changing the staff "mix," often by replacing registered nurse staff with practical nurses and/or care aides (Dick & Bruce, 1994, pp. 99–101).

8. In order to learn more about *how* to address the ethical problems we had identified in earlier studies we embarked on a participatory action research (PAR) study of nursing practice (*Ethics in Action*) conducted in an Emergency Unit and a Medical Oncology Unit (2003–2006). This study (funded by the Social Science and Humanities Research Council and the University of Victoria) involved three years of participant observation, interviews, focus groups, meetings, workshops, and informal work within the two practice settings (Hartrick Doane, Storch, & Pauly, 2009; Rodney, Doane, Storch, & Varcoe, 2006). At each site, the research team included staff nurses and academic investigators working in partnership. Along with qualitative data collection through focus groups and interviews, regular meetings with staff were conducted at each site to discuss, debrief, and to

plan for change. The research process was geared to supporting staff to initiate changes in their workplaces toward ethical practice.

Our PAR work has been continuing. *Building a Moral Community for Collaborative Practice in Ambulatory Oncology Care* was a participatory action study recently completed by an interdisciplinary team in an outpatient oncology clinic (2007–2010), and was funded by the British Columbia Cancer Agency and the Canadian Nurses Foundation. In this study Rodney and her interdisciplinary colleagues at the BC Cancer Agency used qualitative and quantitative methods to assess health care providers' moral climate, work with them to generate strategies for positive change, and evaluate the effectiveness of those changes (Serrano, Martin, & Rodney, 2011). The research team learned how changes in cancer care delivery across Canada have resulted in increasing pressures on all health care providers to deliver complex treatments in rapid-paced outpatient settings. Providers experience moral distress related to their concerns about the significant needs of patients and their family members who are going to have to manage at home, and about how providers delivering services have little input into the restructuring of cancer care delivery services. These same providers have also generated a number of effective strategies to improve the moral climate of their practice.

9. The term "efficient" is placed in quotation marks to draw attention to the fact that the type of efficiency being referred to is only "efficient" in the sense of dealing with more patients in less time, and not in the sense of overall efficiency connected with health outcomes or immediate or long-term benefits for patients. See Stein (2001) for an insightful analysis of how treating efficiency as an end instead of a means erodes effectiveness and accountability.

10. We are intentionally using mixed corporate and military metaphors here. Western biomedicine has been dominated by these two metaphors, which reflect "the quest for control that seems to define both modern medicine and modern politics" (Annas, 1995, p. 747). It is our contention that the quest for control is problematic for nurses, other health care providers, patients, families, and communities.

11. Yyelland (1994) distinguished nurses' emotional labour from their technical labour. We are using the term "emotional labour" as one of many aspects of nurses' work, one that is concerned with promoting the emotional well-being of patients, and harmony among patients and health care professionals.

12. Overlooking the well-being of patients, families, and communities is not the intention of a corporate focus on "outcomes." However, the authors' research and the growing number of other studies we have cited in this chapter warn that it is the result.

13. Acute care has been the focus of most of the research about the impacts of constrained resources on patients and their families. Yet community care is also suffering. Nurses experience anguish when they try to support "high risk" families who are having difficulties with parenting (MacPhail, 1996; Oberle & Tenove, 2000). And home care nurses are deeply concerned about the difficulties they experience meeting their client/family needs because home care resources are so limited (Peter, 2004). Further, in our recent ambulatory oncology care study, nurses and other health care providers expressed concerns about the ability of patients and their families to manage complex illness and treatment protocols with only sporadic outpatient support (Serrano, Martin, & Rodney, 2011).

References

Aiken, L.H., Clarke, S.P., Sloane, D.M., Sochalski, J. and Silber, J.H. (2002). Hospital nurse staffing and patient mortality, nurse burnout, and job dissatisfaction. *JAMA 288*(16), 1987–1993.

Anderson, J.M. (2004). Lessons from a postcolonial-feminist perspective: Suffering and a path to healing. *Nursing Inquiry, 11* (4), 238–246.

Anderson, J. M., Rodney, P., Reimer-Kirkham, S., Browne, A.J., Khan, K.B., & Lynam, M.J. (2009). Inequities in health and healthcare viewed through the ethical lens of critical social justice: Contextual knowledge for the global priorities ahead. *Advances in Nursing Science, 32* (4), 282–294.

Annas, G.J. (1995). Reframing the debate on health care reform by replacing our metaphors. *New England Journal of Medicine, 332*(11), 744–747.

Armstrong, P. (2001). The context for health care reform in Canada. In P. Armstrong, C. Amaratunga, J. Bernier, K. Grant, A. Pederson, A., & K. Wilson (Eds.), *Exposing Privatization: Women and health care reform in Canada* (pp.11–48). Aurora, ON: Garamond Press.

Armstrong, P., & Armstrong, H. (2003). *Wasting away: The undermining of Canadian health care* (2nd ed.) Don Mills, ON: Oxford University Press.

Austin, W., Lemermeyer, G., Goldberg, L., Bergum, V., & Johnson, M.S. (2005). Moral distress in healthcare practice: The situation of nurses. *HEC Forum, 17* (1), 33–48.

Austin, W. (2007). The ethics of everyday practice: Healthcare environments as moral communities. *Advances in Nursing Science, 30* (1), 81–88.

Baylis, F., Kenny, N.P., & Sherwin, S. (2008). A relational account of public health ethics. *Public Health Ethics, 1* (3), 196–209.

Benner, P.A., Tanner, C.A., & Chesla, C.A. (with contributions by Dreyfus, H.L., Dreyfus, S.E., & Rubin, J.) (1996). *Expertise in nursing practice: Caring, clinical judgment, and ethics.* New York: Springer.

Björnsdóttir, K. (2001). From the state to the family: Reconfiguring the responsibility for long-term nursing care at home. *Nursing Inquiry, 9*(1), 3–11.

Browne, A.J. (2001). The influence of liberal political ideology on nursing science. *Nursing Inquiry, 8,* 118–129.

Browne, A.J., Smye, V.L., Rodney, P., Tang, S.Y., Mussell, B., & O'Neill, J. (2011). Access to primary care from the perspective of Aboriginal patients at an urban emergency department. *Qualitative Health Research 21* (3), 333–348.

Campbell, M. (1994). The structure of stress in nurses' work. In B.S. Bolaria & H.D. Dickinson (Eds.), *Health, illness, and health care in Canada* (pp. 592–608). Toronto, ON: Harcourt Brace.

Canadian Nurses Association (2008) *Code of Ethics for Registered Nurses.* Ottawa, ON: Authors.

Canadian Nurses Association and Registered Nurses' Association of Ontario (2010). *Nurse fatigue and patient safety: Research report.* Ottawa, ON: Canadian Nurses Association.

Coburn, D. (2001). Health, health care, and neo-liberalism. In P. Armstrong, H. Armstrong, & D. Coburn (Eds.), *Unhealthy times: Political economy perspectives on health and care in Canada* (pp.45–65). Don Mills, ON: Oxford University Press.

Coburn, D. (2010). Health and health care: A political economy perspective. In T. Bryant, D. Raphael, & M. Rioux (Eds.), *Staying alive: Critical perspectives on health, illness, and health care* (2nd ed.; pp. 65–91). Toronto, ON: Canadian Scholars' Press.

Commission on the Future of Health Care in Canada (2002). *Building on Values: The Future of Health Care in Canada.* Ottawa, ON: Authors.

Coward, H., & Ratanakul, P. (Eds.). (1999). *A cross cultural dialogue on health care ethics.* Waterloo, ON: Wilfrid Laurier University Press.

Dick, J., & Bruce, S. (1994). Cost containment: Doing more with less. In J.M. Hibberd & M.E. Kyle (Eds.), *Nursing management in Canada* (pp. 91–107). Toronto, ON: W.B. Saunders.

Foucault, M. (1978). *The history of sexuality: An introduction.* (R. Hurley, Trans.). New York: Random House. (Original work published 1976.)

Foucault, M. (1980). *Power/knowledge: Selected interviews and other writings (1972–1977).* C. Gordon, (Ed.). New York: Random House.

Frankish, C.J., Hwang, S.W., & Quantz, D. (2005). Homelessness and health in Canada: Research lessons and priorities. *Canadian Journal of Public Health, 96* (S2), S23–S29.

Geertz, C. (2000). *Available light: Anthropological reflections on philosophical topics.* Princeton, NJ: Princeton University Press.

Hamric, A.B., & Blackhall, L.J. (2007). Nurse-physician perspectives on the care of dying patients in intensive care units: Collaboration, moral distress, and ethical climate. *Critical Care Medicine, 35,* (2).

Hartrick Doane, G., Storch, J., & Pauly, B. (2009). Ethical nursing practice: Inquiry-in-action. *Nursing Inquiry, 16*(3), 1–9.

Hartrick-Doane, G., & Varcoe, C. (2005). *Family nursing as relational inquiry: Developing health promoting practice.* Philadelphia, PA: Lippincott, Williams and Wilkins.

Health Council of Canada (2008). *Rekindling Reform: Health Care Renewal in Canada, 2003–2008.* Toronto, ON: Health Council of Canada.

Hiraki, A. (1998). Corporate language and nursing practice. *Nursing Outlook, 46,* 115–119.

Hutchinson, S.A. (1990). Responsible subversion: A study of rule-bending among nurses. *Scholarly Inquiry for Nursing Practice, 4*(1), 3–17.

Jameton, A. (1984). *Nursing practice: The ethical issues.* Englewood Cliffs, NJ: Prentice-Hall.

Lawler, J. (1993). *Behind the screens: Nursing, somology, and the problem of the body.* Redwood City, CA: Benjamin/Cummings.

Liaschenko, J. (1993). *Faithful to the good: Morality and philosophy in nursing practice.* Unpublished doctoral dissertation, University of California, San Francisco.

Lynam, M. J. (2005). Health as a socially mediated process: Theoretical and practice imperatives emerging from research on health inequalities. *Advances in Nursing Science, 28* (1), 25–37.

Lynam, M.J., Henderson, A., Browne, A., Smye, V., Semeniuk, P., Blue, C., Singh, S., and Anderson, J. (2003). Healthcare restructuring with a view to equity and efficiency: Reflections on unintended consequences. *Canadian Journal of Nursing Leadership, 16*(1), 112–140.

MacPhail, S.A. (1996). *Ethical issues in community nursing.* Unpublished master's thesis, University of Alberta, Edmonton.

McCarthy, J., & Deady, R. (2006). Moral distress reconsidered. *Nursing Ethics, 15*(2), 254–262.

Moorhouse, A., & Rodney, P. (2010). Contemporary Canadian challenges in nursing ethics. In M. Yeo, A. Moorhouse, P. Khan & P. Rodney (Eds.), *Concepts and cases in nursing ethics*, (3rd ed.; pp. 73–101). Peterborough, ON: Broadview Press.

Munhall, P.L. (1990). Response to "Responsible subversion: A study of rule-bending among nurses." *Scholarly Inquiry for Nursing Practice, 4*(1), 19–22.

Myrick, F. (2004). Pedagogical integrity in the knowledge economy. *Nursing Philosophy 5,* 23–29.

Oberle, K., & Tenove, S. (2000). Ethical issues in public health nursing. *Nursing Ethics, 7*(5), 425–438.

O'Brien-Pallas, L., Griffin, P., Shamian, J., Buchan, J., Duffield, C., Hughes, F., et al. (2006). The impact of nurse turnover on patient, nurse, and system outcomes: a pilot study and focus for a multicenter international study. *Policy, Politics & Nursing Practice, 7*(3), 169–179.

Pauly, B.M., Storch, J.L., & Varcoe, C. (2010). *Final Report: Moral Distress in Health Care Symposium.* (Unpublished report to the Canadian Institutes of Health Research, University of Victoria, and University of British Columbia). Victoria, BC: Authors.

Pauly, B., Varcoe, C., Storch, J. L., & Newton, L. (2009). Registered nurses' perceptions of moral distress and ethical climate. *Nursing Ethics, 16*(5), 561–573.

Penning, M.J. & Votova, K. (2009). Aging, health, and health care: From hospital and residential care to home and community care. In B.S. Bolaria & H. Dickinson (Eds.), *Health, illness, and health care in Canada* (4th ed.; pp. 349–366). Toronto, ON: Nelson Education.

Peter, E. (2004). Home health care and ethics. In J. Storch, P. Rodney & R. Starzomski (Eds.). *Toward a moral horizon: Nursing ethics for leadership and practice,* (pp. 248–261). Toronto, ON: Pearson Prentice Hall.

Picard, A. (2000). *Critical care: Canadian nurses speak for change.* Toronto: HarperCollins.

Pringle, D. (2009). Alert—Return of 1990s healthcare reform. *Nursing Leadership, 22* (3), 14–15.

QualityWorklife Quality Healthcare Collaborative (2007). *Within our grasp: A healthy workplace action strategy for success and sustainability in Canada's healthcare system.* Ottawa, ON: Canadian Council on Health Services Accreditation.

Rankin, J.M., & Campbell, M. (2006). *Managing to nurse: Inside Canada's health care reform.* Toronto, ON: University of Toronto Press.

Repenshek, M. (2009). Moral distress: Inability to act or discomfort with moral subjectivity? *Nursing Ethics, 16* (6), 734–742.

Rodney, P.A. (1997). *Towards connectedness and trust: Nurses' enactment of their moral agency within an organizational context.* Unpublished doctoral dissertation, University of British Columbia, Vancouver.

Rodney, P., Brown, H., & Liaschenko, J. (2004). Moral agency: Relational connections and trust. In J. Storch, P. Rodney & R. Starzomski (Eds.). *Toward a moral horizon: Nursing ethics for leadership and practice,* (pp. 154–177). Toronto, ON: Pearson-Prentice Hall.

Rodney, P., Doane, G.H., Storch, J. & Varcoe, C. (2006). Workplaces: Toward a safer moral climate.

Rodney, P., Pauly, B., & Burgess, M. (2004). Our theoretical landscape: Complementary approaches to health care ethics. In J. Storch, P. Rodney, & R. Starzomski (Eds.), *Toward a moral horizon: Nursing ethics for leadership and practice* (pp. 77–97). Toronto, ON: Pearson-Prentice Hall.

Rodney, P., & Starzomski, R. (1993). Constraints on the moral agency of nurses. *Canadian Nurse, 89*(9), 23–26.

Rodney, P., & Street, A. (2004). The moral climate of nursing practice: Inquiry and action. In J. Storch, P. Rodney & R. Starzomski (Eds.). *Toward a moral horizon: Nursing ethics for leadership and practice,* (pp. 209–231). Toronto, ON: Pearson-Prentice Hall.

Rodney, P. & Varcoe, C. (2001). Toward ethical inquiry in the economic evaluation of nursing practice. *Canadian Journal of Nursing Research, 33* (1), 35–57.

Rodney, P., Varcoe, C., Storch, J., McPherson, G., Mahoney, K., Brown, H., et al. (2002). Navigating towards a moral horizon: A multisite qualitative study of ethical practice in nursing. *Canadian Journal of Nursing Research, 34*(3), 75–102.

Sanders, K., Pattison, S., & Hurwitz, B. (2011). Tracking shame and humiliation in accident and emergency. *Nursing Philosophy, 12,* 83–93.

Saul, J.R. (2005). *The collapse of globalism and the reinvention of the world.* Toronto, ON: Penguin Canada.

Saul, J.R. (2008). *A fair country: Telling truths about Canada.* Toronto, ON: Viking Canada.

Scanlon, C. (1996–1997). Impact of cost containment on patient welfare concerns nurses. *American Nurses Association Center for Ethics and Human Rights Communique, 5*(2), 1–4.

Serrano, E., Martin, L.A., & Rodney, P. (2011). *Final Report: Building a Moral Community for Collaborative Practice in Ambulatory Oncology*

Care: Toward Improved Patient/Family and Team Outcomes. (Unpublished report to the Canadian Nurses Foundation and the British Columbia Cancer Agency). Vancouver, BC: Authors.

Sherwin, S. (1992). *No longer patient: Feminist ethics & health care*. Philadelphia, PA: Temple University Press.

Sherwin, S. (1998). A relational approach to autonomy in health care. In S. Sherwin et al. (Eds.), *The politics of women's health* (pp. 19–47). Philadelphia, PA: Temple University Press.

Smith, D.E. (1990). *Conceptual practices of power: A feminist sociology of knowledge*. London: Routledge.

Stajduhar, K.I. (2003). Examining the perspectives of family members involved in the delivery of palliative care at home. *Journal of Palliative Care, 19*(1), 27–35.

Stein, J.G. (2001). *The cult of efficiency*. Toronto, ON: Penguin.

Stelling, J. (1994). Nursing metaphors: Reflections on the meaning of time. In B.S. Bolaria & R. Bolaria, *Women, medicine and health* (pp. 205–217). Saskatoon, SK: University of Saskatchewan.

Stephenson, P. (1999). Expanding notions of culture for cross-cultural ethics in health and medicine. In H. Coward & P. Ratanakul (Eds.), *A cross-cultural dialogue on health care ethics*. Waterloo, ON: Wilfrid Laurier University Press.

Storch, J.L. (1996). Foundational values in Canadian health care. In M. Stingl & D. Wilson (Eds.), *Efficiency vs. equality: Health reform in Canada* (pp. 21–26). Halifax, NS: Fernwood.

Storch, J.L. (2005). Patient safety: Is it just another bandwagon? *Nursing Leadership, 18* (2), 39–55.

Storch, J.L. (2010). Canadian healthcare system. In M. McIntyre & C. McDonald (Eds.), *Realities of Canadian nursing: Professional, practice, and power issues,* (3rd ed.; pp. 34–55). Philadelphia, PA: Wolters Kluwer Health.

Storch, J.L., & Meilicke, C.A. (1994). Political, social, and economic forces shaping the health care system. In J.M. Hibberd & M.E. Kyle (Eds.), *Nursing management in Canada* (pp. 19–36). Toronto, ON: W.B. Saunders.

Storch, J., Rodney, P., Pauly, B., Fulton, T., Stevenson, L., Newton, L., & Makaroff, K.S. (2009). Enhancing ethical climates in nursing work environments. *Canadian Nurse, 105* (3), 20–25.

Storch, J., Rodney, P., Varcoe, C., Pauly, B., Starzomski, R., Stevenson, L., Best, L., Mass, H., Fulton, T.R., Mildon, B., Bees, F., Chisholm, A., MacDonald-Rencz, S., McCutcheon, A.S., Shamian, J., Thompson, C., Makaroff, K.S., & Newton, L. (2009). Leadership for ethical policy and practice (LEPP): Participatory action project. *Canadian Journal of Nursing Leadership*, 22(3), 68–80.

Taylor, C. (with Gutmann, A., Rockefeller, S.C., Walzer, M., & Wolf, S.) (1992). *Multiculturalism and "The politics of recognition."* Princeton, NJ: Princeton University Press.

Thomas, J. (1993). *Doing critical ethnography*. Newbury Park, CA: Sage.

Varcoe, C. (1997). *Untying our hands: The social context of nursing in relation to violence against women*. Unpublished doctoral dissertation. Vancouver: University of British Columbia.

Varcoe, C. (2001). Abuse obscured: An ethnographic account of emergency unit nursing practice in relation to violence against women. *Canadian Journal of Nursing Research, 32*(4), 95–115.

Varcoe, C., Doane, G., Pauly, B., Rodney, P., Storch, J. L., Mahoney, K., et al. (2004). Ethical Practice in Nursing—Working the In-betweens. *Journal of Advanced Nursing, 45*(3), 316–325.

Varcoe, C., Pauly, B., & Storch, J. (in review). Nurses' perceptions of and responses to moral distressing situations.

Weiss, S.M., Malone, R.E., Merighi, J.R. & Benner, P. (2002). Economism, efficiency, and the moral ecology of good nursing practice. *Canadian Journal of Nursing Research, 34*(2), 95–119.

Yyelland, B. (1994). Structural constraints, emotional labour and nursing work. In B.S. Bolaria & R. Bolaria, *Women, medicine and health* (pp. 231–240). Saskatoon, SK: University of Saskatchewan.

Air-Support Treatment: A Case Study in the Ethics of Allocating an Expensive Treatment

Benjamin Freedman, James Gilbert, and Lois A. Kaltsounakis

A HOSPITAL UNDER PRESSURE

The first use of air-support treatment in the Jewish General Hospital (JGH) in Montreal gave notice of the sorts of issues—ethical, administrative, and personal—that would be associated with it thereafter. Mrs. S, a patient in her late sixties with advanced senile dementia of the Alzheimer's type, was being treated in orthopedics for a broken hip. In the course of a lengthy convalescence, she developed pressure sores that did not respond to ordinary nursing measures.

A grandson, acting as family spokesperson for Mrs. S, conducted his own investigation into treatment options and launched a successful pressure campaign resulting in the hospital's leasing, and then purchasing, an air-support bed. Surgery to cover Mrs. S's deepest pressure sores with skin grafts, allowing her removal from this expensive apparatus, was refused.

After many months on this bed without healing, the family was informed that Mrs. S would be removed from it so that another patient, in greater need and with greater prospects for improvement, might benefit from it. The family, a demanding group that had often, in the past, used arguments, community pressure, and threats of litigation to get its own way, informed the hospital that it would sue if Mrs. S was not continued on air-support treatment. Among the morals of this story: the hospital needs a rational policy in order to ethically allocate this particular resource.

THE INSTITUTIONAL CONTEXT

The Jewish General Hospital, in common with other hospitals in Canada (and especially Quebec), is a natural laboratory of institutional allocation of health-care resources. A 628–bed McGill University teaching hospital with a very elderly catchment population (of 195,000 patient-days provided last year, 55,000 were for long-term care), it operates within a tight global operating budget. For the year ending March 31, 1990, the JGH's budget was set by the provincial ministry of health at $102 million (in Canadian funds: all following dollar figures refer to Canadian costs unless otherwise noted). From that budget, whose distribution is the hospital's responsibility rather than the government's, all operational needs of the hospital must be satisfied; or in other words, each hospital service and amenity is in budgetary competition with all others. Success in operating within the budget is rewarded: the hospital is permitted to keep any surplus funds and has been given a further grant of around one million dollars as a *cout de système,* an adjustment on behalf of meeting advancing technology and serving an ever-more-needy population. And failure is punished: a deficit is met by a governmentally imposed freeze for the following year on construction, equipment purchase, and the funding of new programs. Given the already fierce competition among existing hospital services, new programs and expensive technologies such as air-support treatment need to be rigorously scrutinized before their introduction into the hospital.

THE AILMENT

As appealing as the prospect of lying in bed for extended periods of time may sometimes be, there are serious side effects to this activity. The only portions of skin on the human body capable of withstanding pressure over 40 mmHg for prolonged periods are the soles of the feet; normal capillary pressure elsewhere ranges from 25 to 35 mmHg. Lying in bed causes the weight to be distributed over other body surfaces with bony prominences (hip, coccyx, heels, and so on) unable to withstand prolonged pressure. With more pressure *on* the capillaries than *in* them, circulation slows, and blood flow is reduced or obstructed. Unless the external pressure is relieved, tissue damage results due to the lack of oxygen.

A dermal ulcer (in prior parlance, decubitus ulcer or pressure ulcer) is the end stage of damage to the skin and its underlying tissue. The risks of developing a dermal ulcer are much greater for seriously ill or debilitated patients because of their immobility that causes pressure on the capillaries, and because their condition (for example, dehydration) may itself contribute to having considerably reduced capillary pressure. It has been estimated that 3 to 5 percent of all patients admitted to hospitals will develop a dermal ulcer; estimated costs of treatment range from $5,000 to $35,000 (US) per ulcer.[1] Over the past year (April 1989 to March 1990) JGH had almost sixty patients who had either stage 3 or stage 4 dermal ulcers, making them priority candidates for the treatment discussed below.

THE THERAPY

As early as 1873, experiments were being conducted on ways to relieve pressure to prevent tissue damage.[2] Over the years, various materials such as moss, straw, feathers, sand, springs, rubber, plastic, foams, and plaster of paris have been used for pressure relief.

In 1961, John Scales started experiments to study the support of the body by temperature controlled air at pressures that would not cause undesirable physiological changes.[3] From this early work it became apparent that patient-support systems, based on the principle of air support but with the air contained and separated from the patient by a membrane permeable to water vapor, could be developed. The low air-loss bed system first came into use at Scales's institution in Stanmore, England, in March 1971.[4] Air-fluidized beds have been available since 1969. These beds contain ceramic beads covered by a closely woven polyester sheet. Warm, pressurized air is forced throughout the particulate mass in order to make the particles behave as a fluid. The patient "floats" on the bed without pressure on the bony prominences. These beds provide an ideal environment for prevention, as well as an excellent treatment for skin breakdown.[5] This therapy may also serve a useful role in the treatment of cancer patients (by providing pain relief) and patients with burns (by permitting skin regeneration). The disadvantage of this therapy, however, is its cost. Air-support therapies vary in technique and technology; purchase price of the beds ranges from $35,000 to $150,000. Maintenance contracts average $3,500 annually. The cost of replacement pillows is $4,142 every second year. The daily rental cost ranges from $65 to $150 depending on the type of bed, and some companies add an installation charge of $100.[6]

These figures put in perspective the issue of allocation posed by air-support beds. The beds are expensive in absolute terms to purchase and maintain, and further problems are posed when an unbudgeted rental is required. These equipment costs are borne by the hospital's budget for nursing, which represents just under half the global hospital budget. However, that nursing budget itself is dominated by personnel costs, which consume well over 85 percent of the total. The average cost per patient-day for the past year was $524, so that a rental at JGH adds 18 percent (based on $100 per day) to the expense of a day of care. Dolezal and his colleagues, estimating air-support therapy to add only 4 to 6 percent to the total hospital bill, state that "the additional expense is justifiable considering the safety of postoperative healing and the comfortable environment provided for these patients."[7] The constraints within which JGH operates do not allow them the latitude to justify costs in this fashion.

Because the JGH has only one air-support therapy bed that has many uses and an increasing patient demand, there is always a queue. In order to ethically decide the order of the queue, a sound policy of allocation of this particular resource is needed.

ETHICAL ALLOCATION I: PATIENT-CENTERED FACTORS

A justifiable scheme for the allocation of medical resources must involve two components. It must provide technically sound patient-centered decisions. That is, it must incorporate a realistic appraisal of the resource in relationship to the needs of the specific patient in question, to ensure that the resource is being used wisely and efficiently. The scheme must also be sensitive to the broad context within which the resource is to be provided. Patients' rights must be respected while the needs and interests of the institution and the population it serves are accommodated. Ethical reasoning is relevant to both of these dimensions of sound allocative policy.

When a patient is admitted to the hospital, a nurse does a skin and wound assessment within the first twenty-four hours. Preventive measures are implemented for patients identified as at risk for dermal ulcer development. Risk factors can be divided into environmental factors (for example, pressure, shear, and friction) and systemic factors (such as age, weight, mobility, nutritional status, moisture problems—incontinence and drainage—and predisposing diseases).

Generally, the greater the number of factors present, the greater the risk. All dermal ulcers are identified according to stage using criteria adapted from Shea.[8] Because tissue breaks down more readily in the presence of systemic risk factors, continued nursing assessment is critical. This initial assessment, along with the factors presented below, forms the basis of what therapy, if any, will be used on the patient. Patients with ulcers at higher stages usually receive priority for air-support treatment.

A resource is wasted unless given to those who need and may benefit from it. Patients who are not bedfast do not need air support; they prevent and heal dermal ulcers by walking around. Likewise, bedfast patients who are not immobile can turn themselves to prevent and heal dermal ulcers. Because air-support therapy is the optimal treatment for and only for bedfast patients who

cannot be positioned off their ulcers, it should be restricted to them.

It is obvious that to qualify for air-support therapy the patient must be able to benefit from it. One class of patients that does not qualify includes those that have the necessary ailments but have such poor nutritional (especially protein) intake that healing cannot take place.[9]

When we talk about a patient "benefiting" from a particular treatment, we usually require that the patient experience the benefit. This is always the case if the benefit received from a treatment is the reduction of pain. It is part of the logic of the word pain that it is experienced. (One cannot say "I am in pain yet I have no sensation of it.") What if the goal of the treatment is simply to heal a dermal ulcer? A patient whose mental status is so compromised that she could not experience the benefit of having her ulcer healed would, in a technical sense, still be benefiting from having the ulcer healed. But unexperienced benefit is of little value: were someone to open up a bank account in a man's name, without his knowing it, and deposit a million dollars in it, he would benefit from this. Even if it never came to his attention that he had this money, he would technically be a millionaire. It would, however, be a useless benefit if, unaware of the transaction, he never spent the money or at least had a chance to revel in the fact that he was so rich. Likewise for the patient who does not experience the benefit of a particular treatment. We therefore choose to exclude patients who cannot and will never experience the benefit of air-support therapy from this costly treatment.

In allocating this particular resource we are forced to address the issue of sometimes conflicting medical goals. Benefit from air-support therapy we have seen can fall into two analytically distinct categories: healing of the dermal ulcer and relief from pain or discomfort. These usually go together, but not always: a stage 4 ulcer causes such extensive neural damage that the patient experiences little or no pain or discomfort. For this patient, benefit from air-support therapy means nothing more than the healing of an ulcer. The reciprocal of this, the patient with an unresponsive ulcer who feels more comfortable on air support, was the case with Mrs. S.

There are many ways of relieving pain other than using air-support therapy. Therefore, policy must ordinarily assign relative priority to the goal of healing. The presence of intractable pain, however, can still be a decisive factor in determining allocation. If two patients are equally qualified for air-support therapy, yet only one of them is experiencing intractable pain that can be relieved by air support, then both reason and emotion dictate that this patient should receive the therapy.

A final principle: a patient that will probably die before the objective of air-support treatment can be realized should be excluded. The justification of this harsh principle follows from the same means-end rationality as has been applied to the nursing evaluation: there is no justification to instituting medical measures from which benefit will not be derived. However, in applying this principle, attention must be paid to the specific treatment goal for which air support is proposed. When air support is proposed as the appropriate comfort measure for a person with, for example, bone metastases, imminent death should not be an exclusion....

ETHICAL ALLOCATION II: ISSUES AND PRINCIPLES OF CONTEXT

The patient-centered level of consideration establishes that the resource may be justified vis-à-vis a particular patient. But without considering the context of the allocation, one could not conclude whether that would represent the best use of the resource, or whether another patient is entitled to the resource. The two-party, doctor–patient model of decisions, so common in medical ethics, is inadequate to this purpose of institutional allocative decisions.

The first issue needing to be addressed is whether any patient has a *right* to the scarce resource, or in other words, is any patient or group of patients *entitled* to air-support treatment? The fundamental importance of this question is expressed in the philosopher's maxim, "Rights are trumps." In our understanding of

ethics and jurisprudence, satisfying a person's right takes precedence over all other claims.

We believe that no patient has a right, legal or moral, to receive air-support treatment. Legally, the ministry does not compel the hospital to make this treatment available to any person. While Canadians by law possess a positive right to "medically necessary treatment,"[10] considerable discretion in describing the boundaries of this concept is provided and necessary. "Medically necessary treatment" in practice extends well beyond the concept of "minimally decent health care," a concept appealed to by American theorists;[11] but it does not encompass a patient's right to optimal treatment, with no regard to cost.

These points, while valid legally and administratively, do not settle the ethical question: is a patient *morally* entitled to air-support treatment? We believe not, for any argument supporting such a right would need to surmount the following obstacle. Precisely because of the peremptory, powerful character of rights, a liberal social scheme must formulate them so that the rights of each are compatible with the right of all. Jurists say, for example, that one's right to freedom of action ends at the tip of someone else's nose—that is, at the point where the exercise of the right infringes the rights of another. The difficulty faced by claiming that a patient has a positive right to some treatment is that the right imposes a correlative duty upon the institution to pay for the satisfaction of that right.

Air-support therapy in our allocative scheme is in competition with all other forms of treatment. Patient candidates are in a zero-sum game with the medical needs of all other patients; one patient's gain is another's loss. With the possible exception of emergency services,[12] no medical treatment within the hospital possesses such a degree of need and urgency as to automatically trump all of its competitors—precisely the condition that would be described were we to say that a patient has a *right* to a particular treatment.

One other possibility, though, requires analysis. Although a patient is not entitled to an air bed paid for by the hospital, he or she may have another source of entitlement. An insurance policy might include this treatment within its coverage, in which case the patient is entitled to have the hospital rent a bed with its costs reimbursed by insurance. Some private health insurers in Canada, such as Blue Cross, have agreed to cover the costs of air-support therapy after case evaluation; similar coverage may be provided by governmental insurers that cover workers' and automobile accidents. This suggests a further criterion of exclusion: the hospital will not pay for air-support treatment on behalf of a person entitled to have it provided from any other source. These persons are to obtain the funding for the treatment from the other source, in effect removing them from the hospital queue.

We have denied that a patient has a right to air-support treatment funded by JGH. Rather, within our understanding, a patient may have a *claim* to that treatment. It is the job of ethics to assess how well grounded is the claim, relative to other claimants.

What if a person is a candidate for, but not yet eligible for, air support provided by the hospital, and he wishes to pay for it out of his own funds? Should he be permitted to buy his way out of the fate shared in common by other patients?

The question has somewhat more bite within the Canadian system, with its egalitarian commitment to the provision of health care, than within the United States. One great political advantage of a universal entitlement to health care is that all are in the same boat—the rich as well as the poor, the politically powerful as well as the disenfranchised—with the former group's self-interest effectively satisfying the latter's needs.

Nonetheless, we tend to favor this exemption. As argued above, there is no entitlement to air-support therapy *per se*; therefore, permitting a patient to buy his way off the queue does not violate universality as it is imperfectly realized at present. And, this exemption is compatible with such egalitarian views as those held by Rawls and his followers.[13] When a patient is allowed to buy his way off the queue, he is being treated in a way that satisfies Rawls's difference principle, allowing unequal treatment that will redound to the benefit of the least advantaged. In our context, the "least advantaged" person in question is the last person on the queue, and his or her situation

is improved because one person ahead has left the line. For these reasons we conclude that one who prepares his own bed—or pays for it—can lie in it.

Even granted that a patient initially has no right to air-support treatment, does the fact that he or she is now in it ground an entitlement to continue? It is often the case that a person is not initially entitled to some good, but, once the good has been offered, the supplier is duty bound to continue. A person has no right to be seen by Dr. Zhivago, but once the doctor has begun to treat her (and perhaps even as soon as he has agreed to see her), a doctor–patient relationship has been established that generally justifies her expectation that it will continue. In general, one who undertakes to supply health care must continue. Does this principle apply to air-support therapy, creating a right to continue on behalf of patients beginning the therapy?

We have decided to the contrary. Just as the patient's rights are not violated when air-support treatment is withheld, so are they not violated when it is withdrawn. This view accords with the general consensus regarding life-support equipment, stated by the President's Commission for the Study of Ethical Problems in Medicine among others, that there is no decisive moral difference between withholding and withdrawing medical treatment.[14] (That there is no difference in principle is assured by the arbitrary way in which we "count" medical treatments. Is each drop in the IV, or each cycle on the respirator, to count as a separate initiation of treatment? In the case of air support, is the treatment reinstituted each time the patient is replaced on the bed after a bath, or after the pillows have been changed?)

Moreover, while there is no significant *moral* difference of principle between withholding and withdrawing a treatment, there are significant *practical* differences that suggest that, in general, the advantage lies with withdrawing rather than withholding the treatment in question. The reason is that a treatment's worth to a specific patient can often only be accurately assessed following a trial period of treatment.

The President's Commission suggested that those institutions that feel comfortable in withholding ventilation from patients, but have difficulty in withdrawing it, are prone to two sorts of errors. First, patients who had been put on ventilation, for whom it is no longer appropriate, continue treatment at a cost of anguish to the patient and at a financial cost to the institution. And second, for fear of being locked into maintaining a patient indefinitely on ventilation, institutions never institute a trial period in others who might in fact have a reversible condition. A regime that permits withholding treatment while prohibiting withdrawing it overtreats the first set of patients while undertreating the second, because it has no way of trying a treatment to see how it goes and deciding on that basis.

The same points apply to air-support therapy. We need to recognize that a treatment that has proven futile may be withdrawn, for the same reason that one that promises to be futile may be withheld. The point in fact applies with even greater force in our case, because of the scarcity of the resource and since the treatment period may be fairly lengthy.[15]

Because there are always several patients in the hospital who could benefit to some degree from air-support therapy, efficiency demands that the bed always be in use, assigned to the patient with the greatest need. In the past, however, the bed has sometimes been unused, for fear that the patient in the greatest need would linger on it indefinitely, locking out other patients whose improvement on air support would be more rapid and assured. This situation should not recur in an institution that allocates the bed rationally, rather than by reference to a fallacious presumption of a right to continue.

One last consideration flows naturally from the above discussion. A bed treating two is more efficient than one helping a single patient, and so some allowance for the stage of the candidates' ulcers needs to be made in the evaluation process. In general, it would seem that priority should be given to Patient A—with stage 4 ulcers (that extend through skin and fat into muscle and/or bone)—*unless* it is the case that patients B and C, with stage 3 ulcers (extending through skin and fat only), could be prevented from progressing to stage 4 in the same treatment interval that it would have taken A to regress back to stage 3.

While rationality seems to demand that we think about the intervention as secondary prevention as well as treatment, inherent prognostic uncertainties, as well as interstaff and interservice political realities, may make it difficult to incorporate this "soft" factor into evaluating priority access.

CONCLUSION

Our attempt to formulate an ethically justified approach to the allocation of air-support treatment presents a means for defining those persons who are eligible for the treatment (those who are "on the queue"), and a basis for considering the relative weight of claim to treatment on the bed of eligible persons.

As a contribution to practical ethics, proposed policy must be clearly useful as well as justified. We feel the deliberation that goes into constructing a policy is itself useful, in forcing the reexamination of preconceptions and the clarification of hospital practice. The points made about defining need and potential for benefit, for example, are nothing more than organized common sense. The same may be said, though, about good nursing or hospital administration; and, there is clearly merit in organizing common sense.

Within our deliberations, we tried first to identify and track the relevant points raised about who should have access to this bed, and then to formalize that within a policy. It is fair to ask, "What advantage is there in having such a policy? Isn't the proposed policy the same old considerations, dressed up so they will appear decent in public?" The objection ignores what may be the chief advantage a policy statement may offer. By definition, the allocation of scarce resources involves conflict, often expressed in interpersonal tension or intrapersonal ambivalence. In the heat of a situation, some principles of choice that had earlier been rejected become appealing once again; others, that had in a calmer moment proven fair, may be forgotten. It is then that a policy is most needed.[16]

The role of philosophy in formulating these sorts of policies is worthy of further thought. In this case, it was most useful playing a critical rather than constructive role, showing that some ideas such as the right of a patient to be treated on air support or the entitlement to continuing treatment were spurious. It might be pleasing to think that the cure for philosophy is more (and better) philosophy; less happy is the thought that the final cure for philosophy might be no philosophy at all.

Yet it seems to us that this criticism asks too much of philosophy. The yearning for constructive principles ultimately rests on the idea that there are right answers to the distribution of scarce resources that philosophy should discover or validate. This may be too much to hope for. Perhaps all that can be done is to eliminate the wrong responses, leaving discretionary choice within a range of equally justified, yet equally problematic answers.

Acknowledgements

The authors appreciate the assistance provided by Charles Kaplan, Director of Finance, Jewish General Hospital, and Patricia Rawlings, Quality Assurance Coordinator, JGH.

Notes

1. C. Van Ness and C.A. Sacramento, "The Implementation of a Quality Assurance Study and Program to Reduce the Incidence of Hospital Acquired Pressure Ulcers," *Journal of Enterosotomal Therapy* 16, no. 2 (1989): 61–64.

2. J. Scales, "Pressure Sore Prevention," *Care Science and Practice* 1 (June 1982): 9–17.

3. J.T. Scales, H.F. Lunn, PA. Leneid, et al., "The Prevention and Treatment of Pressure Sores Using Air Support Systems," *Paraplegia* 12 (August 1974): 118–31.

4. Scales, "Pressure Sore Prevention."

5. Whether these beds would continue to play a necessary role even when optimal nursing care is provided is a matter of professional dispute. See B.L. Moody, J.E. Fanale, M. Thompson, et al., "Impact of Staff Education on Pressure Sore Development in Elderly Hospitalized Patients," *Archives of Internal Medicine* 148 (October 1988): 2241–43.

6. Information on prices as of summer 1990 was provided by the sales office of Kinetic Concepts Inc., whose help is gratefully acknowledged.

7. R. Dolezal, M. Cohen, and R. Schultz, "The Use of Clinitron Therapy Unit in the Immediate Postoperative Care of Pressure Ulcers," *Annals of Plastic Surgery* 14 (January 1985): 36.

8. J.D. Shea, "Pressure Sores: Classification and Management," *Clinical Orthopedics* 112 (1975): 89–100; R. Bennett, M.F. Bettantoni, and J. Ouslander, "Air Fluidized Bed Treatment of Nursing Home Patients with Pressure Sores," *Journal of the American Geriatrics Society* 37, no. 3 (1989): 235–42.

9. R.M. Allman, J. Walker, M. Hart, and C. Laprade, "Air-Fluidized Beds or Conventional Therapy for Pressure Sores: A Randomized Trial," *Annals of Internal Medicine* 107, no. 5 (1987): 641–48. For a contrary view see Bennett, Bettantoni, and Ouslander, "Air Fluidized Bed Treatment."

10. *Statutes of Canada,* "Medical Care Act."

11. See, for example, discussion in H.T. Engelhardt, Jr., *The Foundations of Bioethics* (New York: Oxford University Press, 1986), chap. 8.

12. Were the hospital in the position of a closed system, the sole supplier of service to members of the catchment area, presumably emergency services would definitely trump alternative hospital services. That condition is not present for JGH, which is, for example, permitted to impose an ambulance ban when its allocated emergency services are overloaded, resulting in patients being sent to other hospitals in the Montreal municipal community.

13. J. Rawls, *A Theory of Justice* (Cambridge, MA: Harvard University Press, 1971); R. Green, "Health Care Justice in Contract Theory Perspective," in *Ethics and Health Policy,* ed. R. Veatch and R. Branson (Cambridge, MA: Ballinger, 1976); N. Daniels, "Health Care Needs and Distributive Justice," *Philosophy and Public Affairs* 10, no. 2 (1981): 146–79.

14. President's Commission for the Study of Ethical Problems in Medicine and Biomedical and Behavioral Research, *Decisions to Forgo Life-Sustaining Treatment* (Washington, DC: Government Printing Office, 1983); G. Povar, "Withdrawing and Withholding Therapy: Putting Ethics into Practice," *Journal of Clinical Ethics* 1 (Spring 1990): 50–56; J. Burden, B. Freedman, A. Gelb, "Ethical and Family Management Problems in the Intensive Care Unit—An Illustrative Case," *Canadian Journal of Anaesthesia* 34, no. 3 (1987–1988): 274–79.

15. Shea, "Pressure Sores."

16. B. Freedman, "The Last Bed in the ICU," in *Cases in Bioethics,* ed. C. Levine (New York: St. Martin's Press, 1989), 229–31.

Responsibility and Priority in Liver Transplantation

Walter Glannon

In a provocative 1991 paper, Alvin Moss and Mark Siegler argued that it may be fair to give individuals with alcohol-related end-stage liver disease (ARESLD) lower priority for a liver transplant than those who develop end-stage liver disease (ESLD) from other factors.[1] Like other organs, there is a substantial gap between the available livers for transplantation and the number of people who need liver transplants. Yet, unlike those with end-stage renal disease, who can survive for some time on dialysis before receiving a kidney transplant, those with liver failure will die without a liver transplant. This makes transplantable livers an absolutely scarce resource. As Moss and Siegler claimed, this absolute scarcity "mandates that distribution be based on unusually rigorous standards."[2] At the time they published their paper, they noted that, "in liver transplantation, ARESLD causes more than 50% of the cases of ESLD."[3] They also emphasized that, unlike most diseases, where a causal connection between behavior and a disease is difficult to establish, chronic drinking is a cause of cirrhosis and liver failure.

More recent data show that alcoholic liver disease is the principal diagnosis of 22.1% of liver transplant recipients in the United States, 16.6% in Canada, and 19.9% in the United Kingdom.[4] The figure from the United Kingdom is the highest among recipients there, and it is the second highest (after hepatitis C cirrhosis) in the United States and Canada. So those with ARESLD constitute a significant percentage of all those needing a liver transplant.

We can distinguish individuals with ARESLD from individuals who develop ESLD due to factors beyond their control. The second group includes individuals with congenital biliary atresia, congenital polycystic liver disease, primary biliary cirrhosis, and primary sclerosing cholangitis. In these cases, there is no causal connection between an individual's behavior and the development of liver disease. Because they have no control over the condition, it would be unfair not to give them equal access to a liver transplant. But it may be fair to give lower transplant priority to those with ARESLD. Genetics and social factors may influence a person's behavior, including chronic drinking. However, these factors do not causally determine but underdetermine the outcome of ARESLD. In most cases, an alcoholic's behavior cannot be explained away entirely by genetics or the environment. One may have enough control over one's behavior to play a significant causal role in bringing about liver failure.

I argue for the weaker claim that individuals with ARESLD may be given lower priority for a liver transplant. I defend this claim even if those with ARESLD have transplant outcomes at least as good as those with the conditions I mentioned above. The stronger claim that they should be excluded from transplants is not warranted because it may not be the case that their behavior alone causally determines the outcome. What justifies giving them lower priority for a liver transplant is that they are not only causally but also morally responsible for liver failure. They are causally responsible for this outcome to the extent that they were able but failed to behave in a way that would have prevented it. They are morally responsible because, by having but failing to exercise control over their behavior, they acted negligently and failed to discharge a duty that we owe to others in society. This is the duty to act in such a way as not to increase competition for a scarce life-saving resource. That ARESLD

Glannon, W, "Responsibility and Priority in Liver Transplantation", *Cambridge Quarterly of Health Care Ethics* 18(1), pp. 23–36. Reproduced with permission.

is a preventable outcome for which one can be causally and morally responsible is a reasonable social expectation. It is based on the idea that most of us are capable of acting voluntarily and of knowing the causal connection between chronic drinking and liver failure. The normative claim of moral responsibility rests on the empirical claim of causal responsibility.

Following Robert Veatch, I argue that responsibility for ARESLD can be a "tiebreaker" in liver allocation decisions.[5] This translates into a slight reduction in one's place on the transplant wait list. When two individuals are in equal need of a liver transplant and have an equal chance of a good transplant outcome, responsibility for liver failure can justify giving one person lower priority than the other. My main concern is to give principled reasons for saying that some may have a weaker claim to a scarce life-saving resource than others and that it may be fair to treat people unequally in this regard.

Fairness consists in giving people what they deserve. Intuitively, fairness means that priority for medical treatment should be given to those with the greatest medical needs. But when a medical resource is scarce, whether or to what extent one deserves to receive that resource may depend on how the medical need for it developed. One may be less deserving of that resource and have a weaker claim to it the more control one has over the development of the need. On these grounds, fairness means meeting people's needs in proportion to the strength of their claims to have these needs met. Those who develop diseases they could have prevented have a weaker claim to receive treatment for them. Insofar as ARESLD is a preventable disease, it may be fair to give those with this disease lower priority for a liver transplant than others whose need for a transplant results from factors beyond their control.

CAUSAL AND MORAL RESPONSIBILITY

The argument for responsibility is not an argument about character. It is not about assessing a person in terms of virtue or vice, or the idea that "good" organs should not go to "bad" people. Instead, the argument focuses on the outcome of chronic drinking as one type of action. Daniel Brudney calls this argument "The Principle." In discussing a fictional person "Jane" with ARESLD, Brudney rightly points out that "The Principle does not assert that drinking is *malum in se*. Its focus is on the consequences of Jane's conduct, not on whether that conduct was intrinsically good or bad. If drinking did not destroy livers, Jane's drinking would not trigger the Principle."[6] Although a convicted criminal has waived his or her right to liberty, their criminal behavior theoretically would not imply a weaker claim to an organ transplant unless it causally contributed to their organ failure. Whether one has a weaker claim to and lower priority for a liver transplant depends on the relevant sort of behavior. My argument for responsibility applies only in cases where (1) there is an established causal connection between a particular type of voluntary behavior and a consequence of that behavior, (2) one is capable of knowing that the behavior can lead to that consequence, and (3) where there is absolute scarcity of the good in question—transplantable livers. I do not argue that people should be given lower priority when they have conditions for which treatment is not absolutely scarce and where there is no established causal connection between voluntary behavior and the condition in question. This preempts a "slippery slope" argument that might be extended to other areas of healthcare.

A person can be causally responsible for an outcome when it falls within the knowable risk of certain behavior. We need to distinguish between different types of behavior and their normative significance. Some types of risk-entailing behavior are supported by social expectations. Policing and firefighting fall within this category. Because we expect them to engage in behaviour that poses a risk to their health and lives in order to protect the public, police and firefighters are not penalized for their behavior if they develop health problems as a result of it.[7] Chronic drinking leading to alcoholism and ARESLD is significantly different from police and fire protection because the risk entailed by chronic drinking does not conform to but conflicts with social expectations.

We can spell out the argument for responsibility for ARESLD in five steps:

1. If person A is causally and morally responsible for ARESLD, then A has a weaker claim to and should have lower priority for a liver transplant than person B, who develops end-stage liver disease through no fault of his or her own.
2. A is causally responsible for ARESLD when the disease is causally sensitive to chronic drinking, chronic drinking is sufficiently voluntary, and he or she has the capacity to know that chronic drinking entails a risk of liver failure.
3. A is morally responsible for ARESLD when he or she is causally responsible for it and when he or she is negligent for failing to act on the knowledge that chronic drinking can lead to ARESLD and increased competition for scarce transplantable livers.
4. A is causally and morally responsible for ARESLD.
5. A has a weaker claim to and should have lower priority for a liver transplant than B.

Causal sensitivity can be formulated in counterfactual terms. An outcome is causally sensitive to behavior when that outcome would not have occurred but for the behavior. Causal responsibility presupposes causal control, which consists of voluntariness in one's behavior and knowledge of the probable consequences of that behavior. Each of these volitional and epistemic components of causal control is a capacity that one may or may not exercise in all instances. The normative content in the claim about moral responsibility in (3) rests on social expectations about how people ought to behave toward each other. It rests on social expectations against behavior that increases competition for scarce resources such as transplantable livers.

VOLUNTARINESS

A person behaves voluntarily when he or she is not coerced or compelled to act against the desires and intentions that form his or her motivational states. Coercion and compulsion can impair or undermine voluntariness by interfering with a person's capacity to respond to reasons for or against certain actions. Voluntariness is equivalent to autonomy. A person behaves autonomously when he or she is capable of critically reflecting on and responding to these reasons by acting on or refraining from acting on them.[8] In particular, autonomy requires the capacity to resist the desire to engage in chronic drinking as something contrary to one's best interests and the best reasons for action. Individuals with severe psychiatric conditions such as schizophrenia may not satisfy the criteria of voluntariness, because these conditions are likely to undermine the capacity to control their desires, beliefs, choices, and actions. Accordingly, we can exclude these individuals from judgments of responsibility for their health.

Carl Cohen and Martin Benjamin claim that the voluntariness condition necessary for responsibility in the case at hand cannot be met, because external factors beyond one's control will influence one's behavior and its outcomes.[9] Yet this involves a mistaken inference from the claim that genetic and environmental factors can *influence* one's behavior to the claim that these factors *determine* one's behavior. It is mistaken because, in most cases of ARESLD, the outcome is causally sensitive to one's choices that are not coerced or compelled by external or internal forces. As noted, responsibility for an outcome requires only that the outcome be causally sensitive to one's autonomous choices and actions. It does not require that it be causally sensitive *only* to one's actions and not to any other factors. Genetics and the environment may causally influence but do not causally determine one's choices and actions, in the sense that one could not have chosen and acted otherwise. This is what I meant in saying that one's choices need only be sufficiently voluntary. It allows enough room for the person to causally contribute to and be causally responsible for that outcome. ...

In the early 1990s, researchers discovered an association between the A1 allele of the dopamine D2 receptor gene and alcoholism.[10] More recent search has further clarified the genetic factors alcohol addiction.[11] The research in molecular genetics suggests that people with this allele are more susceptible to developing alcoholism than others who do not have it. But from the fact that a person has a disease with a genetic component, it does not follow that one has no control over and cannot be causally responsible for developing the disease. A gene that makes one susceptible to alcoholism only indicates a higher probability of developing the disease, not that the gene by itself causally determines the disease. At least some of an alcoholic's choices would be a function of his or her own motivational states.

…Simply saying that genetics or a difficult social upbringing predisposes one to alcoholism is not enough to prove that an alcoholic is forced to act against his or her will and therefore cannot alter his or her behavior to prevent liver failure and the need for a liver transplant. Like other addictions, it is presumed that alcoholism undermines voluntariness by compelling one to act against one's considered desires and best interests. Chronic drinking alters brain pathways that ordinarily mediate the desire to drink, converting desire into craving and compulsion. If one accepts this, then one might claim that alcoholics cannot be responsible for developing liver failure because they lack sufficient control over this outcome.

We need to separate two stages of addiction: how one develops it, and how one behaves once one becomes addicted to a particular substance. Addictions usually develop from taking a particular substance repeatedly over time. Taking cocaine, nicotine, or alcohol repeatedly perturbs the dopamine system that regulates the "high" and craving characteristic of addictions. This perturbation makes the system adapt by making dopamine less effective in the relevant brain receptors. Once these receptors assume this defensive maneuver and become less responsive, they are left without normal levels of this neurotransmitter. These changes in the dopamine system cause a person to crave more of the drug. Addiction becomes established as dopamine dependence and produces chronic unpleasant feelings, which triggers the desire to take more

of the drug to feel better.[12] But having an addiction does not explain why a person first takes the substance that results in the addiction. If one is not compelled to begin drinking by genetic or environmental factors beyond one's control, and if one is not so cognitively disabled or immature as not to be capable of knowing the probable addictive consequences of chronic drinking, then one can be responsible for the addiction, as well as for the liver failure that may result from it. The history of how this condition came about may involve enough control for a person to be causally responsible for the addiction and subsequent liver failure.

The fact that many addicts give up their addictions voluntarily shows that the desire for the addictive substance does not always compel an addict to act and does not always undermine autonomy. This suggests that addicts have some degree of control over their behavior. The typical addict goes through withdrawal several or more times. Some deliberately abstain for prolonged periods in order to lower their tolerance for the drug and thereby decrease their need for the high. To the extent that addicts can structure their environment so that the cues that remind them of the drug are absent, they can exercise some restraint over their craving for that drug.[13] The literature on consumptive behavior indicates that compulsions do not explain why addicts exponentially discount the future in taking a substance. They prefer consumption of the drug now and abstention only later.[14] The addict chooses what he or she prefers at the moment, even though the choice is not in his or her long-term best interests. Choosing consumption over abstention does not mean that the addict chooses against his or her will. It is an imprudent, irrational choice, but as such is not a sign of compulsive behavior and not an unfree choice. Thus an addict may be responsible for this choice.…

EPISTEMIC FACTORS

I have claimed that an epistemic condition is necessary in addition to a voluntariness condition to establish causal and moral responsibility for ARESLD. One must have the capacity to know that chronic drinking can result in liver failure and the need for an organ transplant. One must also have the capacity to know that such a claim would increase competition for a scare life-saving resource. Assuming that one has this epistemic capacity, that one's behavior is sufficiently voluntary, and that liver failure is causally sensitive to this behavior, it can be fair to give one lower priority for a liver transplant.

Alcoholics appear to discount the future in the same way other addicts do. But temporal discounting does not excuse one from responsibility for the future consequences of one's voluntary actions....If one is responsible for excessive drinking at an earlier time and is capable of knowing that this behavior entails a risk of developing end-stage liver disease at a later time, then one can be causally responsible for this outcome. Further, if one is causally responsible for ARESLD and knows that chronic drinking and ARESLD can result in a claim to an absolutely scarce life-saving organ and increase competition for it, then one acted negligently and as such is morally responsible for ARESLD. The combination of causal and moral responsibility can give one a weaker claim to a liver transplant.

Brudney argues that this judgment would not be fair to one with ARESLD unless there were a condition of advance notice that excessive chronic drinking could result in a weaker claim to a transplant.[15] He asserts that this "fair warning" condition is necessary because lower priority in this case is functionally equivalent to punishment with a potentially grave consequence. Brudney argues that, because this condition has not been met, the cases in which we could justifiably say that some people are less deserving than others for a liver transplant would be rare.

This argument may have had considerable force 20 years ago. But the connection between chronic drinking and liver failure has been common knowledge for some time. Thanks to the media and public education about health, most people are capable of knowing the risk of their behavior on health outcomes. In particular, most people are capable of knowing that chronic drinking for a period of 10–20 years entails a significant risk of liver failure. They are also capable of knowing that there is a significant gap between the availability of and need for transplantable livers. It would not be unreasonable to expect any competent person to infer from this that behavior resulting in liver failure would increase the number of claims to a limited number of liver transplants. A person who voluntarily engaged in chronic consumption of alcohol and who was capable of knowing the risk of developing liver failure from it would be negligently engaging in conduct that increased competition for transplantable livers. We owe it to each other as social beings to try to avoid this situation. Contrary to what Brudney claims, the cases in which it would be fair to give one lower priority for a liver transplant on the basis of knowledge of the link between drinking and liver failure would not be so rare.

. . .

SUBSTANTIVE RESPONSIBILITY

Many would say that this policy is punitive. It is punitive to give some people lower priority than others with an equal need for a scarce life-saving resource. Let us suppose that it is punitive. The question is whether it is justifiably punitive. The discussion thus far rests on the idea that, even if this policy is punitive, it does not always involve punishing the "victim." Those who can control and are responsible for their actions and their consequences are not victims of them. This reasoning applies to those who are causally responsible for developing diseases they could have prevented as well as to those who are responsible for failing to take steps to control diseases once they have them. We can appeal to Thomas Scanlon's conception of social responsibility for support of the view that it may be fair to give alcoholics with ARESLD lower priority and a weaker claim to a liver transplant.

What Scanlon calls "substantive responsibility" means that, when one is deemed responsible for a certain outcome, "that person cannot complain of the burdens or obligations that result."[16] Although Scanlon does not discuss it, the burden in question here is a weaker claim to a liver transplant. This type of responsibility involves "substantive conclusions of what we owe to each other."[17] For present purposes, the content of this obligation is preventing behavior whose consequences will increase claims on and competition for a scarce life-saving resource. Scanlon's notion of substantive responsibility rests on what he calls the "value of choice," or the ability to choose between alternatives. More specifically, "when a person could have avoided a certain result by choosing appropriately, this fact weakens her grounds for rejecting a principle that would make her bear the burden of that result."[18] For Scanlon, what makes a moral principle justifiable is that it is a principle that no moral agent could reasonably reject. What one could not reasonably reject would be a principle whereby a person deemed causally and morally responsible for liver failure could be given lower priority for a liver transplant. If this person could not reasonably reject and justifiably complain against this principle, then it would not be unfair.

...

LUCK AND THE DOCTOR–PATIENT RELATIONSHIP

Another challenge to the position I am defending appeals to the notion of moral luck in holding some but not other people responsible for an outcome that occurs as a matter of chance. Consider the following hypothetical case. Person A drinks as much alcohol as person B. A's liver is unaffected by his chronic drinking, whereas B develops cirrhosis and liver failure, due, in part, to genetic differences between them. It seems a matter of luck that A does not and B does develop liver failure. Therefore it seems unfair to penalize B by giving him lower priority than others who need a liver transplant. If drinking played no causal role in B's liver failure, then it would indeed be unfair to give him lower priority than others in need of a transplant. However, if B's drinking did play such a role, then his disease would have fallen within the knowable risk of his drinking. If he was capable

of knowing this risk, then he would have cognitive control over the sequence of events resulting in his need for a transplant. A person's knowledge of what risky behavior entails enables him or her to influence the probability of developing a condition such as liver failure by engaging in or avoiding the behavior. It would not be entirely a matter of luck, and, accordingly, it would not be unfair to give that person a weaker claim to a liver transplant.

This is a situation in which A and B play a type of lottery by engaging in risk-entailing behavior. As such, their behavior leaves something to chance.[19] If A drinks and does not develop liver failure, then he wins the lottery. If B drinks and develops liver failure, then he loses the lottery. But it is not entirely up to chance. Provided that B's choices are voluntary, that the outcome is causally sensitive to these choices, and that he has the capacity to know what the outcome might be, B has some causal control over and can be responsible for the outcome. In this regard, it would not be unfair to give B lower priority than others for a liver transplant. What *does* seem unfair is to deny a transplant to individuals who lack the social support to ensure adherence to immunosuppressive drugs following transplantation. Individuals can be excluded from transplants for this reason. Yet it is entirely a matter of luck whether they have or lack the social support to ensure a successful outcome. It is entirely beyond their control, which intuitively seems more punitive than giving people with at least some volitional and epistemic control over ARESLD lower priority for a transplant.

Some might object that adopting the principle I have defended would mean that doctors could deny life-saving treatments to patients. Yet the issue of whether responsibility should be a criterion in the allocation of scarce medical resources is not limited to but goes beyond the doctor–patient relationship. Doctors have duties to society as well as to patients. They are part of an expansive system of healthcare that has to be managed responsibly. Doctors have to be good stewards of that system and not just practitioners working with individual patients. The question of how a scarce resource can be allocated fairly requires a deliberative process that involves not only physicians and their patients but also society at large. In the United States, UNOS and regional transplant agencies play a critical role in allocation decisions, and these decisions are made by a broad range of healthcare professionals with public input. Decisions about how public goods such as transplantable livers should be allocated are social decisions. The practice of medicine, including organ transplantation, cannot be divorced from the broader social network that influences how it is practiced. Questions about priority in access to organ transplant pertain not only to the relationship between the patient and the doctor but also to the relationship between the patient and society.

Autonomy and responsibility are mutually entailing concepts. Autonomy involves the capacity to take responsibility for one's choices, actions, and their consequences. Responsibility for choices, actions, and their consequences presupposes autonomy. To say that people cannot be responsible for ARESLD because alcoholism is a disease threatens to separate autonomy from responsibility. If people can make autonomous choices about lifestyle that have adverse health consequences, then they can be responsible for these consequences, even if they include serious diseases. People can make imprudent choices that are nonetheless autonomous and for which they can be responsible. To say that people cannot be responsible for their health risks a return to paternalism and the idea that people are incapable of knowing what is in their best interests and taking responsibility for what they do. If we are to uphold autonomy, then we must also uphold personal responsibility for the health consequences of our autonomous choices.

...

CONCLUSION

In most cases, individuals with ARESLD have sufficient control over their behavior to be causally responsible for their condition. They may be morally responsible for ARESLD if they act negligently by failing to prevent this outcome

and increasing competition for scarce transplantable livers. This can justify giving them lower priority for a liver transplant. "Most cases" leaves open the possibility that some individuals who drink may not have the requisite control over their behavior and thus may not be responsible for alcoholism and its consequences. There may be extenuating environmental factors that would effectively constitute a form of coercion or compulsion and thus undermine control and excuse individuals from responsibility for liver failure. People living in extreme poverty or extreme social isolation might fall within this category.... The onus is on those claiming that lower priority would be unfair to some people with liver failure to show that these responsibility-undermining factors are present. They would have to argue that one's actions are not sufficiently voluntary and that one does not have the capacity to know the medical and social consequences of chronic drinking. The arguments that have been advanced for this position have not been persuasive.

If we affirm the interdependence of autonomy and responsibility, then we can be responsible for a disease we contract when we are able but fail to exercise control over the events that cause the disease. This may mean giving lower priority to some people regarding claims to scarce life-saving medical resources such as transplantable livers. But provided that these decisions are based on a clearly defined and reasonable conception of causal and moral responsibility, it may be fair to treat people unequally on these grounds.

Notes

1. Moss A, Siegler M. Should alcoholics compete equally for liver transplantation? *JAMA* 1991;265: 1295–8.
2. See note 1, Moss, Siegler 1991:1296.
3. See note 1, Moss, Siegler 1991:1296.
4. Stell D, McAlister V, Thorburn D. A comparison of disease severity and survival rates after liver transplantation in the United Kingdom, Canada, and the United States. *Liver Transplantation* 2004;10:898–902, at p. 900.
5. Veatch R. *Transplantation Ethics.* Washington, DC: Georgetown University Press; 2000:311–21.

6. Brudney D. Are alcoholics less deserving of liver transplants? *Hastings Center Report* 2007;37:41–7, at p. 42.

7. Veatch R. Voluntary risks to health: The ethical issues. *JAMA* 1980;243:50–5; see note 5, Veatch 2000.

8. See Fischer JM, Ravizza M. *Responsibility and Control: A Theory of Moral Responsibility.* New York: Cambridge University Press; 1998:62–91.

9. Cohen C, Benjamin M. Alcoholics and liver transplantation. *JAMA* 1991;265:1299–301; see also Benjamin M. Transplantation for alcoholic liver disease: The ethical issues. *Liver Transplantation and Surgery* 1997;3:337–42.

10. Blum K, Noble EP, Sheridan PJ, Montgomery A, Ritchie T, Jagadeeswaran P, et al. Allelic association of human dopamine D2 receptor gene in alcoholism. *JAMA* 1990;263:2055–60.

11. Young R, Lawford BR, Nutting A, Noble EP. Advances in molecular genetics and the prevention and treatment of substance misuse: Implications of association studies of the A1 allele of the D2 dopamine receptor gene. *Addictive Behaviors* 2004;29:1275–94.

12. For discussion of the pathophysiology of addiction, see Ahmed S. Addiction as compulsive reward prediction. *Science* 2004;306:1901–2;

Kalivas P, Volkow N. The neural basis of addiction. *American Journal of Psychiatry* 2005;162:1403–13; Hyman S. The neurobiology of addiction: Implications for voluntary control of behavior. *American Journal of Bioethics—AJOB Neuroscience* 2007;7:8–11.

13. Neil Levy makes these points in Levy N. Autonomy and addiction. *Canadian Journal of Philosophy* 2006;36:427–47.

14. See note 14, Levy 2006:433–37; see also Ainslie G. A research-based theory of addictive motivation. *Law and Philosophy* 2000;19:77–115; Ainslie G. *Breakdown of Will.* Cambridge: Cambridge University Press; 2001; Loewenstein G. Willpower: A decision theorist's perspective. *Law and Philosophy* 2000;19:51–76; Elster J. *Strong Feelings: Emotion, Addiction and Human Behavior.* Cambridge, MA: MIT Press; 1999.

15. See note 6, Brudney 2007:44.

16. Scanlon T. *What We Owe to Each Other.* Cambridge, MA: Harvard University Press; 1998:248.

17. See note 25, Scanlon 1998:248, 290.

18. See note 25, Scanlon 1998:256.

19. David Lewis proposed this idea in Lewis D. The Punishment That Leaves Something to Chance. *Philosophy & Public Affairs* 1989;18:53–67.

Social Contract Theory and Just Decision Making: Lessons from Genetic Testing for the BRCA Mutations

Bryn Williams-Jones and Michael M. Burgess

The intersection of health insurance coverage and intellectual property arrangements such as patent protection is an international phenomenon. Every health care insurance system, whether private or public, spreads the cost of health care services across a population. The fact that intellectual property protection affects the costs and, therefore, the availability of health care services is relevant to all insurance systems. But unique aspects of culture, politics, and economics shape the responses of various components of a health care insurance system, and local responses are distinguishable from, although not independent of, national and global responses. Thus, the intersection of health

Williams-Jones, Bryn and Michael M. Burgess. "Social Contract Theory and Just Decision Making: Lessons from Genetic Testing for the BRCA Mutations". *Kennedy Institute of Ethics* 14:2 (2004), 115–142. © 2004 The Johns Hopkins University Press. Reprinted with permission of the Johns Hopkins University Press.

care accessibility and intellectual property protection is best studied through examination of a local experience and tracking the relevant influences. The present analysis is based on the doctoral research of one of the authors (Williams-Jones), which entails a close study of one Canadian provincial health insurance system's response to the Myriad Genetics patents and its implications for accessibility (Williams-Jones 2002a).

The majority of Canadians who access genetic services do so through the public health care system, but for those with the means, private purchase also is an option. The rapid expansion of the Internet and the creation of a "global marketplace" have made it possible for Canadians to purchase genetic testing through international sources (Williams-Jones 2003). With an agreement in 2000 between the U.S. biotechnology company Myriad Genetics and the Canadian diagnostic company MDS Laboratory Services, Canadians were able to purchase genetic testing locally for conditions such as hereditary breast or colorectal cancer (Myriad Genetics 2000a & b). This development is not without controversy, and there is ongoing public debate about whether the Canadian health care system should prohibit, permit, or encourage provision of and access to private health care services (Evans 2000; Mazankowski 2001; Romanow 2002).

In the context of genetic testing, the situation is further complicated by gene patents that confer to biotechnology companies controlling rights over genes, mutations, and susceptibility tests.[1] Gene patents can increase the cost of testing and restrict provision to particular licensees (Merz et al. 2002; Williams-Jones 2002b; Cho et al. 2003). Licensees that are private companies have an interest in marketing their products to patients to build demand for testing services (Hull and Prasad 2001; Gollust, Hull, and Wilfond 2002). If successful, marketing stimulates pressure to expand insurance or permit the growth of privately accessible services. In either case, a consequence of increased demand and use of genetic testing is an increased burden on publicly supported ancillary health care services, such as genetic counseling. Patents also may restrict downstream research into better, cheaper, or more accurate tests and therapeutics

(Borger 1999; Knoppers, Hirtle, and Glass 1999; Heller and Eisenberg 1998). The potential costs raise serious concerns for continued expansion of public health care insurance to cover a growing number of genetic tests. The clear challenge to the ability of public health insurance to reduce or eliminate inequities based on access to health care services is a good reason to evaluate the benefits of strong intellectual property protection. It is critical to investigate the potential for restricting access to genetic services outside of the public system, evaluate which services are sufficiently beneficial to warrant coverage as part of public health care insurance, and explore the ethical role of public consultation and accountability in these evaluations. In using the case of BRCA testing in Canada, our intent is not to provide a definitive argument for or against the coverage of BRCA testing as part of public health care insurance, but instead to explore the elements necessary for such a decision-making process to be considered just.

JUSTICE IN ACCESS TO SERVICES AND PRIORITY SETTING

A common objection to access to private health care services is that it is unfair. Health, it is argued, is fundamental to the enjoyment of other important goods, such as the freedom to make life plans about one's career or education, thus it is the responsibility of a just society to ensure that all citizens have access to needed health care.[2] This view is a fundamental tenet of universal public health insurance schemes, namely that citizens should have equal access to needed health care services regardless of ability to pay. Such an egalitarian ethic is enshrined in Canadian legislation: According to the *Canada Health Act* (CHA), citizens are entitled to health insurance that is publicly administered, comprehensive, universal, portable, and accessible (Canada Health Act, R.S. 1985, c. C-6). Health care services covered under the CHA may not be made available for private purchase, and the federal government is empowered to withhold health transfer payments to provinces that permit such private services until those provinces comply with the CHA (Deber et al. 1998).[3]

Provincial legislation in 6 of 10 provinces also prohibits private insurance for medically necessary hospital and physician services (Flood and Archibald 2001).

At first glance, federal and provincial legislation appear to guarantee public provision of all needed health care services and prohibition of private purchase. But these requirements apply only to an agreed upon set of "listed" hospital and physician services (Flood 1999). For "non-listed" services—such as dental care, many reproductive technologies, and most pharmaceuticals used outside hospitals[4] (Giacomini, Hurley, and Stoddart 2000)—commercial provision and private purchase is permitted. Despite the requirements for "comprehensiveness" and "universality" found in the CHA, some beneficial health care services continue not to be publicly insured and so are available only to people with sufficient wealth or private health insurance. In 2002, private spending on health care, including pharmaceuticals, complementary care, dental care, in Canada totaled C$32.9 billion (Canadian Institute for Health Information 2003).

Decision making about resource allocation in the context of public health insurance often occurs in a complex and interest-driven fashion, influenced by a range of social, economic, and political factors (Flood 1999). The *ad hoc* nature of such decision making and the existing uneven distribution of benefits means that injustices occur—some people receive the medical services they need while others do not (Sherwin 1996; Caulfield et al. 2001). Just access to health care might be thought to entail equal access to every needed medical service, but taken literally and especially if "need" is construed broadly, this approach is unworkable. The current political reality is characterized by limited financial resources available for health care and the need to fund other important goods such as social services, education, and public works.

The cost of health care in Western countries continues to increase, in part as a result of pressure from a range of interests, including consumer groups, clinicians, and industry, to introduce new and often expensive medical diagnostics and treatments (Daniels 2001). In Canada, total public health care expenditures (in current dollars) increased from C$9 billion in 1975 to C$79 billion in 2002, corresponding to a rise in percent GDP from 7.3 percent in 1981 to 9.3 percent in 2001 (Canadian Institute for Health Information 2003). Recent budget surpluses and mounting public pressure to reform health care have been met by increased federal government cash transfers to the provinces and a new Health Reform Fund, totaling C$34.8 billion over five years (Department of Finance (Canada) 2003). But even this large investment may not be enough. For example, in the wake of the difficulties in containing the Severe Acute Respiratory Syndrome (SARS) outbreak in February 2003, the Canadian Medical Association (2003) has called for a further C$1.5 billion to address extraordinary health emergencies.

Whatever share of public funds governments spend on health care, the amount still will be insufficient to support all potentially beneficial services.[5] Decisions will be required to determine which services should be funded, and whether and how private purchase of services should be permitted (Evans et al. 2000; Deber et al. 1998; Caulfield et al. 2001). Before discussing how one might make such decisions, it is helpful to explore the issues that arise in the provision of a particular health care service, namely genetic susceptibility testing for hereditary breast and ovarian cancer.

PROVISION OF BRCA TESTING IN CANADA

The discovery and sequencing in the early 1990s of two genes associated with hereditary breast and ovarian cancer (BRCA1 and BRCA2) helped to make possible genetic susceptibility testing for patients to determine their risk status. This information may facilitate life planning, anxiety reduction, and access to specialized surveillance and prevention strategies. Treatments such as prophylactic surgery (Lynch, Lynch, and Rubinstein 2001; Hartmann et al. 2001) and tamoxifen (King et al. 2001) can significantly reduce (but not eliminate) the risk of developing cancer, and access to BRCA testing will be an important part of clinical management (Robson 2002).

In most provinces in Canada, BRCA testing is provided through public health care institutions—such as the Hereditary Cancer Program (HCP) at the B.C. Cancer Agency in Vancouver, British Columbia—as part of coordinated clinical oncology programs. These public programs have guidelines restricting access to patients with risk factors, such as a strong family history (multiple cases of breast or ovarian cancer), early age of onset (pre-menopausal), or membership in a specific ethnic group (e.g., Ashkenazi Jewish, French Canadian) (Carter 2001). Testing is not available to "patients off the street" with little or no family history of disease. But with the granting in 2000 and 2001 of four Canadian patents on the BRCA genes to Myriad Genetics, the continued public provision and control of genetic testing services has been jeopardized.

Myriad licensed MDS Laboratory Services— one of Canada's largest medical diagnostics companies—to be the exclusive Canadian provider of Myriad's patented *BRACAnalysis* test (Myriad Genetics 2000b), and began a campaign to convince Canadian health care institutions to comply with the patents and refer all tests to MDS or Myriad (Canadian Press 2001; Kent 2001a). This move generated strong professional and government opposition across Canada (Williams-Jones 2002b), and only British Columbia complied with Myriad's demands and ceased in-house testing. (Québec performs some mutation testing locally but sends index testing to Myriad for full analysis.)

In the spring of 2001, the B.C. Ministry of Health Services, on advice from legal counsel, informed HCP and the B.C. Cancer Agency that should they wish to continue providing BRCA testing, HCP would have to purchase testing from Myriad out of its existing operating budget. The cost of BRCA testing at HCP is approximately C$1,200 per test (Kent 2001a). The purchase of testing from Myriad at triple the cost—C$3,850/US$2,400 for full sequencing—would quickly exhaust HCP's budget and undermine its ability and mandate to provide services to patients at risk for a variety of hereditary cancer syndromes. HCP halted BRCA testing in July 2001.

By complying with the Canadian BRCA patents, even when other provinces had rejected Myriad's patent claims and continued to provide in-house testing (Eggertson 2002), the B.C. Ministry of Health Services arguably took a stand in favor of protecting intellectual property rights. But given this position, to not then increase funding to HCP to cover the difference in cost of purchasing Myriad's test made the B.C. government complicit in the discontinuation of publicly provided BRCA testing in the province. In effect, the Ministry engaged in *de facto* priority setting, placing IP protection ahead of equitable access and establishing two categories of patients, those who could and those who could not afford the test. In February 2003, the B.C. Minister of Health Services authorized the resumption of in-house BRCA testing, in line with a reversal of the government's position on gene patenting. According to the Minister: "B.C. women and other future patients have a right to all the information they need to stay healthy. It is completely unethical to use patents based on genetic sequencing to block patients' access to their own genetic information, particularly when we already have the knowledge, ability and equipment to provide women with this information" (British Columbia Ministry of Health Services 2003). The Minister also called on the federal government to follow the lead of countries such as France and the Netherlands and oppose the Myriad patents, and to review the patenting of DNA more generally.

At the national level—and strictly speaking in contravention of the *Canada Health Act*— patients, for a period of two years, were treated differently depending on the province where they lived. Although this may be a somewhat inevitable feature of a provincially managed national health insurance system, the financial basis for the discrepancy and the establishment of two groups of patients within the province is an injustice. Since the Canada Health Act is the relevant social contract for fair distribution of health services, it is worth exploring how a social contract can be renegotiated or enforced.

SOCIAL CONTRACT THEORY

One approach to deliberating about fair allocation of health care resources is social contract theory, most notably elucidated in John Rawls's (1971) *A Theory of Justice,* in which society is organized in accordance with mutually beneficial principles of justice. We can adapt Rawls's approach to imagine how a group of rational, self-interested decision makers would develop principles for a just health care system. These decision makers, in an ideal bargaining situation, do not know their current or future positions in society—e.g., social class, education, health status and needs—and can be trusted not to pursue their own interests at the expense of others. Of a range of principles that such decision makers might identify, Norman Daniels's version of the equality of opportunity principle has achieved some prominence in theorizing about just health care and priority setting (Daniels 1985, 2001).

Equality of Opportunity

The principle of equality of opportunity is rooted in a conception of justice that focuses on the creation of a "fair or level playing field" and requires not only the elimination of discrimination, but also efforts to ameliorate social factors that limit opportunity. Poverty and lack of education, as well as illness and disease, can have profound negative consequences for people's ability to pursue their life goals freely. One purpose of providing health care (or social assistance or public education) is to help people have a fair chance at pursuing their life goals and objectives so they can participate as full members of society (Daniels 1985; Sherwin 1996). A just society, then, should "remove the barriers to opportunity that are due to disease" (Buchanan et al. 2000,

p. 16) through the provision of health care, so that people who are disadvantaged can become normally functioning members of society.

The principle of equality of opportunity provides a strong basis for an entitlement to health care, something that most Canadians support, but does not imply the unrealistic claim to all possible health care services. In using this principle as part of resource allocation decision-making processes about public health care services, one would support only those services that effectively help individuals maintain their health; other services could reasonably be denied public funding, although this would not necessarily restrict private purchase.

...

Accountability for Reasonableness

Equality of opportunity may be a sufficiently robust principle for Daniels, but he also is concerned that in a pluralistic liberal democratic society, there will be differing views of what should constitute the substantive principles of justice for health care decision making. In collaboration with James Sabin, Daniels proposes a procedural approach to just decision making that is open to a wider range of principles and reasoning and is publicly accountable. Specifically, decision-making processes should be "accountable for reasonableness" and based on appeals to reasons that are "not only ... publicly available, but [also] those that 'fair-minded' people can agree are relevant to pursuing appropriate patient care under necessary resource constraints" (Daniels and Sabin 1998, p. 51). Four conditions must be met for a process to be accountable for reasonableness: (1) Publicity: Rationales for coverage of new technologies must be transparent and publicly accessible; (2) Relevance: Rationales must be reasonable, that is based on appeals to evidence or principles that fair-minded parties accept as relevant; (3) Appeals: There must be mechanisms for challenges, ongoing review, and revision of decisions as new information develops or the context changes; and (4) Enforcement: Decision-making processes must be publicly regulated to ensure that the first three conditions are met (Daniels and Sabin 1998, p. 57).

By grounding decision-making processes on accountability for reasonableness, Daniels and Sabin explicitly invoke a rationalist, expert-driven model. Decision makers must be "fair minded" and willing to reason openly, seek mutually acceptable rules to narrow and resolve disagreements, and aim for the common good. The hope of this procedural justice approach to decision making is that even if a particular priority-setting decision does not please all stakeholders, such as particular groups of patients, it still will have been arrived at in a manner that is open, transparent, and based on sound reasoning that is publicly accountable. Patients who are excluded from care need to know that their exclusion is reasonable and not the result of arbitrary cost-cutting decisions.

Daniels and Sabin hope that patients and clinicians will judge such a transparent and publicly accountable process to be fair and acceptable. However, they acknowledge that a decision-making process that is accountable for reasonableness—i.e., meets their four conditions—does not supplant the need for broader public democratic deliberation about the overall goals and objectives of public health care. Instead, decisions resulting from such a process should become part of larger democratic public deliberation. In the following section, we apply the concepts of equality of opportunity and accountability for reasonableness to the case of BRCA testing in Canada's national health insurance system and explore the types of information, reasons, and principles that are needed to evaluate whether this service should be covered by public health care insurance.

RATIONALES FOR COVERAGE OF BRCA TESTING

Prevalence & Test Accuracy

In 2003, an estimated 21,200 Canadian women were diagnosed with breast cancer—a cumulative lifetime risk of 1 in 9—with 5,300 women predicted to die from the disease (Canadian Cancer Society 2003). Of these women, only 5 to 10 percent are likely to have inherited an allele associated with increased risk of developing the disease (Szabo and King 1997; Carter 2001; Narod 2002). Mutations in the BRCA1 and BRCA2 genes have been strongly associated with hereditary breast cancer, conveying a cumulative lifetime risk of 40 to 85 percent for breast cancer, and 16 to 40 percent for ovarian cancer, depending on the mutation and one's family history (Carter 2001).[6] But even for very accurate testing methods, only 20 to 25 percent of patients with a strong family history—e.g., early age of onset or multiple affected family members—will have a positive BRCA mutation; a 2002 study by researchers at Myriad Genetics detected BRCA mutations in only 17.2 percent of 10,000 individuals (of whom 5,503 indicated a personal history of breast or ovarian cancer) analyzed over a 3–year period (Frank et al. 2002).

In other words, for 75 to 80 percent of breast cancer patients, the heritable component of their cancers remains unknown. There are almost certainly other, yet to be discovered, genes that affect breast cancer risk in families negative for BRCA mutations.... Social and environmental factors clearly also influence the risk of developing breast cancer (Narod 2002). Interpretation of test results, thus, is closely tied to a detailed evaluation of the patient's family history, so BRCA testing is not a useful screening test for the general population. Most people without a family history of cancer will not have any detectable BRCA mutations. The test will provide clinically relevant information only to those people with a strong family history of breast cancer and where the family mutation is found (in an index case) and can then be used to determine occurrence of the mutation in other family members. However, for most people with a strong family history of the disease, no family mutation will be identified (the heritable component remains unknown) and thus the tests results will be "uninformative"—these people remain at high risk based on their family histories.

Benefits & Costs

Patients with a family history of hereditary breast cancer live with the anxiety of being at risk, as well as the objective risk of developing the disease. They may have to undergo regular high-risk screening, care for affected family members, and deal with the personal trauma of early disease onset as well as the death of family members from the disease. Living with this condition in one's family may seriously compromise an individual's (and family members') equality of opportunity. Studies of families at risk for hereditary cancers, such as breast, ovarian, or colorectal cancers, show that even in the absence of cures, access to genetic testing information can be extremely important for a variety of psychosocial reasons (Prospero et al. 2001; Hutson 2003). Genetic information may be used to facilitate life planning, to initiate family discussions of issues such as social and psychological support, guilt, and responsibility for other family members (Burgess and d'Agincourt-Canning 2002), or to help people make changes in career plans.

A strong family history by itself should be sufficient to initiate regular monitoring—as well as counseling and other support services—as part of high risk cancer screening clinics. A positive result from BRCA testing—i.e., a result that indicates a deleterious mutation—will confirm a patient's putative high-risk status and may convince some physicians to monitor patients with a family history more aggressively (d'Agincourt-Canning 2003). This, in turn, may facilitate access to other health care services that can significantly reduce a patient's risk of developing the disease, such as preventative drug therapies or prophylactic measures (Lynch, Lynch, and Rubinstein 2001; Hartmann et al. 2001; King et al. 2001), and have a positive effect on risk-reduction behavior and earlier diagnosis of tumors (Scheuer et al. 2002). Although some patients who receive negative test results are not reassured, those patients found not to have the identified family mutation are considered

to be no longer at high risk—i.e., they have the same background risk as the general population—and thus can avoid frequent, expensive, and unpleasant monitoring. BRCA testing thus can be an important means of helping at-risk families to have more normal lives and access to a fair range of opportunities.

However, although genetic testing for hereditary breast cancer appears to provide tangible clinical results, it also can have negative physical, social, and psychological sequelae. Drug treatments or prophylactic surgery are not cures and may be difficult to apply given insufficient knowledge concerning the optimum time to undergo surgery or the desirability or length of time for using tamoxifen in particular populations—e.g., childless women or women with early/late menarche (Narod 2002). Positive test results may lead to fatalistic attitudes about developing cancer or increase fear and anxiety. Genetic information presents patients with potentially difficult choices about whether and how to discuss their results with other family members and whether they should be advocates for promoting testing in the family (Hallowell et al. 2003). In the case of testing for specific mutations associated with increased prevalence in certain communities—e.g., the three "Ashkenazi Jewish" mutations—an individual choice may contribute to stigmatization of and discrimination against the larger community (Evans, Skrzynia, and Burke 2001; Koenig et al. 1998).

. . .

The availability of BRCA testing for private purchase introduces other long-term social costs. People may seek genetic testing even when medical professionals do not deem them to be at sufficient risk, because the information is valued for "non-clinical" uses, such as anxiety reduction or initiation of family dialogues (Burgess and Hayden 1996; Cox and McKellin 1999). Some patients also may opt for private purchase when the service is not provided through the public health care system. The reasons for using the technology and the way it is provided have begun to "drift" (Williams-Jones and Graham 2003), and these reasons may be manipulated by direct-to-consumer (DTC) advertising. Myriad is marketing its *BRACAnalysis* test both to physicians and to the general public through TV, print media, and the Internet (Myriad Genetics 2002). Critics argue that this advertising campaign exploits a climate of genetic determinism and public anxiety in an effort to convince members of the general public that they need and should either purchase or demand from their physicians an expensive genetic test that is unlikely to be clinically useful (Moreno 2002; Krasner 2003; Gollust, Hull, and Wilfond 2002).

Although DTC advertising is not permitted in Canada, the globalization of media (TV, radio, Internet) means that Canadians can access advertising about Myriad's genetic test. Since Myriad has an interest in selling its services to as large a market as possible, it should not be surprising that the company's access criteria—i.e., that a physician determine that his/her patient would benefit from testing, e.g., has a single family member with breast cancer—are less restrictive than those in the public health care system (Birmingham 1997; Smith 1997). When patients need only convince their physicians that they should have the test—after all they are paying out-of-pocket—the public health care system loses its former ability to constrain utilization and to ensure that tests are only made available to those people for whom the tests will provide accurate and useful information (Carter 2001; Holtzman and Shapiro 1998). Direct purchase could increase costs to the health care system, as more people would require genetic counseling (usually to be told that they are not at risk), a service not included in the price of direct purchase. In addition, those few people found to have positive test results then become eligible for other health care services and monitoring, costs that are legitimately covered by public health care insurance.

...

PUBLICLY ACCOUNTABLE PROCESSES

There is substantial public pessimism about the way government representatives and policy makers are involved in decision-making processes, as well as the influences that shape their decisions. The *ad hoc* nature and opacity of the decision making is not conducive to public trust or support—decisions are made in a "black box" and usually only the results are available for public inspection. For Daniels and Sabin, rational decisions about health care resource allocation, even if based on "reasonable" evidence or principles, will be insufficient if the decisions rendered *and* their rationales are not also publicized. Transparency—which Daniels and Sabin call condition 1: Publicity—is essential for public accountability.

In the case of access to BRCA testing in British Columbia, the B.C. Ministry of Health Services did not publicize its reasoning for complying with the Myriad patents in face of opposition to those patents by other provinces. The Ministry simply told the B.C. Cancer Agency and the Hereditary Cancer Program to comply with the patent and purchase testing from Myriad. HCP, however, did publicize its decision to terminate the provision of BRCA testing. Letters were sent to all patients enrolled in the program—and a note was posted on the B.C. Cancer Agency website—explaining that, due to the Ministry, HCP could no longer afford to provide BRCA testing to its patients because purchasing testing from Myriad would triple the cost of the services and undermine the program's ability to provide other services to patients with a diversity of hereditary cancers. HCP would continue to offer counseling support for patients and facilitate referrals to Myriad or MDS should patients wish to purchase testing themselves (Coldman 2001).

...

Transparency and relevance, however, are insufficient for public accountability (or accountability for reasonableness). Daniels and Sabin also require mechanisms for appeal, dispute resolution, as well as ongoing review and revision of decisions. This condition does not require public input into the initial decision—a decision-making process is fair and accountable for reasonableness if it is open to challenges and disputes of particular funding arrangements. Openness ensures the opportunity to revise decisions in light of new evidence and to be responsive to changing social and political realities of health care and technology development. Once again, in the absence of transparency, and the consequent inability to assess the relevance of the reasoning, it is difficult to determine the extent to which the B.C. Ministry of Health Services' policy reversal was the result of appeals. In any event, the official route for appeals to the Ministry is not well publicized, which leads to another discrepancy in that only well-informed individuals know how to register their concerns.

Enforcement is the final condition of accountability for reasonableness. Although public administrators and elected officials claim that the "public" interest is their primary focus, only a decision that is transparent, relevant, and open to appeal meets the conditions for accountability for reasonableness. The final condition of enforcement requires public regulation to ensure that these other conditions are met. Although the decisions in B.C. related to the support of the BRCA patents and subsequent restriction of in-house testing were made by public officials, there was no mechanism to hold them accountable to the first three conditions.

. . .

CONCLUSION

Adult genetic testing will have to meet high standards to be included among funded Canadian health care services when compared to other beneficial services such as hospital care, wheelchairs, or pharmaceuticals (Caulfield et al. 2001). The case of BRCA testing in Canada is useful for illustrating the difficulty of integrating technical or practical considerations with more theoretical discussions. We have not argued for or against the public provision of BRCA testing in light of the Myriad patents, but instead have sought to elucidate the relevant factors needed to make such a decision. . . .

Acknowledgements

We thank Timothy Caulfield, Janice Graham, Patricia Baird, Chris MacDonald, Wayne Norman, Oonagh Corrigan, and John McMillan for their constructive comments on various drafts of this paper; the staff of Hereditary Cancer Program of the B.C. Cancer Agency for background information about the science and politics of providing genetic testing for hereditary breast cancer; and the *Journal* reviewers for their helpful critiques. Many of the ideas here benefited from ongoing discussion with the Genetics and Ethics Research Group at the W. Maurice Young Centre for Applied Ethics, University of British Columbia. Williams-Jones was supported by fellowships from the Canadian Health Services Research Foundation, the Social Sciences and Humanities Research Council of Canada, the Québec Fonds pour la Formation de Chercheurs et l'Aide à la Recherche, and the W. Maurice Young Centre for Applied Ethics. Burgess's research into moral experience of hereditary breast cancer was supported by the Canadian Breast Cancer Foundation, and collaboration with the members of the HCP made the research possible.

Notes

1. The protection of strong intellectual property rights (IPR) in new technologies increasingly is seen as fundamental to continued technological and economic growth. Without strong IPR, it is maintained, companies would not be able to recoup the costs of (or make a profit from) investments in research, thereby undermining the development of new and beneficial biotechnologies. Nevertheless, there is also substantial debate about whether patenting of genes and biological materials is ethically acceptable (see, e.g., McGee 1998; Caplan 1998; Eisenberg 2002). The ethical permissibility of human gene patents is beyond the scope of this paper, and we focus instead on analyzing the implications of gene patents for access to health care services. For a broader discussion, see (Nuffield Council on Bioethics 2002; Royal Society 2003).

2. Some advocates for universal health care insurance will make a stronger claim for equal access based on social solidarity (Bergmark 2000; Houtepen and ter Meulen 2000). Personal wealth should not permit some people to obtain better or preferential treatment, and if not all useful health care services can be made available to all citizens then only those services that can be made available to all should be permitted. Other commentators use a more nuanced—e.g., relational—view of justice that goes

beyond mere distribution to include consideration of the broader costs of providing particular services, such as lost opportunity costs in not being able to fund other services (Sherwin 2001). Nevertheless, one should bear in mind that health care services are not as important to health, or at least population health, as broader social changes that address issues such as income disparity, employment and job stress, or diet (Evans, Barer, and Marmor 1994; Kaplan et al. 1996; Mechanic 1999).

3. During the last decade, federal government fiscal constraints have resulted in a steady reduction in transfer payments from the federal government to the provinces (Flood 1999), although this has to some extent been reversed by new federal funding initiatives (Department of Finance (Canada) 2003). The reduction in funding has significantly compromised the power of the federal government to constrain the privatization of health care. Provinces are less dependent on transfer payments that constitute ever smaller portions of provincial health care budgets (which are nevertheless growing steadily), and there is less money for the federal government to withhold as punishment. The result is a noticeable growth in patient-paid access to health care services across the country, such as private MRIs, PET scans, and laser eye clinics in British Columbia, Ontario and Québec (see Kent 2001b; Pinker 2000).

4. Some financial support from provincial governments is provided to subsidize the costs of obtaining prescription drugs—e.g., PharmaCare in British Columbia covers costs for anyone spending more than 3 percent of his/her income, with full coverage for the indigent and a 2 percent deductible for the elderly.

5. This is a controversial assertion, since one might argue that reorganization and better management of service delivery—e.g., discarding services with no proven benefit and eliminating expensive pharmaceuticals that are no more effective than cheaper competitors—might enable the public funding of all services of proven benefit. However, if medical technological and pharmaceutical development continues unabated and these products prove effective (but also costly), it will not be feasible to fund them all. This issue requires substantial evidence-based research, and the economic limits to adoption of all efficacious health care may be inevitable.

6. Much of the research on the incidence of breast cancer and penetrance of the BRCA mutations is drawn from studies of large families with many affected individuals. There is some evidence that risk figures may overestimate and not accurately reflect the levels of risk in families with less extreme incidences of cancer or in the general population (Robson 2002; King, Marks, and Mandell 2003).

References

Bergmark, A. 2000. Solidarity in Swedish Welfare—Standing the Test of Time? *Health Care Analysis* 8: 395–11.

Birmingham, K. 1997. News: Myriad's Rationale for Wider Testing. *Nature Medicine* 3: 709.

Borger, Julian. 1999. Rush to Patent Genes Is Hampering Medical Research. *The Guardian* (15 December). Available at *http://www.organicconsumers.org/ Patent/rushpatent.cfm*. Accessed 20 April 2004.

British Columbia Ministry of Health Services. 2003. Federal Leadership Urged as Genetic Testing Resumes. *Press Release* (14 February). Available at *http-.ll www2.news.gov.bc.ca/nrm_news_ releases/2003 HSER0009-000160.htm*. Accessed 20 April 2004.

Buchanan, Allen; Brock, Dan W.; Daniels, Norman; and Wikler, Daniel. 2000. *From Chance to Choice: Genetics and Justice.* New York: Cambridge University Press.

Burgess, Michael M., and d'Agincourt-Canning, Lori. 2002. Genetic Testing for Hereditary Disease: Attending to Relational Responsibility. *Journal of Clinical Ethics* 12:361–72.

Burgess, Michael M., and Hayden, Michael R. 1996. Patients' Rights to Laboratory Data: Trinucleotide Repeat Length in Huntington Disease. *American Journal of Medical Genetics* 62: 6–9.

Canadian Cancer Society. 2003. *Canadian Cancer Statistics.* Available at *http:// www.cancer.ca/vgn/ images/portal/cit_776/61/38/56158640niw_stats_ en.pdf*. Accessed 20 April 2004.

Canadian Institute for Health Information. 2003. *Health Care in Canada, 2003.* Available at *http://secure. cihi.ca/cihiweb/dispPage.jsp?cw_ page=PG_27_E&cw_topic=27&cw_rel=AR_43_ E.* Accessed 20 April 2004.

Canadian Medical Association. 2003. CMA President Unveils a National Public Health Action Plan. *Press Release* (25 June). Available at *http://www.cma.ca/ cma/menu/displayMenu.do?tab=422&skin- 432&pMenuId=2&pSub MenuId=6&pageId=/ staticContent/HTML/N0/l2/advocacy/ news/2003/06–25.htm*. Accessed 20 Apri 2004.

Canadian Press. 2001. Ontario Defies U.S. Gene Company over Cancer Test, Arguing Health Care at Risk. *Excite News* (19 September). Available at *http:// lists.essential.org/pipermail/ip-health/ 2001–September/001885.html.* Accessed 20 April 2004.

Caplan, Arthur. 1998. What's So Special About the Human Genome? *Cambridge Quarterly of Healthcare Ethics 7:* 422–24.

Carter, Ronald F. 2001. BRCA1, BRCA2 and Breast Cancer: A Concise Clinical Review. *Clinical & Investigative Medicine* 24 (3): 147–57.

Caulfield, Timothy A.; Burgess, Michael M.; Williams-Jones, Bryn; et al. 2001. Providing Genetic Testing through the Private Sector: A View from Canada. *ISUMA: Canadian Journal of Policy Research* 2 (3): 72–81.

Cho, Mildred K.; Illangasekare, Samantha; Weaver, Meredith A.; et al. 2003. Effects of Patents and Licenses on the Provision of Clinical Genetic Testing Services. *Journal of Molecular Diagnostics* 5(1): 3–8.

Coldman, Andrew J. 2001. Policy Change for Testing of Breast Cancer Susceptibility Genes: BRCA1 and BRCA2. *Press Release* (24 August), B.C. Cancer Agency.

Cox, Susan M., and McKellin, William. 1999. "There's This Thing in Our Family": Predictive Testing and the Construction of Risk for Huntington Disease. *Sociology of Health & Illness* 21: 622–46.

d'Agincourt-Canning, Lorraine. 2003. *Advanced Warning: A Gift or a Yoke? Experiential Knowledge, Moral Agency and Genetic Testing for Hereditary Breast/Ovarian Cancer.* Ph.D., Interdisciplinary Studies, University of British Columbia, Vancouver.

Daniels, Norman. 1985. *Just Health Care.* New York: Cambridge University Press.

———. 2001. Justice, Health, and Health Care. *American Journal of Bioethics* 1 (2): 2–16.

———, and Sabin, James. 1998. The Ethics of Accountability in Managed Care Reform. *Health Affairs* 17 (5): 50–64.

Deber, Raisa; Narine, Lutchmie; Baranek, Pat; et al. 1998. The Public-Private Mix in Health Care. In *Striking a Balance: Health Care Systems in Canada and Elsewhere,* ed. National Forum on Health, pp. 423–545. Sainte-Foy, QC: Éditions MultiMondes.

Department of Finance (Canada). 2003. *Investing in Canada's Health Care System.* 18 February. Available at *http://www.fin.gc.ca/budget03/ booklets/bkheae.htm.* Accessed 20 April 2004.

Eggertson, Laura. 2002. Ontario Defies US Firm's Genetic Patent, Continues Cancer Screening. *Canadian Medical Association Journal* 166: 494.

Eisenberg, Rebecca S. 2002. How Can You Patent Genes? *American Journal of Bioethics* 2 (3): 3–11.

Evans, James P.; Skrzynia, Cécile; and Burke, Wylie. 2001. The Complexities of Predictive Testing. *British Medical Journal* 322: 1052–56.

Evans, Robert G. 2000. The Role of Private and Public Health Care Delivery in Alberta. Paper read at Health Forum, 5 February, Edmonton, AB.

———; Barer, Morris L.; Lewis, Steven; et al. 2000. *Private Highway, One-Way Street: The Deklein and Fall of Canadian Medicare?* Centre for Health Sciences and Policy Research, University of British Columbia, Vancouver, B.C., pp. 1–56. Available at *http://www.chspr.ubc.ca/hpru/pdf/20003D.PDF.* Accessed 20 April 2004.

———; Barer, Morris L. and Marmor, Theodore R., eds. 1994. *Why Are Some People Healthy and Others Not? The Determinants of Health of Populations.* New York: Aldine de Gruyter.

Flood, Colleen M. 1999. The Structure and Dynamics of Canada's Health Care System. In *Canadian Health Law and Policy,* ed. J. G. Downie and T. A. Caulfield, pp. 5–50. Toronto, ON: Butterworths.

———, and Archibald, Tom. 2001. The Illegality of Private Health Care in Canada. *Canadian Medical Association Journal* 164: 825–30.

Frank, Thomas S.; Deffenbaugh, Amie M.; Reid, Julia E.; et al. 2002. Clinical Characteristics of Individuals with Germline Mutations in BRCA1 and BRCA2: Analysis of 10,000 Individuals. *Journal of Clinical Oncology* 20: 1480–90.

Giacomini, M.; Hurley, J.; and Stoddart, Greg L. 2000. The Many Meanings of Deinsuring a Health Service: The Case of *In Vitro* Fertilization in Ontario. *Social Science & Medicine* 50: 1485–1500.

Gollust, Sarah E.; Hull, Sara C.; and Wilfond, Benjamin S. 2002. Limitations of Direct-to-Consumer Advertising for Clinical Genetic Testing. *JAMA* 288: 1762–67.

Hallowell, N.; Foster, C.; Eeles, R.; et al. 2003. Balancing Autonomy and Responsibility: The Ethics of Generating and Disclosing Genetic Information. *Journal of Medical Ethics* 29 (2): 74–79. [Discussion follows on pp. 80–83.]

Hartmann, Lynn C.; Sellers, Thomas A.; Schaid, Daniel J.; et al. 2001. Efficacy of Bilateral Prophylactic Mastectomy in BRCA1 and BRCA2 Gene Mutation Carriers. *Journal of the National Cancer Institute* 93: 1633–37.

Heller, Michael A., and Eisenberg, Rebecca S. 1998. Can Patents Deter Innovation? The Anticommons in Biomedical Research. *Science* 280: 698–701.

Holtzman, Neil A., and Shapiro, David. 1998. The New Genetics: Genetic Testing and Public Policy. *British Medical Journal* 316: 852–56.

Houtepen, R., and ter Meulen, R. T. 2000. The Expectation(s) of Solidarity: Matters of Justice, Responsibility and Identity in the Reconstruction of the Health Care System. *Health Care Analysis* 8: 355–76.

Hull, Sara C, and Prasad, Kiran. 2001. Reading Between the Lines: Direct-to-Consumer Advertising of Genetic Testing in the USA. *Reproductive Health Matters 9* (18): 44–48.

Hutson, S. P. 2003. Attitudes and Psychological Impact of Genetic Testing, Genetic Counseling, and Breast Cancer Risk Assessment among Women at Increased Risk. *Oncology Nursing Forum* 30: 241–46.

Kaplan, George A.; Pamuk, Elsie R.; Lynch, John W.; et al. 1996. Inequality in Income and Mortality in the United States: Analysis of Mortality and Potential Pathways. *British Medical Journal* 312: 999–1003.

Kent, Heather. 2001a. Patenting Move Ends BC's Gene-Testing Program. *Canadian Medical Association Journal* 165: 812.

King, Mary-Claire; Marks, Joan H.; and Mandell, Jessica B. 2003. Breast and Ovarian Cancer Risks Due to Inherited Mutations in BRCA1 and BRCA2. *Science* 302: 643–46.

King, Mary-Claire; Wieand, Sam; Hale, Kathryn; et al. 2001. Tamoxifen and Breast Cancer Incidence among Women with Inherited Mutations in BRCA1 and BRCA2. *JAMA* 286: 2251–56.

Knoppers, Bartha Maria; Hirtle, Marie; and Glass, Kathleen Cranley. 1999. Commercialization of Genetics Research and Public Policy. *Science* 286: 2277–78.

Koenig, Barbara A.; Greely, Henry T.; McConnell, L. M.; et al. 1998. Genetic Testing for BRCA1 and BRCA2: Recommendations of the Stanford Program in Genomics, Ethics, and Society. *Journal of Women's Health 7:* 531.

Krasner, Jeffrey. 2003. Marketing of Cancer-Gene Test Raises Ethical, Medical Concerns. *The Boston Globe* (26 March).

Lynch, Henry T.; Lynch, Jane F.; and Rubinstein, Wendy S. 2001. Prophylactic Mastectomy: Obstacles and Benefits [Editorial]. *Journal of the National Cancer Institute* 93: 1586–87.

Mazankowski, Don. 2001. *A Framework for Reform: Report of the Premier's Advisory Council on Health.* December. Available at *http://www. premiers advisory.com/reform.html.* Accessed 20 April 2004.

McGee, Glenn. 1998. Gene Patents Can Be Ethical. *Cambridge Quarterly of Healthcare Ethics* 7: 417–21.

Mechanic, David. 1999. Issues in Promoting Health. *Social Science & Medicine* 48: 711–18.

Merz, Jon F.; Kriss, Antigone G.; Leonard, Debra G. B.; and Cho, Mildred K. 2002. Diagnostic Testing Fails the Test. *Nature* 415: 577–79.

Moreno, Jonathan. 2002. Selling Genetic Tests: Shades of Gray in Your DNA. *ABCNEWS.com.* Available at *http://abcnews.go.com/sections/living/ DailyNews/ ONCALL_DTC_brca_tests020923.html.* Accessed 20 April 2004.

Myriad Genetics. 2000a. Myriad Genetics Launches Colaris[(Tm)] in Canada: MDS to Market Colaris Colon Cancer Product Throughout Canada. *Press Release* (19 October). Available at *http://www. corporate-ir.net/ireye ir_site.zhtml?ticker=mygn& script=411 &layout=9&item_id=212127.* Accessed 20 April 2004.

———. 2000b. Myriad Genetics Launches Molecular Diagnostic Testing in Canada—MDS Laboratory Services to Provide BRACAnalysis Throughout Canada. *Press Release* (9 March). Available at *http://www.corporate-ir.net/ireye/ir_site. zhtml?ticker=mygn&script=411 &layout=9&item_ id=212154.* Accessed 20 April 2004.

———. 2002. Myriad Genetics Launches Direct to Consumer Advertising Campaign for Breast Cancer Test. *Press Release* (12 September). Available at *http:/www.corporate-ir.net/ireye/ir_site. zhtml?ticker=mygn& script=413 & layout=9&item_ id=333030.* Accessed 20 April 2004.

Narod, Steven A. 2002. Modifiers of Risk of Hereditary Breast and Ovarian Cancer. *Nature Reviews Cancer 2:* 113–123.

Nuffield Council on Bioethics. 2002. *The Ethics of Patenting DNA: A Discussion Paper.* July. Available at *http://www.nuffieldbioethics.org/filelibrary/pdf/ theethicsofpatentingdna.pdf* Accessed 20 April 2004.

Pinker, Susan. 2000. Private MRI Clinics Flourishing in Quebec. *Canadian Medical Association Journal* 163: 1326.

Prospero, Lisa; Seminsky, Maureen; Honeyford, Joanne; et al. 2001. Psychosocial Issues Following a Positive Result of Genetic Testing for BRCA1 and BRCA2 Mutations: Findings from a Focus Group and a Needs-Assessment Survey. *Canadian Medical Association Journal* 164: 1005–9.

Rawls, John. 1971. *A Theory of Justice.* Cambridge, MA: Belknap Press.

Robson, Mark E. 2002. Clinical Considerations in the Management of Individuals at Risk for Hereditary Breast and Ovarian Cancer. *Cancer Control* 9: 457–65.

Romanow, Roy J. 2002. *Final Report: Building on Values: The Future of Health Care in Canada.* 28 November. Available at *http://www.hc-sc.gc.ca/english/care/romanow/index1.html.* Accessed 20 April 2004.

Royal Society. 2003. *Keeping Science Open: The Effects of Intellectual Property Policy on the Conduct of Science.* April. Available at *http://www.royalsoc ac.uk/files/statfiles/document-221.pdf.* Accessed 20 April 2004.

Scheuer, Lauren; Kauff, Noah; Robson, Mark; et al. 2002. Outcome of Preventive Surgery and Screening for Breast and Ovarian Cancer in BRCA Mutation Carriers. *Journal of Clinical Oncology* 20: 1260–68.

Sherwin, Susan. 1996. Theory Versus Practice in Ethics: A Feminist Perspective on Justice in Health Care. In *Philosophical Perspectives on Bioethics,* ed. L. W. Sumner and J. Boyle, pp. 187–209. Toronto, ON: University of Toronto Press.

———. 2001. *Towards an Adequate Ethical Framework for Setting Biotechnology Policy.* January. Available at *http://cbac-cccb.ca/epic/internet/incbaccccb.nsf/vwapj/BioPolicy_Sherwin_e.pdf/$FILE/BioPolicy_Sherwin_e.pdf.* Accessed 20 April 2004.

Smith, O. 1997. News: Breast Cancer Susceptibility Tests Still Valid, Companies Argue. *Nature Medicine* 3: 709.

Szabo, Csilla I., and King, Mary-Claire 1997. Population Genetics of BRCA1 and BRCA2. *American Journal of Human Genetics* 60: 1013–20.

Williams-Jones, Bryn. 2002a. *Genetic Testing for Sale: Implications of Commercial BRCA Testing in Canada.* Ph.D., Individual Interdisciplinary Studies Graduate Program, University of British Columbia, Vancouver, B.C.

———. 2002b. History of a Gene Patent: Tracing the Development and Application of Commercial BRCA Testing. *Health Law Journal* 10: 121–44.

———. 2003. Where There's a Web, There's a Way: Commercial Genetic Testing and the Internet. *Community Genetics* 6 (1): 46–57.

———, and Graham, Janice E. 2003. Actor-Network Theory: A Tool to Support Ethical Analysis of Commercial Genetic Testing. *New Genetics & Society* 22:271–96.

Debate: Should Canada Allow Direct-to-Consumer Advertising of Prescription Drugs?

YES

Durhane Wong-Rieger

It is time to end the debate in Canada. The greater risk to Canadian patients is not the drug advertisements from American-sourced media, but rather the lack of access to prescription drug information. As a patient advocate, a mother of 2 children with health conditions, and a wife of someone with multiple chronic conditions, I know the frustration of trying to get information about new therapies. In Europe, where similar barriers exist, a survey of 268 nonprofit patient organizations found that one-fifth of respondents reported they could "never" access high-quality prescription drug information, three-fifths said they "sometimes" could, while only 13% said they "always" could.[1]

In Canada, the discussion of direct patient access to drug information has been derailed by the debate over US-style advertising. Critics

Wong-Rieger, D. (2009) "Should Canada Allow Direct-to-Consumer Advertising of Prescription Drugs? YES." *Canadian Family Physician* 55(2): pp. 130, 132.

often extend concerns with direct-to-consumer advertising (DTCA) to direct-to-consumer information, despite the lack of evidence.[2]

Supporting Points

This paper discusses 4 points that support patient direct access to information about prescription drugs:

Drug or disease ads contribute to public health by increasing appropriate consultation for undiagnosed or untreated health conditions. Most studies agree that "disease awareness" or "drug awareness" ads lead to increases in consultations for targeted conditions.[3] Critics complain that healthy patients seeking physician advice are a waste of health care resources;[4] however, there is scant evidence that these consultations are inappropriate.[5]

In a survey by the US Food and Drug Administration, physicians reported that the majority (88%) of patients asking about specific drugs after seeing advertisements did indeed have the conditions for which the drugs were intended.[6] About one-fourth of patients whose visits were prompted by ads received new diagnoses, some for preventable conditions such as hypertension, diabetes, high cholesterol, and depression.[7] And nearly three-fourths of physician respondents reported that the campaigns improved the quality of their discussions with patients. Overall, advertising can help redress the "health deficit" whereby serious conditions are underdiagnosed and undertreated.

Ads do not lead to patients getting inappropriate medications. Prescription drugs are among the few substances requiring approval of a learned intermediary, which tends to limit rather than promote access. While physicians report being asked by patients about advertised drugs, more than half of the physicians surveyed by the Boston Consulting Group said formularies had a major effect on their prescribing practices and one-third said they would not discuss treatments not covered by insurers.[8]

A longitudinal study comparing English-speaking Canadians exposed to (illicit) American ads about 3 drugs with French-speaking Canadians not exposed to such ads concluded that the ads did not affect prescribing rates for 2 of the drugs and led to only a short-term increase in the prescribing rates of the third.[9]

Similarly, the US Government Auditing Office concluded that only 27% of those who saw drug ads actually requested and received prescriptions for those drugs.[10] Three-fourths of patients who sought physician advice after seeing a drug advertised reported that the doctors discussed health and lifestyle changes; more than half were prescribed a generic alternative, while 51% received suggestions about nonprescription treatments.

Direct-to-consumer information about pharmaceutical products serves an unmet patient need. Not only do most Canadians (68%) support direct-to-consumer prescription drug information, but most believe that DTCA is allowed.[11]

Similarly, the European Commission has been pressed by the public to allow pharmaceutical companies to provide information (not advertising) directly to consumers through public media, including broadcasting, print media, and the Internet.[12] Most European cancer patient groups surveyed said they could not rely on their specialists to provide sufficient information and many felt doctors' prescribing practices were governed by restrictive health authority budgets.[13] In another survey, patient groups felt they should have the right to directly approach pharmaceutical companies for product information.[14]

Direct-to-consumer drug information must be balanced, screened, and monitored. In April 2008, the European Commission, while retaining the ban on advertising, proposed a framework supporting direct information on prescription drugs through public media and audiovisual and written material, subject to prescreening and monitoring by an independent body.[15] Information could not be "misleading by omission" and required "balanced representation" of both benefits and risks so consumers could make informed decisions.

Health Canada's guide for advertising nonprescription drugs recognizes that consumers should be provided with fair and balanced information about the benefits and risks associated with medications in order to make informed decisions. It acknowledges that the public is ignorant about package inserts or product monographs but does pay attention to product advertising. Therefore, balanced information to patients through advertising can promote appropriate use of drugs, with concomitant benefits to the health care system.[16]

I propose extending the same rationale and guidelines to prescription medicines. Information must be evidence-based and not exceed what has been approved for the product monographs. All substantive benefits and risks must be included and all communications prescreened and approved. Inaccurate communications must be corrected or removed, and misleading information should lead to penalties.

Last Words

It is illogical and irresponsible to allow a free-flow of DTCA across the border while restricting the more appropriate information created in Canada, which would be vetted and monitored by Canadian authorities. A patient-centred approach can be found to meet the need for balanced, high-quality, comprehensive information about prescription drugs that neither misleads patients nor promotes inappropriate medication use.

Closing Arguments

- Drug or disease advertisements contribute to public health by increasing appropriate consultation for undiagnosed or untreated health conditions.
- As prescription medications require approval of a learned intermediary, advertisements do not lead to patients getting inappropriate medications.
- Patient surveys suggest that direct-to-consumer information about pharmaceutical products serves an unmet patient need.
- Direct-to-consumer drug information that is balanced, screened, and monitored can promote the appropriate use of drugs.

Notes

1. Medicines and Healthcare Products Regulatory Agency (MHRA). MHRA public consultation with patient representatives: medicines information and advertising. Powys, UK: PatientView;

2005. Available from: www.patient-view.com/ 3.%20Main%20Report%20to%20MHRA%20 Public%20Consultation%20with %20Patient%20 Representatives,%20Sept%202005.pdf. Accessed 2008 Dec 18.

2. Moynihan R, Henry D. The fight against disease mongering: generating knowledge for action. *PLOS Med* 2006;3(4):e191. Epub 2006 Apr 11.

3. Mintzes B, Barer ML, Kravitz RL, Bassett K, Lexchin J, Kazanjian A, et al. How does direct-to-consumer advertising (DTCA) affect prescribing? A survey in primary care environments with and without legal DTCA. *CMAJ* 2003;169(5):405–12.

4. Mintzes B, Kazanjian A, Bassett K, Lexchin J. *Pills, persuasion and public health policies. Report of an expert survey on direct-to-consumer advertising of prescription drugs in Canada, the United States and New Zealand.* Vancouver, BC: Health Policy Research Unit, University of British Columbia; 2001. Available from: www.chspr.ubc. ca/node/215. Accessed 2008 Dec 18.

5. DeLuca C. *Direct to consumer advertising of prescription medicines: assessing the impact of consumer directed drug advertisement and the legality of current prohibitions.* Toronto, ON: University of Toronto Health Law and Policy Group; 2005. Available from: www.law. utoronto. ca/HEALTHLAW/docs/student_DeLuca-DTCA. pdf. Accessed 2008 Dec 18.

6. Aikin KJ, Swasy JL, Braman AC. *Patient and physician attitudes and behaviors associated with DTC promotion of prescription drugs. Summary of FDA survey research results.* Washington, DC: Food and Drug Administration, Center for Drug Evaluation and Research; 2004. Available from: www.fda.gov/cder/ddmac/Final%20Report/ FRFinalExSu1119042.pdf. Accessed 2008 Dec 19.

7. Weissman JS, Blumenthal D, Silk AJ, Newman M, Zapert K, Leitman R, et al. Physicians report on patient encounters involving direct-to-consumer advertising. *Health Aff* (Millwood) 2004;Suppl Web Exclusives:W4–219–33. Available from: http:// content.healthaffairs.org/cgi/reprint/hlthaff. w4.219v1. Accessed 2008 Dec 19.

8. Wynia MK, VanGeest JB, Cummins DS, Wilson IB. Do physicians not offer useful services because of coverage restrictions? *Health Aff* (Millwood) 2003;22(4):190–7.

9. Law MR, Majumdar SR, Soumerai SB. Effect of illicit direct to consumer advertising on use of etanercept, mometasone, and tegaserod in Canada: controlled longitudinal study. *BMJ* 2008;337:a1055.

10. U.S. Government Accountability Office. *Prescription drugs: improvements needed in FDA's oversight of direct-to-consumer advertising.* Washington, DC: Government Accountability Office; 2006. Available from: www.gao.gov/ products/GAO-07–54. Accessed 2008 Dec 19.

11. Alliance for the Access to Medical Information. *How do Canadians feel about direct-to-consumer advertising of prescription medicines? A summary of the Ipsos-Reid survey results.* Ottawa, ON: Canadian Association of Broadcasters; 2002. Available from: www.cab-acr.ca/english/ research/02/ipsoreadsummary_jan3102.pdf. Accessed 2008 Dec 19.

12. European Commission Enterprise and Industry Directorate-General. *Key ideas of a legal proposal on information to patients. Summary of the public consultation responses.* Brussels, BE: European Commission; 2008. Available from: http:// ec.europa.eu/enterprise/pharmaceuticals/patients/ docs/summary_publ_cons_220508.pdf. Accessed 2008 Dec 19.

13. Gooderham C, Nead C, Wyke A. Information on prescription medicines for cancer patients: an unmet need. *Cancer Futures* 2003;2:33–5. Available from: www.cancerworld. org/CancerWorldAdmin/images/ static_modules/images/1428/CF_1_ Vol2_33.pdf. Accessed 2008 Dec 19.

14. PatientView. *Prescription drug information for the public: a strategy document.* London, UK: PatientView; 2002. Available from: www.patient-view.com/projects4. htm#4. Accessed 2008 Dec 19.

15. European Commission Enterprise and Industry Directorate-General. *Public consultation. Legal proposal on information to patients.* Brussels, BE: European Commission; 2008. Available from: http:// ec.europa.eu/enterprise/pharmaceuticals/pharmacos/ docs/ doc2008/2008_02/info_to_patients_con-sult_200802.pdf. Accessed 2008 Dec 19.

16. Health Canada. *Issue paper: Health Canada's approach to the inclusion of risk/safety information communication (Section 2.21) in the revised consumer advertising guidelines for marketed health products (for nonprescription drugs including natural health products).* Ottawa, ON: Health Canada, Health Products and Food Branch; 2006. Available from: www.hc-sc.gc.ca/dhp-mps/advert-publicit/ report-rapport/hc-sc_issue_ paper-document_ reference_section_221–eng.php. Accessed 2008 Dec 19.

NO

Barbara Mintzes

Direct-to-consumer advertising (DTCA) of prescription drugs has increased enormously over the past decade in the United States and New Zealand, the 2 countries where it is legal. In 2005, more than $4.2 billion (US) was spent on DTCA in the United States,[1] and Americans spent an average of 16 hours watching televised drug advertisements—far more time than they spent with family doctors.

Market research company IMS Health reviewed the returns on investment in DTCA for 49 brands from 1998 to 2003 and found that for "blockbuster" drugs, such as rofecoxib, companies on average obtained $3.66 per dollar invested.[2] The key controversy is not whether DTCA stimulates sales, but whether or not this is good or bad for health, health care quality, and total health care costs.

Direct-to-consumer advertising of prescription drugs is prohibited in Canada as a health protection measure. Manufacturers cannot advertise prescription-only drugs directly to the public because of their toxicity and the potential for harm from medically unnecessary or inappropriate use. Any debate over DTCA, however, must address enforcement. Despite its illegality, exposure to cross-border and, increasingly, "made-in-Canada" ads is widespread. Just because such ads are allowed in the United States, cross-border DTCA on US cable television is not inevitable. It is technically simple to replace US ads with local advertising. Similarly, "made-in-Canada" DTCA

Mintzes, B. (2009) "Should Canada Allow Direct-to-Consumer Advertising of Prescription Drugs? NO." *Canadian Family Physician* 55(2): pp. 131, 133. Reprinted by permission of the publisher.

could be prevented under current laws—the question is one of political will. Succumbing to heavy pressure, Health Canada reinterpreted a 1975 price advertising regulation to allow one type of DTCA, branded "reminder" advertising, in 2000.[3]

Negative Effects

In a Vancouver, BC, study of primary care, patient requests for advertised drugs affected prescribing volume and choice (albeit less strongly than in a US setting, a reflection of lowered exposure).[4] In a 2002 survey of health professionals in Canada (N = 1975), 67% of GPs reported sometimes or often feeling pressured to prescribe advertised drugs.[5] By portraying various medicines as a 100% effective solution to an array of life problems, DTCA turns doctors into gatekeepers for desired brands.

The 2006 tegaserod ad for irritable bowel syndrome is emblematic of the hazards of prescription drug advertising. The eye-catching ad featured women baring their bellies to reveal slogans. Closing shots panned women of many different ages and races, suggesting widespread use. Relief of vague symptoms along with a comparison to fibre and laxatives implied use for mild problems. But key information on safety concerns, limited effectiveness, and the limited appropriate patient population was lacking. In 2007, the drug was withdrawn from the market because of cardiovascular risks. The first Food and Drug Administration safety warning, on risks of ischemic colitis, dated back to 2004. Tegaserod prescriptions rose by 56% in a US Medicaid population and 42% in English speaking Canada following exposure to US DTCA campaigns.[6]

The 2004 market withdrawal of rofecoxib had already raised red flags about DTCA's ability to rapidly stimulate sales of new drugs with emergent serious risks. Rofecoxib led to an estimated 88 000 to 140 000 heart attacks in the United States, 44% of which were fatal.[7] It was among the most heavily advertised drugs for 4 years after the first large-scale clinical trial showed evidence of cardiac risks. In a Kaiser Permanente study, 20% of initial users of cyclooxygenase-2 inhibitors had requested prescriptions after seeing ads.[8]

These users were 4 times as likely as other users to be inconsistent with treatment guidelines.

Because of its focus on new, expensive drugs, DTCA drives up consumer costs. In New Zealand, DTCA for fluticasone asthma inhalers fueled broad substitution for beclomethasone, which is equally effective and less costly. More than $1 billion (US) was spent on US DTCA for esomeprazole; yet the same treatment effects can be achieved with generic omeprazole. Most new drugs have no therapeutic advantage over existing alternatives, and new serious risks are often discovered in the early postmarketing period. From a public health perspective, caution, not rapid uptake, is needed.

Social Control

Is opposition to DTCA paternalistic? Independent consumer groups reject this claim, arguing that DTCA fails to provide the unbiased, comparative information needed for shared and informed treatment choices. Key information, such as the probability of treatment success, is usually missing. Instead, emotive messages dominate: in a sample of television ads, drug use was associated with happiness in 95% of ads, control over one's life in 85%, and social approval in 78%.[9] The US regulatory experience is also instructive—of 135 ads violating US law from 1997 to 2005, 84% minimized risks or exaggerated benefits.[10]

Direct-to-consumer advertising of prescription drugs affects prescribing volume and choice.[11] In one study, physicians prescribed most DTCA drugs patients requested, but were 8 times more likely to judge those drugs as only "possible" or "unlikely" choices for similar patients than "very likely" choices.[4] In an experimental study, patient requests led to twice as many antidepressant prescriptions for patients with depression and a 5–fold increase for patients with "adjustment disorder," which does not require drug treatment.[12] Patient requests were a stronger predictor of prescriptions than symptoms.

Undertreatment of depression is often cited as a problem DTCA could help solve, as population surveys have identified many untreated people who meet *Diagnostic and Statistical Manual of Mental Disorders,* 4th edition, criteria. A Canadian survey compared people with depression taking antidepressants with those not taking antidepressants (N = 9508).[13] Half of those not taking antidepressants recovered within 5 weeks. Mean episode duration was 11 weeks versus 19 weeks for those taking antidepressants. Bottom line, many of the so-called "under-treated" patients might not actually require drugs.

Direct-to-consumer advertising can and does cause harm. Any benefits could be better achieved through public health campaigns. The law prohibiting DTCA remains valid, but needs better enforcement. A simple start is to repeal the price advertising regulation to eliminate reminder ads.[3]

If money is power, DTCA is indeed empowering. The question is, for whom and at what cost to the public and to medication as a social good?

Closing Arguments

- Direct-to-consumer prescription drug advertising can cause damage by instigating rapid, widespread stimulation of use of new drugs before harmful effects are fully known.
- Advertisements exaggerate treatment benefits and use emotive messages to target people with milder health problems, many of whom are unlikely to benefit from the drugs advertised.
- Advertising leads to higher drug costs and overall health care costs through substitution of new, expensive drugs without treatment advantages.
- Better enforcement of direct-to-consumer advertising laws in Canada is needed.

Notes

1. Donohue JM, Cevasco M, Rosenthal MB. A decade of direct-to-consumer advertising of prescription drugs. *N Engl J Med* 2007;357(7):673–81.
2. Gascoigne D. *DTC at the crossroads: a "direct" hit ... or miss?* Plymouth Meeting, PA: IMS Health; 2004.
3. Gardner D, Mintzes B, Ostry A. Direct-to-consumer prescription drug advertising in Canada: permission by default? *CMAJ* 2003;169(5):425–7.
4. Mintzes B, Barer ML, Kravitz RL, Bassett K, Lexchin J, Kazanjian A, et al. How does direct-to-consumer advertising (DTCA) affect prescribing? A survey in primary care environments with and without legal DTCA. *CMAJ* 2003;169(5):405–12.
5. Environics Research Group Limited. *General public favours advertising of prescription drugs, but health care professionals have strong doubts.* Toronto, ON: Environic Research Group Limited; 2002. Available from: http://erg. environics.net/ practice_areas/pharma/pdf/advertising_drugs.pdf. Accessed 2008 Dec 22.
6. Law MR, Malumdar SR, Soumerai SB. Effect of illicit direct to consumer advertising on use of etanercept, mometasone, and tegaserod in Canada: controlled longitudinal study. *BMJ* 2008;337:11055.
7. Graham DJ, Campen D, Hui R, Spence M, Cheetham C, Levy G, et al. Risk of acute myocardial infarction and sudden cardiac death in patients treated with cyclo-oxygenase 2 selective and non-selective non-steroidal anti-inflammatory drugs: nested case-control study. *Lancet* 2005;365(9458):475–81.
8. Spence MM, Teleki SS, Cheetham TC, Schweitzer SO, Millares M. Direct-to-consumer advertising of COX-2 inhibitors: effect on appropriateness of prescribing. *Med Care Res Rev* 2005;62(5):544–59.
9. Frosch DL, Krueger PM, Hornik RC, Cronholm PF, Barg FK. Creating demand for prescription drugs: a content analysis of television direct-to-consumer advertising. *Ann Fam Med* 2007;5(1):6–13.
10. United States Government Accountability Office. *Prescription drugs. Improvements needed in FDA oversight of direct-to-consumer advertising.* Washington, DC: Government Accountability Office; 2006. Available from: www.gao.gov/new.items/d0754.pdf. Accessed 2009 Jan 5.
11. Gilbody S, Wilson P, Watt I. Benefits and harms of direct to consumer advertising: a systematic review. *Qual Saf Health Care* 2005;14(4):246–50.
12. Kravitz RL, Epstein RM, Feldman MD, Franz CE, Azari R, Wilkes MS, et al. Influence of patients' requests for direct-to-consumer advertised antidepressants: a randomized controlled trial. *JAMA* 2005;293(16):1995–2002.
13. Patten SB. The impact of antidepressant treatment on population health: synthesis of data from two national data sources in Canada. *Popul Health Metr* 2004;2(1):9.

The Ethical Physician Encounters International Medical Travel

G. K. D. Crozier and Françoise Baylis

International medical travel occurs when patients cross national borders to purchase medical goods and services. Discussions of international medical travel once tended to focus on patients travelling from less-developed to more-developed countries for safe, high-quality medical care not otherwise available in their home countries. Consider, for example, the highly publicised case of conjoined twins Lin and Win Htut[1] who were separated at the Hospital for Sick Children in Canada because of insufficient medical expertise and limited financial resources in their home country of Burma.[2]

Subsequently, discussions of international medical travel turned to cases of patients travelling between equally developed countries for more accessible or more affordable care. For example, the bi-directional movement of patients between Canada and the US saw considerable attention in the media during the 1990s: Canadians travelling south to avoid waiting lists, and Americans travelling north for less costly healthcare.

But now, with the ease of international communication, travel and marketing, international medical travel has become an increasingly attractive option for patients travelling from more developed to less-developed countries. Often, this travel is for elective procedures such as laser eye surgery or cosmetic procedures. However, it can also be for procedures with considerable impact on quality of life and longevity, such as hip replacement surgery, kidney transplantation, or fertility treatment. Consider, for example, the case of Ranjit and Jagir Hayer, a 60–year-old Canadian couple of Indian origin. After having been denied access to fertility treatments in Canada, the Hayers travelled to India in the summer of 2008 where they procured eggs from a woman much younger than Mrs Hayer (possibly purchasing them a practice which is illegal in Canada). The fertilised eggs were transferred to Mrs Hayer, who then returned to Canada for the gestation and birth of twin boys, who were delivered prematurely in a Calgary hospital in February 2009.[3] The high cost of maternal and neonatal care was paid for by the Canadian public healthcare system.[4] This led many commentators to reflect on the benefits and harms of medical travel for both the individuals involved and for the healthcare system.

THE SCOPE OF INTERNATIONAL MEDICAL TRAVEL

We will start by suggesting some very basic ways of looking at the global industry of international medical travel in terms of the number of customers and the revenue reported for various countries. These figures suggest that this market is a significant one; however, as we will subsequently discuss, quantifying its extent in relative terms has proven challenging.

A number of destination countries are actively cultivating the medical travel industry as a lever for economic growth. For example, Asian markets are growing at a rate of 20% per year, and alone they could generate about US$4 billion annually by 2012.[5] Half of this market is expected to be in India, where predicted revenue of US$2.2 billion by 2012[5] would represent roughly 1% of that country's gross domestic product (GDP).[6] In an effort to capitalise on this

Crozier G.K., Baylis F. (2010) "The Ethical Physician Encounters International Medical Travel." *Journal of Medical Ethics*. 2010 May; 36(5): pp. 297–301.

potential market, India has established a visa specifically for medical travellers.

Another Asian country that is a major destination point for medical travel is Thailand. According to the Kasikorn Research Center, which publishes statistics on hospitals in Thailand, 1.2 million foreigners were treated in Thai hospitals in 2005 generating an estimated revenue of $850 million US,[7] roughly 0.5% of GDP. This revenue represents a large portion of the health industry in Thailand, where total expenditure on healthcare in 2005 represented only 4% of GDP, and private healthcare expenditure totalled only 1% of GDP.[8] Although it is unclear what percentage of these patients travelled to Thailand for the main purpose of accessing medical care, large institutions such as Bumrungrad Hospital and Samitijev Hospital have been aggressively promoting services for medical travellers.

If we consider examples outside of Asia, the Czech Republic's medical travel industry is reportedly worth over US$182 million, close to 1% of GDP. In all, 35 000 medical travellers visited Israel in 2009 and contributed US$100 million in revenue, close to 0.05% of GDP.[9] Costa Rican healthcare professionals treated roughly 150 000 medical travellers in 2007, mostly for cosmetic and dental procedures.[10] In 2007, 200 000 medical travellers sought treatment in Cuba.[10] (Estimates on the dollar value of these markets are not available.) According to Medical Tourism Association president, Jonathan Edelheit, within this decade over half of US medical travellers will choose Latin American destination points, spending nearly US$40 billion per year in these countries alone by 2017.[11]

Given these basic figures, the industry in international medical travel clearly matters. It is expected that competition among countries for a share of this lucrative market will become increasingly fierce. But while these figures indicate that the international medical travel industry is significant, and will become increasingly so in the future, it is very difficult to quantify its importance in relative terms.

Empirical information on the scope and financial importance of international medical travel is limited, and what information is available is generally subject to wide variations. For example, the 2008 Deloitte Medical Tourism Study[12] estimates a massive industry, projecting that the US alone will send six million medical travellers abroad in 2010, which potentially represents lost revenue to US healthcare providers of just under US$16 billion. In sharp contrast, Ehrbech and colleagues, in a report prepared for the consulting firm McKinsey and Company[13] estimate that the international medical travel industry is negligible in size, with as few as 60 000 travellers per year.

The small number of medical travellers cited in the McKinsey report is due in no small part to the use of a highly restrictive definition of medical travel.[14] For example, the study excludes outpatient procedures such as dentistry and some cosmetic procedures, which are very popular draws for 'medical tourists'. Most researchers find it useful to include these cases in overall estimates, and thus conclude that this study significantly underestimates the size and significance of the medical travel industry. Given this limitation, the McKinsey report has garnered relatively little attention in either news reports or academic articles on medical travel. Meanwhile, although the accuracy of Deloitte's estimates have been questioned by critics[15]—who contest both the survey methodology and the background research on which the extrapolations were based—these estimates have been widely cited by influential media outlets such as the Economist and CNN. But wherein lies the truth about the size and influence of the international medical travel industry?

In a 2006 publication, Carrera and Bridges[16] estimated a global industry of US$500 billion per year. More recently, in 2009, Grail Research[17] estimated that by 2012 the global market would be worth US$100 billion per year.[18] These are impressive (and confusing) differences. In 2009, Youngman[14] assessed the global industry at five million patients per year, considerably less than the six million patients per year from the US alone, originally estimated by Deloitte in their influential 2008 report. Deloitte's follow-up 2009 Survey of Health Care Consumers is more conservative in its estimates of the size of the international medical travel industry of just over three million patients per year from the US.[19,20] Its 2008 publication *Medical tourism: the Asian chapter* was also more conservative, reporting that only half a million patients from the US travelled abroad for treatment in 2007.[21]

Empirical investigations of the international medical travel industry can be expected to continue to produce divergent conclusions. For one thing, as mentioned above, there is no consensus on the definition of medical travel. Additionally, researchers vary with respect to the types of evidence they draw upon, consequently producing different results. For example, some statistics might be skewed by subtle political manipulations, such as over-inflated figures from a country or hospital that wants to promote itself as a destination point for international medical travel. As Youngman[14] writes: "A typical example last year was an Asian country, where one week one minister stood up and said his country had 100 000 medical tourists, while the next week saw another minister claiming it was 200 000…almost every official figure is flawed. They are often badly collected, imperfectly collated and spun to infinity. Some hospitals inflate figures by counting the number of patient visits rather than number of patients."

In light of variations in data about the scope of the industry and the consequent opaqueness of the effects of various aspects of this industry, how can individual physicians in home countries make headway in promoting ethical markets and restricting unethical ones?

PATIENT DECISION SPACES

On occasion, physicians in home countries will be the last point of domestic contact for patients seeking healthcare information before they travel abroad for care. When this is the case, physicians have a unique opportunity to inform patients about their options and help guide them towards ethical practices.[22] This opportunity brings to the fore an important question: what role should physicians in more-developed home countries play in promoting or constraining international medical travel towards less-developed destination countries?

In our view, a useful starting point for evaluating the proper response of physicians to various forms of international medical travel is critical attention to patients' decision spaces. An agent's *decision space* is characterised by the extent of various categories of constraints, such as personal (including financial) circumstances, socia-cultural cues, and legal constraints—that inform decision-making.[23,24] We explore some of these decision spaces, as might be described by identifiable patients and/or discerned by their physicians, in an effort to better understand when physicians should attempt to facilitate medical travel for their patients, and when as a matter of professional ethics they should actively dissuade their patients from travelling abroad for medical treatment.

There are various dimensions to each patient's decision space, including the degree of necessity of a desired medical procedure, the cost of the procedure relative to the patient's available income, as well as legal and socio-cultural constraints on the availability of the procedure. While there are many decision spaces in which patients opt to engage in international medical travel, we focus on four broad categories of such spaces which are among the most likely to be encountered by, and raise ethical questions for, physicians in more-developed home countries. These are situations where patients pursue:

A. Elective procedures that are expensive in their home country, and which are available at a fraction of the cost in destination countries;

B. Medically necessary procedures for which there are long domestic waiting lists;

C. Medical interventions unavailable in their home country because they have not yet been shown to be safe and effective; and

D. Medical interventions that are illegal in their home country because they harmfully exploit vulnerable third-parties.

Each of these categories of patient decision spaces raises a different set of ethical considerations, and may demand a different response from physicians. Of course, a particular patient's decision space may fall into more than one of these categories, but for clarity we have chosen to discuss them as though they were isolated.

Price

Many of the cases of international medical travel that physicians in home countries will encounter occur in the context of significant cost differentials between home and destination countries. Some popular 'elective' procedures—such as cosmetic surgery[25] and dental care[26]—are prohibitively expensive for many in more-developed countries such as the US, Canada and the UK, and can be accessed at a fraction of the cost in less developed countries such as Thailand, the Czech Republic and Tunisia.

All other things being equal, this seems to be a fairly innocuous form of medical travel. If so, the most appropriate response may be to leave this category of travel to the free market—un-facilitated and unencumbered. As with all medical travel, however, we should be concerned about the socio-economic consequences of various markets for third parties. For example, clinics and hospitals abroad may be less selective about the efficacy and quality of care, ultimately burdening the individual patient or the home country's public healthcare system with significant costs in corrective and follow-up procedures. Also, some markets may negatively affect access to medical interventions for non-consumers in both home and destination countries. We discuss these, and other, important confounding factors below.

Waiting Lists

Another category of patient decision spaces includes situations wherein patients' access to necessary medical procedures, such as orthopaedic surgery or cancer treatments, is constrained by long waiting lists.[27] For example, consider the case of Mr Dolinsky who, in the spring of 2007, travelled to India for hip surgery. Mr Dolinsky was in serious pain because of osteoarthritis and was unwilling to wait a year in Canada for the recommended hip resurfacing procedure.[28]

All other things being equal, physicians should facilitate this category of medical travel when patients' needs cannot be efficiently addressed in the home country. It is preferable that patients access medical procedures that can significantly improve their quality of life in a timely fashion. Additionally, to the extent that medical travel shortens the queue in home countries, it is desirable for patients to go abroad. Collaterally, medical travel might ease pressure on public care waiting lists by moving some of the patients to a different system, without at the same time removing physicians from the public system of home countries.

On a larger socio-political scale, in some cases, home countries might even be obligated to fund travel for medically necessary interventions so that all citizens can access them without incurring debt: for example, where the capacity to supply a particular service lags behind a spike in demand for this service. Additionally—excepting in cases such as rare procedures, where there is benefit in promoting regional specialisations—home countries should simultaneously be working to shorten domestic waiting lists for medically necessary procedures so that patients are not forced to go abroad for them. For those nations that are committed to government-funded universal healthcare, there is an obligation to ensure that international travel for medically necessary procedures does not become the status quo.

Unproven Medical Interventions

When medical travel is undertaken for the purpose of accessing unproven medical interventions, physicians may be warranted in adopting a more interventionist response. For example, it has recently been reported that UK children with congenitally underdeveloped optic nerves have travelled to China for unproven and costly stem cell transplantation. Belfast couple Darren and Wilma Clarke paid £30 000 for their 3–year-old daughter Dakota to receive six injections of stem cells. She obtained these injections in February 2009 in Qingdao, northeast China.[29] Welsh couple Joanna and Anthony Clark paid £40 000 for their 16-month-old son Joshua to receive a stem cell transplant in April 2009 in Hangzhou, near Shanghai.[30]

Stem cell transplantations such as these are not permitted in the UK because they are deemed unsafe and ineffective. The concern with medical travel for unproven interventions is the risk of serious harm to patients—a risk recently reported in relation to another case involving stem cell transplantation where "an Israeli boy developed benign tumours in the brain and spinal cord after being injected with foetal neural cells at a Moscow clinic in Russia."[31] International medical travel for "unproven stem-cell treatments that lack appropriate oversight or patient monitoring or use poorly characterised cells" is explicitly condemned by the International Society for Stem Cell Research.[32]

Beyond a concern about harm, there are concerns about false hope and exploitation. A commitment to patient autonomy dictates that if patients understand and freely consent to purchase a desired medical procedure, we ought not to interfere with their plans. But what about the vulnerable positions in which these patients and their families often find themselves? They may be subject to tremendous pressures to exhaust all available means to cure the illness in question, thus rendering them easy marks for exploitation. Even if physicians should not directly intervene by preventing travel for unproven interventions sought by competent patients, this does not mean that they should support it. Arguably, at the very least, physicians should deter patients from seeking unproven procedures abroad (through education and counselling), when there is good reason to believe that the sought after interventions are likely to do more harm than good.

With the cases cited above, the ethical challenges are greater by virtue of the fact that the procedures in question were performed on children. Considerations of patient autonomy are considerably more complicated when the patient is a child and the purchaser is a guardian who may be exposing her child to harm. In such situations, a stronger interventionist approach might be warranted.

Legal Prohibitions

When patients' decision spaces are characterised by the illegality of the desired procedure in the home country—in particular because the procedure is exploitative—this raises a different set of ethical considerations. These situations include medical interventions such as transplantation involving the purchase of a kidney[33] or fertility treatments involving payment for ova.[34]

Consider medical travel to Pakistan by patients from countries such as Saudi Arabia, Kosovo, Turkey and Bulgaria for the purchase and transplantation of human kidneys. Despite the fact that the sale of organs is legally prohibited in Pakistan, this country remains a leading destination for foreigners seeking to purchase kidneys. In June of 2009, the Supreme Court of Pakistan confirmed that the sale of kidneys for transplantation continues despite the legal prohibition.[35]

A kidney patient might be tempted to go abroad for transplant surgery because of the shortage of kidneys in her country of origin, which results from domestic legal prohibition on the buying and selling of organs. Home country governmental prohibitions on the commodification of kidneys (and other human bodily resources) are motivated in part by a desire to protect members of vulnerable groups from exploitation. Surely the exploitation of destination-country organ providers is no more ethically acceptable than would be the exploitation of home-country organ providers. Therefore, when home-country legislation prohibits a certain medical practice in order to protect vulnerable persons, there is an ethical obligation to engage in serious conversation and counselling—and possibly also to deter patients from travelling abroad—in an effort to prevent the exportation of harmful exploitation.

Now some might argue that in situations where the domestically prohibited activity is not illegal in the destination country a softer approach to dissuading patients may be warranted. Perhaps, but this assessment will depend upon a careful analysis of the nature of the activity that is legally prohibited in the home country. Activities that are prohibited in an effort to protect the vulnerable from exploitation are decidedly different from activities that are prohibited on the basis of presumed social mores and customs. An example of the latter is the legal prohibition in Italy on access to fertility treatment for those who are not legally married heterosexual couples. If common law partners, single women, lesbian couples, or others who do not fit the description of 'legally married heterosexual couples' want to access fertility treatment in a foreign country where such treatment is legally available to them, there might be few grounds on which to deter patients from travelling abroad. The same might not be true with respect to medical travel for ova sales and surrogacy contracts where women in the destination countries—for example, India and the US—are at risk of exploitation.

CONFOUNDING FACTORS

There are a variety of ethically relevant considerations that are not captured in the analysis provided thus far. These include the potential costs to the health of travellers,[36] the internal 'care drain' of healthcare professionals from public and rural hospitals to private and urban hospitals that do not service the public healthcare needs of the domestic populations, and the undermining of public healthcare systems in home and destination countries by challenging the core value of equal access to healthcare. To say the least, many of these considerations are highly complex.

For example, while international medical travel motivated by a desire to avoid long waiting lists might be ethically uncontroversial from a patient perspective, especially when the

patient is wealthy and willing to pay for the travel, the ethics assessment is somewhat more complicated from a health-systems perspective. To the extent that international medical travel shortens the queue for medical procedures in home countries, it is desirable for patients to go abroad. In this way, international medical travel eases pressure on public care waiting lists by moving some of the patients to a different system, without at the same time removing healthcare providers from the public system. But this strategy for shortening wait lists is ethically problematic—especially when the procedures are medically necessary (as opposed to elective) and the cost of the medical travel must be borne by the patients. At a minimum, this introduces an advantage for the wealthy who can buy their way off the waiting list. Now for some, this is not ethically problematic; there are many things the rich can buy that the poor must do without. But for those who believe in government-funded healthcare, this is a significant ethical issue—medical travel for necessary medical treatment undermines a core value of equal access.

From another perspective, it is worth considering the impact of medical travel on access to healthcare for local patients in resource-poor destination countries, when the effort and energy of local healthcare providers is directed at the needs of foreign travellers. On the one hand, the medical travel industry threatens to exacerbate the internal 'care drain' by acceleration the depletion of an already scarce supply of healthcare providers from the critical public healthcare sector. On the other hand, this market could provide a means for attracting, retaining, and training doctors and nurses who might otherwise seek employment abroad. Additionally, the funds that medical travellers pay to hospitals, clinics and medical professionals can, in some cases, be used to subsidise the healthcare of local populations—for example, with the dedication of a percentage of hospital beds to patients within the public healthcare system. For resource-poor destination countries that are experiencing a shortage of medical resources and healthcare providers, medical travel has the potential to either help or harm their public healthcare systems.

CONCLUSION

It is easy to empathise with those who are (potential) international medical travellers. They want timely and affordable medical interventions that are not readily available to them domestically. In many cases the patients believe the desired interventions will allow them to lead the kinds of lives they envision for themselves and will significantly benefit their health. In a smaller number of cases, the patients see international medical travel as their only hope of survival. Chastising or punishing patients for travelling abroad is not the right response, but this leaves unanswered two pivotal questions: when, if ever, should patients participate in international medical travel, and when, if ever, should physicians facilitate or hinder their efforts to do so?

In an ideal world, governments with publicly funded healthcare systems should organise their systems to provide needed healthcare for all citizens at home. In the real world, this is not always possible, however, which accounts for the burgeoning international industry in medical travel.

All things considered, physicians should not inhibit their patients' access to international medical travel where the decision spaces of the travelling patients are characterised by relative expense (A) or by long domestic wait lists (B). Beyond this, one might even argue that physicians should facilitate such travel by offering appropriate referrals and directing patients to appropriate educational resources. At the same time, physicians should advocate for policy and practice changes in their home country, so that medically necessary services are controlled by the domestic public healthcare system for the benefit of all citizens. This is especially important given the underlying

belief with most publicly funded healthcare systems; namely, that healthcare should be provided in a timely fashion on the basis of need, not ability to pay.

Matters are notably different, however, when the international medical travel involves the element of harmful exploitation. Where the patient decision space is characterised by domestic bans on unproven medical interventions (C) or medical interventions that are domestically illegal because they take advantage of vulnerable third parties (D), a more restrictive approach is warranted. Where the potential victims of the harmful exploitation are the patients themselves, as in (C), the role of the physician may legitimately involve directive counselling aimed at dissuading the patient from travelling. At the very least, however, patients should be provided with full information about potential harms and available alternatives. When vulnerable third parties are the potential victims, as in (C) where the patients are children, or (D), the physician's efforts at discouraging international medical travel should be all the more assertive.

International medical travel is an ethically challenging aspect of globalisation. In our view, consideration of patient decision spaces is a useful analytical tool for illuminating the moral dimensions of medical travel, particularly in light of the scarcity of robust empirical data on various aspects of this burgeoning industry. It may also be a useful approach for physicians in deciding whether to facilitate or hinder patient efforts to engage in international medical travel. The four categories of decision spaces discussed in this article raise different ethical considerations; the weightiest of these concern the pursuit of interventions that are unproven (C), or illegal in the home country (D). Ultimately, in these contexts, the home country's obligation to protect its citizens from unnecessary harm and to promote the health and safety of vulnerable persons in source and destination countries are ethical considerations that must be given priority.

Acknowledgements

This research was developed, in part, under the Canadian Institutes of Health Research (CIHR) grant 'Ethics of Health Research and Policy'. For insightful feedback on drafts of this essay, the authors are grateful to the members of the Novel Tech Ethics research team, especially Andrew Fenton, and also to Jim Sabin and David Badcott. Any oversights or errors remain the authors' own.

Notes

1. Sweeting T, Patterson P. Lin and Win Htut: the conjoined twins from Burma. *Can Nurse* 1984;80:18–20.

2. Hospital for Sick Children. Sick kids evaluates conjoined twins for separation surgery. *Hospital for Sick Children Press Release* 2004. http://www.sickkids.ca/AboutSickKids/News-Room/Past-News/2004/SickKids-evaluates-conjoined-twinsfor-separation-surgery.html (accessed 2 Feb 2010).

3. Nolan S. Desperate mothers fuel India's baby factories. *Globe and Mail* 13 Feb 2009.

4. Baylis F, Crozier GKD. Postmenopausal reproduction: in whose interests? *J Obstet Gynaecol Can* 2009;31:457–8.

5. Staff writer. Health tourism in Asia, 2009. http://www.healthtourisminasia.com (accessed 2 Feb 2010).

6. The figures in this passage regarding percentage of country GDP derived from medical travel have been calculated from the cited figures of industry dollar value and on reports of country GDP published by the World Bank.[8]

7. Thaiwebsites.com. Medical tourism in Thailand: internationally-oriented hospitals. http://www.thaiwebsites.com/medical-tourism-thailand.asp (accessed 2 Feb 2010).

8. World Bank Group. World development indicators, 2009. Washington DC: World Bank Group.

9. Staff writer. Israel: hospitals look to medical tourism as a revenue source. *International Medical Travel Journal* 2009. http://www.imtj.com/news/?EntryId82=149400 (accessed 2 Feb 2010).

10. Understanding medical tourism. Medical tourism statistics. http://www.understanding-medical-tourism.com/medical-tourism-statistics.php (accessed 2 Feb 2010).

11. Venquist DG, Valdez E, Morrison B. Medical tourism economic report: Latin America versus Asia. *Medical Tourism Magazine* 2009. http://www.medicaltourismmag.com/issue-detail.php?item=214&issue=10# (accessed 2 Feb 2010).

12. Deloitte. *Medical tourism: consumers in search of value.* Washington DC: Deloitte Center For Health Solutions, 2008. http://www.deloitte.com/assets/Dcom-UnitedStates/Local%20Assets/Documents/us_chs_MedicalTourismStudy(3).pdf (accessed 2 Feb 2010).

13. Ehrbech T, Guevara C, Mango PD. Mapping the market for medical travel. *McKinsey Quarterly* 2008.

14. Youngman I. Medical tourism statistics: why McKinsey has got it wrong. *International Medical Travel Journal* 2009. http://www.imtjonline.com/articles/2009/mckinsey-wrong-medical-travel (accessed 2 Feb 2010).

15. DeNoble D. Deloitte's medical tourism fallacy. *Asia Health Care Blog* 2009. http://www.asia-healthcareblog.com/2009/04/06/deloittes-medical-tourism-fallacy/ (accessed 2 Feb 2010).

16. Carrera P, Bridges JFP. Globalization and healthcare: understanding health and medical tourism. *Expert Rev Pharmacoecon Outcomes Res* 2006;6:447–54.

17. Grail Research. *The rise of medical tourism.* LLC, 2009. http://www.grailresearch.com/pdf/ContenPodsPdf/Rise_of_Medical_Tourism_Summary.pdf. (accessed 2 Feb 2010).

18. Zaracostas J. Rising cost of care in rich countries is driving patients to seek treatment in developing nations. *BMJ* 2009;339:b3541.

19. Deloitte. *Survey of health care consumers.* Washington DC: Deloitte Center For Health Solutions, 2009.

20. Of 4001 survey respondents, 1% reported having travelled outside the US to access medical services. The figure of 3.05 million US medical travellers is based on this figure and on a US population in 2009 of roughly 305 million.

21. Yap J, Chen SS, Nones N. *Medical tourism: the Asian chapter.* Deloitte Consulting Pte Ltd, 2008. http://www.deloitte.com/assets/Dcom-Global/Local%20Assets/Documents/Medical%20Tourism%20–%20Asia%20Report%20–%20Web(1).pdf (accessed 2 Feb 2010).

22. Physicians are not the only healthcare providers who may have an opportunity to discuss the ethics of international medical travel with prospective travellers. In many cases, nurses, technicians, and others will be better situated to share relevant information with, and glean the relevant information from, patients.

23. Bossert T. Analyzing the decentralization of health systems in developing countries: decision space, innovation, and performance. *Soc Sci Med* 1998;47:1513–27.

24. Bossert TJ, Beauvais JC. Decentralization of health systems in Ghana, Zambia, Uganda and the Philippines: a comparative analysis of decision space. *Health Policy Plan* 2002;17:14–31.

25. Horowitz MD, Rosensweig JA, Jones CA. Medical tourism: globalization of the healthcare marketplace. *MedGenMed* 2007;9:33. http://www.pubmedcentral.nih.gov/articlerender.fcgi?artid=2234298 (accessed 2 Feb 2010).

26. Turner L. Cross-border dental care: 'Dental tourism' and patient mobility. *Br Dent J* 2008;204:553–4.

27. Turner L. Medical tourism: family medicine and international health-related travel. *Can Fam Physician* 2007;53:1639–41.

28. Ward D. A scalpel and a willing doctor: the new tourist attraction. *Vancouver Sun*, 2007. http://www.canada.com/nationalpost/story.html?id=c08b3dbc-c91a-4f69–a477–15f59d94f596 (accessed 2 February 2010).

29. BBC. Stem cell appeal reaches target. *BBC News* 2009. http://news.bbc.co.uk/2/hi/uk_news/wales/mid_/7989545.stm (accessed 2 Feb 2010).

30. BBC. The hunt for a stem cell miracle. *BBC News* 2009. http://news.bbc.co.uk/go/pr/fr/-/2/hi/uk_news/8052227.stm (accessed 2 Feb 2010).

31. MacReady N. The murky ethics of stem-cell tourism. *Lancet Oncol* 2009;10:317–18.

32. Nature. Stem-cell Society condemns medical tourism. *Nature News* 2008;453:969.

33. Prasad GVR, Shukla A, Huang M, et al. Outcomes of commercial renal transplantation: a Canadian experience. *Transplantation* 2006;82:1130–5.

34. Leigh S. Reproductive 'tourism'. *USA Today* 2005. http://www.usatoday.com/news/health/2005–05–02–reproductive-tourism_x.htm (accessed 4 May 2009).

35. INTJ Blog. Pakistan wants medical tourists, but not illegal transplants. *International Medical Travel Journal*, 2009. http://www.imtjonline.com/news/?EntryId82=140663 (accessed 2 Feb 2010).

36. McKelvey A, David AL, Shenfield F, et al. The impact of cross-border reproductive care or 'fertility tourism' on NHS maternity services. *BJOG* 2009;116:1520–3. doi:10.1111/j.1471–0528.2009.02294.x.

CASES

Cameron v Nova Scotia (Attorney General)(1999), 204 NSR (2d) 1, 1999 CanLII 7243 (CA)

Summary prepared by Josephine Johnston

Mr. Cameron and Dr. Smith, husband and wife, were unable to conceive a child due to the husband's "severe male factor infertility" (reduced sperm count). In an effort to conceive a child, they had both undergone surgery before they were referred by their physicians for intracytoplasmic sperm injection (ICSI). ICSI is a specialized form of in vitro fertilization (IVF) in which a single sperm is injected into an egg and the resulting fertilized egg is transferred to the woman for implantation and gestation. ICSI is considered the treatment of choice for severe male factor infertility.

The couple had four cycles of ICSI (two in Toronto and two in Calgary) and Dr. Smith received two frozen embryo transfers.

Reprinted by permission of the author.

None of the procedures were successful and the couple incurred approximately $40,000 in costs for treatments, drugs, travel, and lodging. They were unable to recover any of these costs from Maritime Medical Care, Inc. (MMC) because MMC said that the services accessed were not considered insured services in Nova Scotia.

Among other remedies, the couple sought recovery of their out-of-province fertility treatment costs, a declaration that they were entitled to coverage for any further treatment, and an order directing the Nova Scotia Minister of Health to establish a mechanism for payment for IVF and ICSI procedures. They argued that the services they accessed in Toronto and Calgary (and IVF generally) were "medically necessary" services and so ought to be covered under the Nova Scotia medical plan.

Discussion Questions

1. Is being a parent of a genetically related child a right that society should recognize and support financially?
2. Given that there never will be enough public money to pay for all potentially beneficial health care services, how should funding priorities for these services be determined?
3. How much responsibility for promoting health and providing health care should society accept, and how much should individual persons assume?

NOTE: At the time of writing, only two Canadian provinces pay for IVF. Ontario pays for three IVF cycles for women with bi-lateral blocked fallopian tubes. Quebec pays for three stimulated (or six natural) IVF cycles for all infertile women of childbearing age.

Auton (Guardian ad litem of) v British Columbia (Attorney General), 2004 SCC 78, [2004] 3 SCR 657

Summary prepared by Lisa Shields

The parents of children with autism or autism spectrum disorder (ASD) brought a legal action against the government of British Columbia seeking funding for treatment of their children's conditions and a declaration that the government's refusal to provide such treatment was a violation of ss. 7 and 15 of the *Canadian Charter of Rights and Freedoms*. Autism or ASD is a neurobehavioural syndrome that leads to behavioural impairments in social interaction and communication. Without appropriate therapy, almost all individuals with autism or ASD will lead a life of isolation and may be institutionalized.

The parents sought coverage for a specific type of early, intensive behavioural therapy called the "Lovaas Autism Treatment." This method of therapy

had been credited with increasing the independence and level of functioning of autistic children. The parents argued that the treatment provided their children with the greatest possible opportunities in life and consequently significantly contributed to the children's well-being. Each of the children involved had already shown notable improvements using the Lovaas method. Unfortunately, the treatment was extremely expensive.

The government refused to fund the Lovaas Autism Treatment because of a concern that providing treatment for autism or ASD would lead to other similar demands for coverage, thereby placing too great a financial strain on the provincial health care system. The government also questioned the efficacy of the Lovaas Autism Treatment.

Reprinted by permission of the author.

Discussion Questions

1. What kind and how much evidence about the effectiveness of a new treatment is required in order for it to be publicly funded?

2. Is it possible to make judgments about the comparative importance of treatments that enhance the quality of life and treatments that save or prolong life?

Useful Resources

ONLINE

Canadian Policy Research Networks (CPRN)

Contains numerous research reports on a variety of topics, including reports on caring for nurses and improving the working conditions of Canadian nurses and on managing waiting lists.

REPORT

Canadian Bar Association Report

Task Force on Health Care, The Canadian Bar Association. (1994). *What's law got to do with it? Health care reform in Canada.* Ottawa, ON: The Canadian Bar Association. This report examines whether there is a legal right to health care in Canada and reviews legal and ethical issues arising from health care resource allocation.

READINGS

Calabresi, G., & Bobbitt, P. (1978). *Tragic choices.* New York: Norton.

Daniels, N., & Sabin, J. E. (2008). *Setting limits fairly: Can we learn to share medical resources fairly* (2nd ed.). New York, NY: Oxford University Press.

Ham, C., & Pickard, S. (1998). *Tragic choices in health care: The case of Child B.* London: King's Fund Publishing.

Klein, R., Day, P., & Redmayne, S. (1996). *Managing scarcity: Priority setting and rationing in the National Health Service.* Philadelphia, PA: Open University Press.

Rhodes, R., Battin, M. P., & Silvers, A. (2002). *Medicine and social justice: Essays on the distribution of health care.* New York, NY: Oxford University Press.

HEALTH LAW

Eldridge v British Columbia (Attorney General), [1997] 3 SCR 624, 1997 CanLII 327 (SCC).

Three persons who were born deaf and whose preferred means of communication is sign language argued that the absence of interpreters impaired their ability to communicate with health care providers and thus increased the risk of misdiagnosis and ineffective treatment.

Flora v Ontario (Health Insurance Plan, General Manager), 2008 ONCA 538, 91 OR (3d) 412.

Mr. Flora was diagnosed with liver cancer. He was told that he had a life expectancy of six to eight months and that he was not a candidate for a liver transplant. He received a living-donor liver transplantation in London, England at a cost of approximately $450,000. He sought to have this expense reimbursed by the Ontario Health Insurance Plan.

CanWest MediaWorks Inc v Canada (Minister of Health) and Attorney General of Canada, 2008 FCA 2007, 78 Admin LR (4th) 1.

CanWest MediaWorks challenged a provision of the *Food and Drugs Act* that limits "Direct to Customer Advertising" of prescribed drugs in Canada by prohibiting advertisements that claim a drug treats, prevents, or cures medical conditions and diseases listed in the Act, and by restricting representations of drugs to facts about names, price, and quantity.

CanLII

CanLII is a non-profit organization managed by the Federation of Law Societies of Canada. CanLII's goal is to make Canadian law accessible for free on the Internet.

Chapter 4 PUBLIC HEALTH

INTRODUCTION

The term "public health" encompasses a wide range of activities that share a focus on protecting or promoting the health of populations, not individuals per se. In 2004, the Canadian government created the Public Health Agency of Canada with a mandate to promote health, prevent and control chronic diseases and injuries, prevent and control infectious diseases, prepare for and respond to public health emergencies, and strengthen public health capacity in a manner consistent with a shared understanding of the determinants of health and of the common factors that maintain health or lead to disease and injury. To fulfill this comprehensive mandate, the agency must engage in disease surveillance, undertake initiatives that will prevent disease and injury, act to protect and promote health, prepare for health emergencies, and conduct relevant research. There are many difficult ethical questions associated with each of these activities.

For example, disease surveillance raises questions of privacy and confidentiality whether the disease in question is a sexually transmitted disease or a frightening new virus (e.g., HIV or SARS). Legislation requiring seat belt or helmet use or prohibiting smoking in public places is effective at preventing injury and disease but at the cost of constraining personal freedom. In addition, many questions arise regarding the types of intervention that can be pursued by government agencies as public health practitioners struggle to deal with health threats such as obesity, violence, and homelessness. Health emergencies posed by pandemics, terrorist attacks, or natural disasters require public health officials to act quickly and decisively in ways that may violate individual rights and traditional freedoms, create or worsen discrimination against particular social groups, or require rationing of scarce, lifesaving resources, while transforming conventional relationships between patients and their health providers.

In this chapter, we look closely at a few important topics in the emerging field of public health ethics. We explore ethics questions related to theory, practice, and policy. We begin with a discussion of some key theoretical underpinnings for ethics appropriate for public health. Nuala Kenny, Susan Sherwin, and Françoise Baylis warn against the temptation to generate a public health ethics by simply modifying bioethics principles that were created for dilemmas that arise in the very different contexts of clinical ethics and research ethics. They propose an approach to public health ethics that extends far beyond the specific issues that arise in the midst of a public health crisis such as a serious pandemic. The theory they recommend is described as a relational approach, in that it highlights the importance of attending to social and political relations within the populations that are the target of public health activities.

Ted Schrecker proposes a strategy for addressing a very common problem that arises in the context of public health management of crises that seem connected to matters of scarcity. He considers problems associated with "health disparities" where members of economically disadvantaged groups face significantly elevated risks of harm. Focusing on the loss of life among the very poor in a 1995 Chicago heat wave and the catastrophic 2005 Hurricane Katrina, he discusses the social forces that created the conditions that proved so hazardous to human health. He argues that the scarcities that are at the heart of health disparities are neither natural nor inevitable but are the result of political choices that could and should be otherwise.

The chapter then turns to debate regarding some specific policies and practices in central areas of public health responsibility: epidemics and pandemics. Vaccination is a very important tool of public health efforts at disease prevention and, in most cases, the development of a vaccine to reduce the incidence of a common and serious disease is a cause for celebration. Abby Lippman identifies a series of concerns regarding the development and rapid introduction of a vaccine to prevent major forms of the human pappillomavirus (HPV) in adolescent girls demonstrating how difficult it can be to set public policy in the face of such an opportunity. HPV is primarily of concern because of its apparent connection to cervical cancer years later. Lippman agrees that cervical cancer is a serious threat to women's health and that the spread of HPV is a public health problem worthy of attention, but she worries that reliance on a new vaccine may not provide adequate long-term protection, will obscure other effective forms of prevention and treatment of cervical cancer, and will exacerbate health disparities around this disease.

Alison Thompson and colleagues present an ethical framework for pandemic influenza planning. Recognizing the many ethical questions that arise in the context of a pandemic outbreak, they argue for the importance of including an ethics framework as part of the work of pandemic preparedness. The particular framework presented was developed in light of lessons learned from the outbreak of SARS in Southern Ontario in 2003 when health care institutions were caught unprepared by the many ethical issues that rapidly emerged. The authors identify a number of ethical issues that require response in the face of a serious influenza outbreak and stress the importance of having a general ethics framework in place to help guide decision-making as issues arise. They name 10 key ethical values that they believe should guide the formation of the ethics framework and decision-making in a pandemic and propose three procedural elements for the development and application of a pandemic ethics framework.

Nathan Ford and colleagues expand the focus of public health ethics from local or national populations to the international context. They look at some of the thorny questions faced by the humanitarian health organization Médecins Sans Frontières (MSF or Doctors Without Borders) as it struggles to provide health care in the midst of dangerous crises with severely inadequate resources. They explore questions of process and substance regarding the need to decide on the appropriate deployment of resources and the levels of risk staff can be allowed or requested to assume when addressing health emergencies in foreign lands.

Re-visioning Public Health Ethics: A Relational Perspective

Nuala P. Kenny, Susan Sherwin, and Françoise Baylis

Canada has a proud tradition of making substantial conceptual advances in public health. With the renewed global interest in public health generated by the H1N1 pandemic, Canada is poised to make significant contributions to the development of a new public health ethics that is firmly grounded in a commitment to the health of populations and communities and to

Kenny, N., Sherwin, S., & Baylis, F. (2010) "Re-visioning Public Health Ethics: A Relational Perspective." *Canadian Journal of Public Health* 101(1): pp. 9–11. Reprinted with permission.

the reduction of health inequalities. However, we are concerned that this opportunity may be squandered by an inordinate focus on issues of emergency-preparedness to the exclusion of the full range of public health concerns[1,2] and an ongoing reliance on bioethical analysis steeped in the individual rights/autonomy discourse of clinical and research ethics.[3–5]

In this paper, we describe some concerns regarding the focus on pandemic ethics in isolation from public health ethics; identify inadequacies in the dominant individualistic ethics framework; and summarize our nascent work on the relational concepts that inform our re-visioning of public health ethics.[6]

PANDEMIC ETHICS: A NARROW VISION

The 2003 Canadian experience of the SARS near-pandemic brought home the reality of fundamental ethical concerns in times of emergency threats to public safety. Among the issues that were identified are restrictions of civil liberties, privacy, the duty of care, the right of health care workers to refuse dangerous work, the right of non-infected patients to access care facilities, the fair distribution of scientific credit for research discoveries, and patent protection.[7,8] While these are important issues, we have argued that,

> "[f]rom the perspective of pandemic planning and public health, this is an odd and limited list of concerns a list that likely would not have been generated but for the fact that the analysis remains steeped in an individual rights discourse inherited from clinical ethics and research ethics, and consonant with the dominant moral and political culture."[6]

Indeed, this analysis situates pandemic as a largely *personal health care issue* when it is in fact a global *public health issue*.

To date, the principle-based approach to ethics generated for clinical care and research, and involving respect for autonomy (of individuals), beneficence, non-maleficence and justice[9] has dominated ethical reflection in all health areas. With this approach, the interests and well-being of individual patients or research subjects are a primary concern. When a health risk affects a population, however, of necessity, the emphasis must shift from individual to collective interests. As the Public Health Agency of Canada recognizes: "When a health risk affects a population, ... public health ethics will predominate and a high value will be placed on the collective interests".[10] We join with the Public Health Agency of Canada and others[3,11,12] who call for a social starting point for public health ethics that recognizes community as foundational, and from this perspective caution against pandemic planning in the absence of a robust, population-focused ethic for public health.

At this time, there is no consensus regarding the appropriate theory and method for public health ethics.[2,13,14] It is widely understood, however, that the familiar autonomy-centred principles of contemporary bioethics are clearly inadequate when mapped to the agenda of public health.

Public health ethics requires an approach that is itself "public" rather than individualistic, i.e., one that understands the social nature and goals of public health work. It must make clear the complex ways in which individuals are inseparable from communities and populations and build on the need to attend to the interests of communities and populations as well as individuals.

A RELATIONAL ACCOUNT OF PUBLIC HEALTH ETHICS

We propose an alternative approach to public health ethics that is rooted in a relational understanding of persons. Public health deals with the health needs of communities and populations through actions that are taken at a social and political level. As such, it requires a conception of persons as embedded within communities in particular ways; it should recognize and respond to their fundamental social and political nature, and be attentive to ways in which patterns of systematic discrimination (or privilege) operate in terms of the goals and activities of public health.[15] Where traditional bioethics treats persons as self-contained, self-interested, and self-directing creatures, relational ethics insists that persons be treated as the social, interdependent beings that they are. Relational persons develop and deploy their values within the social worlds they inhabit, conditioned by the opportunities and obstacles that shape their lives according to the socially salient features of their embodied lives (e.g., their gender, race, class, age, disability status, ethnicity).[16]

Relational Autonomy

Autonomy remains an important value because public health involves actions aimed at the common good and the health of populations and it is easy to lose track of the rights and interests of individuals. However, relational autonomy embraces (rather than ignores) the fact that persons are inherently socially, politically, and economically-situated beings. A relational approach to autonomy directs us to attend to the many and varied ways in which competing policy options affect the opportunities available to members of different social groups (for example, quarantine may have a very different impact on those with significant disabilities than it will on those who can look after their own bodily needs), and to make visible the ways in which the autonomy of some may come at the expense of others. Relational autonomy encourages us to see that there are many ways in which autonomy can be compromised. It allows us to see that sometimes autonomy is best promoted through social change rather than simply protecting individuals' freedom to act within existing structures.

Relational Social Justice

The traditional bioethics principle of justice is primarily concerned with non-discrimination and distributive justice (the fair distribution of quantifiable benefits and burdens) among discrete individuals, including allocation of scarce resources such as vaccines or hospital beds. On a relational account, the concern falls more heavily on matters of social justice, involving fair access to social goods such as rights, opportunities,

power, and self respect.[17] This view of social justice directs us to explore the context in which certain political and social policies and structures are created and maintained. It asks us to look beyond effects on individuals and to see how members of different social groups may be collectively affected by practices that create inequalities in access and opportunity. Social justice enjoins us to correct *patterns* of systemic injustice among different groups, seeking to improve rather than worsen systematic disadvantages in society. It requires attention to the need[s] of the most disadvantaged. We join with Powers and Faden in believing that social justice is "the foundational moral justification for public health".[12]

Relational Solidarity

Public health involves efforts to attend to the needs of all, especially the most vulnerable and systematically disadvantaged members of society; as such, it should promote the value of solidarity.[1,7,17] Conventional solidarity refers to common interests purposes, or sympathies between discrete individuals or among members of a group.[18] Sometimes the emphasis is on altruism and helping relationships, particularly with the needy and disadvantaged. At other times, the emphasis is on reciprocity (with a focus on communality and mutuality) and the benefits of social cohesion. This conventional understanding of solidarity, however, is limited in its usefulness for public health ethics because of its ultimate reliance on the oppositional categories "us" and "them" based on identification with a common cause, a collective identity, and anticipation of mutual advantage among the "us" (usually defined in opposition to some excluded "others"). This understanding of solidarity fails to capture the wider public, many of whom may be among the vulnerable and systematically disadvantaged.

A relational concept of solidarity, built on a relational understanding of personhood and autonomy, aims to expand the category of "us" to "us all" and to do away with the binary opposition at work with the notions of "us" and "them". Relational solidarity values interconnections without being steeped in assumption: about commonality or collective identity in contrast to some other group. What matters in public health is a shared interest in survival, safety and security—an interest that can be effectively pursued through the pursuit of public goods understood as "non-excludable" and "non-rivalrous".[19] There are few pure public goods and health *per se* is not among them. However, there are numerous public goods *for* health, including; scientific knowledge, communicable disease control (including vaccination), and control of antibiotic resistance. Indeed, it is in this function of public health to promote public goods that we can best appreciate the role of solidarity at work. In this sense, the meaning of solidarity is found *within* public health itself.

RELATIONAL ETHICS IN THE REAL WORLD OF PUBLIC HEALTH POLICY

Public health ethics must expand as well as modify the traditional principles of bioethics.

In an earlier paper, we developed an extensive theoretical account of the principles of relational autonomy, relational social justice and relational solidarity,[6] and while there is still much work to be done to further refine these principles, we believe they have an important role to play in the practical and pressured policy world.

Specifically, we believe that these principles can help to reclaim and centre the common and collective good at risk in pandemic and other emergency situations. Indeed, since discussions of common and shared resources are almost impossible to raise in the environment of personal health care, public health may be the only viable source for reflections about our interdependence in times of need.

Minimally, these principles for a relational public health ethic carry with them important procedural and substantive demands. They require a policy-making process that is truly transparent, fair and inclusive, which requires that it be sensitive and responsive to the workings of systemic inequalities. Substantively, these relational principles also require public recognition of the fact that we enter any crisis with varying degrees of inequity and that the public policy response to the crisis must not forseeably increase existing inequities. These are modest demands but they are easily overlooked within a framework that focuses solely on the rights of individuals apart from their social context.

Public health joins a few other key public goods (e.g., universal education, prevention of further contributions to climate change, avoidance of nuclear war) in helping all to appreciate the reality of our mutual interest in survival, safety and security on the one hand, and our mutual vulnerability to disease, violence and death on the other. Because public health is an essential tool for promoting these very interests, we must come to appreciate the importance in recognizing our common vulnerabilities and needs and see the importance of a commitment to relational public health ethics as the means to achieve the necessary public goods.

Notes

1. Childress JF, Faden RR, Gaare RD, Gostin LO, Kahn J, Bonnie RJ, et al. Public health ethics: Mapping the terrain. *J Law Med Ethics* 2002;30:170–78.
2. Kass NE. An ethics framework for public health. *Am J Public Health* 2001;91(11):1776–82.
3. Beauchamp DE. Community: The neglected tradition of public health. *Hastings Center Report* 1985;15:28–36.
4. Rogers WA. Feminism and public health ethics. *J Med Ethics* 2008:32:351–54.
5. Jennings B. Public health and civic republicanism: Toward an alternative framework for public health ethics. In: Dawson A, Verweij M (Eds.), *Ethics, Prevention and Public Health*. New York. NY: Oxford University Press, 2007.
6. Baylis F, Kenny NP, Sherwin S. A relational account of public health ethics. *Public Health Ethics* 2008;l(3):196–209.
7. Singer PA, Benatar SR, Bernstein M, Abdallah SD, Dickens BM, MacRae SK, et al. Ethics and SARS: Lessons from Toronto. *BMJ* 2003;327:1342–44.
8. University of Toronto. Joint Centre for Bioethics Pandemic Influenza Working Group. Stand

on Guard for Thee: Ethical Considerations in Preparedness Planning for Pandemic Influenza. November 2005. Available at: http://www.joint-centreforbioethics.ca/publications/documents/stand_on_guard.pdf (Accessed February 19, 2009).

9. Beauchamp TL, Childress JF. *Principles of Biomedical Ethics*, 4th ed. New York: Oxford University Press, 2004.

10. Public Health Agency of Canada. The Canadian Pandemic Influenza Plan for the Health Sector. Section Two: Background, 2006. Available at: http://www.phac-aspc.gc.ca/cpip-pclcpi/pdf-e/section_2–eng.pdf (Accessed February 19, 2009).

11. Callahan D. Individual good and common good: A communitarian approach to bioethics. *Perspect Biol Med* 2003;46:496–507.

12. Powers M, Faden R. *Social Justice: The Moral Foundations of Public Health and Health Policy.* New York: Oxford University Press, 2006.

13. Roberts MJ, Reich MR. Ethical analysis in public health. *Lancet* 2002:359:1055–59.

14. Upshur RE. Principles for the justification of public health intervention. *Can J Public Health* 2002:93(2): 101–3.

15. Sherwin S, and The Canadian Feminist Health Research Network (Eds). A relational approach to autonomy in health care. In: Sherwin S, *The Politics of Women's Health: Exploring Agency and Autonomy.* Philadelphia, PA: Temple University Press, 1998.

16. Young IM. *Justice and the Politics of Difference.* Princeton., NJ: Princeton University Press, 1990.

17. Taubet AI. Medians, public health and the ethics of rationing. *Perspect Biol Med* 2002;45:16–30.

18. Houtepen R, ter Muelen R. The expectation(s) of solidarity and identity in the reconstruction of the health care system. *Health Care Analysis* 2006b;8:355–76.

19. Labonté R, Schrecker T. Globalization and social determinants of health: Promoting health equity in global governance (Part 3 of 3). *Globalization and Health* 2007;3, doi:10.1186/1744–8603–3–7. Available at: http://www.globalizationandhealth.com/content/3/1/7 (Accessed February 19, 2009).

Denaturalizing Scarcity: A Strategy of Enquiry for Public-Health Ethics

Ted Schrecker

WHY "DENATURALIZING SCARCITY"?

In 1995, a heat wave resulted in the deaths of more than 500 people in Chicago, United States of America (USA). Eric Klinenberg's "social autopsy" of this episode points out that "the processes through which Chicagoans lost their lives followed the entrenched logic of social and spatial divisions that governs the metropolis".[1] People in Chicago's poorest neighbourhoods, also with some of the highest proportions of African-Americans as the result of a history of racial segregation, were least likely to have, or be able to afford, air conditioning. In particular, realistic fear of crime kept the elderly socially isolated and barricaded into their homes, while a downsized city government failed to link residents with services that could have saved their lives. In 2005, the impact of hurricane Katrina on New Orleans brought to worldwide attention the deadly mix of racial and economic segregation, failure to invest in adequate flood-control measures despite ample warnings, and the presumption that everyone could afford to get in a car and drive to safety. When the storm hit, those who did not have this option, overwhelmingly poor and African-American, were effectively abandoned as refugees in their own country.[2,3]

Schrecker, T. (2008) "Denaturalizing Scarcity: A Strategy of Enquiry for Public-Health Ethics." *Bulletin of the World Health Organization* 86: pp. 600–605. http://www.who.int/bulletin/volumes/86/8/08-050880/en/

The impacts of the heat wave and the hurricane were not natural, any more than the inability of people in wheelchairs to get around buildings without ramps and elevators is natural. Here, I adapt the title of Klinenberg's study (*Denaturalizing Disaster*)[1] to the study of scarcities of resources to provide health care or to remove causes of illness by addressing social determinants of health. These scarcities are rarely natural, in the sense that they originate in circumstances outside human control. Far more common, in the words of Calabresi & Bobbitt's *Tragic Choices*,[4] are situations in which "scarcity is not the result of any absolute lack of a resource but rather of the decision by society that it is not prepared to forgo other goods and benefits in a number sufficient to remove the scarcity". The starting point of my argument is that to conduct responsible policy analysis: "We must determine where if at all in the history of a society's approach to the particular scarce resource, a decision substantially within the control of that society was made as a result of which the resource was permitted to remain scarce. ... Scarcity cannot simply be assumed as a given".[4] Denaturalizing scarcity is a strategy for applying this insight to research, policy analysis and advocacy.

ON THE AFFORDABILITY OF SAVING (AND TAKING) LIVES

What kinds of scarcities are at issue? In the context of high-income countries, consider the USA's failure to provide health insurance for more than 40 million people, with predictable medical and financial consequences. On one estimate, providing health coverage for the uninsured would cost US$ 100 billion a year: a huge sum, yet just half the annual cost of the country's military adventure in Iraq.[5] Using a measure designed for cross-national comparisons, the prevalence of child poverty in the USA is 10 times as high as it is in Norway.[6] The difference matters for public health, not only because of the long-term importance of early childhood development[7] but also because an economic gradient

in health status is evident even in the richest societies, although generally less steep in more egalitarian ones.[8,9] Such situations direct our attention to national choices and priorities that make resources scarce for some purposes, but abundant for others.

However, this paper concentrates on even more dramatic global contrasts between scarcity and abundance and their implications for public health. Per capita spending on health care varies by two orders of magnitude between rich and poor countries, from US$ 15 per capita in the least developed countries (as defined by the United Nations) where 770 million people live, and US$ 24 per capita in low-income countries (as defined by the World Bank) where 2.4 billion people live, to US$ 3687 per capita in high-income countries.[10] In low-income countries, much health-care spending is out of pocket, may not benefit those whose health is poorest or most precarious, and may have catastrophic financial consequences for the household even when it does. The estimated US$ 40 minimum cost of providing basic health care per person per year is out of reach for many low-income countries, and will remain so for some time without major infusions of external resources.[11]

Another illustration of the impact of scarcity comes from researchers associated with the Bellagio Study Group on Child Survival, who estimate that a package of interventions costing US$ 5.1 billion per year would save the lives of 6 million children per year in 42 countries that account for 90% of the global toll of under-5 child mortality.[12] This figure is imprecise (it could be as high as US$ 8 billion) and it is an underestimate because it includes direct costs but not the costs of maintaining, rebuilding or expanding health systems that in many developing countries are fragile or collapsing. Nevertheless, it suggests an affirmative answer to the question: "Can the world afford to save the lives of 6 million children each year"?[12]

Health-threatening resource scarcities are equally conspicuous with respect to social determinants of health. The World Bank estimates that a billion people worldwide live below its

"US$ 1 a day" poverty line and 2.6 billion, or two-fifths of the world's people, below the "US$ 2 a day" threshold.[10] Many commentators argue that these poverty lines substantially understate the true extent of serious deprivation.[13,14] Approximately 850 million people suffer from chronically insufficient caloric intake.[15] Apart from undernutrition, poverty creates situations in which the daily routines of living are themselves hazardous. More than 850 million people now live in slums, where they are routinely exposed to multiple health hazards;[16] rapid urbanization will increase the number to 1.4 billion in 2020 in the absence of effective policy interventions.[17] Indoor pollution from cooking fires is a major contributor to respiratory disease among the world's poor,[18] as is lack of safe drinking water and sanitation to infectious diarrhoea and a variety of parasitic diseases.[19] These are just selected demonstrations that "many of the most devastating problems that plague the daily lives of billions of people are problems that emerge from a single, fundamental source: the consequences of poverty and inequality".[20]

WHY CARE ABOUT SCARCITY IN THE CONTEXT OF PUBLIC HEALTH?

Why should we care about resource scarcities that distribute the chance to live a long and healthy life unequally within and among societies? In oversimplified terms, two lines of reasoning, which are not mutually exclusive, can be identified.

First, widespread persistence of unmet basic needs related to health may be regarded as creating at least a prima facie case for allocating resources in a way that gives priority to meeting those needs. Henry Shue[21] captured the essence of this argument with the observation that: "One person's desire for an additional jar of caviar is not equal in urgency to another person's need for an additional bowl of black beans". If the quantum of resources available were such that reducing the availability of caviar to a few would not have a meaningful effect on access to black beans (or basic health care,

or other social determinants of health) for all, then Shue's observation would have limited relevance. However, this is not the case. The US$ 5.1 billion annual cost of child-saving interventions referred to above corresponds to less than four days' US military spending, and is less than the personal incomes of the United States' two highest-earning hedge fund managers in 2007.[22] Redistributing just 0.9% of the global economic product would be sufficient to raise the income of all the world's poor above the World Bank's US$ 2 a day threshold.[23] Such comparisons can be dismissed as polemical, but in addition to serving as a resource for ethical reflection they underscore an observation by economist Jeffrey Sachs, who directed a multinational research effort on how to achieve the United Nations' Millennium Development Goals:[24] "[I]n a world of trillions of dollars of income every year, the amount of money that you need to address the health crises is easily available".[25]

The position that priority should be given to meeting basic health-related needs gains force from the moral arbitrariness of accidents of birth[26] that determine (for instance) whether one will be born in Canada, where life expectancy at birth is 80 years, or in Zambia, where it is 38 years. It loses force, for some, because it fails to specify the basis for an obligation to mitigate the consequences of such accidents, especially across national borders. A second line of reasoning, which responds to this challenge, starts from factual evidence of multiple causal connections that link the situations and futures of rich and poor. This position is most closely associated with the work of Thomas Pogge,[23,27,28] for whom moral responsibility follows causal responsibility (for poverty and other deprivations) within and across national borders, so long as a plausible alternative set of social arrangements or institutions that would be less inimical to poverty reduction and meeting other basic needs is available.

As shown in the next section of this paper, such plausible alternative arrangements can readily be imagined. The strategy of enquiry is important because unless one rejects a priori the position that remediable health-threatening scarcities of resources are a matter of ethical concern, denaturalizing scarcity is in some respects at least *logically prior* to the effort to construct an ethical argument in support of obligations to reduce or eliminate scarcities, within or across national borders. Only after resource scarcities have been identified as the consequence of either specific policy choices or more general social arrangements can appropriate ethical arguments be constructed.

DENATURALIZING SCARCITY AND GLOBALIZATION

Denaturalizing scarcity in the international frame of reference starts with understanding globalization: the increasingly dense web of trade and investment flows and institutional relationships that connects people in rich and poor countries.[29] Those flows and relationships are "asymmetrical" in multiple dimensions.[30]

Trade policy provides the most familiar example. Because the relative size of industrialized- and developing-country markets creates major disparities in bargaining power, developing countries may have to give up a great deal in return for market access, especially in the context of bilateral and regional agreements;[31] for instance, the United States is trying to incorporate provisions that undermine hard-won flexibilities with respect to patent rights and access to essential medicines.[32] More generally, global reorganization of production across multiple national borders facilitated by trade liberalization, but long predating the establishment of the World Trade Organization has created a situation in which countries must compete for foreign direct investment and outsourced contract production. Although effects on health are not always or unequivocally destructive, the World Bank's observation that global reorganization of production "mercilessly weeds out those centers with below-par macroeconomic environments, services, and labor-market flexibility"[33] is indicative of the constraints involved.

Many developing countries found themselves unable to service their external debts starting in

the early 1980s, for reasons largely outside their control. The International Monetary Fund (IMF), along with the World Bank, offered "structural adjustment" loans to facilitate rescheduling these debts, but the loans were predicated on a package of macroeconomic policies designed primarily to protect recipient countries' ability to repay external creditors.[34-36] Structural adjustment also had the effect, probably intentional, of promoting the broader, market-oriented agenda of key Group of Seven (G7) nations at the time.[36] The resulting economic dislocations and austerity measures often had destructive effects on health-care spending and social determinants of health noted as early as 1987 by a United Nations Children's Fund (UNICEF) study calling instead for "adjustment with a human face"[37] and were often met with widespread popular resistance.

Although the IMF is now less important as a lender, its influence remains pervasive. Private investors view IMF approval of a country's macroeconomic policies as an indispensable endorsement, and the IMF and World Bank must sign off on a country's policies as a condition for many forms of development assistance, including debt relief under the Multilateral Debt Relief Initiative. This process appears to reproduce many earlier forms of conditionality, with an emphasis on rapid integration into the global marketplace.[38-40] Recently, the IMF's demand for public-sector wage expenditure ceilings has been criticized for preventing the hiring of badly needed health personnel and teachers, even when the funds are available from development assistance. The IMF first disputed these criticisms, but internal and external assessments confirmed in 2007 that public-sector wage-bill ceilings were often recommended; that IMF projections of future development assistance were consistently low, leading to excessive caution with respect to public expenditure; and that in 29 sub-Saharan countries, IMF strictures meant that just 27 cents of every incremental US dollar in development assistance was budgeted for new programmes, with the balance being used for repaying domestic debt and accumulating foreign-exchange reserves.[41,42] This is correct as textbook public finance, but potentially destructive of health and education systems that are already fragile.

A more subtle dynamic of "implicit conditionality"[43] operates when governments are constrained by capital hypermobility in global financial markets. Economic crises that reduce the value of national currencies by 50% or more, and spread unemployment and economic insecurity, exemplify what a former managing director of the IMF has called the "swift, brutal and destabilizing" consequences that ensue when policies are not "deemed basically sound" by investors.[44] Less dramatically, financial markets' anticipation of redistributive domestic policies can lead the governments in question, e.g. Brazil's during the first term of the Workers' Party and South Africa's post-1994, to accept high unemployment and limited social expenditure[45,46] "dismal development and excellent macroeconomic outcomes", in the words of one observer of South Africa.[47] Thus, a sophisticated researcher warns that "those societies most in need of egalitarian redistribution may have, in terms of external financial market pressures, the most difficulty achieving it".[48] The global financial marketplace further facilitates patterns of capital flight that contribute to shortages of resources for development in entire regions, such as sub-Saharan Africa.[49,50]

These dynamics, and many others described more extensively elsewhere,[29,51] suffice to demonstrate that in today's global economy, resource scarcities that threaten health are like those in the specific contexts of the Chicago heat wave and the New Orleans hurricane anything but natural. They are the outcomes of decisions that could have been made differently and, in particular, of social institutions that could be designed differently.[23]

INFORMING PHILOSOPHY AND PRACTICE

Some philosophers concede that health-related resource scarcities give rise to ethical obligations within national borders, yet argue that despite the moral arbitrariness of the accidents of birth referred to earlier, obligations that would entail global redistribution of resources can only exist within a previously established framework of institutional associations and political accountabilities analogous to the nation-state. They further assert that no such framework exists on a global scale.[52]

Moellendorf counters persuasively that both the historical record (for instance of colonialism and its legacies) and today's multiple cross-border economic connections, such as foreign direct investment flows and the reach of the IMF, constitute a "global association" sufficient to give rise to claims of distributive justice across borders.[53] Indeed, it is perverse in the extreme to reject the existence of health-related ethical obligations that cross national borders simply *because* no mechanisms exist to hold powerful social institutions, and the key actors within them, accountable for scarcities they cause or perpetuate, perhaps half a world away. The situation would seem, rather, to call for an intensified effort to create such mechanisms where they do not exist, and improve the effectiveness of the imperfect institutions of international governance (such as the framework of human rights law)[54] that are available. Expanding on these possibilities would require a separate paper.

Certainly, accepting the existence of duties of international justice related to the causes of health disparities does not define the scope of the relevant obligations. Denaturalizing scarcity will not resolve that debate, but can contribute usefully in the context of increased policy attention to health equity: the absence of disparities in health that are unfair, unavoidable and systematically related to social (dis)advantage.[55] Critical and informed study of policies and institutions that affect the distribution of opportunities to lead a healthy life, both within and across national borders, lends strong support to the position of the Commission on Social Determinants of Health that: "The vast majority of inequalities in health, between and within countries, are avoidable and, hence, inequitable".[56] Mainstream health ethics usually accept scarcity as given and adaptation as imperative: for instance, by proposing substantive criteria or procedural algorithms for setting priorities in "resource-poor settings". Denaturalizing scarcity asks, instead, why some settings are consistently and fatally resource poor and others are not. It is therefore an indispensable foundation for a public-health ethics that lives up to the historical tradition of public-health practice by searching for the root causes of illness and injury.

Notes

1. Klinenberg E. Denaturalizing disaster: a social autopsy of the 1995 Chicago heat wave. *Theory Soc* 1999;28:239–95. doi:10.1023/A:1006995507723

2. Dreier P. Katrina and power in America. *Urban Aff Rev Thousand Oaks Calif* 2006;41:528–49. doi:10.1177/1078087405284886

3. Hartman C, Squires GD, eds. *There is no such thing as a natural disaster: race, class, and hurricane Katrina.* New York: Routledge; 2006.

4. Calabresi G, Bobbitt P. *Tragic choices.* New York: WW Norton; 1978. pp. 22, 150–1.

5. Leonhardt D. What $1.2 trillion can buy. *New York Times* 2007: 17 Jan. Available from: http://www.nytimes.com/2007/01/17/business/17leonhardt.html [accessed on 9 June 2008].

6. *Child poverty in rich countries 2005.* Florence: UNICEF, Innocenti Research Centre; 2005.

7. Irwin LG, Siddiqi A, Hertzman C. 7. *Early child development: a powerful equalizer final report of the Early Child Development Knowledge Network* [to the WHO Commission on Social Determinants of Health]. Vancouver: Human Early Learning Partnership, University of British Columbia; 2007. Available from: http://www.who.int/social_determinants/resources/ecd_kn_report_07_2007.pdf [accessed on 9 June 2008].

8. Siddiqi A, Kawachi I, Berkman L, Subramanian SV, Hertzman C. Variation of socioeconomic gradients in children's developmental health across advanced capitalist societies: analysis of 22 OECD nations. *Int J Health Serv* 2007;37:63–87. PMID:17436986 doi:10.2190/JU86-457P-7656-W4W7

9. Phipps SA, Burton PS, Osberg LS, Lethbridge LN. Poverty and the extent of child obesity in Canada, Norway and the United States. *Obes Rev* 2006;7:5-12. PMID:16436098 doi:10.1111/j.1467-789X.2006.00217.x

10. HNPStats [on-line]. World Bank Health Nutrition & Population Program. Available from: http://web.worldbank.org/WBSITE/EXTERNAL/TOPICS/EXTHEALTHNUTRITIONANDPOPULATION/EXTDATASTATISTICSHNP/EXTHNPSTATS/0,menuPK:3237172~pagePK:64168427~piPK:64168435~theSitePK:3237118,00.html [accessed on 9 June 2008].

11. Ooms G, Damme WV, Baker BK, Zeitz P, Schrecker T. The "diagonal" approach to global fund financing: a cure for the broader malaise of health systems? *Globalization and Health* 2008;4:6. Available from: http://www.globalizationandhealth.com/content/4/1/6 [accessed on 9 June 2008].

12. Bryce J, Black RE, Walker N, Bhutta ZA, Lawn JE, Steketee RW. Can the world afford to save the lives of 6 million children each year? *Lancet* 2005;365:2193-200. PMID:15978927 doi:10.1016/S0140-6736(05)66777-3

13. Reddy SG, Pogge TW. *How not to count the poor,* version 6.2. New York: Columbia University; 2005. Available from: http://www.undp-povertycentre.org/publications/poverty/HowNOTtocountthepoor-SANJAYREDDY.pdf [accessed on 9 June 2008].

14. Satterthwaite D. The Millennium Development Goals and urban poverty reduction: great expectations and nonsense statistics. *Environ Urban* 2003; 15:179–90. doi:10.1177/095624780301500208

15. *The state of food insecurity in the world 2006.* Rome: United Nations Food and Agriculture Organization; 2006. Available from: ftp://ftp.fao.org/docrep/fao/009/a0750e/a0750e00.pdf [accessed on 9 June 2008].

16. Unger A, Riley LW. Slum health: from understanding to action. *PLoS Medicine* 2007;4:e295. Available from: http://medicine.plosjournals.org/perlserv/?request=get-document&doi=10.1371/journal.pmed.0040295&ct=1 [accessed on 9 June 2008].

17. UN Millennium Project Task Force on Improving the Lives of Slum Dwellers. *A home in the city.* London: Earthscan; 2005.

18. Rehfuess E. *Fuel for life: Household energy and health.* Geneva: WHO; 2006. Available from: http://www.who.int/entity/indoorair/publications/fuelforlife.pdf [accessed on 9 June 2008].

19. Prüss A, Kay D, Fewtrell L, Bartram J. Estimating the burden of disease from water, sanitation, and hygiene at a global level. *Environ Health Perspect* 2002;110:537-42. PMID:12003760

20. Paluzzi JE, Farmer PE. The wrong question. *Development* 2005;48(1):12–18. doi:10.1057/palgrave.development.1100114

21. Shue H. Environmental change and the varieties of justice. In: Hampson F, Reppy J, eds. *Earthly goods: environmental change and social justice.* Ithaca, NY: Cornell University Press; 1996. pp. 9–29.

22. Taub S. Alpha's top moneymakers. *Alpha Magazine* 2008, 15 April. Available from: http://www.iimagazine.com/Article.aspx?articleID=1914971&HideRelated=1&SearchResult=1 [accessed on 9 June 2008].

23. Pogge T. Severe poverty as a human rights violation. In: Pogge T, ed. *Freedom from poverty as a human right: who owes what to the very poor?* Oxford: Oxford University Press; 2007 pp. 11–53.

24. *Investing in development: a practical plan to achieve the Millennium Development Goals.* UN Millennium Project. London: Earthscan; 2005.

25. Sachs J. Achieving the Millennium Development Goals: health in the developing world. Speech at the: *Second Global Consultation of the Commission on Macroeconomics and Health.* Geneva: WHO; 2003. Available from: http://www.earth.columbia.edu/sitefiles/File/about/director/pubs/CMHSpeech102903.pdf [accessed on 9 June 2008].

26. Ruger JP. Ethics and governance of global health inequalities. *J Epidemiol Community Health* 2006;60:998-1002. PMID:17053290 doi:10.1136/jech.2005.041947

27. Pogge T. Human rights and human responsibilities. In: De Greiff P, Cronin C, eds. *Global justice and transnational politics.* Cambridge, MA: MIT Press; 2002. pp. 151–95.

28. Pogge T. Recognized and violated by international law: the human rights of the global poor. *Leiden J Int Law* 2005;18:717-45. doi:10.1017/S0922156505002980

29. Labonté R, Schrecker T. Globalization and social determinants of health: the role of the global marketplace (part 2 of 3). *Globalization and Health* 2007;3:6. PMID:17578569 doi:10.1186/1744-8603-3-6

30. Birdsall N. *The world is not flat: inequality and injustice in our global economy.* WIDER Annual Lecture 9. Helsinki: World Institute for Development Economics Research; 2006. Available from: http://www.wider.unu.edu/publications/annual-lectures/en_GB/annual-lectures/ [accessed on 9 June 2008].

31. Shadlen KC. Exchanging development for market access? Deep integration and industrial policy under multilateral and regional-bilateral trade greements. *Rev Int Polit Econ* 2005;12:750–75. doi:10.1080/09692290500339685

32. *U.S. trade policy guidance on WTO declaration on access to medicines may need clarification,* GAO-07–1198. Washington, DC: United States Government Accountability Office; 2007. Available from: http://www.gao.gov/new.items/d071198.pdf [accessed on 9 June 2008].

33. *World development report 1999/2000: entering the 21st century.* New York: Oxford University Press; 1999. p. 50.

34. Milward B. What is structural adjustment? In: Mohan G, Brown E, Milward B, Zack-Williams AB, eds. *Structural adjustment: theory, practice and impacts.* London: Routledge; 2000. p. 24–38.

35. Babb S. The social consequences of structural adjustment: recent evidence and current debates. *Annu Rev Sociol* 2005;31:199-222. doi:10.1146/annurev.soc.31.041304.122258

36. Woods N. *The globalizers: the IMF, the World Bank, and their borrowers.* Ithaca, NY: Cornell University Press; 2006.

37. Cornia GA, Jolly R, Stewart F, eds. *Adjustment with a human face, vol.1: Protecting the vulnerable and promoting growth.* Oxford: Clarendon Press; 1987.

38. Cheru F. *Economic, social and cultural rights: the highly indebted poor countries (HIPC) initiative: a human rights assessment of the Poverty Reduction Strategy Papers* (PRSP), E/CN.4/2001/56. Geneva: UN Economic and Social Council; 2001. Available from: http://www.unhchr.ch/Huridocda/Huridoca.nsf/0/d3b348546ad5fb91c1256a110056aca4/$FILE/G0110184.pdf [accessed on 9 June 2008].

39. Gore C. MDGs and PRSPs: are poor countries enmeshed in a global-local double bind? *Global Social Policy* 2004;4:277-83. doi:10.1177/1468018104004400302

40. Brock K, McGee R. *Mapping trade policy: understanding the challenges of civil society participation.* IDS working paper 225. Brighton, Sussex: Institute for Development Studies; 2004. Available from: http://www.ids.ac.uk/ids/bookshop/wp/wp225.pdf [accessed on 9 June 2008].

41. *The IMF and aid to sub-Saharan Africa.* Washington, DC: Independent Evaluation Office, International Monetary Fund; 2007.

42. Working Group on IMF Programs and Health Spending. *Does the IMF constrain health spending in poor countries? Evidence and an agenda for action.* Washington, DC: Center for Global Development; 2007.

43. Griffith-Jones S, Stallings B. New global financial trends: implications for development. In: Stallings B, ed. *Global change, regional response: the new international context of development.* Cambridge: Cambridge University Press; 1995. pp. 143–73.

44. Camdessus M. *The IMF and the challenges of globalization the fund's evolving approach to its constant mission: the case of Mexico.* Address at Zurich Economics Society. Washington, DC: International Monetary Fund; 1995. Available

from: http://www.imf.org/external/np/sec/mds/1995/mds9517.htm [accessed on 9 June 2008].

45. Evans P. Neoliberalism as a political opportunity: constraint and innovation in contemporary development strategy. In: Gallagher K, ed. *Putting development first: the importance of policy space in the WTO and IFIs.* London: Zed Books; 2005. pp. 195–215.

46. Koelble T, Lipuma E. The effects of circulatory capitalism on democratization: observations from South Africa and Brazil. *Democratization* 2006;13:605–31. doi:10.1080/13510340600791913

47. Streak JC. The GEAR legacy: did GEAR fail or move South Africa forward in development? *Dev South Afr* 2004;21:271–88. doi:10.1080/0376835042000219541

48. Mosley L. Constraints, opportunities, and information: financial market–government relations around the world. In: Bardhan P, Bowles S, Wallerstein M, eds. *Globalization and egalitarian redistribution.* New York and Princeton: Russell Sage Foundation and Princeton University Press; 2006. pp. 87–119.

49. Ndikumana L, Boyce JK. Public debts and private assets: explaining capital flight from sub-Saharan African countries. *World Dev* 2003;31:107–30. doi:10.1016/S0305-750X(02)00181-X

50. Collier P, Hoeffler A, Pattillo C. Flight capital as a portfolio choice. *World Bank Econ Rev* 2001;15:55–80. doi:10.1093/wber/15.1.55

51. Labonte R, Blouin C, Chopra M, Lee K, Packer C, Rowson M, et al. *Towards health-equitable globalisation: rights, regulation and redistribution.* Final report of the Globalization Knowledge Network [to the WHO Commission on Social Determinants of Health]. Ottawa, ON: Institute of Population Health, University of Ottawa; 2007. Available from: http://www.who.int/social_determinants/resources/gkn_final_report_042008.pdf [accessed on 9 June 2008].

52. Nagel T. The problem of global justice. *Philos Public Aff* 2005;33:113–47. doi:10.1111/j.1088-4963.2005.00027.x

53. Moellendorf D. *Cosmopolitan justice.* Boulder, CO: Westview; 2002. pp. 31–9.

54. Nygren-Krug H. *25 questions and answers about health and human rights.* Geneva: WHO; 2002. Available from: http://www.who.int/hhr/NEW37871OMSOK.pdf [accessed on 9 June 2008].

55. Solar O, Irwin A. *A conceptual framework for action on the social determinants of health.* Geneva: WHO (Commission on Social Determinants of Health); 2007. Available from: http://www.who.int/entity/social_determinants/resources/csdh_framework_action_05_07.pdf [accessed 9 June 2008].

56. *Achieving health equity: from root causes to fair outcomes* [interim statement]. Geneva: WHO (Commission on Social Determinants of Health); 2007. pp. 2. Available from: http://libdoc.who.int/publications/2007/interim_statement_eng.pdf [accessed on 9 June 2008].

Human Papillomavirus (HPV) Vaccination and the Development of Public Policies

Abby Lippman

Through heavy, profit-driven marketing, cervical cancer has been (re)constructed in the past couple of years in North America almost solely as an independent vaccine-preventable disease. With the heady mix of young girls and their sexual behaviour as background, and an open-ended advertising budget providing memorable catchphrases,[1] the powerful major story-tellers (pharmaceutical companies, physicians and their organisations, the media) have constructed a gripping story comprising a feared disease (cancer), a unique product (the human papillomavirus (HPV)

Reproduced from the *Journal of Epidemiology and Community Health*, Lippman, A., Volume 62, "Human papillomavirus (HPV) vaccination and the development of public policies", pp. 570–571. Copyright © 2008 with permission from BMJ Publishing Group Ltd.

vaccine, Gardasil[2]) to address it, and hyped promises of prevention. This presentation has all too often silenced, or at least marginalised, other ways of talking about cervical cancer (and HPV infection), at the same time arousing controversies, confusions and conundrums in the minds of many.

In July 2006, the Canadian regulator for vaccines officially approved Merck's HPV vaccine, Gardasil. In February 2007, NACI (the federal National Advisory Committee on Immunizations) released its report recommending the use of the vaccine for females aged 9–13. Immediately thereafter, in March 2007, the federal government announced in the budget speech an allocation of CDN$300 million for the express purpose of purchasing Gardasil to immunise young girls.

This hastily made decision parallels the Gardasil phenomenon in the USA, which has been characterised by a headlong rush to establish mandatory vaccination programmes for as many young girls as possible, as quickly as possible. Western European countries have been more leisurely, although many have already adopted some vaccination policy. Interestingly, Australia only did so after negotiating down the price and getting assurances that costs would be covered if a booster were ever to be needed.[3] But while the question could be asked in both Canada and the USA "why the hurry?" especially when there is no epidemic of infection and the mortality rates from cervical cancer have been in decline the responses to the rush diverge markedly. Unlike the USA, where concern about the sexuality/sexualisation of young girls and mandatory immunisations have usually been placed at the centre of the debates, in Canada (and Spain), the loudest voices criticising mass vaccination programmes have come from women's health advocates/activists and this possibly counterintuitive response stems from these groups' concerns about both how public health policies are developed and implemented in a neoliberal environment and how (and by whom) boundaries between biomedical and biosocial domains are drawn.[4–7] Moreover, these groups recall other "quick fixes" proposed to prevent women's health problems (eg diethylstilbestrol

(DES) for "recurrent" miscarriages; hormone replacement therapy (HRT) for menopause-related cardiac conditions) that turned out to be quite harmful. Thus, their hesitations and cautionary words have an evidence base, and others[8] have recently advanced very similar critiques.

In many ways, the HPV vaccine is a microcosm in which multiple women's health issues are represented: the rapid introduction of a new (not fully tested) "preventive" intervention, the narrow medicalisation of a larger issue of sexual health and the individualising of risk factors in the face of a problem with structural determinants are but three of them.

In telling the "Gardasil story", cancer control and prevention, as well as sexually transmitted infection (STI) control and prevention, have all been conflated. As well, and as is true of many new pharmaceutical products, a "one shot" approach to a problem (HPV infection) framed as an independent risk is emphasised. This sidelines issues about how HPV is transmitted and emphasises women's individualised and privatised need to respond for their own, and their daughters', well being. Worse, perhaps, ongoing marketing frames girls/women as responsible for ensuring they (or their daughters) are vaccinated and "protected", thereby ignoring the responsibility of the health system for ensuring the elimination of *its* failures that lead to the absence of Pap testing, follow-ups, etc., failures that, for example, appear to underlie at least 50% (Canada[9]) and 80% (Spain[8]) of the cases of invasive cervical cancer and explain inequities in the distribution of the disease everywhere. The vaccine may provide some still unknown number of years of protection against infection with four HPV types for girls who are immunised, but is this narrow medicalisation of HPV infections sufficient for meeting girls' and women's broader and often unmet sexual health needs, needs that cry out for more holistic approaches?

In presenting the vaccine, researchers, physicians and the media have made much of how the two "high risk" HPV types covered by Gardasil are associated with "70–80%" (the numbers vary from author to author) of cases of cervical cancer.

But, while this appears accurate, it is a one-sided version of reality that omits the equally accurate information about the great capacity of healthy, immuno-competent (especially young) women spontaneously to clear up to 90% of HPV infections, infections almost all will one day acquire, within 1–2 years. Nor do the main stories discuss how cervical cancer develops only for a small minority of women when infection persists and is not detected through screening.

Although cervical cancer is very strongly associated with HPV infections, the converse is not true: those with HPV infections are highly unlikely to develop invasive cervical cancer. Moreover, while vaccine proponents emphasise the many thousands of women who participated in clinical trials of the product, they gloss over how few young girls in the age range (9–13 years) targeted specifically for school-based immunisations were included as well as how only the very short-term immunogenicity and safety, and not the efficacy, of Gardasil was studied.[10] Why are these stories not being told?

Similarly missing from the media and marketing stories of Gardasil has been mention that surrogate endpoints, not cervical cancer, have been used to measure efficacy in the clinical trials of the product.[11] That this is, in general, an ethical approach is unarguable; no one would want to wait to see cervical cancer develop in participants. But the general failure to mention that the precancerous lesions chosen for study are not only potentially removable, and that most (those that are CIN 2) would probably have resolved on their own without any intervention, *is* arguable—as is the absence of attention to how efficacy in a clinical trial does not necessarily translate into effectiveness in the real world. Public health programmes have an obligation to fully inform and educate people in appropriate, unbiased ways.

HPV infection is more than an independent, individual risk to be managed. As with other STIs, it is a public health problem that too often reflects the cracks in society that follow place, class and race differences created by political and economic decisions of the state. If we are to address invasive cervical cancer in developed countries in enduring ways that acknowledge the realities of women's lives, we need—at the least—to stop scaring people and avoid being rushed prematurely into vaccination programmes using products about which the long-term effects (benefits and harms, expected and unexpected) as well as the full costs, including lost opportunity costs, remain unknown. Instead, we need now to reinforce ongoing Pap testing and follow-up programmes—and develop stronger systematic screening processes; to engage clinical professionals and the population in discussion and analysis of issues that are not coloured by marketing techniques; and to obtain independent data about the effectiveness and duration—and risks—of vaccine protection—including information about any changes in behaviour by practitioners or girls and women that themselves might contribute to maintaining current rates of cervical cancer.

Advertisements vaunt the vaccine as meaning there will be "one less" (case of cancer) unless one gets the shots. But, to prevent cervical cancer, more needs to be considered than merely maximising uptake of school-based immunisations. The story about the importance of acting at multiple levels[12] and of carrying out primordial prevention to address the societal and structural determinants of STIs and cervical cancer needs to be marketed urgently not only so that those being solicited to be vaccinated can give truly informed consent, but so that there can be a full and open debate about the goals of public health and the values—equity, justice, solidarity and accountability—that should underlie any population-based programme.

Cervical cancer in developed countries is a disease of marginalisation, and simplistic approaches to its control will not suffice. If women's health truly is a priority in these resource-rich countries, we might better push for a responsive and effective public system of care and for holistic health promotion and protection policies, rather than take on one disease that is first demonised at a time. It is true that mass vaccination of schoolgirls would itself be an equitable approach to reducing the differential rates of cervical cancer if all those in the chosen grade are immunised, but this avoids the question: is reducing the rates of cervical cancer, a non-crisis condition for which there are already methods of prevention, the first priority in seeking health equity in resource-rich countries?

Whether or not the recent calls for a moratorium on vaccination programmes will influence policies, it is important that they have been issued—and supported; we must listen to the stories from these groups. They remind us that setting public health policies and reducing health inequities are—and must remain—societal matters, and that these must be kept completely separate from the interests of private profit and the scare tactics of promoters. "Health and illness [have] emerged as a fertile new field for corporate profitability" in a "culture of prevention and precaution"[13] and HPV vaccines conform to this framing. Our challenge, therefore, is to create other frames that lead to ways of seeing problems that prevent private interests from determining health policies or short-circuiting public health needs.

Notes

1. Angelmar R, Angelmar S, Kane L. Building strong condition brands. *J Med Marketing* 2007;7:341–51.
2. Although two HPV vaccines have been developed, only one of these, Gardasil, has been approved for use in Canada and the USA and so I focus on it here.
3. Australian Government, Department of Health and Ageing: Fact Sheet: Government funding of Gardasil, Updated 28 November 2006. http://www.health.gov. au/internet/main/publishing.nsf/ Content/ 4754B33584405E06CA2572220008CFA 8/$File/Gardasilfunding-factsheet.pdf (accessed 15 Apr 2008).
4. CWHN. HPV, Vaccines, and Gender: Policy Considerations. Posted 25 June 2007 http://www. cwhn.ca/PDF/CWHN_HPVjuly30.pdf (accessed 1 Feb 2008).
5. Lippman A. Melnychuk R, Shimmin C, et al. Human papillomavirus, vaccines and women's health. *Can Med Assoc* J 2007;177:484–7.
6. Lippman A, Boscoe M, Scurfield C. Debate: Do you approve of spending $300 million on HPV vaccination? No. *Can Fam Phys* 2008;54:175–7.
7. Declaracion. Razones para una moratoria en la aplicación de la vacuna del virus del papiloma humano en Espa a. 2007. http://www.caps.pangea. org/ declaracion/ (accessed 6 Apr 2008).
8. Gérvas J. La incierta prevencion del cancer de cuello de utero con la vacuna contra el Virus del Papiloma Humano. *Rev Port Clin Geral* 2007;23: 547–55.
9. Decker K, Demers AA, Chateau D, et al. Cervical cancer in Manitoba: evaluating Pap test utilization, cancer risk, and opportunity to be screened. *Open Med* (in press).
10. Reisinger KS, Block SL, Lazcano-Ponce E, et al. Safety and persistent immunogenicity of quadrivalent human papillomavirus types 6, 11, 16, 18 L1 virus-like particle vaccine in preadolescents and adolescents: a randomized controlled trial. *Pediatr Infect Dis* J 2007;26:201–9.
11. Rambout L, Hopkins L, Hutton B, et al. Prophylactic vaccination against human papillomavirus infection and disease in women: a systematic review of randomized controlled trials. *Can Med Assoc* J 2007;177:469–79.
12. Krieger N. Proximal, distal, and the politics of causation: What's level got to do with it? *Am J Publ Health* 2008;98:221–30.
13. Rose N. Molecular biopolitics, somatic ethics and the spirit of biocapital. *Soc Theory Health* 2007;15: 3–29.

Pandemic Influenza Preparedness: An Ethical Framework to Guide Decision-Making

Alison K. Thompson, Karen Faith, Jennifer L. Gibson, and Ross E.G. Upshur

BACKGROUND

As the world prepares for the emergence of a pandemic strain of influenza, trans-national, national and local organisations and agencies are designing plans to manage community outbreaks. In addition, the medical community is identifying scientific research priorities and needs related to the anticipated pandemic.[1-5] There is also a need to examine the ethical issues that arise from planning for a public health crisis of this magnitude. Who should get the limited supply of antivirals? Are health care workers duty-bound to care for the ill in a pandemic when they may have competing familial obligations? Who will be prioritized for scarce ventilated hospital beds? When should hospitals cancel elective surgeries or restrict hospital visitation? To date, the bioethics community has been slow to respond to public health issues in general,[6,7] and pandemic influenza planning in particular.[8,9] In this paper we discuss the need for ethics in pandemic influenza planning and discuss the ethical framework we developed to guide pandemic planning in hospitals.

In the only article we could find that has an in-depth analysis of the ethics of pandemic planning, Kotalik offers an ethical analysis of the pandemic plans of three countries. His arguments are primarily about the ethics *of* pandemic planning efforts, as opposed to the ethics *in* pandemic planning. For example, he argues persuasively that it is problematic that all three countries' plans accept particular conditions of resource scarcity as planning assumptions.[10] While Kotalik has raised important issues about the ethics *of* pandemic planning in his article, our ethical

framework focuses specifically on providing guidance to decision-makers about ethical issues *in* pandemic planning. This includes providing guidance on how to design an ethical process for decision-making, and providing guiding ethical values for the consideration of substantive issues.

The framework here proposed is an example of practical ethics that attempts to provide decision-makers with an introduction to and articulation of generally accepted ethical principles or values. The significance of this ethical framework is a) in the unique collaborative approach taken to its development that involved ethicists with different areas of expertise and a variety of health care stakeholders, and b) that it fills an important need in pandemic planning for an ethical framework to guide decision-making that has been unmet in most pandemic planning processes world wide.

The Importance of Ethics in Pandemic Planning

One of the characteristics of a public health crisis is that health needs overwhelm available human and material resources. Difficult decisions must be made about how, where and to whom resources should be allocated. Medical science provides valuable information to help make these decisions. However, science alone is insufficient. Now consider that resource allocation decisions are just one kind of decision decision-makers face in preparing for, and getting through an influenza pandemic.[9] As a few scholars have begun to point out, pandemic planning needs to take ethical considerations

Thompson, A., Faith, K., Gibson, J., Upshur, R. "Pandemic influenza Preparedness: an Ethical Framework to Guide Decision-Making". From *BMC Medical Ethics* 7(12) © 2006 Biomed Central. Reprinted with permission.

seriously, and not allow the urgency of logistical and scientific needs to sideline a discussion of ethical considerations.[10,11]

Kotalik argues that as "every discourse about health care has not only a scientific but also a moral dimension, [pandemic influenza] plans also presuppose certain ethical values, principles, norms, interests and preferences".[10] It is important to make these presuppositions explicit, because, as the SARS experience in Toronto taught health care organisations, the costs of not addressing the ethical concerns are severe: loss of public trust, low hospital staff morale, confusion about roles and responsibilities, stigmatization of vulnerable communities, and misinformation.[12–14] Another key insight from SARS that we overlook at our peril was that in times of crisis, "where guidance is incomplete, consequences uncertain, and information constantly changing, where hour-by-hour decisions involve life and death, *fairness is more important, rather than less* [emphasis added]"[14] As we shall argue, fairness considerations are both procedurally and substantively important: there is a need for fair decision-making processes, as well as equitable distributions of scarce human and material resources.

Take the example of triaging ventilated beds in an ICU. In theory, decision-makers rely on scientific evidence to determine how best to maximise benefit in the allocation of ventilated beds, but science cannot tell us whether or not the initial decision to maximise benefit is just. Because the notion of maximising benefit is derived from a reflection on values, ethical analysis is required to determine why a utilitarian approach to triage though maximisation of benefit is preferable to the assignment of ventilated beds on a different basis, for example that of greatest need. Even if the utilitarian maximisation of benefit is thought to be ethically sound, how to implement a system based on this criterion is not ethically straightforward, and requires ethical reflection about what counts as good stewardship, and about the moral obligation to demonstrate transparency, accountability,

fairness and trustworthiness in the allocation of scarce resources.

The importance of ethics to pandemic planning is in the "the application of value judgements to science",[15] especially as they are embedded in planning assumptions, and within the practice of medicine itself. For example, while ethics might have little to contribute to understanding the mechanism of influenza virus transmission, it can make a significant contribution to debates such as what levels of harm the public are prepared to accept, how the burdens of negative outcomes should be distributed across the population and whether or not more resources should be invested in stockpiling antiviral medications.

The use of ethical frameworks to guide decision-making may help to mitigate some of the unintended and unavoidable collateral damage from an influenza pandemic. As Kotalik argues, the incorporation of ethics into pandemic plans can help to make them "instruments for building mutual trust and solidarity at such time that will likely present a major challenge to our societies".[10] Using ethical frameworks to help guide decisions can offer greater assurance that the values instantiated within them, such as accountability, transparency and trust, will be carefully thought about in decision-making and when reviewing decisions with stakeholders.

DISCUSSION

Development of the Ethical Framework

One of the key lessons from the Toronto SARS experience was that health care institutions and their staff could benefit from the development of ethical frameworks for decision-making.[12] The intention of this section is not to systematically derivate from normative theory the values and principles in the framework. This paper has a more narrow focus—it is an example of applied/practical ethics that attempts to introduce and articulate values that are already commonly accepted. It is not our intention to comprehensively defend the values in the framework, but rather to show from which areas of scholarship they were drawn, articulate their relevance to pandemic planning, and to demonstrate their discursive legitimacy through a process of stakeholder engagement and vetting. To our knowledge, no other pandemic planning process has attempted to a) develop an ethical framework to guide pandemic influenza planning and b) assess an ethical framework's robustness and resonance in the community of its intended users. Thus, the significance of the procedural elements of the development of the framework is not to be minimized, nor are the insights we have gleaned from implementing the framework in health care organisations and in a governmental setting.

Building on key lessons from SARS[12–14] and the "emergency ethics" literature and drawing on our expertise in clinical, organisational, and public health ethics, we identified key ethical processes and values that are relevant for health care organisations. These values were presented to and vetted by a variety of health care stakeholders. Thus, this framework is the product of an iterative and inclusive process.

Formation of a Working Group In Ontario the need for guidance on the ethical issues pertaining to an influenza pandemic has been widely acknowledged. As word of our work on an ethical framework for Sunnybrook and Women's College Health Science Centre (S & W) became known, we were invited to join other hospitals' pandemic planning efforts. There was also broader sectoral interest in ethics, and we were invited to join the Ontario Ministry of Health and Long Term Care's (MOHLTC) efforts to design a pandemic plan.

Our working group was formed in response to the pandemic planning initiative that took place at S & W in early 2005. The hospital's Clinical Ethics Centre was invited to provide ethics support in this planning initiative. It soon became apparent that the scope of the issues went beyond the purview of clinical ethics to include organisational and public health ethics. Expertise in organisational and public health ethics was

quickly procured through the University of Toronto Joint Centre for Bioethics which is a partnership between the University and sixteen affiliated healthcare organizations that includes S & W among its partners. S & W was subsequently de-amalgamated into Sunnybrook Health Sciences Centre and Women's College Hospital, thus the ethical framework is currently being implemented at Sunnybrook HSC.

As the framework took shape, we were invited to join the MOHLTC planning efforts. We began to work with the Vaccine and Antiviral working group at the MOHLTC, and we adapted our work to meet the related but distinct challenges facing government. While our work with the MOHLTC began with the Vaccine and Antiviral working group, the ethical framework we developed for the MOHLTC was eventually included in the *Ontario Health Pandemic Influenza Plan*[16] not as an annex to the section on vaccines and antivirals as we had originally anticipated, but as an ethical framework for the plan as a whole.

Review of Clinical Ethics and Public Health Ethics Literature Expertise in clinical ethics was important to the development of this framework because of the knowledge, skills and experience clinical ethicists need to address dilemmas or challenges found in the daily clinical arena. An obvious challenge was how to integrate expertise in public health ethics into a framework designed to guide decision-making in clinical health care settings. A related challenge was to thoughtfully integrate generally accepted principles and values from clinical ethics with those in public health ethics. In order to meet this challenge, the authors turned not only to the respective ethics literature, but also to the SARS experiences of Toronto hospitals and health care providers. A review of the SARS literature, and that of public health ethics more generally, guided the integration of the public health and the clinical ethics perspectives.[6,9,10,12–14,17–19] The Toronto experience with SARS demonstrated that organisations faced unique ethical challenges when dealing with a public health crisis, and much of the ethics literature identified a need for greater forethought in how organisations can foster ethical decision-making in times of crisis.[12–14] We reasoned that the legitimacy of this framework would be enhanced by including insights from the analysis of a recent public health crisis like SARS.

Lessons from Emergency Ethics Not surprisingly, the literature on clinical ethics has little to say about disaster preparedness and how to make decisions about such things as triage under extraordinary circumstances. The ethics literature on bioterrorism and battle-field triage informed our thinking and called our attention to important issues such as the duty to care, reciprocity, equity and good stewardship.[20–25] The importance of having ethically robust criteria and policies developed in advance of a pandemic influenza outbreak is underscored in this literature, for "critical decisions like these should not be made on an individual case-by-case basis" and "physicians should never be placed in a position of individually deciding to deny treatment to patients without the guidance of policy or protocol".[22] Robust disaster preparedness requires practising preventive ethics.

Stakeholder Vetting The ethical framework was vetted through S & W's Pandemic Planning Committee, the Joint Centre for Bioethics' Clinical Ethics Group (comprised of the affiliated health care organizations' clinical ethicists), the MOHLTC Vaccine and Antiviral Working Group, and the MOHLTC pandemic planning committee. Through this process, we refined the framework and we are grateful to these groups for their valuable insights.

The Ethical Framework

The ethical framework is intended to inform decision making, not replace it. It is intended to encourage reflection on important values, discussion and review of ethical concerns arising from a public health crisis. It is intended also as a means to improve accountability for decision making and may require revision as feedback and circumstances require.

The framework is divided into two distinct parts, and begins with the premise that planning decisions for a pandemic influenza outbreak ought to be 1) guided by ethical decision-making processes and 2) informed by ethical values. Ethical processes can help to improve accountability and it is hoped that, to the extent that it is possible for ethical processes to produce ethical outcomes, the substantive ethical quality of decisions will be enhanced. Recognising, however, that ethical processes do not guarantee ethical outcomes, we have identified ten key ethical values to guide decision-making that address the substantive ethical dimensions of decision-making in this context.

Ethical Processes In planning for and throughout a pandemic influenza crisis, difficult decisions will be made that are fraught with ethical challenges. Our framework around ethical processes is based upon the "accountability for reasonableness" model developed by Daniels & Sabin[26] and adapted by Gibson, Martin & Singer.[27] This model provides a useful means of identifying the key elements of ethical decision-making processes. An extensive literature has developed around Daniels' and Sabin's accountability for reasonableness framework. The Daniels and Sabin framework has broad applicability across institutional settings and priority setting situations.[28–35] Because the Daniels and Sabin framework applies deliberative theories of democratic justice to the specific problem of health care priority setting, and because it is unique in this regard, we felt it promoted the kind of deliberative approach to pandemic planning that this ethical framework is intended to support. Table 1 outlines the characteristics of an ethical decision-making process. Stakeholders will be more able to accept difficult decisions during a pandemic influenza crisis if the decision-making process has, and is perceived to have, ethical legitimacy.

Ethical Values The second part of the framework identifies ten key ethical values that should inform the pandemic influenza planning process and decision-making during an outbreak. These values are intended to provide guidance, and it is important to consider that more than one value may be relevant to a situation. Indeed, the hallmark of a challenging ethical decision is that one or more value(s) are in tension and that there is no clear answer about which one to privilege in making the decision. When values are in tension with one another, the importance of having ethical decision-making processes is reinforced (see above.)

The values identified in our ethical framework were based initially on previous research findings on ethics and SARS at the University of Toronto Joint Centre for Bioethics (JCB). This work was funded by a Canadian Institutes of Health Research grant in 2004 through 2006 and has led to several key publications on the ethical dimensions of SARS.[14,36-39] In particular, Singer et al., in their seminal British Medical Journal article begin to identify key

Table 1

Ethical Processes (Listed in Alphabetical Order). Adapted from Daniels, N. Accountability for reasonableness. *BMJ* 2000, 321:1300–1301.

Value	Description
Accountability	There should be mechanisms in place to ensure that ethical decision-making is sustained throughout the crisis.
Inclusiveness	Decisions should be made explicitly with stakeholder views in mind and there should be opportunities for stakeholders to be engaged in the decision-making process. For example, decision-making related to staff deployment should include the input of affected staff.
Openness & Transparency	Decisions should be publicly defensible. This means that the process by which decisions were made must be open to scrutiny and the basis upon which decisions are made should be publicly accessible to affected stakeholders. For example, there should be a communication plan developed in advance to ensure that information can be effectively disseminated to affected stakeholders and that stakeholders know where to go for needed information.
Reasonableness	Decisions should be based on reasons (i.e., evidence, principles, values) that stakeholders can agree are relevant to meeting health needs in a pandemic influenza crisis and they should be made by people who are credible and accountable. For example, decision-makers should provide a rationale for prioritising particular groups for antiviral medication and for limiting access to elective surgeries and other services.
Responsiveness	There should be opportunities to revisit and revise decisions as new information emerges throughout the crisis as well as mechanisms to address disputes and complaints. For example, if elective surgeries are cancelled or postponed, there should [be] a formal mechanism for stakeholders to voice any concerns they may have with the decision.

ethical values that were of relevance during the SARS epidemic in Toronto. These values were then further articulated by our working group and adapted for the pandemic influenza planning context. Through a discursive process of stakeholder consultation with public health specialists, ministry officials, S & W's pandemic influenza committee, and the Clinical Ethics Group at the JCB, we augmented the values to include two new values (stewardship and trust[40,41]) and refined the definitions of each value in light of the anticipated demands of a pandemic influenza crisis compared to a hospital-based epidemic such as SARS. The substantive values identified and articulated in the framework are not intended to be an exhaustive set, and they may underdetermine how best to achieve the *overall* goals of pandemic planning, which generally include the minimization of morbidity, mortality, and societal disruption. Nevertheless, this is not to say that a procedural engagement about the overall goals of a pandemic response would not benefit from using the ethical framework to guide and shape debate. A description of the values that should guide decision-making can be found in Table 2.

Included in the framework are "hot button" ethical issues that we identified through our work with Toronto hospitals and the MOHLTC. These issues were as follows:

a) Targeting and prioritizing populations for vaccines and antivirals
b) Intensive Care Unit and hospital bed assignment
c) Duty to care
d) Human resources allocation and staffing
e) Visiting restrictions
f) Communications and how reviews of decisions will be handled

These "hot button" issues are not intended to be exhaustive, but rather they serve to illustrate how the values in the ethical framework can be used to identify key ethical aspects of decision-making.

Let us take the issue of targeting and prioritizing populations for vaccine and antivirals to illustrate how the values in the ethical framework can help guide decision-making. The values of solidarity and protecting the public from harm would require that priorities be set to maximize the capacity to help society ensure that the ill are cared for during a pandemic. Furthermore proportionality would require that decision-makers consider who within the community are most vulnerable to the contagion as well as who are most likely to benefit from immunization. A well-informed public conversant with the values in the ethical framework and aware of the expertise that informed the ranking of priorities for immunisation would be consistent with value of trust and the principle of transparency.

Lastly, while knowing how to use the framework to inform decision-making is vital, there is more to ensuring that the framework will be used or useful.

Lessons for Implementing an Ethical Framework

We have identified three necessary, if not exhaustive elements to the successful integration of ethics into hospital pandemic planning processes. These elements are 1) sponsorship of the ethical framework by senior hospital administration; 2) vetting of the framework by key stakeholders and; 3) decision review processes.

Sponsorship by Senior Administrators Whether or not an ethical framework is used to inform decision-making in a health care institution depends to a large extent on people in senior positions of an organisation seeing its relevance to the decision-making process. In part, this is [dependent] on how robust the framework is, but it also requires the willingness to frame (at least some) pandemic planning issues as normative in nature.

Some may argue that the values in the framework are too stringent or impractical to implement under crisis conditions, especially those

Table 2		
Ethical Values to Guide Decision-making (Listed in Alphabetical Order)		
Value	*Description*	*Example*
Duty to Provide Care	The duty to provide care and to respond to suffering is inherent to all health care professionals' codes of ethics. In an influenza pandemic, demands on health care providers and the institutions in which they work will overwhelm resources. Health care providers will have to weigh demands from their professional role with other competing obligations to their own health, to family and friends. Health care workers will face significant challenges related to resource allocation, scope of practice, professional liability, and workplace conditions. *Decision makers should*: • Work collaboratively with stakeholders and professional colleagues in advance of an influenza pandemic to establish practice guidelines • Work collaboratively to develop fair and accountable processes to resolve disputes • Provide supports to ease this moral burden of those with the duty to care • Develop means through which institutions will handle appeals or complaints, especially with regards to work exemptions, or the vaccination/prophylaxis of staff	Health care workers who are at increased risk because they are caring for patients with influenza must weigh familial obligations, and obligations to self with their professional duty to care. In addition, they may also have to comply with vaccination or antiviral regimens for prophylaxis which may conflict with their individual liberty.
Equity	The principle of equity holds that, all things being equal, all patients have an equal claim to receive needed health care. During [an] influenza pandemic, however, tough decisions will need to be made about which health services to maintain and which to defer because of extraordinary circumstances. Measures taken to contain the spread of a deadly disease will inevitably cause considerable collateral damage. In an influenza pandemic, this will extend beyond the cessation of elective surgeries and may limit the provision of emergent or necessary services. *Decision-makers must strive to*: • Preserve as much equity as possible between the interests of patients [afflicted with the influenza] and those who need urgent treatment for other diseases • Ensure procedural fairness in decision-making	In allocating scarce resources, the value of equity could guide in developing fair criteria for allocation while consideration is given also to compensation for those who will not meet inclusion criteria yet are entitled to receive care.

(continues)

Table 2 (continued)

Value	Description	Example
Individual Liberty	Individual liberty is a value enshrined in health care practice under the principle of respect for autonomy. Under usual circumstances, health care providers balance respect for individual autonomy with a duty to protect individual patients from harm. In a public health crisis, however, restrictions to individual liberty may be necessary to protect the public from serious harm. Patients, staff, and members of the public may all be affected by such restrictions. *Restrictions to individual liberty should:* • Be proportional to the risk of public harm • Be necessary and relevant to protecting the public good • Employ the least restrictive means necessary to achieve public health goals • Be applied without discrimination	Social distancing strategies that employ visitor restrictions in hospitals must be necessary for the protection of the public and must be proportionate to the threat being allayed.
Privacy	Individuals have a right to privacy in health care. In a public health crisis, it may be necessary to override this right to protect the public from serious harm. A proportionate response to the need for private information requires that it be released only if there are no less intrusive means to protect public health. *Decision makers should*: • Disclose only private information that is relevant to achieve legitimate and necessary public health goals • Release private information only if there are no less intrusive means to protect public health • Determine whether the good that is intended is significant enough to justify the potential harm that can come from suspending privacy rights, (e.g. the harm from stigmatization of individuals or particular communities) • Provide public education to correct misconceptions about disease transmission and to offset misattribution of blame to particular communities	The need to conduct contact tracing of possibly infected people might require that particular groups or even individuals are identified publicly. The need to do so must be weighed against the potential harm of exposing communities and individuals to stigmatization.
Proportionality	Proportionality requires that restrictions to individual liberty and measures taken to protect the public from harm should not exceed what is necessary to address the actual level of risk to, or critical need of, the community. *Decision makers should*: • Use least restrictive or coercive measures in limiting or restricting liberties or entitlements	The decision to close an emergency room must consider if the potential harm in keeping the emergency room open is significant

	• Use more coercive measures only in circumstances where less restrictive measures have failed to achieve appropriate public health ends.	enough to warrant its closure.
Protection of the Public from Harm	A foundational principle of public health ethics is the obligation to protect the public from serious harm. This principle requires that citizens comply with imposed restrictions in order to ensure public wellbeing or safety. To protect the public from harm, hospitals may be required to restrict public access to service areas (e.g. restricted visiting hours), to limit availability of some services (e.g. elective surgeries), or to impose infectious control practices (e.g. masks or quarantine). *When making decisions designed to protect the public from harm, decision makers should*: • Weigh the medical and moral imperative for compliance • Ensure stakeholders are made aware of the medical and moral reasons for public health measures • Ensure stakeholders are aware of the benefits of compliance & the consequences of non-compliance • Establish mechanisms to review these decisions as the public health situation changes and to address stakeholders concerns or complaints	When making the decision to quarantine individuals, protection of the public from harm must be weighed against individual liberty. Note that while the ethical value of individual liberty is often in tension with the protection of the public from harm, it is also in individuals' interests to minimize harm to others.
Reciprocity	Reciprocity requires that society supports those who face a disproportionate burden in protecting the public good and takes steps to minimise their impact as far as possible. In an influenza pandemic, measures to protect the public good are likely to impose a disproportionate burden on health care workers, patients, and their families. Health care workers may face expanded duties, increased workplace risks, physical and emotional stress, isolation from peers and family, and in some cases, infection leading to hospitalization or even death. Similarly, quarantined individuals or families of ill patients may experience significant social, economic, and emotional burdens. *Decision-makers and institutions are responsible for*: • Easing the burdens of health care workers, patients, and patient's families in their hospitals and in coordination with other health care organizations • Ensuring the safety of their workers, especially when redeploying staff in areas beyond the usual scope of practice	The provision of antiviral medication and/or vaccination to hospital staff for prophylaxis is one way hospitals can ensure the safety of their workers who may be exposed to greater than usual risks in discharging their duty to care.

(continues)

	Table 2 (continued)	
Value	*Description*	*Example*
Solidarity	SARS heightened the global awareness of the interdependence of health systems and the need for solidarity across systemic and institutional boundaries in stemming a serious contagious disease. An influenza pandemic will not only require global solidarity, it will require a vision of solidarity within and between health care institutions. *Solidarity requires*: • Good, open and honest communication • Open collaboration, in a spirit of common purpose, within and between health care institutions • Sharing public health information • Coordinating health care delivery, transfer of patients, and deployment of human and material resources	Territoriality between hospital departments and between health care institutions needs to be overcome with good communication and sense of common purpose in order to provide equitable care across jurisdictions.
Stewardship	In our society, both institutions and individuals will be entrusted with governance over scarce resources, such as vaccines, antivirals, ventilators, hospital beds and even health care workers. During a pandemic influenza outbreak, difficult decisions about how to allocate material and human resources will have to be made, and there will be collateral damage as a result of these allocation decisions. Those entrusted with governance roles should be guided by the notion of stewardship. Inherent in stewardship are the notions of trust, ethical behaviour, and good decision-making. *Decision makers have a responsibility to*: • Avoid and/or reduce collateral damage that may result from resource allocation decisions • Maximize benefits when allocating resources • Protect and develop resources where possible • Consider good outcomes (i.e. benefits to the public good) and equity (i.e., fair distribution of benefits & burdens)	A hospital's decision to stock-pile antiviral medication must consider whether this is an effective way of protecting staff from infection, where the money for stockpiling will come from, and whether that money could be put to better use elsewhere.

| Trust | Trust is an essential component in the relationships between clinician and patient, between staff and the organization, between the public and health care providers, and between organizations within a health system. In a public health crisis, stakeholders may perceive public health measures as a betrayal of trust (e.g. when access to needed care is denied) or as abandonment at a time of greatest need. Decision-makers will be confronted with the challenge of maintaining stakeholders' trust while at the same time stemming an influenza pandemic through various control measures. It takes time to build trust. *Decision-makers should*:
• Take steps to build trust with stakeholders before the crisis hits not while it is in full swing
• Ensure decision making processes are ethical and transparent to those affected stakeholders | Early engagement with stakeholders may go some distance to justify stakeholder confidence in decision-makers' trustworthiness. In part, the value of trust is respected and promoted by following the ethical *processes* outlined above. |

found in the Ethical Processes part of the framework (see Table 1). Certainly, crisis conditions may place constraints on the extent to which each principle can be acted upon. However, efforts should be made to put them into action to the fullest extent possible under the circumstances and in our experience this is only possible with the support of senior administrators.

The senior administration at S & W (many of whom were part of the Pandemic Planning Committee) had previous experience with the accountability for reasonableness framework for decision-making, and thus their pandemic influenza planning committee was already familiar with the Ethical Processes part of the framework, and they were receptive to the idea of being guided by an ethical framework. Senior administrators may also have been receptive to the ethical framework because, as they learned from SARS, organisations that did not have decision-making processes that honoured the values for ethical process during SARS have been dealing with a legacy of collateral damage to staff and patients in the form of distrust and low morale.[12] For these reasons, the senior administrators at S & W played an important role in vetting the ethical

framework. Ensuring that institutional "sponsors" are in favour of adopting an ethical framework is important for gaining widespread support for using an ethical framework in decision-making, and for ensuring that the ethical framework does not become something that looks good but remains unused.

Vetting of the Ethical Framework by Key Stakeholders In order to obtain support for, or "buy in" to an ethical framework, it is important that key stakeholders in an institution vet the framework. This requires careful consideration of who the key stakeholders are in an institution. Not only should this include those with responsibility for decision-making, but also those who will be affected by decisions taken. For the vetting process is not just intended to create "buy in" but also to decrease the likelihood that interests and issues that are (morally) relevant to pandemic planning will be neglected or overlooked, thereby enhancing the moral legitimacy of the values in the framework. In addition, a process of stakeholder vetting increases the likelihood that the values instantiated in the framework resonate with the stakeholder community.

It has been our experience that the values in the framework did resonate with the pandemic planners with whom we have shared this ethical framework. The primarily pragmatic justification for the selection of the values in the framework means that the framework is provisional so it ought to be subject to revision in light of compelling argument, empirical evidence and further stakeholder feedback. It is important to note, however, that the iterative and inclusive process through which the values in the framework were deliberated amongst the various stakeholder groups lends them a form of discursive ethical legitimacy and helps to justify their inclusion in the ethical framework. We intend that the framework invite further dialogue about its legitimacy and its adequacy. We will return to this issue in the final section of this paper.

Ideally, the vetting process would include people who can represent the interests of patients, families and volunteers who are part of the hospital's constituency. Although patient relations, human resources and occupational health representatives from S & W provided guidance and feedback in the development of the framework, direct input from patients and family representatives was not obtained. One limitation of our framework is that [it] has yet to be vetted by these important stakeholders.

The importance of solidarity to the management of a public health crisis would also suggest that the public and other health care organisations be considered stakeholders in hospital pandemic planning. While it may not be pragmatic for hospitals to undertake broad public consultation and vetting processes for their pandemic plans in general, and their ethical frameworks in particular, solidarity and equity suggest that these broader stakeholder interests are relevant to pandemic planning. Consequently, opportunities for broader ethical dialogue about pandemic planning need to be encouraged.

Decision Review Processes In order to ensure that the support of key stakeholders is maintained through an outbreak, there need to be effective communication mechanisms in place. An important aspect of responsive decision-making processes is ensuring that there are formal opportunities to revisit and revise decisions as new information emerges. As part of our ethical framework, we formulated a template for decision review processes, (adapted from, Gibson, JL: *Formal decision review process template.* Unpublished; 2003) that aids organisations in identifying existing and establishing new mechanisms that can be used for the formal reviews of decisions. We believe decision review mechanisms are an essential part of ethical decision-making in a public health crisis, and are one way to put the values in the ethical framework in to action.

Formal mechanisms for reviewing decisions are needed in order to capture feedback from stakeholders on key decisions, and to resolve disputes and challenges. These processes are important for ensuring that decisions are the best possible under the circumstances given changing information and for engaging stakeholders constructively around the difficult decisions that must be made. Given the unpredictable nature of public health emergencies and the difficulty this poses for those in charge of planning and decision-making, it is reasonable to assume that decisions will be revised throughout the pandemic influenza crisis. Disputes or challenges may arise from the restrictions or requirements imposed on staff, patients and families during a pandemic influenza outbreak. Thus, decision review processes are essential. Again, while some may argue that this is too stringent a measure for a time of crisis, we argue that reviews of decisions will be taking place regardless (most likely in an *ad hoc* manner), and that to formalize this process is to increase its fairness and moral legitimacy. Indeed, there may be existing mechanisms which can handle these kinds of reviews.

Scope of the Ethical Framework

It is important to distinguish between different types of ethical analyses in order to explain the approach that was taken to the development of the ethical framework discussed herein. Callahan and Jennings draw a useful distinction between *applied* ethics and *critical* ethics.[7] Our ethical framework is an example of applied ethics because the framework identifies and relies on "general principles that can be applied to real-world examples of professional conduct or decision-making"[7] and because it is "designed to give professionals guidance and to give clients and the general public standards to use in assessing professional conduct".[42] While there is certainly a need for critical ethical analysis that pays attention to problems that are the "result of institutional arrangements and prevailing structures of cultural attitudes and social power",[7] one would not expect a[n] ethical framework designed to guide clinical decision-making to explicitly address these kinds of issues.

This is not to say that this ethical framework *cannot* address the kinds of issues that a critical ethical analysis might address. For example, the framework promotes values and processes that seek to redress the power disparities within institutions. The section of the framework that deals with ethical processes in particular is a challenge to how institutional decisions are typically made. For example, the value of "inclusiveness" as a process principle is essential for redressing power differences amongst key stakeholders.[27] Thus, while the ethical framework is the product of applied ethical analysis, and should be evaluated in light of this, one of its strengths is that it can also redress what Callahan and Jennings would characterize as "critical" ethics problem of power disparities within institutions.

CONCLUSION

Cultural Limitations and Future Directions

Within pluralistic societies, there are many different ethical perspectives that exist simultaneously on issues about global, public and individual health. An ethical framework to guide decision-making is robust to the extent that it reflects the values and beliefs of the decision-makers who refer to it and the values and beliefs of those affected by the decisions being taken.

Our framework relied heavily on the Toronto experience with SARS to surface and examine the ethical values that are important for a public health crisis. An influenza pandemic is likely to present us with particular ethical challenges that are different from SARS due to the predicted severity of the contagion and its spread to the community. It would therefore be important not to uncritically adopt such a framework but rather to use it as a basis for continued reflection and re-evaluation to ensure its relevance and responsiveness during the unfolding health crisis. It is also important to consider the extent to which an ethical framework is reflective of the community in which it is to be used. Lessons from SARS as it was experienced in China would likely surface some different ethical values, or emphasise different aspects of our framework. As Callahan and Jennings have argued:

> We submit that a rich discourse on ethics and public health cannot be advanced without relating it to the background values of the general society, and the particular communities, in which it will be carried out.[7]

Indeed, as previously maintained, there are many issues related to pandemic influenza planning particularly those raised by a *critical* ethical analysis that require broad public debate. While these kinds of issues require public debate that takes place at the societal level, ethical pandemic planning requires that organisations and agencies foster internal dialogue about the values instantiated in an ethical framework. For it is imperative that the values outlined in a framework resonate with the members of an organisation, and the community it serves. The procedural aspects of the framework provide a means to ensuring that the values of the community are reflected in decision-making through the procedural principles of inclusiveness and responsiveness.

It is important, too, to recognise that values are not static, and that circumstances will evolve rapidly during a pandemic influenza outbreak. Ethical frameworks will also require re-evaluation and revision. The challenge will be to continue to recognise the importance of moral reflection under circumstances that are not conducive to it and to encourage a process of re-evaluation that strives to assess whether resulting decisions are consistent with those values the framework is intended to promote. For this reason, it is imperative to start the ethical dialogue in advance, and to find ways to encourage consideration of ethical issues at all stages of decision-making. We hope that this paper will go some way towards advancing this objective, and that this paper stimulates discussion of the ethical issues and values that pervade pandemic planning.

We believe that this framework is unique in its blending of clinical, public health, and organizational ethics. One of its strengths is that it draws on lessons from the recent public health crisis of SARS in Toronto, and it is to some extent empirically grounded. Another strength is that it is the product of an inclusive process of development that included stakeholder vetting. It is also unique in its attempt to provide guidance to decision-makers facing a public health crisis. We hope that the framework's acceptance by hospitals and the provincial government in Ontario signals a change in the way that decisions are taken by institutions that are charged with making decisions that have life and death consequences for the public.

Acknowledgements

We should like to thank the Pandemic Influenza Planning Committee at Sunnybrook and Women's College Health Sciences Centre, the Clinical Ethics Group at the University of Toronto Joint Centre for Bioethics, and the Vaccine and Antivirals Working Group of the Ontario Ministry of Health and Long Term Care. This framework was vetted through these groups and was bettered from their feedback. Ross Upshur is supported by the Canada Research Chair in Primary Care Research. We also thank our three peer reviewers, Angela Bate, Ezekiel Emanuel and Akria Akabayashi for their helpful insights and comments.

Notes

1. Stohr K: Avian influenza and pandemics: research needs and opportunities. *N Engl J Med* 2005, 352:405–407.

2. Osterholm MT: Preparing for the next pandemic. *N Engl J Med* 2005, 352:1839–1842.

3. Tam T, Sciberras J, Mullington B, King A: Fortune favours the prepared mind: a national perspective on pandemic preparedness. *Can J Public Health* 2005, 96:406–408.

4. Reichert TA: Preparing for the next influenza pandemic. *The Pediatric Infectious Disease Journal* 2005, 24:S228–S231.

5. Wong S, Yuen K: Avian influenza virus infections in humans. *Chest* 2006, 129:156–168.

6. Beauchamp E, Steinbock B: *New Ethics for the Public's Health*. New York, Oxford University Press; 1999.

7. Callahan D, Jennings B: Ethics and public health: forging a strong relationship. *American Journal of Public Health* 2002, 92:169–176.

8. Kotalik J: Preparing for an influenza pandemic: ethical issues. *Bioethics* 2005, 19:422–431.

9. Zoloth L, Zoloth S: Don't be chicken: bioethics and avian flu. *The American Journal of Bioethics* 2006, 6:5–8.

10. Kotalik J: Addressing issues and questions relating to pandemic influenza planning: final report and recommendations. Health Canada; 2003.

11. Tracy SC, Upshur R, Daar A: Avian influenza and pandemics. *N Engl J Med* 2005, 352:1928.

12. Berstein M, Hawryluck L: Challenging beliefs and ethical concepts: the collateral damage of SARS. *Critical Care* 2003, 7:269–271.

13. Singer P, Benatar S, Berstein M, Daar A, Dickens B, MacRae S, Upshur R, Wright L, Zlotnick Shaul R: Ethics and SARS: lessons from Toronto. *BMJ* 2003, 327:1342–1344.

14. Bell J, Hyland S, DePelligrin T, Upshur R, Berstein M, Martin D: SARS and hosptial priority setting: a qualitative case study and evaluation. *BMC Health Services Research* 2004, 4.

15. Perhac R: Comparative risk assessment: where does the public fit in? *Science, Technology and Human Values* 1998, 23:221–241.

16. MOHLTC: Ontario Health Pandemic Influenza Plan. Toronto; 2005.

17. Upshur R: Principles for the justification of public health intervention. *Can J Public Health* 2002, 93:101–103.

18. Gostin LO: Public health, ethics, and human rights: a tribute to the late Johnathan Mann. *J Law Med Ethics* 2001, 29:121–130.

19. O'Neill O: Public Health or Clinical Ethics: Thinking beyond Borders. *Ethics & International Affairs* 2002, 16.

20. Wynia MK, Gostin LO: Ethical challenges in preparing for bioterrorism: barriers within the health care system. *Am J Public Health* 2004, 97(7): 1096–1102.

21. Iserson K, Pesik N: Ethical resources distribution after biological, chemical or radiological terrorism. *Cambridge Quarterly of Healthcare Ethics* 2003, 12:455–465.

22. Pesik N, Keim M, Iserson K: Terrorism and the ethics of emergency medical care. *Annals of Emergency Medicine* 2001, 37:642–646.

23. Veatch R: Disaster preparedeness and triage: justice and the common good. *Mt Sinai J Med* 2005, 72(4):236–241.

24. Kipnis K: Overwhelming casualties: medical ethics in a time of terror. *Accountability in Research* 2003, 10:57–68.

25. Marer S, Sutjita M, Rajagopalan S: Bioterrorism, bioethics and the emergency physician. *Topics in Emergency Medicine* 2004, 26:44–48.

26. Daniels N: Accountability for reasonableness. *BMJ* 2000, 321:1300–1301.

27. Gibson J, Martin D, Singer P: Priority setting in hospitals: fairness, inclusiveness and the problem of institutional power differences. *Social Science and Medicine* 2005, 61:2355–2362.

28. Ham C: Tragic choices in health care: lessons from the Child B case. *British Medical Journal* 1999, 319:1258–1261.

29. Norheim OF: Procedures for priority setting and mechanisms of appeal in the Norwegian health care system: Amsterdam; 2000.

30. Daniels N, Sabin J: Setting limits fairly: can we learn to share scarce resources? Oxford, Oxford University Press; 2002.

31. Martin DK, Giacomini M, Singer P: Fairness, accountability for reasonableness and the views of priority setting decision-makers. *Health Policy* 2002, 61:279–290.

32. Martin DK, Shulman K, Santiago-Sorrell P, Singer P: Priority setting and hospital strategic planning: a qualitative case study. *Journal of Health Services Research and Policy* 2003, 8:59–68.

33. Gibson J, Martin DK, Singer P: Setting priorities in health care organisations: criteria, processes, and parameters of success. *BMC Health Services Research* 2004, 4.

34. Gibson J, Martin DK, Singer P: Priority setting in hospitals: fairness, inclusiveness, and the problem of institutional power differences. *Social Science and Medecine* 2005, 61:2355–2362.

35. Mitton C, Donaldson C: Health care priority setting: principles, practice and challenges. *Cost Eff Resour Alloc* 2004, 2(1):3.

36. Nickell LA, Crighton EJ, Tracy CS, Al-Enazy H, Bolaji Y, Hanjrah S, Hussain A, Makhlouf S, Upshur R: Psychosocial effects of SARS on hospital staff: survey of a large tertiary care institution. *Canadian Medical Association Journal* 2004, 170:793–798.

37. Ruderman C, Tracy CS, Bensimon CM, Bernstein M, Hawryluck L, Zlotnick Shaul R, Upshur REG: On pandemics and the duty to care: whose duty? who cares? *BMC Medical Ethics* 2006, 7.

38. Singer P, Benatar S, Bernstein M, Daar A, Dickens B, MacRae S, Upshur R, Wright L, Zlotnick Shaul R: Ethics and SARS: lessons from Toronto. *British Medical Journal* 2003, 327:1342–1344.

39. Wilson K, McDougall C, Upshur R, Joint Centre for Bioethics SARS Global Health Ethics Research Group: The new International Health Regulations and the federalism dilemma. *PLoS Med* 2006, 3(1):e1.

40. Saltman RB, Feroussier-Davis O: The concept of stewardship in health policy. *Bulletin of the World Health Organization* 2000, 78.

41. Goold SD: Trust and the ethics of health care institutions. *The Hastings Centre Report* 2001, 31:26–33.

42. Jennings B: Frameworks for ethics in public health. *Acta Bioethica* 2003, 9:165–176.

Defining the Limits of Emergency Humanitarian Action: Where, and How, to Draw the Line?

Nathan Ford, Rony Zachariah, Ed Mills, and Ross Upshur

For doctors used to practicing medicine in the well-resourced Western world, humanitarian emergencies are extraordinary situations. Health professionals who normally rely on a panoply of routine diagnostic tests, therapeutic options and specialist colleagues are transported to highly impoverished areas with collapsed health services, limited human resources and an excessive burden of infectious and chronic diseases. In extreme situations of isolation and insecurity, a modest team of expatriate health workers equipped with a limited supply of essential medicines and clinical algorithms may represent, for the limited duration of their presence, the only health professionals in the area. In zones of active conflict—the traditional terrain of humanitarian assistance—the provision of relief is further complicated by unpredictable violence and insecurity. Decisions about how to target medical assistance are fraught with dilemmas ranging from non-availability of basic tools, to massive demographic and epidemiological shifts, to the possibility of having to evacuate at any moment.

The starting point for any decision about how, where, and when to intervene in a humanitarian crisis is the institutional mandate that defines the scope of humanitarian assistance provided by a particular organization. Mandates can vary enormously in the breadth of activities they lay out, from the all-encompassing to the specific. So while Oxfam aims to 'find lasting solutions to poverty and injustice' Médecins Sans Frontières (MSF) defines itself as an organization that 'delivers emergency aid to people affected by armed conflict, epidemics, healthcare exclusion and natural or manmade disasters'.

From an operational perspective institutions are obliged, due to capacity constraints and a multiplicity of competing priorities, to select specific sites of intervention and clearly define their objectives and the beneficiaries of their actions. This is essential to ensuring that operations are focused and have the best chance of achieving the expected results, while ensuring maintaining capacity to intervene in other crises. Operational interventions are thus clearly guided by a priori choices before getting to the field. For an international humanitarian organization, a decision to assist cholera patients in Juba is not only a decision to single out a particular disease (Devakumar, 2008). It is also a decision to intervene in Juba (a region in Sudan), as opposed to other areas in Sudan; to deploy human and financial resources in Sudan instead of other counties in crisis; and to provide health care as opposed to other humanitarian services (water, shelter, nutrition).

At what point does a crisis become a humanitarian intervention? The science is far from perfect. A decision to intervene is often based on little more than a crude measurement of population-level mortality; a doubling of existing mortality rates is often used as an arbitrary threshold for declaring an emergency situation (Sphere Project, 2004). But often, mortality per se provides insufficient justification for a particular NGO to intervene in a given context,

Ford, N., Zachariah, R., Mills, E., Upshur, R., *Public Health Ethics* 2009, Vol. 3, Issue 1, pp. 68–71, by permission of Oxford University Press.

and the presence of other associated factors, e.g., vulnerable groups (children, the elderly), exclusion from access to health care, media or donor pressure and political choices can all influence the decision to intervene (Checchi et al., 2007).

The primary causes of mortality—violence, malnutrition and infectious diseases—may define the initial operational response, but when other life-threatening conditions are confronted, and if the means are available, it would seem fairly clear that a health professional is duty-bound to respond. But again, the means that are available are often conditioned by organizational a priori choices. The case study from Juba accepts that certain interventions like surgery could not be done, but is this any more acceptable than referring non-cholera cases? How much surgical disease is required before the lack of surgical care becomes an ethical dilemma and should this automatically become the responsibility of an NGO who may be in the area with a completely different operational mandate? An emergency intervention can become even more complicated when health teams are faced with a pressing burden of chronic disease. In most humanitarian contexts in Africa, health care workers will inevitably be confronted with HIV, a life-threatening disease requiring treatment for life. In the absence of some limiting criteria, a time-bound emergency cholera intervention could evolve into a programme providing surgical care and anti-retroviral therapy. Health professionals reacting to the 'moral duty' to treat could rapidly exceed the organizations' technical and financial capacity, preventing action in other crisis areas.

The reality is that there is very poor guidance for decision-making about resource allocation at a public health level (Kass, 2001). Because of this, health workers most often appeal to medical ethics, viewing these dilemmas exclusively at the level of the doctor–patient relationship. But when a doctor working for an international agency in a remote part of Africa is confronted with a pathology they cannot respond to for technical reasons, or reasons of limited mandate, this situation is not simply a medical ethical

dilemma. Rather, the situation is conditioned by dynamics that run from the micro-level (bedside) to the meso- and macro-level (institutions and health systems) (Sreenivasan and Benater, 2006).

These dynamics can run in both directions. It is not only a matter of a doctor in a remote area situating themselves within the broader landscape of international humanitarian needs—the stream of influence can run from the bottom up. It was the voice of frustration of doctors not being able to treat HIV that convinced MSF to launch treatment programmes across Africa. To be able to treat patients on the ground, the organization had to first engage in a considerable number of macro-level fora, including lobbying pharmaceutical companies to lower the price of their drugs, convincing UN agencies that treatment should be provided as well as prevention, pushing donor governments to put money into HIV programmes, and convincing national governments to allow pilot programmes to proceed. Indeed, it is often this advocacy work that allows humanitarian workers to live with the relative imperfections of operational decision-making. NGOs can often not do more than make a temporary contribution to saving lives and restoring the dignity of a small number of individuals, but by demonstrating that action is possible, and holding others to account, it may be possible to ensure that a broader, more sustainable improvement in peoples' lives is made.

The provision of anti-retrovirals in Africa provides one of the few examples where attempts have been made to define criteria for decision taking on resource allocation at the international public health level (Daniels, 2005). The decision of who to treat rests primarily on clinical grounds, with patients with lower immunity prioritized. While the use of clinical criteria as a basis for rationing care appears to make sense at first glance, clinical criteria have been used in the past to mask moral and social judgments made in the rationing of penicillin, liver transplants and renal dialysis (McGough et al., 2005). Any single criterion is going to be imperfect, so the process of defining criteria, and the involvement of a broad range of stakeholders, [are] essential (Rosen et al., 2005). But as the cholera case study notes, community members are generally not parties to MOUs and rightly perceive the possibility of care when they see red crosses and other indicators of the presence of health care providers. Raising community awareness on the rationale and mandate for a given humanitarian intervention particularly when it is selective (in this case cholera) would seem a minimum and worthwhile responsibility. Communities should not be the agents bearing responsibility for any misperception of mandates.

Limit setting is one of the greatest ethical challenges in health care delivery (Coulter and Ham, 2000). The fact that humanitarian organizations have to set limits to their actions is not controversial; rather, the process of defining the limits raises ethical questions. It has been proposed that such a process should take into account the following issues: limit setting should be discussed in the context of practice, and not in isolation; they can give rise to true ethical dilemmas, where the best available option is the 'least worst' and not an ideal solution; and they can give rise to disagreement and this should be respected given the absence of a universally accepted ethical framework (Hurst, 2005). All three conditions are present in MSF's operational decisions-making processes. Frameworks for resource allocation, for example to help determine how much operational activity should be devoted to responding to conflicts versus chronic diseases like HIV/AIDS, are subject to constant reflection and reiteration, and perspectives are sought at all levels, from implementers at the programme level to operational directors at headquarters. While decisions regarding resource allocation are ultimately taken by headquarters, the perspectives of programmes staff tend to hold considerable weight as it is understood that they have the best necessary knowledge and experience with particular communities to assess the degree of vulnerability and need, and they are also the people who ultimately have to give explanations to beneficiaries when changes or closures are going to be instituted

(Fuller, 2006). Thus, debate and disagreement is actively encouraged, but the objective is to ensure transparency, accountability and justification in decision-making; consensus seeking does not supersede the need to act.

Finally, humanitarian agencies have a responsibility to [ensure] that their workers are better prepared to reflect on these dilemmas and challenge the status quo when it costs lives. Global health has matured to the point that developed world clinicians working on the front line in the developing world should not be surprised by the vast health needs outside the mandate of their program. Indeed, planning for interventions in under-resourced areas should now factor in such possibilities as part of their interventions, and providers need pre-departure briefing on expected conditions informed by epidemiology in order to mitigate, to some extent, the distress caused by the mismatch between the organizational mandate and the ground realities. While this issue has been ethically problematic in research contexts as witnessed by the debate on ancillary care obligations, it bears thorough foresight on the part of organizations pledged to serving health needs in humanitarian crises.

Institutional mandates are important for managing resources and setting limits for action, which is an essential way to ensuring that an organization maintains capacity to respond to a range of crises. But ultimately, mandates are self-endowed and therefore revisable. If they repeatedly fail to stimulate or even hinder an adequate response to the priority health needs of populations in crisis, then they should be called into question.

References

Checchi, F., Gayer, M., Freeman Grais, R. and Mills, E. (2007). *Public Health in Crisis-Affected Populations. A Practical Guide for Decision-Makers.* Humanitarian Practice Network, Network Paper 61. London: Overseas Development Institute.

Coulter, A. and Ham, C. (2000). *The Global Challenge of Health Care Rationing.* Buckingham: Open University Press.

Daniels, N. (2005). Fair Process in Patient Selection for Antiretroviral Treatment in WHO's Goal of 3 by 5. *Lancet*, 366, 169–171.

Devakumar,D. (2008). Cholera and Nothing More. *Public Health Ethics*, 1–2.

Fuller, L. (2006). Justified Commitments? Considering Resource Allocation and Fairness in Medecins sans Frontieres-Holland.*Developing World Bioethics*, 6, 59–70.

Hurst, S. (2005). What Limits to the Responsibilities of Humanitarian Medicine? A Few Pointers for Difficult Ethical Questions. In: *My Sweet La Mancha*. Geneva: MSF, 2006.

Kass, N. (2001). An Ethics Framework for Public Health. *American Journal of Public Health*, 91, 1776–1782.

McGough, L., Reynolds, S., Quinn, T. and Zenilnian, J. (2005). Which Patients First? Setting Priorities for Antiretroviral Therapy Where Resources Are Limited. *American Journal of Public Health,* 95, 1173–1180.

Rosen, S., Sanne, I., Collier, A. and Simon, J. (2005). Rationing Antoretroviral Therapy for HIV/AIDS in Africa: Choices and Consequences. *Plos Medicine,* 2, 1098–1104.

Sphere Project. (2004). *Humanitarian Charter and Minimum Standards in Disaster Response*. Geneva: The Sphere Project.

Sreenivasan, G. and Benater, S. (2006). Challenges for Global Health in the 21st Century: Some Upstream Considerations. *Theoretical Medicine & Bioethics*, 27, 3–11.

Cases

Abarquez v Ontario, 2009 ONCA 374, 310 DLR (4th) 726

Summary prepared by Lorraine Lafferty

SARS is a communicable disease. In March 2003, facing an outbreak of SARS in Toronto, the province of Ontario declared an emergency pursuant to provincial emergency legislation. The Minister of Health issued Directives to hospitals in the Greater Toronto Area that included, among other things, controlling the entrance and movement of staff and patients within health care facilities, wearing of protective equipment, and creating isolation areas for SARS patients. In late April 2003, when the province began to relax the Directives, a second wave of SARS occurred. All hospitals were ordered to reinstate heightened infection-control procedures. By May 17, 2003 the outbreak was declared under control and the declaration of emergency ended.

Fifty-three registered nurses who were employees in Toronto-area hospitals and who contracted SARS (including the estate of one nurse who died) sued the government of Ontario alleging it issued inadequate Directives, exposed them to the risk of contracting the disease, and failed to ensure their health and safety in the workplace. They also alleged the Directives were prematurely relaxed for an improper motive (to remove a travel warning issued by the World Health Organization). The nurses claimed damages in negligence and for breach of their rights to life, liberty, and security of the person under section 7 of the *Canadian Charter of Rights and Freedoms*. Ninety-five family members of the nurses also sued the government for loss of care, guidance and companionship under the *Ontario Family Law Act.*

Reprinted by permission of the author.

Discussion Questions

1. What obligations should governments have to protect the health and safety of health care providers in an emergency situation?
2. Should nurses and other health care providers have the right to remain at home (with or without pay) when there is an outbreak of a potentially deadly infectious disease?
3. How should governments balance economic interests and health interests in the management of emergency situations?

RJR-MacDonald Inc v Canada (Attorney General), [1995] 3 SCR 199, 127 DLR (4th) 1

Summary prepared by Clark Colwell

In 1988, the federal Parliament passed the *Tobacco Products Control Act,* which, amongst other measures, prohibited nearly all advertising and promotion of tobacco products. It also prohibited their sale unless the packaging included a prescribed, unattributed health warning and a list of toxic ingredients.

The tobacco industry brought several constitutional challenges to the new legislation, including a claim that the forced inclusion of unattributed warnings violated their right to freedom of expression. Further, they argued that the Government had failed to show that less-restrictive measures would not be able to accomplish its public health goals.

The Government, in opposition to the challenge, conceded that the law violated the industry representatives' rights to freedom of expression. It argued, however, that given the prominent public health goals of the legislation, the violation was justified under section 1 of the *Canadian Charter of Rights and Freedoms* as a "reasonable limit, demonstrably justified in a free and democratic society," and that less aggressive measures would not be suitable to meet its public health objectives.

Discussion Questions

1. How much weight should be given to a business's concerns about freedom of expression? Should governments always be able to dictate what information businesses must include in their product packaging?
2. To what extent should a public health initiative justify interference with individual freedoms? Does a "public" right always trump an individual one? Should there be any limitations?
3. Would the analysis be any different if the required health warnings were attributable to another entity, for example, Health Canada?

Useful Resources

ONLINE

Addressing Ethical Issues in Pandemic Influenza Planning

A report prepared for the World Health Organization regarding preparedness for an influenza pandemic (2006).

A New Perspective on the Health of Canadians: A Working Document

A report released by Marc Lalonde (Minister of Health and Welfare for Canada) in 1974. It is one of the founding documents on health promotion and is highly regarded both nationally and internationally for challenging traditional thinking about health.

Ottawa Charter for Health Promotion

Drafted at the first international conference on health promotion, held in Ottawa in 1986. An important document in the World Health Organization's campaign to achieve "Health for All by the year 2000."

Public Health Ethics (Journal)

First journal dedicated to issues in public health ethics. Initial issue in April 2008.

Stand on Guard for Thee: Ethical Considerations in Preparedness Planning for Pandemic Influenza

Report issued by the University of Toronto Joint Centre for Bioethics Pandemic Influenza Working Group in the wake of the SARS epidemic of 2003–2004.

What Determines Health?

Discussion of the 12 key determinants of health according to current Canadian analysis; this report is available on the website of the Public Health Agency of Canada.

World Health Organization (WHO), Links to Bioethics Resources on the Web

The WHO website's ethics section provides links divided into five categories: Collaborating Centres in Bioethics, United Nations Organizations, International Organizations, Regional and National Organizations, and Related Health Topics.

HEALTH LAW

Toronto (City, Medical Officer of Health) v Deakin, [2002] OJ no 2777 (QL) (Ct J)

A Toronto area man was infected with contagious tuberculosis. He was not cooperative, and resisted outpatient treatment measures. The Medical Officer of Health applied for and received a temporary order from a judge to detain and treat him. The patient continued to be uncooperative, and after periodic violent outbursts and one successful escape, he was housed in a magnetically sealed room, placed under guard, and occasionally forcefully restrained. When the initial order expired, the Medical Officer of Health applied to the court for a four-month extension. The patient contested, claiming the measures violated his Constitutional rights to life, liberty, and security of the person, as well as the right not to be arbitrarily detained or imprisoned.

Eliopoulos Estate v Ontario (Minister of Health and Long-Term Care), 82 OR (3d) 321, 276 DLR (4th) 411 (CA)

Mr. Eliopoulos was bitten by a mosquito and infected with West Nile Virus. He subsequently died. His estate and family sued the government of Ontario for failing to prevent the outbreak of West Nile Virus.

CanLII

CanLII is a non-profit organization managed by the Federation of Law Societies of Canada. CanLII's goal is to make Canadian law accessible for free on the Internet.

Chapter 5   PATIENTS AND PROVIDERS

INTRODUCTION

It is a feature of most of our lives that we will occasionally find ourselves in the care of a health care provider, whether it is for an acute condition such as an ear infection or broken arm, a chronic condition such as asthma or diabetes, or long-term or palliative care as we approach the end of our lives. We often encounter health care providers at significant moments in our lives and the lives of our loved ones—at births and deaths, for instance—and we entrust them with our care when we are at our most vulnerable. The relationship between patients and health care providers is one marked by an imbalance of power and knowledge, and which in itself may be a healing or destructive force, independent of any particular cures, treatments, or advice offered to the patient. What sorts of principles or rules ought to guide these relationships? How might different types of interactions between patients and providers be characterized and assessed?

Traditionally, medical practice was characterized by a paternalistic approach, in which physicians made decisions for patients, in patients' best interests. Modern medicine has for the most part rejected this approach in favour of respecting patient autonomy, or decision-making capacity, but this in itself doesn't tell us what new model of health care has been, or should be, adopted in place of the paternalistic models of the past. In fact, one concern is that the pendulum might swing too far—that health care providers might place so much value on patient autonomy that they fail to act beneficently (for the well-being of the patient). They might, for instance, become merely technical advisors or providers of information rather than advocates for health. Insofar as beneficence is the core

ethical value in medicine, this shift may be worrisome. Further, in spite of widespread recognition of the importance of placing higher value on patient autonomy, even the much-maligned paternalistic approach to medicine seems to be justified in some health care contexts, for instance emergency care. The first article, by Janet Storch, offers a critical perspective on a number of different models and metaphors that have been proposed to characterize various patient–provider relationships. Storch focuses on the nurse–patient relationship and advises us that every model or metaphor must be used cautiously, since it has the potential to mislead as much as it enlightens. Her lessons are broadly applicable, and explore a number of different characterizations of the patient–provider relationship. Many of the most enduring ethical problems in medicine come down to the debate over the relative weight assigned to beneficence and respect for autonomy in particular cases, and the different models and metaphors outlined by Storch each implicitly identify different balancing points between these principles.

If we want to understand the patient–provider relationship, we need to pay close attention to the characteristics and experiences of patients, who are often vulnerable in many different ways when they encounter a health care provider. In the second article, Barry Hoffmaster asks what vulnerability means and attempts to answer the question by taking a closer look at the vulnerability of his aging parents. He then explores whether and how vulnerability might feature more prominently in bioethical discussions, arguing that it might help us understand the limits of individualism, the role of the body, and the role of feelings in our moral lives. Vulnerability is also one of the reasons why trust is so important in patient–provider relationships. Carolyn McLeod offers a careful analysis of trust in the next article. She argues that trust forms the ethical foundation of any healthy patient–provider relationship, and that this trust must be built and maintained over time. According to McLeod's analysis, trust involves optimism about the competence of the person being trusted and two expectations: that the person in whom trust is placed is motivated by moral integrity, and that she or he interprets the character of the relationship in the right way. McLeod suggests a few practical ways in which providers can cultivate the trust of patients, including displaying competence and integrity, honouring commitments to patients, stating their values and, where necessary, indicating a willingness to make a referral to another health care provider when expectations clash.

In the next article Franklin Miller and Luana Colloca explore the healing power of elements of the patient–provider relationship itself. In particular, they consider the ethics of recommending placebo treatments to patients. Placebo treatments are those treatments that are not believed to have any specific efficacy in the treatment of the condition for which they are offered. They can take many forms (including the "sugar pills" that likely come to mind). One of the strongest ethical arguments against the use of placebos in clinical practice is that they seem to require deception on the part of the health care provider—she or he would have to lie about the placebo treatment and suggest that it had known efficacy for the patient's condition. This looks like it would be in tension with a commitment to respecting patient autonomy, and we might worry that it could undermine patient trust if patients were to find out that they had been lied to. However, Miller and Colloca explore whether placebos might be offered without deception. They argue that when the research evidence suggests there is clinically significant benefit to placebos compared to other available treatments, and when deception is avoided without undermining this benefit, health care providers may be justified in recommending placebo treatments to patients.

The final article by Nuala Kenny, Jocelyn Downie, and Christine Harrison focuses on the particular features of the relationship children have with health care providers, and offers some guidance on how decision-making with children might proceed in a way that both recognizes their variable vulnerability and fosters trust. Kenny and colleagues suggest that respectful involvement of children in decision-making requires that they be informed and included in discussions about their care even when they aren't fully autonomous. The authors provide an overview of debates about how to respect the decisions made by three groups: infants and young children, primary-school children, and adolescents. While the article by Hoffmaster focuses on the challenges of ensuring respectful caregiving for the elderly, the article from Kenny and colleagues reminds us that similar challenges exist for the care of children.

Moral Relationships Between Nurse and Client: The Influence of Metaphors

Janet L. Storch

Metaphors have been commonly used to characterize the nature of the health professional–client relationship, with particular attention to the moral dimensions of that relationship. Metaphors often highlight significant aspects of a relationship, providing us with concrete ways of thinking about the nature of the relationship. However, any metaphor must be used with caution, recognizing that it has the capacity to enlighten, to mislead, and to constrain our thinking. Given the power that metaphors can exert on our practice, critical reflection on how they can shape the moral dimensions of the client–professional relationship is essential.

In this essay, an overview of the types of nurse–client relationships described in the literature through the use of metaphors is provided. The ways in which various metaphors can assist us with or detract us from a clear understanding of our moral agency and our moral duties to our clients/patients are then examined by considering metaphors that are limiting, misguided, or helpful in clarifying the nature of that moral relationship. Finally, a synopsis of key aspects of this special relationship concludes the essay. In an era when health care delivery is beset by a variety of sociopolitical ideologies, it is timely for nursing to embrace metaphors that articulate the values inherent in its practice.

METAPHORS AND MODELS TO DEFINE RELATIONSHIPS

Before embarking on the discussion, a brief commentary on the use of metaphors is in order. A metaphor is defined as a figure of speech in which one thing is compared to another thing by being spoken of as if it were the other. Although metaphors are commonly used in poetry and in lyrics, as well as in ordinary conversation to embellish discourse, they can be most useful in helping us to see some aspects of life, such as interpersonal relationships, in a way that enhances our understanding. Thus, we are directed to see and to think about that relationship in a particular way. That is, metaphors lead us to emphasize certain aspects of the relationship and minimize others. At the same time, metaphors offer alternative views or ways of seeing a relationship. In this way, metaphors can have a powerful influence on our language, on how we think, and on how we come to understand that aspect of life. In many respects, this influence is positive and enlightening. At the same time, this emphasis can lead to a distortion in thinking because it can overemphasize one view at the expense of other equally valid views that become excluded from consideration. That exclusion itself is significant because it allows us to "not see" the whole picture (Morgan, 1997).

Veatch (1972) and Callaban (1988) are two ethicists who have employed metaphors to facilitate understanding of health professional–patient relationships. Several models and metaphors have been identified in health care and health ethics literature. They are captured in the table on the following page (Table 5.1). Some of these metaphors focus on the comparison of physicians to engineers, to priests, or to contractors (see Veatch, 1972). These metaphors portray medicine as among the first of professions. A more recent discussion, by Emanuel and Emanuel (1992), is based on various approaches

From Storch, J.L. (1999) "Moral Relationships Between Nurse and Client: The Influence of Metaphors." In Kluge, E.-H. (ed.) *Readings in Biomedical Ethics: A Canadian Focus*, Second Edition. Reprinted by permission of the author.

Table 5.1

MODELS AND METAPHORS IDENTIFIED IN THE LITERATURE

Physician–Patient Relationships and Health Professional–Patient Relationships

VEATCH 1972	MAY 1975	BAYLES 1981
1. Engineering (Employer)	1. Contract	1. Agency
2. Priestly	2. Covenant	2. Contract
3. Collegial		3. Friendship
4. Contractual		4. Paternalistic
		5. Fiduciary

CALLAHAN 1988	EMANUEL & EMANUEL 1992
1. Contract	1. Paternalistic
2. Covenant	2. Informative
3. Advocate	3. Interpretive
4. Fiduciary	4. Deliberative

Nurse-Client Relationships

SMITH 1950	BROCK 1580
1. Nurse as surrogate mother	1. Nurse as parent surrogate
2. Nurse as technician	2. Nurse as physician surrogate
3. Nurse as contracted clinician	3. Nurse as healer
	4. Nurse as patient advocate or protector
	5. Nurse as educator
	6. Nurse as contracted clinician

WINSLOW 1984
I. Military metaphor
2. Legal metaphor (Advocacy)

FOWLER 1984	MITCHELL 1990
1. Mercantile	1. Domestic (servant)
2. Indentured servant	2. Family (mother surrogate)
3. Engineering	3. Medical (physician extender)
4. Priestly	4. Business (employee)
5. Collegial	5. Advocacy (patient advocate)
6. Contractual	6. Contractual (contracted clinician)
7. Friendship (Artistotelian)	7. Friendship (friend)
8. Covenantal	

in one's relationships with clients rather than on strictly metaphorical comparisons. Consideration of these approaches seems to have been directed towards moving the medical profession forward to keep pace with the changed expectations of the public to be served.

In the discourse about nurse–client relationships that uses metaphorical thinking, there is clearly some "borrowing" of approaches from the literature describing other health professional–patient relationships through model and metaphor. There are also significant contrasts in the types of models and metaphors utilized to understand the nature of the relationship between physicians and patients when compared with those used to characterize nurse–client relationships. In general, nurse–client models and metaphors are more concrete and, therefore, more explicit in their characterization of nursing (e.g., mother, servant). This concreteness can create particular problems for the nursing profession. The nursing profession can be characterized so clearly that images are difficult for the public, other professions, and nurses themselves to shed with ease. It may even be difficult to recognize the distortions the metaphors convey.

METAPHORS AND NURSE–CLIENT RELATIONSHIPS

It seems unlikely that any other vocation or profession has experienced the diversity of imagery and metaphor that nursing has encountered in the Western world over the past century. Initially the depiction of nursing was through pictures (painted or sketched), often with metaphors as captions (e.g., Angels of Mercy). More recently, the use of written metaphors to describe and analyze nurses and nurse–client relationships has been common. One can only surmise that the penchant for "picturing" the nurse historically is related to a fascination with the female figure. Physicians have also experienced imagery of their roles and relationships with patients, but the images and metaphors of physicians have not been so varied, so gender related, nor so extensive. As noted earlier, the concrete nature of nursing metaphors, such as those depicted in Table 5.1, is also significant. Many of the conclusions about nursing embedded in the minds of readers or viewers have been based upon these metaphors and have been difficult for nursing to overcome. These metaphors are rooted in longstanding historical images.

Historical Images of Professional Nursing

In 1996, the International Council of Nurses, the International Red Cross, and the Red Crescent Museum in Geneva developed an exhibition to capture in images, text, and testimonials the first 30 years (1900–1930) of "… nursing's rise as an intellectual, socially responsible endeavor" (*Profession: Nurse* 1995, p. 11). This exhibition included a wide range of posters, postcards, drawings, paintings, and photographs that depicted nurses and conveyed a sense of the nurse's role and relationship to patients and to society.

The pictures and other material provided images of nurse as mother, sister, friend, lover, guardian angel, or army sergeant. In the accompanying publication, produced by the International Red Cross and Red Crescent Museum, the authors note that these images of nursing (these metaphors of nursing) were widely used during the First World War for purposes of raising funds for the war effort, raising morale, and stimulating patriotic zeal. "A mother figure to all the wounded, the needy and children, a nurse—with or without the red cross or crescent on her uniform—was often perceived as a savior in the glow of fervent patriotism…. Nurses were viewed as moral figures above all suspicion and were therefore used for propaganda purposes …" (*Profession: Nurse,* 1995, p. 26).

Following World War I, as the image of the universal mother and guardian angel gave way to Post War realities, nurses began to be depicted as fighters or soldiers who fought the residual ills of the War and epidemics, and worked in communities with social welfare officers to fight social ills.

The World Wars, and wars of the previous century, had a profound influence on the development of nursing. Florence Nightingale's work in founding nursing as a profession was given impetus by the Crimean War. And the influence of military models of health care delivery and hospital organization directed the manner in which nursing unfolded as an independent entity. Only in the latter three decades of the twentieth century has the influence of some of these metaphors begun to fade from view. In fact, some of these historical images or metaphors of nursing continue to have a profound effect on the public's view of nurses, fellow health professionals' understanding of nurse–client relationships, and the views of nurses themselves. Some of these views or perceptions have served to limit the significance of professional nursing.

Limiting Metaphors: Nurse As Parent, Nurse As Servant, Nurse As Friend

Assuming the majority of people hold positive perceptions of parents, and of mothers in particular, the metaphor of *nurse as parent surrogate* or *nurse as mother surrogate* to describe the nurse–client relationship allows us to see some fundamental foundations of that relationship. It is a relationship based upon trust, integrity, promise-keeping, dedication, and nurturance. Taking that metaphor of mother or parent further, one can understand the nurse–client relationship to involve some degree of protection of the client in care, an attempt to help clients gain or regain independence, and a commitment to never abandon a client in need. Inasmuch as this metaphor serves to enlarge understanding about these moral features of the relationship, it is well used.

However, in highlighting some similar characteristics, there can be a tendency to overgeneralize. All features of the nurse–client relationship come to be seen as "parenting" or "mothering" relationships. The ways in which this might distort the nature of the relationship are many. Nursing comes to be seen as largely women's work and as a selfless endeavour. Like mothering, nursing then comes to be viewed as something that anyone can do. In making these assumptions, it becomes easy to discount nursing knowledge, skill, and expertise. The "tender loving care" provided by nurses may appear to be just like mother's care and concern, with little more knowledge required than what arises from trying to be caring and helpful to another.

Mitchell (1990) has labeled the mother/parent metaphor a *family metaphor*. She identifies a primary concern within the metaphor of surrogate mother to be found in "… the arrangement of health care services and relationships according to family roles, with the physician as father, nurse as mother, and patients as dependents …" (page 5). In

this scenario the nurse is expected to work (likely harder than anyone else) to maintain harmony in the home, i.e., the hospital. Further, the nurse as helpmate is not accorded power for decision making. This has significant implications for the nurse's ability to exercise his or her moral agency.

The *friendship metaphor* has positive parallels to the family metaphor, including expectations that clients can depend upon nurses and that nurses would value truth-telling and fidelity. It is misleading, however, in that the nurse–client relationship cannot be a relationship of equals, like friendship. Clients are often in a vulnerable state during their health care encounter and there is, by reason of that vulnerability and by reason of the different type and level of knowledge about the client's condition, an asymmetry of power in the healing relationship.

Finally, the *nurse as servant metaphor* adds one level of clarity to the nurse–client relationship, but at the price of potentially serious misconceptions about the relationship. From a positive view, the servant metaphor emphasizes service to others, and in this way captures the moral ideal of service critical to professional roles. In this case, nurses as professionals use their knowledge and skills in service to others The misleading aspects of the metaphor include the implication that nurses will do anything that needs to be done at work, including domestic work (Mitchell, 1990). This has led to the serious exploitation of nurses in the past and to a significant extent in the present. Nurses' responses to such exploitation have been to establish unions for some protection from the arbitrariness of employers. Through unions they have set limits on the work they are required to do and the times in which they will do it. Nevertheless, in our current era of health care cost constraint, nurses are all too often expected to fill in the gaps when resources are cut.

A serious distortion of the metaphor of nurse as servant is the characterization of the nurse as an *indentured servant* who just "follows orders" (Fowler, 1984). This understanding of the nurse's role and relationship within the health care team led to obedience, in which the nurse cedes his or her moral agency to institutional directives, with the result that both nurse and client suffer. From this indentured servant metaphor, the long history of nurse as handmaiden to the physician has also been prominent. This places the client in a secondary position relative to the nurse–physician, then nurse–client relationship. Indeed, the Nightingale pledge that many nurses took at either capping ceremonies or graduations in times past included the phrase "… with loyalty will I endeavor to aide the physician in his work and devote myself to the welfare of the patient" (Storch, 1982, p. 202). In this sense, devotion to the patient was considered to be realized through loyally aiding the physician (Fowler, 1984). It was not until the middle of the twentieth century that those two commitments (to physician and to patient) were disentangled. By the early 1970s the International Council of Nurses Code of Ethics stated with unmistaken clarity that "The nurse's primary responsibility is to those people who require nursing care" (Storch, 1982, p. 201). Yet, amongst physicians, health administrators and the public, there are still many who wonder why nurses are not "doing nursing" anymore (e.g., Stein, 1990). Whether their puzzlement is written or stated, the source of concern often can be traced to the query about why nurses are not there to "aid" physicians any longer or to follow orders without question(s).

Misguided Metaphors

Use of the *metaphor of technician* or *nurse as engineer* to describe the nurse–patient relationship emphasizes the task aspect of nursing roles. The strength of this metaphor rests in its emphasis on technical competence. Competence is a highly valued dimension of the nurse-patient relationship since "… caring without knowledge remains simply a matter of good intentions …" (Falk Raphael, 1996). Unless the nurse meets the level of technical competence to carry out her tasks, "… the whole relationship begins with a lie" (Pellegrino, 1979, p. 48).

However, emphasizing the technical and task aspects of nursing captures only a fraction of nursing knowledge and skill, and the metaphor of technician limits understanding about the work that nurses do. As "re-engineering" of care-giver roles has become fashionable (Schweikhart and Smith-Daniels, 1996), this distortion of role has led to the devaluing of wholistic nursing practice and, alarmingly, to simplistic solutions to nursing replacement. Since many can see only the "tasks" nurses do, the rest of nursing work remains invisible. For example, in the giving of a medication, what is observed is a pill moving from the nurse's hand to the client's mouth. What is unobserved is the nurse's assessment of the client's condition while that simple act is in progress—respirations, pallor, comfort, degree of mobility, ease of swallowing, skin turgor, evidence of edema, etc.—the mental note taken of a plan of care on-course or one in need of modification (based on expert knowledge of the condition, the drug, and environmental stressors). Verbal and non-verbal communication occur in that simple but highly complex interaction. Opportunities arise to engage in client teaching, support, guidance, and reassurance. Perhaps, most important, is the sense of presence the expert nurse brings to the encounter—a way of being with the client that reflects the depth of care and concern, laced with competence to deliver, for that one individual. Thus, the concrete task observed is not the real work of nursing: the real work of nursing requires knowledge and skill that is all but invisible to the observer. The type of care expert nurses provide must begin with considerable investment in the relationship, involves the use of self, and involves attention to the uniqueness of that client.

These same misguided task-oriented conclusions are operative in the *physician extender* and *physician surrogate* metaphors. While there are aspects of medical tasks and medical work that nurses are able to perform, even in performing those tasks nursing work is different. Taking on specific tasks of medicine does not equate to being either a physician extender or a physician surrogate, or a physician for that matter. Nursing roles and relationships are different, with different goals and different processes of care. For example, both physicians and nurses will monitor arterial blood gas results. The physician monitors those results to diagnose cardio-pulmonary dysfunction; the nurse monitors the same results to plan activity, rest, and comfort.

Nursing knowledge increasingly involves many ways of knowing, beyond empirical knowledge and technical skill. It includes knowledge gained through empirics, but also knowledge drawn from ethics, personal knowledge, aesthetics, and sociopolitical knowing (Carper, 1978; White, 1995), Different knowledge and skill lead to different ways of approaching care, and to a different form of nurse–client relationship, including greater attention to "ways of being" in relationship with the clients (Silva, Sorrell and Sorell, 1995).

Helpful Metaphors: Nurse As in a Covenantal Relationship, As Healer, As Advocate

Among the many metaphors applied to nurse–client relationships are several that stand out as characterizing more clearly than others the ideals of what these relationships should be. Use of the metaphor of a *covenantal relationship* emphasizes that nurse and client are "… bound to one another in many ways, not the least of which is morally" (Fowler, 1984, p. 338). As members of a community, and within that community a health care system, nurses are expected to be faithful and to keep their promise of profession, i.e., to use their knowledge and skills to minimize harm and to benefit others.

> A convenantal model calls attention to the reciprocal indebtedness of the public and the profession, suggesting that professional power is a gift from the public to the profession given in exchange for its expertise and orientation to the service of others (Bernal, 1992, p. 22).

In emphasizing concepts of relatedness and reciprocity, the covenantal model underscores nursing practice priorities of the 1990s.

The image of *nurse as healer* is a long standing metaphor utilized since the early 1900s to emphasize the healing powers of the nursing presence. Whether a nurse is fully present with a client through the painful journey of being a critically ill patient in ICU or CCU, through

an outpatient experience of chemotherapy, or through a long period of rehabilitation at home recovering from a stroke, the professional nurse's ongoing presence can facilitate the individual to move towards restoration and healing. In this way the nurse has a different but complementary role to that of physician.

The *nurse as client advocate* was introduced in the early 1970s and was based on a clearer understanding of nurses' direct accountability (legal and ethical) to clients. Considerable attention in nursing literature (see for example, Donahue, 1978; Abrams, 1978; Curtin, 1979; Gadow, 1980; Kohnke, 1982; Fowler, 1989; Bernal, 1995) has been directed towards identifying the role of advocacy and types of advocacy (e.g., intervening, protecting, informing, supporting, speaking for, coordinating, empowering, etc.) as well as problems for nurses in fulfilling a role as client advocate.

In 1984, Winslow analyzed the shift from a nursing practice based on a military model (characterized by hierarchy and obedience) to one based on a legal model that focused on advocacy for the client in health care. He identified several issues surrounding the nurse as patient or client advocate, including lack of clarity of the concept, the need to revise nursing practice acts to allow for this type of nursing role, the question as to whether clients and their families were prepared to accept advocacy as a nursing role, the potentially adversarial nature of advocacy, and the potential conflicting interests and loyalties inherent in advocacy. Advocacy has served as a powerful metaphor for nursing, although often with only superficial understanding of its real power.

As long as advocacy is confined to legal metaphor it is limiting. However, when it is viewed as "… not simply one more alternative to be added to the list of past and present concepts of nursing … but as embracing all of them …" (Curtin, 1979, p. 2), its real meaning is understood. Benner (1994) characterized client advocacy as involving openness and engagement in moral and clinical reasoning. Drawing upon the work of Gadow (1980), who conceptualized "existential advocacy," Benner contrasts the "narrow legal sense of advocacy" (page 49) with a deeper and more meaningful form of advocacy.

She describes this type of advocate as one who "stands alongside, who interprets, and understands ..." (page 49)—language congruent with a covenantal relationship. She suggests that this enriched metaphor of client advocacy is manifest in the following way: managing and coordinating services to a client so that all services are directed toward an agreed upon intent to ensure client and family well-being, "... standing in for someone to give them voice ... getting appropriate medical intervention for [clients] ... and presencing and acknowledging loss and grief" with one who is dying (page 51).

These metaphors of nurse in a covenantal relationship, nurse as healer, and nurse as advocate, approach more closely than the previous metaphors the morally significant aspects of the nurse–client relationship. Their emphasis is on the moral commitment of the nurse to be a comforting presence to clients through difficult health situations; to be in relationship with clients; and to intervene, inform, support, and facilitate their empowerment. This emphasis provides insight into the "special" nature of the nurse–client relationship.

What Metaphors Enable Us to See and Learn

Metaphors used to describe the nurse–client relationship can be instructive and they can be limiting. Their limitations include their potential to further devalue nursing knowledge and skill, to perpetuate stereotypical notions of nurse–client and physician-client relationships, to mislead by suggesting equal partnership in that relationship, to perpetuate the task-oriented view of nursing, and to conflate nurse and physician roles. The strength of metaphors applied to nursing rests in the ability to understand more readily the historical shifts in nursing roles and nurse–client relationships and to appreciate both constancy and change in nurse–client relationships over time. Further, metaphors help to articulate the values in nursing practice in an era when roles are under threat from an economic imperative.

The constant themes of the nurse–client relationship accessed through metaphor are relationships based on the moral foundations of trust,

integrity, respect, truth-telling, and promise-keeping. These themes are fundamental to nursing. The covenantal metaphor emphasis on reciprocity and connectedness makes more visible the foundation of the relationship. Metaphors have also served a useful purpose in drawing distinctions between medicine and nursing over time. When used with care, metaphors enable us to see and learn much about the nature of nursing and the nature of the nurse-patient relationship. Most importantly, the moral foundations of that relationship can become more visible and less difficult to articulate and defend.

Acknowledgements

The author wishes to thank Dr. Gwen Hartrick, Dr. Patricia Rodney, and Dr. Rita Schreiber for their critical review of this essay and for their helpful suggestions.

References

Abrams, Natalie (1978). "A contrary view of the nurse as patient advocate," *Nursing Forum* 17(3): 258–267.

Bayles, Michael D. (1981). *Professional Ethics.* Belmont: CA. Wadsworth Publishing Co.

Baylis, Francoise, Downie, Jocelyn, Freedman, Benjamin, Hoffmaster, Barry, and Sherwin, Susan, eds. (1996). *Health Care Ethics in Canada.* Toronto: Harcourt Brace and Company.

Benner, Patricia (1994). "Caring as ways of knowing and not knowing." In *The Crisis of Care* (pp. 42–62). Edited by Susan Phillips and Patricia Benner. Washington D.C.: Georgetown University Press.

Bernal, Ellen W. (1992), "The nurse as patient advocate." *Hastings Center Report* 22(4): 18–23.

Brock, Dan W. (1980). "The nurse-patient relation: Some rights and duties." In *Nursing: Images and Ideals* (pp. 102–124). Edited by Stuart F. Spicker and Sally Gadow. New York: Springer Publishing Co.

Callahan, Joan, ed. (1988). *Ethical Issues in Professional Life.* New York: Oxford University Press.

Carper, Barbara (1978). "Fundamental patterns of knowing in nursing." *Advances in Nursing Science* 1(1): 13–23.

Curtin, Leah (1979). "Nurse as advocate: A philosophical foundation for nursing." *Advances in Nursing Science* 1(3): 1–10.

Donahue, M. Patricia (1978). "The nurse: A patient advocate?" *Nursing Forum* 17(2): 143–151.

Emanuel, Ezekiel J. and Emanuel, Linda L. (1995). "Four models of the physician-patient relationship." In *Health Care Ethics in Canada* (pp. 163–179). Edited by Francoise Baylis et al. Toronto: Harcourt Brace and Company.

Fowler, Marsha (1984). Ethics and Nursing, 1893–1984: The Ideal of Service, the Reality of History. Doctoral Dissertation, University of Southern California.

_____ (1989). "Social advocacy." *Heart and Lung* 18(1): 97–99.

Gadow, Sally (1980). "Existential advocacy: Philosophical foundations of nursing." In *Nursing: Images and Ideals* (pp. 79–101). Edited by Stuart F. Smith and Sally Gadow. New York: Springer Publishing Company.

Kohnke, Mary (1982). *Advocacy: Risk or Reality.* Toronto: C.V. Mosby.

May, William F. (1975). "Code and covenant or philanthropy and contract." *Hastings Center Report* 5(6): 29–38.

Mitchell, Christine (1990). "The nurse-patient relationship: A source of some moral duties." In Humanities and the Health Professions, Occasional Papers of the Connecticut Humanities Council, No. 8, 3–16.

Morgan, Gareth (1997). *Images of Organizations.* Thousand Oaks: Sage Publications.

Profession: Nurse, Images 1900–1930 (1995). Geneva: Musée International de la Red Cross et du Red Crescent.

RNABC (1997). *The Role of the Nurse in Advocacy.* Vancouver: Registered Nurses Association of British Columbia.

Schweikhart, Sharon Bergman, and Smith-Daniels, Vicki (1996). "Reengineering the work of caregivers: Roles redefinition, team structures, and organizational redesign." *Hospital and Health Administration* 41(1): 19–35.

Silva, Mary, Sorrell, Jeanne, and Sorrell, Christine (1995). "From Carper's ways of knowing to ways of being: An ontological shift in nursing." *Advances in Nursing Science* 18(1): 1–13.

Smith, Sheri (1980). "Three models of the nurse-patient relationship." In *Nursing: Images and Ideals* (pp. 176–188). Edited by Stuart F. Spicker and Sally Gadow. New York: Springer Publishing Company.

Stein, Leonard, Watts, D.T., and Howell, T. (1990). "The doctor-nurse game revisited." *New England Journal of Medicine* 60(5): 812–816.

Storch, Janet L. (1982). *Patients' Rights: Ethical and Legal Issues in Health Care and in Nursing.* Toronto: McGraw Hill.

Veatch, Robert M. (1972). "Models for ethical medicine in a revolutionary age." *Hastings Center Report* 2(3): 5–7.

White, Jill (1995). "Patterns of knowing: Review, critique and update." *Advances in Nursing Science* 17(4): 78–86.

Winslow, Gerald R. (1984). "From loyalty to advocacy: A new metaphor for nursing." *Hastings Center Report* 14(3): 32–40.

What Does Vulnerability Mean?

Barry Hoffmaster

Vulnerability does not mean much for our contemporary morality. It is antithetical to our emphasis on individualism and rationality; it requires that we attend to the body and to our feelings. Yet only by recognizing the depth and breadth of our vulnerability can we affirm our humanity.

Vulnerability is one of those general notions we bandy about confidently but carelessly, assuming that we know what it means and that it means the same thing for everybody. Were we challenged to explain it, though, we might admit to some unclarity and puzzlement. What does vulnerability actually mean?

Hoffmaster, B. "What does vulnerability mean?" from the *Hastings Center Report* 36(2). 2006.

A dictionary provides multiple definitions. One meaning of "vulnerable" is to be susceptible to something, a bad something naturally, such as disease or infection. People living in a war-torn country where the water and sewer systems have been destroyed are, for example, vulnerable to contracting malaria. A second meaning of "vulnerable" is to be capable of being physically or emotionally wounded. A child born with a physical or mental handicap, for instance, could be devastated by the unceasing jeers and taunts of brutal schoolmates. A third meaning of "vulnerable" is to be capable of being persuaded or tempted. A young woman burdened by university debt might be enticed, for example, to reply to an advertisement that offers substantial remuneration for egg donation. And a fourth meaning is to be liable to increased penalties, as any bridge player whose team has won a game in a rubber knows. The real meaning of vulnerability is richer than these sketchy definitions, however. To understand it, we must appreciate what it means to live with vulnerability. People who are old, particularly those who reside in nursing homes or other long-term care facilities, are vulnerable in many ways. What does vulnerability mean for them?

To try to answer that question, I have to describe the vulnerability of two people I know. The first is my eighty-five-year-old father. As this is written, my father most likely is sleeping in a bed in a nursing home. Forty years ago my father stopped playing basketball with me and a friend of mine, went inside our house, lay down on our living room couch, and had a heart attack. Two days later my mother threw open the back door of our house, rushed in crying, and told me that my father had had a stroke in the hospital. I did not know what that meant at the time; it turned out that he did not have just any stroke, but what is aptly and ominously called a "catastrophic" stroke. His entire right side was paralyzed. From then on, he could not use his right arm and hand, and he could walk only with a cane and a brace.

His speech was impaired, and he always struggled—most often unsuccessfully— to find the word he wanted and to complete the sentence he had started.

Now, forty years later, ravaged by the misfortunes of stroke and old age, my father epitomizes what it is to be vulnerable. He contracts multiple infections and diseases. He has recurring urinary tract infections, each of which renders him weaker and pushes him to an ever-lower plateau. He has some form of dementia on top of the cognitive impairment caused by the stroke. His left hand shakes, so he might have Parkinson's. In the nursing home, he fell prey to vancomycin-resistant enterococcus, which put him in a private room. Because he cannot swallow, he is fed through a peg-tube. When the tube is washed out, sometimes fluid builds up in his lungs, and he is transferred to the hospital to be treated for congestive heart failure.

My father has been physically devastated. He can still be further wounded, however. Other than when he is transferred to a recliner and wheeled into the hall, he spends all his time in bed, so he gets bed sores. One sore on his ankle refused to heal and exposed bone, necessitating surgery and a subsequent skin graft. Despite this intervention, the wound persists.

My father can also be wounded emotionally. After one hospital stay he was transferred to a different nursing home, and when I went to see him there, I found him in a lineup of wheelchairs across from a nurses' station. Even from a distance, I could see that his azure eyes were blazing. When I approached and he recognized me, he began waving his left arm and talking, spewing sounds full of fury but devoid of sense. I had rarely seen him angry, and throughout my entire life I had never seen him that angry. He did not want to be there, but he was helpless. At last, probably out of desperation, he was raging against a fate that he had endured with patience, determination, and equanimity for half his life.

As the days pass, though, he seems less and less capable of being emotionally wounded. And he no longer is capable of being persuaded or tempted, even by food—perhaps the last pleasure he had. Nor, although he and my mother were avid bridge players, is he any longer capable of playing a hand, let alone of winning a game.

The second person is my eighty-four-year-old mother. For forty years she has cared for my father. In addition to all the usual spousal duties assumed by a woman of her time and background, she has attended to the details of his care and his extra needs, even when he was still at home in a rented hospital bed, and she knew she did not have the size and the strength to get him into a wheelchair or to turn him in bed. After he entered what became a series of nursing homes, she visited him at least once a day, helped him eat, shaved him, cleaned his dental plate, and took his laundry home to wash. She was vigilant in detecting lapses in his care and aggressive in reporting those failings to anybody who could do something about them. She understood, intellectually at least, that there were many other patients in the nursing homes who required care, and that there were routines and schedules that had to be followed. Yet her advocacy on behalf of my father was unstinting and unsparing. As a result, she had tumultuous relationships with the staff and the administrators, and she was undoubtedly regarded as a "difficult" spouse.

My mother remains in amazingly good physical health, lives in a house by herself, drives a car, goes shopping, cooks and cleans, pays the bills, and gardens. Only recently has she started to have problems with her short-term memory. How, then, could she be regarded as vulnerable?

Let me approach that question indirectly because I believe the ways in which my mother is vulnerable are, although not as palpable as the ways in which my father is vulnerable, nevertheless regrettably familiar. One of the articles I use when I teach bioethics discusses the plight of a hospitalized ninety-one-year-old man who is profoundly demented and, after a stay in the intensive care unit, is at risk for a precipitous decline.[1] A new attending physician, who

believes a return visit to the intensive care unit would be "futile," asks the house staff about the patient's code status. They report that they have tried, without success, to talk to the patient's eighty-seven-year-old wife about her husband's poor prognosis, and that she has refused to consent to a "do not resuscitate" order and wants her husband to receive all "aggressive measures." They describe the wife as "demanding and difficult."

When the new attending physician talks to the wife, he discovers that she has cared for her husband at home for fifteen years, up until six weeks ago, when she had to transfer him to a nursing home. The wife is tearful about the transfer; she says that "he had been fine until he went there." In subsequent conversations she explains that the house staff seem too rushed and distracted to talk with her. The residents speak to her in hallways with clipboards in their hands, and they are interrupted by pages. When the attending physician talks to her in the comparative quiet and comfort of a solarium, she begins to express her feelings and reveal her own need to grieve and to be healed. After providing devoted care for many years, she now feels excluded from decisions about her husband's care and wellbeing. Eventually, the attending physician comes to see the wife's desire for "aggressive" management as a product of her continuing sense of responsibility and obligation to her husband:

> In a reparative way, she felt obliged to rescue her husband. To … [her], aggressive care was not an intervention approaching medical futility. Instead, the use of medical technology was a means of demonstrating the integrity of their marriage covenant. As she had cared for her husband at home for years, she now would mobilize all of the hospital's resources in the service of her husband. Simply put, she was making amends for a misplaced sense of spousal abandonment. When the clinician suggested to … [her] that she felt responsible for her husband's

situation, she broke down and cried. She confessed that she felt responsible for his current situation because she had not kept him at home.[2]

This woman has been emotionally wounded beyond what the house staff have the time, and perhaps the interest or the capacity, to comprehend. She tended lovingly and dutifully to a husband until that simply became impossible. When she finally had to give up, she lost control of what happened to her husband. She felt guilty about what she perceived as her own failings. She felt ignorant because she could not obtain the information she needed so badly. And because of her ignorance, she felt powerless to affect her husband's destiny and to provide the care and comfort she owed him. Yet she had to remain faithful to her husband and find ways of assuaging her guilt when she felt she had failed. The only way she could see to do that was to insist on continued "aggressive" care. And that made her "difficult and demanding."

Change the details of the husband's history and present condition and change the hospital to a nursing home, and you have my mother. My mother had supported and cared for a husband with a catastrophic stroke for half her life. When she finally had to give up—a decision recommended to her for a long time by many people and beset by some reversals—it was with enormous struggle and agony.

And now she has lost control of what happens to her husband. The person to whom she has scrupulously attended and whom she has striven to help and protect is abandoned to and at the mercy of strangers. She feels guilty. She attributes my father's loss of the strength to walk and the ability to swallow food and drink water to being in a nursing home. She excoriates staff—usually, but not always, to my brother and me—for not providing care as good as the care she had provided at home. More than once she has had a point. On several occasions, with her keen and practiced senses, she has detected worrisome deteriorations in my father's condition that went unnoticed by staff. One time her

insistent concern led to a rapid transfer of my father to a hospital. She never seems able to obtain the information she desperately wants, and consequently she, too, feels powerless. She complains that she cannot talk to my father's doctors, either in the nursing home or when he is transferred to the hospital. She complains that the staff in the nursing home either do not have the time to talk to her or are not willing to talk to her.

In some sense and to some extent, she understands why information is so hard to come by. She realizes that the nurses, aides, and social workers in a nursing home are responsible for many people and are busy coping with inordinate, unceasing demands on their time. She realizes that it is the doctor who ultimately is responsible for my father's care, who knows my father's condition best, and who makes decisions about his medical treatment. She realizes that nurses and aides might not fully know what is being done to my father, nor why it is being done, nor what the expected outcome is. And she realizes that rather than provide incomplete, inaccurate, or misleading information, it is better that they provide no information. Nevertheless, her ignorance and her powerlessness foster feelings of guilt, inadequacy, and infidelity. She, too, has suffered deep and irreparable emotional wounds.

My father's and my mother's vulnerabilities are linked, of course. When my father was still at home, my mother could have injured her back trying to turn him in bed or help him sit up. When my father entered a nursing home, my mother was plagued by fears and anxieties about how he was doing there and how he was being treated. As my father becomes progressively more withdrawn and silent, my mother loses even the partial interaction and the incomplete, uncertain communication she has had with him. She becomes more isolated, and her worries magnify because her guesses about what he wants and how he is feeling are even more speculative. For a long time my mother has completed sentences for my father and done things for him when he was struggling. She has fewer opportunities for that now, but she has always believed, quite sincerely, that she is helping him. And after years of helping him in countless unremitting ways, it is easy to understand why she would want to make it a little easier and quicker for herself. But the words she spoke for him, the decisions she made for him, and the things she did for him made him even more vulnerable because they highlighted what he could not do for himself. They also made it impossible for him to do more for himself, and, on occasion, undoubtedly made it impossible for him to get what he really wanted. He was aware of that, and he could be frustrated and angered by that. It was obvious when he simply gave up.

There are also, of course, differences between my father's and my mother's vulnerabilities. My father's vulnerability is largely the result of natural causes and is much more comprehensive because of the extensive physical damage he has suffered. Many functions of the tissues, organs, and systems of his body have been disrupted or destroyed, and harm to those biological functions has cascaded into his physical and mental functions. Paralysis and progressive weakness have rendered him immobile and unable to eat or drink. Destruction of tissues in his brain has impaired his alertness, his perceptiveness, and his comprehension. And the loss of physical and mental functions has virtually eliminated his social functioning. His exchanges with other people are limited, brief, and transitory. When vulnerability is the result of natural causes, there is little, if any, difference between being "vulnerable" and being "at risk." One could instead describe my father as at risk of having another urinary tract infection, of getting aspiration pneumonia, of developing bed sores.

My mother's vulnerability is, in contrast, more limited and more selective. It derives primarily from blocked or impeded social functioning. For that reason it is largely the result of human causes and human creations. Some of those causes are individual: the incapacity or unwillingness of individuals to provide the information she needs or to provide it in a manner she can comprehend

and retain. Some of those causes are cultural. My mother, like many people, has a deep and abiding belief in the myths of medicine. She expects medicine to discover the cause of every new illness, infection, ailment, and complication, and she expects medicine to have a cure for every new problem. Those expectations, as unrealistic as they are, are not entirely her own creation. They have been fostered and encouraged by the scientifically and technologically oriented, progress-preoccupied society she inhabits, by the cure and research missions of the medical community and the fund-raising organizations that support them, by the rampant advertising of drug companies, and by the deeply rooted cultural injunction that associates responsibility with action rather than with acceptance, to cite just a few factors. And some of those causes are organizational or institutional: the structures, staffing, and schedules of hospitals and nursing homes, and the public and private arrangements for providing and funding health care services.

Despite those differences, though, there is a crucial similarity between the vulnerability of my father and the vulnerability of my mother. What does not come out explicitly in the dictionary definitions of "vulnerable," but what is most important about vulnerability, is what my father and my mother experience the most: the loss of power that vulnerability imposes and signifies, and the attendant loss of control that ensues. We fear vulnerability most immediately because of the particular harms we seek to avoid. But we fear vulnerability most profoundly because of the power we seek to retain.

Rollo May, a psychologist and psychoanalyst who used to be read a lot but is not read much anymore, once said, "no human being can stand the perpetually numbing experience of his own powerlessness."[3] My father's powerlessness extends almost as far as it can. When I speak to my mother, she regularly tells me: "Your father's not good. He hardly speaks, and all he does is sleep." In my view sleep is one of his last blessings. My mother's powerlessness, although less extensive, is more agonizing because she is acutely aware of it. She appreciates what my father has lost and how little she now can do for him. She appreciates what she has lost and what they together have lost. She sees the lives that other people have, and she knows that their kinds of past, present, and future opportunities were foreclosed to my father and her, never to be recovered and never to be rectified. More than once, my mother has said to me, "This is not much of a life," but it is the only life she has.

And she has to think about the future. What kind of life will she have after my father dies? Perhaps she will be liberated to do things for herself, to have fun and enjoy life in ways that heretofore have not been possible. Less optimistically, perhaps she will struggle to find a new orientation and focus for her life, and the depredations of aging will add deep physical wounds to her already deep emotional wounds. Like the wife of the ninety-one-year-old, severely demented man, my mother has much for which to grieve and much about which to worry.

How do we respond to such sweeping, debilitating vulnerabilities? Vulnerability gives us much to fear, and we respond to it as we do to other fears: we try to suppress and ignore it. A familiar strategy for fleeing from fear and discomfort is to become task-oriented. Rather than focusing on the person for whom a task is being performed, focus on the task itself. That strategy is alluring because it offers the reward of efficiency when many tasks are accomplished and the reward of satisfaction when those tasks are accomplished well. But its greatest reward is distance from fear and discomfort. With that reward comes a danger, however. The person lying in the bed can be depersonalized and objectified. Cheerfulness, encouragement, and familiarity are, of course, gifts to those for whom one is providing care, and they should not be foregone. Yet they are brief and episodic, and their scheduled repetition might only expose their ultimate hollowness. They can be incorporated into a routinized way of making it through a shift or a day, but they cannot dispel the intractable realities of debilitation and dependence. When those realities are pervasive, the only way to cope might be to immerse oneself in the demands of

the job, to disengage from what overwhelming vulnerability does to a person.

There is another strategy for responding to the fear of vulnerability: denial. That is what enabled me to cope. Despite my father's cane, braces, walker, and wheelchair; despite the chair-lift that was installed on the stairs; and despite the handicapped license plates on the car, I did not think of my father as disabled. There were, of course, times when the impact of his condition was too vivid and too concrete to be ignored, but I quickly dismissed and suppressed those unwelcome intrusions. Being disabled or handicapped was something—*had* to be something— that happened to other people. My father's struggles were, for me, an ordinary part of life. Notwithstanding the overwhelming evidence to the contrary, I did not regard him as different, and I did not regard my family as different.

So what does vulnerability mean for those who are vulnerable? The philosopher Alfred North Whitehead once said that human beings have "a three-fold urge: (i) to live, (ii) to live well, and (iii) to live better."[4] Vulnerability means loss to all three: loss of opportunities to live better, loss of abilities to live well, and, at its extreme, loss of living. My father's stroke deprived my father and my mother of opportunities to live better and severely constrained their abilities to live well. Vulnerability can impair living well and can destroy the good life. Ethics, from the time of Plato and Aristotle, has been about living well, about the good life. Shouldn't ethics therefore be concerned about vulnerability, and if so, what does vulnerability mean for morality?

The sad answer to that question, as of now, is "not much." There are three reasons for this, I think. The first is that vulnerability is antithetical to the ethos of individualism that pervades and dominates the moralities of Western societies. The individualistic ideal is to make one's own way in the world, to make one's mark on the world through one's accomplishments, and to be rewarded for those accomplishments by happiness. In pursuit of that ideal, individualism seeks and requires self-sufficiency and insulation from the risks that vulnerability poses. Respect for autonomy is, in large measure, a moral proxy for that individualistic ideal. Vulnerability threatens individualism, however, because it is enveloped in contingency and chance, the elements of life that caught the attention of Greek writers. The tragedy and suffering that vulnerability can bring mean dependence, and dependence means the failure of self-sufficiency.

The sociologist Arthur Frank recognizes this incompatibility when he explains how Inanna's journey to the underworld exemplifies Joseph Campbell's view that heroism is not a matter of overcoming adversity but of enduring suffering. Frank points out that, in Campbell's interpretation of the myth, Inanna's heroism is "heroism as perseverance," and he makes the connection to today: "The notion of fate that pervades Inanna's heroism seems increasingly intolerable to more individualistic notions of the person."[5] Frank explains why:

> Campbell's heroic model is more feminine than masculine, finding its earliest paradigm in the journey of Inanna to the underworld. Inanna undertakes the journey, suffers helplessly, is rescued by helpers from the world she has left, and returns to sort out matters with those who did not contribute to her rescue. She wields no weapons; her strength is her perseverance. This trope of heroism as perseverance is most useful to people who are ill and dying.[6]

Inanna is vulnerable because she suffers "helplessly" and because she depends on the help of others for her rescue. She cannot do it on her own. Campbell's interpretation of the myth makes sense of her suffering and gives it a moral point. That sense and that point are foreign to the ethos of individualism, though, and Frank rightfully worries about how Inanna's struggle with her vulnerability is misrepresented by that ethos:

> I am troubled by what happens when Campbell's notion of the heroic is transformed into self-help prescriptions for

a happy life; reconstructing the myth within a contemporary spiritual narrative loses the heroic. Though Inanna increases her power and her divinity through her journey, she does not enter the underworld to have a personal growth experience. She goes because it is her fate to go. She is called to the underworld as preparation to become the goddess whom she can become only by making that journey and incurring such suffering. The cosmic order requires her becoming and thus her journey. Neither the journey nor its aftermath makes her happy by most human standards. Inanna does increase in wisdom and stature, but this "growth" is neither personal nor linked to pleasure.[7]

Vulnerability means that one is controlled by, rather than in control of, the world. Vulnerability marks the limits of individualism, but the ethos of individualism doggedly refuses to acknowledge those limits and instead construes vulnerability to fit its assumptions and goals.

The second reason that vulnerability doesn't mean much to morality is that vulnerability is missing from moral philosophy, our intellectual endeavour to understand and enhance morality, because moral philosophy ignores the body. Moral theories, at least in the tradition of Western analytic philosophy, are grounded in reason, and the purer that reason can be—the more it can emulate the reason of logic and mathematics—the better it is. A paradigm of this strongly rationalistic approach is Immanuel Kant's classic work, *Groundwork of the Metaphysic of Morals*,[8] which has shaped the course of moral philosophy ever since it appeared in 1785. Kant's challenge in the *Groundwork* is to explain how imperatives—directives that tell us what we *ought* to do—are possible and, in turn, how the supreme principle of morality, which Kant calls the "Categorical Imperative," is possible. Kant's answer is that a categorical imperative can exist only if there is something that is an "end in itself "—that is, is not valuable as a means to something else but has intrinsic, unconditional value. The only thing that has such intrinsic, unconditional value, in Kant's view, is rationality. Kant famously distinguishes nonrational beings, which have "only a relative value as means and are consequently called *things*," from rational beings, which "are called *persons* because their nature already marks them out as ends in themselves—that is, as something which ought not to be used merely as a means—and consequently imposes to that extent a limit on all arbitrary treatment of them (and is an object of reverence)."[9] In this tradition of moral philosophy, rationality gives human beings their unique moral status and their incomparable moral worth.

Human beings are rational, but human beings also have bodies, and because they have bodies, they are vulnerable. In fact, vulnerability is an even more basic feature of our human constitution than rationality because, while all human beings are vulnerable, not all human beings are rational or even possess the potential to become rational. All human beings are born into vulnerability and remain deeply vulnerable for some time, but human beings who are born without certain portions of their brains or with extreme mental impairments never will become rational. Moreover, our universal vulnerability resonates with moral significance. For one thing, it is our very vulnerability that creates the need for morality. The legal philosopher H.L.A. Hart links the fundamental moral and legal prohibitions on killing and inflicting harm to our common vulnerability. That people are "prone to, and normally vulnerable to, bodily attack" is, Hart says, a truism:

> [T]hings might have been, and might one day be, otherwise. There are species of animals whose physical structure (including exoskeletons or a carapace) renders them virtually immune from attack by other members of their species and animals who have no organs enabling them to attack. If men were to lose their vulnerability to each other there would vanish one obvious reason for the most characteristic provision of law and morals: *Thou shalt not kill*.[10]

None of us is invincible; all of us are vulnerable, in similar ways at the beginning of our lives and later in different ways at different times in different circumstances. All of us, therefore, need the protection—and legal enforcement—of morality.

For another thing, we cannot understand the persons we are, and thus how to live well, without recognizing vulnerability as an ineluctable feature of our embodied humanity. In his Paul Carus Lectures, the philosopher Alasdair MacIntyre criticizes himself for making the error of "supposing an ethics independent of biology to be possible,"[11] and he criticizes Western moral philosophy, from Plato through Kant to G.E. Moore in the twentieth century, for ignoring the vulnerabilities inherent in that biology:

> Consider how both physical and mental disability are afflictions of the body and how therefore habits of mind that express an attitude of denial towards the facts of disability and dependence presuppose either a failure or a refusal to acknowledge adequately the bodily dimensions of our existence.[12]

Our vulnerabilities and concomitant dependencies are, as MacIntyre puts it, "so evidently of singular importance that it might seem that no account of the human condition whose authors hoped to achieve credibility could avoid giving them a central place."[13] Yet human vulnerabilities and dependencies have no place, let alone a central place, in philosophical approaches that equate morality with rationality and moral agency with rational agency.

The third reason vulnerability doesn't figure in our understanding of morality is that, like vulnerability, feelings have no place in rationalistic conceptions of moral philosophy and morality. Nevertheless, vulnerability engages our feelings as much as, if not more than, our reason. My father taught me that. During my family's last visit to see my father and mother, I spent a lot of time in my father's room watching him sleep. Sometimes he was sleeping when I arrived and sleeping when I left; I would come back later, and he still would be sleeping. But there were exceptions. On one occasion, shortly after I arrived, my father looked at me and said, "That's a nice shirt." Before our visit, my mother had wanted to put some goldfish in my father's room to give him something to look at, but his nursing home does not allow pets. My wife then had the inspiration of using some colored glass fish we had bought in Nova Scotia instead. The fish are tied to glass balls that float on top of the water, so it looks as if they are swimming. While I was spending time with my father, my wife scattered brightly colored stones on the bottom of a goldfish bowl, added water, and then carefully arranged three fish inside the bowl. She set the bowl on a window ledge where my father could see it. He gazed at it for a while, then said, "That's very neat." What amazed me was that my father had uttered two complete, articulate sentences. Often the sounds he makes as he struggles to speak are garbled and incoherent, or he will get out a few words that begin a sentence but be unable to complete it. I cannot remember the last time I heard a coherent sentence from my father. When he spoke those two sentences, and for a long time afterwards, I had no idea why they suddenly and unexpectedly emerged.

Now I have a suspicion. My suspicion is that it was because they expressed feelings. Rollo May says that although care goes beyond feeling, it begins with feeling: "It is a feeling denoting a relationship of concern, when the other's existence matters to you; a relationship of dedication, taking the ultimate form of being willing to get delight in or, in ultimate terms, to suffer for, the other."[14] I think that in complimenting my shirt my father was telling me that I mattered to him, and that in complimenting the fish bowl he was telling me that he was happy that he mattered to us.[15] And I think he was able to utter those sentences because feeling is more basic than reason. Listen to Rollo May again:

> When William James says, "Feeling is everything," he means not that there is nothing more than feeling, but that everything starts there. Feeling commits one, ties one to the object, and ensures action. But in the decades after James made this

"existentialist" statement, feeling became demoted and was disparaged as merely subjective. Reason or, more accurately, technical reason was the guide to the way issues were to be settled. We said "I feel" as a synonym for "I vaguely believe," when we didn't *know*— little realizing that we cannot know except as we *feel*.[16]

The denial that MacIntyre castigates and the denial that shrouded me is so powerful, and the habit of mind that promulgates denial is so entrenched, that, as May insists, we cannot *know* vulnerability except as we *feel* vulnerability.

We need to feel our vulnerability to affirm our humanity. While we are not invincible, neither are we superhuman. When we recognize the depth and the breadth of our vulnerability, we realize how much we need the help of others to protect us from our weaknesses and our infirmities. How well my father has coped for four decades has depended, in large measure, on my mother. His plight reflects, as MacIntyre observes, a general truth about the human condition: "It is most often to others that we owe our survival, let alone our flourishing, as we encounter bodily illness and injury, inadequate nutrition, mental defect and disturbance, and human aggression and neglect."[17] Vulnerability is a source of our concern for others, but it also is a source of our interest in and reliance on others. Our common vulnerability bonds us and binds us to other people. The demented, helpless individual lying in a bed might still be capable of feeling, but, perhaps more important, that person is capable of making us feel. We can feel compassion for that person's losses and that person's suffering. We also can feel our common humanity—our own fragility and our own dependency. If we do, we truly can care for that person and for ourselves. That is what vulnerability means for us.

Acknowledgements

The first draft of this paper was written for a conference on "Vulnerability in Later Life: Challenges and Possibilities for Supporting Persons 'At Risk,'" the 20th Annual McMaster Summer Institute on Gerontology, organized by the McMaster Centre for Gerontological Studies, Hamilton, Ontario, and held on June 2, 2003. I thank the organizers for the invitation to speak and the participants for their helpful questions and supportive comments. I thank Sylvie Lamer and Kathryn Desai for reading drafts of this paper and for their valuable suggestions. I thank Arthur Frank for his detailed, acute assessments of several versions of this paper, his wealth of knowledge, and his encouragement. And I thank the *Hastings Center Report*'s anonymous referees for their perceptive comments and criticisms.

Notes

1. J.J. Fins, M.D. Bacchetta, and F.F. Miller, "Clinical Pragmatism: A Method of Moral Problem Solving," in *Pragmatic Bioethics*, ed. Glenn McGee (Nashville, Tenn.: Vanderbilt University Press, 1999), 30–44. The précis of the case is taken from 32–39.
2. Ibid., 37–38.
3. R. May, *Love and Will* (New York: Dell Publishing Co., 1969), 14.
4. A.N. Whitehead, *The Function of Reason* (Boston, Mass.: Beacon Press, 1929), 8.
5. A.W. Frank, "Narratives of Spirituality and Religion in End-of-Life Care," in *Narrative Research in Health and Illness*, ed. B. Hurwitz, T. Greenhaigh, and V. Skultans (London, UK: Blackwell Publishing and BMJ Books, 2004), 141.
6. Ibid., 140–41.
7. Ibid., 141.
8. I. Kant, *Groundwork of the Metaphysic of Morals*, tr. H.J. Paton (New York: Harper & Row, 1964).
9. Ibid., 96 (pages 428 and 65 in the edition issued by the Royal Prussian Academy in Berlin and in the second edition, respectively).
10. H.L.A. Hart, *The Concept of Law* (New York: Oxford University Press, 1961), 190 (emphasis in original).
11. A. MacIntyre, *Dependent Rational Animals* (Chicago, Ill.: Open Court, 1999), x.
12. Ibid., 4.
13. Ibid., 1.
14. May, *Love and Will*, at 303.
15. Richard Zaner makes this point about people who are dying: "Some … are haunted by whether or not their lives made any difference, whether they mattered. Others want especially to let us know they care for us, that we who remain alive matter to them, that our lives have been worthy." R.M. Zaner, *Troubled Voices* (Cleveland, Oh.: The Pilgrim Press, 1993), 144.
16. May, *Love and Will*, at 303 (emphasis in original).
17. MacIntyre, *Dependent Rational Animals*, at 1. See also Zaner, *Troubled Voices*, at 145.

Understanding Trust

Carolyn McLeod

Current health care practitioners are in a different situation than their predecessors when it comes to patient trust. One Canadian physician is quoted as saying, "The profession had more respect [in the past]. Your opinion doesn't count as much with patients any more" (*The Globe and Mail*, F4, 23/11/2002). Physicians and other practitioners cannot take the trust of patients in their opinions for granted.[1] Yet trust provides the moral foundation for any healthy patient–practitioner relationship.[2] The problem is serious. Now how do we solve it? Well, part of the solution (and only part of it[3]) is to teach practitioners how to build and maintain patient trust. This step in turn requires a clear understanding of what trust is; otherwise, advice on how to promote it would surely be empty. My intention here is to provide such understanding, along with a rough guide on how practitioners could use it to foster trust in their relationships with patients.

A THEORY OF TRUST[4]

What is it that we trust in other people? What about them makes us willing to trust? A general answer, for which there is some consensus in ethics, is their competence to do what we trust them to do and their motivation for doing it; surely, we would not trust people unless we thought they had the necessary competence and desire to do what we want them to do. However, controversy exists around the question of how we want people we trust to be motivated to act. Following Annette Baier,[5] many ethicists assume that the relevant motivation is goodwill: we want those whom we trust to be motivated by goodwill towards us. But not all philosophers agree, and some fail to give a clear answer to that question.[6] It is important not to be ambiguous in answering it because part of what makes trust unique from other attitudes, such as mere reliance, *is* the kind of motivation we expect from people we trust. I propose that what we expect is not goodwill, but moral integrity. This virtue involves consistently doing what "one takes oneself to have the most moral reason to do."[7] Moreover, we would want them to generally share our understanding of what counts as a good moral reason.

Thus, our attitude about how we want people we trust to be motivated to act targets both their moral integrity and what they stand for. But there is more still: sometimes that attitude also concerns their perception of their relationship with us. Sometimes, for us to be optimistic that other people will be motivated to honour our trust, we have to expect that they perceive their relationship with us similarly to the way that we perceive it.

THE COMPETENCE OF THE ONE TRUSTED

The idea that trust involves optimism about the competence of the other is not controversial; but let me discuss it nonetheless, specifically as it relates to patient trust. For such trust to occur, optimism about the competence of the practitioner is essential. Consider a sample relationship in this domain.

For years, Todd has had the same family physician, Dr. Young. He has always depended on Dr. Young to provide him with good medical advice and to perform medical procedures competently. He has kept her as his family physician for so long partly because Dr. Young gives him a lot of information about potential harms and benefits of different procedures or treatments. It is important to Todd that he be informed as much as possible about his health care so that he can be sure he truly wants what he gets.

Todd clearly relies on the competence of Dr. Young. He is optimistic that she is competent to perform medical procedures and to give Todd sound advice as well as detailed information about his health care options. If such optimism were to fade away, so would Todd's trust.

Trusters such as Todd are often unaware of what people they trust have to do to display their competence, and the former are vulnerable as a result. Todd trusts Dr. Young to give him competent advice, even though Todd probably could not tell good medical advice from bad. Bioethicists emphasize the need for patients to trust their practitioners because of the knowledge gap that normally exists between them.[8] Patients are vulnerable in medical encounters in part because of that gap.[9]

Patients trust not only the technical competence of health care professionals, but also their moral competence. One dimension of moral competence is knowing what is morally required in different situations. And another is acting on what is required: that is, being morally virtuous. The latter overlaps with moral integrity as a feature of trust, which I discuss below. The former—moral understanding—is relevant to trust in the competence of health care practitioners in the following ways. Minimally, patients expect practitioners to understand the moral importance of honouring a commitment to provide them with health care. However, many expect greater moral understanding than that. For example, Todd is representative of a growing segment of Western society that trusts physicians to understand the need to respect patient autonomy (along with related issues such as the responsibility to disclose information to patients). It is not enough that health care practitioners have the necessary technical skills and scientific knowledge to be competent practitioners. Even patients who assume that physicians should be paternalistic trust physicians to understand the moral importance of acting in their best interests.

Thus, patients trust health care practitioners to have some moral understanding, or competence, which is part of their more general optimism about the competence of their practitioners to do what they trust them to do.

THE MOTIVATION OF THE ONE TRUSTED

We want people we trust to have not only the ability to do what we trust them to do, but also the motivation to do it. People can be motivated to do things in many different ways. What is the relevant motivation in trust relations? Baier argues that it can neither be something sleazy (e.g., pure selfishness) nor something that implies total indifference to others' welfare. For example, I might think that a surgeon will perform surgery on me competently not because I believe he has any concern for me or because he has moral integrity, but because I know that he does not want to get sued. The language of trust would be out of place in describing my attitude toward him. I do not trust the surgeon; I merely rely on him. Reliance is an attitude toward another's competence where, as long as that person is motivated to do what he is competent to do, it is irrelevant to us what kind of motivation he has for acting. With trust, this issue is not at all irrelevant.

What we trust in others is not simply kindly feeling towards us, however. We can trust others even without being optimistic that they feel kindly toward us; e.g., we may trust them without expecting them to have specific concern for us. For example, it is conceivable that a patient could trust a nurse to be motivated by a commitment to provide her with good health care without assuming that the nurse has kindly feelings for her. Particularly in trust relations between patients and specialists, such as surgeons, kindly feelings need not be a feature of the relationship.

Even if someone does have kindly feelings toward us, knowing that may not be a good reason to trust that person. Suppose that not only is Todd optimistic that Dr. Young respects his autonomy, Dr. Young is committed to doing so (where that requires that she disclose information to Todd about his health status and his health care options). If Dr. Young were to develop reliable and kindly feelings toward Todd and be motivated because of those feelings to be dishonest with him about his health status, she would be betraying Todd's trust. She would be failing to inform him of any potentially serious health problems not because she thinks it is her moral duty to prevent Todd from experiencing distress (Dr. Young is committed to promoting patient autonomy), but because she has a strong desire not to cause Todd any distress. In that case, Dr. Young would be acting on kindly feelings without doing what Todd trusts her to do. Todd's trust in her therefore could not be grounded in kindly feelings.

Trust is usually incompatible with serious forms of deception unless deception is necessary to shield the trusting person from severe harm. If Todd became clinically depressed and suicidal, it might be compatible with his trust in Dr. Young for Dr. Young to withhold information from him about a serious illness, at least temporarily. But even when it is not necessary to deceive others to protect their welfare, kindly feelings can encourage deception if those feelings are strong enough. What we want, ultimately, from people we trust are not kindly feelings, but *a commitment to doing what is right in the circumstances*. In the scenario above, the right thing for Dr. Young to do, both from her perspective and from Todd's, is to disclose information to Todd in a way that is respectful of his autonomy.

One might think it is a bit overblown to say that what we want from people we trust is for them to "do the right thing." It may be that we just want them to make considered judgments in determining how to best serve our interests, as opposed to having their kindly feelings motivate them in ways that might subvert our interests. We might still trust their goodwill but only if it is informed by their judgment. The idea that goodwill of this sort is a component of trust is compelling; nonetheless, it fails to capture one aspect of trust relations. Consider a situation where someone we trust uses her considered judgment to determine our interests and she acts accordingly, but she ignores her responsibilities to others in the process. For example, what if Dr. Young were good at respecting Todd's autonomy, but she also gave preferential treatment to Todd, even over patients who were suffering more than him and who had arrived at Dr. Young's office first? Many people in Todd's place would be appalled, or at least concerned, and insist that was not what they had trusted the physician to do. Presumably, then, I have misconstrued Todd's interests by implying that Dr. Young could satisfy them simply by respecting Todd's autonomy. Assuming that Todd is a decent guy, his interest could not be to have others suffer for his own sake. But even if he were not at all decent, it would not be in his interests to see his physician treating her patients unfairly; Todd may be disturbed by such treatment if only because it suggests to him that one day Dr. Young might treat *him* unfairly! Either way, what Todd trusts Dr. Young to do *is* the right thing. He trusts her to be motivated by judgments that are not merely considered but are also moral.

In summary, we want those we trust to be motivated by moral integrity. We want them to have an enduring commitment to act in a morally respectful way toward us and we want their actions to accord with that commitment. Having integrity means that your actions are integrated with what you stand for, while having moral integrity means that they are integrated with what you stand for morally speaking. When Dr. Young fails to disclose important information to Todd about his health status, she compromises her own moral integrity, and in doing so, betrays Todd's trust.

What the Trusted One Stands for

Because people can stand for very different things, it cannot only be moral integrity that we expect from people we trust. We care about what they stand for, not just about whether they will act on what they stand for. Todd does not trust Dr. Young simply to act on whatever values Dr. Young accepts as the right values. He expects her to endorse specifically the value of respect for patient autonomy. A further feature of trust, therefore, is an expectation that what the one trusted stands for, morally speaking, is similar enough to what we stand for (as far as we know what that is) that we can count on her to do what we trust her to do.

To trust others, we usually require some sense of what they stand for so that we can know whether they are likely to act in the way that we would expect them to. And what that way is depends on what we perceive to be morally acceptable ways to act. For example, what Todd expects from health care practitioners he trusts is respect for patient autonomy because he believes that is important in health care.

But perhaps it is unrealistic to claim that before patients can trust practitioners, they have to have some idea of what they stand for. Patients often deal with practitioners whom they have never met. How could they assume anything about where their moral commitments lie? But surely they could presume that practitioners will respect the values of their own profession, which, among other things, include benefiting patients and respecting their autonomy. Such a presumption is rebuttable, of course—not *all* health care practitioners embrace those values; however, it is not unreasonable because of how practitioners are taught to behave.

One could add that trust tends to grow or diminish as our knowledge of what others stand for increases. Further, the amount of evidence we need about how similar their values are to our own likely depends on what is at stake for us by trusting them. For example, there is more at stake in trusting a physician to treat us for cancer than in trusting one to give us a flu shot. Presumably, we would want to know more about the values of the physician in the first case than we would in the second before trusting that physician.

The Trusted One's Perception of Our Relationship

A final feature of trust is that we expect people we trust to interpret the nature of our relationship similarly to the way we do. If they conceive of our relationship differently, they may not welcome our trust (just as practitioners may not welcome patients trusting them in certain ways). Adding this feature takes care of cases of unwelcome trust, and it concerns our attitude specifically toward *whether*, as opposed to *how*, people we trust will be motivated to act.

When people do not welcome our trust, they do not object to our optimism about their competence, their moral integrity, or about the fact that we admire what they stand for. Rather, they object to our expectation that they do something for us.[10] For example, practitioners who do not welcome the trust of patients do not wish to do what these patients trust them to do (e.g., make house calls or perform unnecessary procedures).

While some moral commitments demand that we respect the interests of everyone (e.g., our duty not to commit murder), others require only that we behave in a certain way toward people with whom we are in a special kind of relationship. Although I may have a duty to be honest on some level with everyone, I am not morally required, I do not think, to be as honest about my feelings with everyone as I am with people with whom I am intimate. Similarly, I am not morally obligated to be as concerned for the welfare of others as I ought to be for my own family members and close friends. Often what we trust in others, including parents, lovers, and professional people, is that they do something for us that they would not do for just anyone. In other words, we trust them to act on relationship-specific commitments.

Unwelcome trust is a potential problem only in relationships where one expects the other to have what I call *special concern*. When we trust others to have specific concern that they are committed to having toward everyone, unwelcome trust should not be an issue. If we trust them to have special concern—that is, to do only what they are committed to doing in certain kinds of relationships—our trust may be unwanted. It would be unwanted specifically if we expected the trusted person to interpret our relationship differently than the way she does. For example, if a patient trusts a health practitioner to be emotionally attentive in the way that a lover would, but the practitioner does not think of (and does not want to think of) his relationship with the patient as an intimate relationship, the patient's trust would be unwanted. Yet by having such trust in her practitioner, the patient must expect him to think of their relationship as more like an intimate relationship than a patient-practitioner one. Without that expectation, she could not be optimistic that he would be emotionally supportive in the way that he would with a lover.

SUMMARY AND NOTES ON FOSTERING PATIENT TRUST

With that last expectation, we come to a rather complex understanding of trust. It involves optimism about the trusted person's competence and moral integrity, together with two expectations, which concern what that person stands for and her perception of our relationship. This analysis might seem so complex as to be implausible given how pervasive trust is and how easily some of us seem to be able to trust other people. However, it is important to realize that a trusting attitude, and each feature of it, need not be conscious for trust to exist. Because trust *is* so pervasive—we trust people in a myriad of ways every single day—there must be "such a thing as unconscious trust" (Baier 1995, 99).

We are most conscious of what the key elements of trust are when trust is missing; we realize what is important to us in trust relations when we contemplate why we *dis*trust someone. On my account, such reflection should lead to one or more of the following conclusions: that we are pessimistic rather than optimistic about the other's competence or moral integrity;[11] and that we suspect that person does not have certain values in common with us or does not share our perception of our relationship. These seem to be clear avenues toward distrust, and they originate in the theory I have outlined here.

So how can health care practitioners use this theory to try to promote patient trust? The answer is straightforward: they need to make room for each element of trust in their relationships with patients. First, they need to allow for optimism about their own competence and moral integrity by continually displaying each with patients. Of course, they must maintain their competence as health practitioners and also be able to convey to patients that they are competent. The relevant competence includes a kind of moral competence, which practitioners should have to begin with or learn through some training in bioethics. They need to know, for example, how to respect the autonomy of their patients, which is one of the core moral values of all health professions.

Displaying moral integrity with patients requires that practitioners honour their commitments to patients. And since moral integrity involves a general promise to do what is *right*, the commitments they honour cannot be substantially different for patients in similar circumstances. Rightness entails treating like cases alike. Further, if practitioners fail for whatever reason to meet a specific commitment to a patient, they must take some responsibility for the harm or disappointment they have caused.[12] People with integrity take their commitments seriously, which means that they try to remedy situations in which those commitments have been violated.

Second, practitioners must try to encourage the two expectations involved with trust. They could probably promote the expectation of shared values by clearly stating what they value about patient care. For example, they could assure patients that they are committed to promoting their welfare and to respecting their autonomy. And if procedures exist which they would refuse to perform because their conscience prohibits them, they could make those procedures known to patients, thereby setting the boundaries of their trust relationship. At the same time, however, they need to assure patients that they would refer them to practitioners who would consent to the relevant procedures, which is a requirement of most medical associations including the CMA. Exceptions, of course, are cases where the relevant procedures (e.g., prenatal diagnosis for the purposes of sex selection) violate fundamental norms of our society.

To promote the expectation about the nature of their relationship with patients, practitioners could assure patients that they perceive that relationship to be professional. Patients can more easily trust practitioners to honour the sorts of commitments one can reasonably expect them to fulfill (depending on their specific profession) if the practitioners ensure that their relationships with patients remain on a professional level.

Note that caution is necessary in establishing trust when practitioners know or suspect that a patient is in an abusive relationship or has a history of physical or sexual abuse. Survivors of abuse often have problems with trusting, or distrusting, because they have trusted another whom they should have been able to trust, but who betrayed them severely.[13] Rather than perpetuate damage to their trust skills, practitioners should not expect trust from those patients until they give the patients ample evidence that they themselves are trustworthy.[14] Here is an example of what that might mean in practice: in performing a physical examination or procedure, the practitioner could ask the patient frequently if she is all right, rather than simply expect that she will be all right and will not fear being violated again.

Particularly in cases where the ability of patients to trust others has been damaged, the call for practitioners to try to promote patient trust may seem unreasonable. And it may in fact be unreasonable in some cases. But surely that is not always true. And hopefully understanding trust and the different components of it makes it clear what practitioners could do to encourage trust from patients, which is of fundamental importance because of the moral value of trust.

Notes

1. For detailed discussion of the decline in patient trust, see Edmund Pellegrino's "Trust and Distrust in Professional Ethics," *Ethics, Trust, and the Professions*, eds. Pellegrino, Robert Veatch, and John Langan (Washington: Georgetown University Press, 1991), and Onora O'Neill's *Autonomy and*

Trust in Bioethics (Cambridge UK: Cambridge University Press, 2002).

2. Without trust, other morally relevant aspects of these relationships (e.g., beneficence and respect for autonomy) would not exist. See Caroline Whitbeck, "Trust," *The Encyclopedia of Bioethics* (2nd ed. New York: MacMillan, 1995).

3. I do not pretend that the burden of a solution should lie entirely with health care practitioners. Other measures, such as using the media to inform the public of the benefit that many practitioners provide to patients on a daily basis, are also necessary. See O'Neill's *Autonomy and Trust in Bioethics* on using the media to communicate actual information to the public about the work of practitioners.

4. This theory was first published in "Our Attitude Towards the Motivation of Those We Trust," *Southern Journal of Philosophy* 38(3), 2000: 465–479. It reappears in my book, *Self-Trust and Reproductive Autonomy* (Cambridge, Mass: MIT Press, 2002). I wish to thank both *The Southern Journal* and the MIT Press for their permission to reprint parts of these works. The theory I present here is a shortened version of the original.

5. See Baier, "Trust and Anti-Trust," *Ethics* 96 (1986): 231–260.

6. Disagreement comes from Richard Holton, in "Deciding to Trust, Coming to Believe," *Australasian Journal of Philosophy* 72 (March): 63–76. Ambiguity about the relevant motivation with trust exists in Trudy Govier's *Dilemmas of Trust* (Montreal: McGill-Queen's University Press, 1998). She writes that when we trust someone, "we believe in his or her basic integrity; we are willing to rely on

him or her," (91) and that when we trust ourselves, we have a firm belief in our "own good character and good sense" (95), or at least a "positive sense of our own motivation" (99). So do we want the trusted one to act with integrity, with good sense, with any kind of positive motivation, or with any motivation compatible with relying on someone?

7. Cheshire Calhoun, "Standing for Something," *The Journal of Philosophy* 92(5): 249.

8. Edmund Pellegrino, "Trust and Distrust in Professional Ethics"; Richard Zaner, "The Phenomenon of Trust and the Patient-Physician Relationship," in *Ethics, Trust, and the Professions*; and Caroline Whitbeck, "Trust."

9. Another important reason is their illness.

10. See Karen Jones, "Trust as an Affective Attitude," *Ethics* 107:4–25.

11. Jones (ibid.) argues that distrust is an attitude of pessimism rather than optimism about the motivation or competence of others.

12. I discuss in detail this backward-looking element of integrity in the longer versions of this paper. See also Margaret Urban Walker's "Picking Up Pieces: Lives, Stories, and Integrity" (*Moral Understandings: A Feminist Study in Ethics.* New York: Routledge, 1998).

13. See Judith Herman, *Trauma and Recovery* (New York: Basic Books, 1992), especially pp. 51, 52.

14. Diane Lepine, "Ending the Cycle of Violence: Overcoming Guilt in Incest Survivors," *Healing Voices: Feminist Approaches to Therapy with Women,* eds. Toni Ann Laidlaw, Cheryl Malmo, and Associates (San Francisco: Jossey-Bass, 1990).

The Legitimacy of Placebo Treatments in Clinical Practice: Evidence and Ethics

Franklin G. Miller and Luana Colloca

Prior to the era of modern therapeutics, physicians routinely prescribed 'inert' agents or tonics believed to lack any specific pharmacologic potency but presented to patients as real medications (Shapiro and Shapiro 1997). Physicians thereby gratified their patients' desire for prescribed treatment, which provided reassurance and comfort and may have promoted a placebo effect. This practice fell

"The Legitimacy of Placebo Treatments in Clinical Practice: Evidence and Ethics" by Franklin G. Miller and Luana Colloca. *The American Journal of Bioethics* 9(12), 2009 Taylor & Francis. Reprinted by permission of the publisher (Taylor & Francis Group, http://www.informaworld.com).

out of favor as physicians gained access to powerful drugs for curing disease and relieving symptoms and as the law and medical ethics embraced respect for patient autonomy and informed consent (Brody 1982). Yet recent survey data indicate that physicians continue to recommend 'placebo treatments', believed to lack specific efficacy in treating patients but to have the potential to promote a beneficial 'placebo effect' (Hrobjartsson and Norup 2003; Sherman and Hickner 2008; Tilburt et al. 2008). Is this practice ethical?

The resolution of many ethical problems in biomedicine is characterized by dilemmas posed by competing ethical considerations. For the most part, this is not true of the ethical problem of the use of placebo treatments in clinical practice. The major ethical issues relevant to this problem are not inherently unclear or controversial. As in the case of all treatments prescribed by physicians, there should be adequate evidence that they offer patients a favorable benefit-to- risk ratio compared with available alternatives. In addition, these treatments should be prescribed in the context of communication with patients that satisfies the requirement for informed consent. The *application* of these norms to "placebo treatments," however, is uncertain and subject to controversy. In order to make progress in assessing the ethics of placebo treatments in clinical practice, it is necessary to draw attention to two key empirical questions: (1) is there rigorous evidence indicating clinically significant benefit from placebo treatments? and (2) can placebo treatment be effective without deception? To date, the ethical discussion of placebo treatments in clinical practice has not paid sufficient attention to the range of pertinent empirical data and the need for future research relevant to answering these questions.

The concept of a placebo is elusive and confusing (Grunbaum 1986; Miller and Kaptchuk 2008). Therefore, before launching this inquiry, it is salutary to clarify some of the terminology that relates to the use of placebos. What makes an intervention count as a placebo is its lack of specific pharmacological or physiological efficacy for a patient's condition. In other words, there is nothing about the internal or characteristic

properties of the intervention that is capable of producing therapeutic benefit for patients with a particular medical condition (Grunbaum 1986). Traditionally, commentators have distinguished between 'pure' and 'impure' placebos (Brody 1982). Pure placebos consist of 'inert' interventions, such as a sugar pill or saline injection, which are typically presented (deceptively) to the patient as a real medication. These interventions are not strictly speaking inert, but the sugar and the saline have no beneficial (or harmful) biological effects across a wide range of conditions. Impure placebos consist of biologically 'active' treatments, typically (but not necessarily) having specific efficacy for some condition but used as a placebo for another condition. Based on current evidence, a wide range of recommended treatments may qualify as impure placebos: for example, vitamins for various patient complaints, antibiotics for probable viral infections, and various complementary and alternative medicine treatments, such as saw palmetto for urinary symptoms, glucosamine for osteoarthritis of the knee, and acupuncture for types of chronic pain. A major motivation for placebo treatments may be to promote 'the placebo effect'—therapeutic benefit produced by the context of the clinical encounter, including the ritual of treatment, rather than by the efficacy of an interventional agent.

It is important to recognize that the placebo effect does not depend on the administration of a placebo intervention, whether a purely inert or impure placebo treatment (Miller and Kaptchuk 2008). The context of the clinical encounter plays a crucial role in triggering a placebo effect. All medical treatments are administered within a context that surrounds the clinical encounter (Di Blasi et al. 2001; Benedetti 2002), which is made up of clinicians' words, attitudes, and behavior, as well as the appearance and method of administrating treatment interventions. The power of context in facilitating cognitive and emotional modulation of a therapeutic response definitively emerges from experiments demonstrating different therapeutic outcomes after an open or hidden administration of the same treatment (Colloca et al. 2004). This experimental paradigm is noteworthy because it permits isolating a placebo effect even though no placebo has been given. Comparing the responses of patients in open versus hidden administration of treatment obviates the potential to mistakenly attribute the placebo response to the inertness of a placebo. We discuss the open/hidden paradigm in greater detail below.

PLACEBOS IN CONTEMPORARY CLINICAL PRACTICE

Two recent surveys of physicians illuminate the practice of physicians with respect to placebo treatments. Hrobjartsson and Norup (2003) surveyed a randomly selected sample of Danish physicians concerning their use of placebo treatments defined as "an intervention not considered to have any 'specific effect' on the condition treated, but with a possible 'unspecific' effect" (155). With a response rate of 65%, the survey included data on 182 general practitioners, 185 hospital-based physicians, and 136 private specialists. Of the general practitioners, 86% reported using placebo interventions during the past year (48% doing so 10 or more times); 54% of the hospital-based physicians and 41% of the private specialists reported placebo use during the past year (with 10% of both groups indicating using placebo interventions more than 10 times). These physicians most frequently prescribed "impure" placebos. During the past year antibiotics were prescribed as a placebo intervention by 70% of general practitioners, 33% of hospital-based physicians, and 18% of private specialists. The respective proportions of reported placebo use were 59%, 24%, and 13% for physiotherapy; 45%, 24%, and 10% for sedatives; and 48%, 10%, and 9% for B vitamins. Pure placebos, such as saline injections, were very rarely employed. Interestingly, the most frequent reported reason for placebo interventions was to "follow the wish of the patient and avoid conflict" (159). However, substantial proportions of the physicians indicated that they were motivated to "take advantage of an effect of placebo" (159), (48% of the general practitioners, 22% of hospital-based physicians, and 32% of private special-

ists). Surveyed physicians were mixed in their attitudes about the ethics of placebo treatments: 46% regarded them as ethically acceptable and 40% as unethical (14% reported that they did not know or did not answer the question).

Tilburt and colleagues (2008) surveyed a random sample of 1200 United States internists and rheumatologists, with a response rate of 57% (334 internists and 345 rheumatologists). The physicians were asked to indicate which of several placebo treatments they had used in the past year, defined as "a treatment whose benefits derive from positive patient expectations and not from the physiologic mechanism of the treatment itself" (1–2). Of these physicians, 55% reported having recommended at least one of a list of interventions as a placebo treatment during the past year: 41% recommended use of over-the-counter analgesics, 38% vitamins, 13% sedatives, and 13% antibiotics. Only 5% reported using pure placebos, such as sugar pills and saline injections. There was no significant difference between the two medical specialties in the propensity to recommend placebo treatments. When asked about their frequency of recommending a therapy "primarily to enhance patient expectation" (3), 46% reported doing so at least two to three times per month. Of those physicians who reported recommending one or more placebo treatments in the past year, 68% described this recommendation to their patients as "a medicine not typically used for your condition but may benefit you" (3).

On the whole, it appears from these two surveys (and comparable smaller surveys) that use of placebo treatments is common among contemporary physicians, typically taking the form of "impure" placebos (Nitzan and Lichtenberg 2004; Sherman and Hickner 2008). Physicians generally report positive attitudes about using treatments for the purpose of promoting a placebo effect in patients. Disclosure to patients about the nature of placebo treatments seems less than transparent. A distinctive limitation of the published physician surveys is that they provide no data on the specific medical conditions or patient complaints for which physicians recommend placebo treatments. Without such data, risk-benefit assessment of current practice relating to placebo treatments is speculative.

ETHICAL CONCERNS

The use of placebo treatments in clinical practice raises a variety of ethical concerns. We review these ethical issues briefly to set the stage for focusing on key empirical questions that are important to assessing the ethics of recommending treatments for the primary purpose of promoting placebo effects. First, the use of placebo treatments has been criticized as unprofessional practice (Hrobjartsson 2008). According to standards of evidence-based medicine, superiority to placebo is considered to be the minimal requirement for validating therapies, making it suspect for physicians to recommend or administer treatments for the sole purpose of promoting a placebo effect. This perspective however, is debatable. If the placebo effect is a real phenomenon and there is consistent evidence from randomized controlled trials that placebo treatments produce significantly improved outcomes, then there may be a legitimate place within contemporary medicine for using interventions to promote the placebo effect (Miller et al. 2004). The legitimacy of placebo treatments, thus rests, at least in part, on an empirical question relating to evidence of clinically significant benefit—a question examined below.

However, prescribing placebos merely to please patients or comply with patient demands for treatment may be convenient but clearly seems incompatible with medical professionalism. For different reasons, use of antibiotics as placebo treatments poses a genuine ethical concern relating to professional practice. Owing to side effects from antibiotics, they lack a favorable risk-benefit ratio, especially given the absence of solid evidence of placebo efficacy in treatment of viral conditions. Moreover, the societal risk of promoting drug-resistant bacteria makes this type of intervention a poor candidate for placebogenic treatment.

A second, more subtle, ethical problem relating to placebo treatments is the contribution of this practice to medicalization of common somatic complaints that bring many patients to visit doctors in the absence of detectable disease (Hadler 2008). To respond by prescribing a placebo treatment reinforces the belief that 'there is a pill for every ill'. Nevertheless, the mission of medicine to relieve suffering supports the use of placebo treatments, provided that they are known to be harmless or low risk and such use is backed by solid evidence of efficacy in producing symptomatic relief.

Third, the strongest ethical concern about placebo treatments is the use of deception that they involve (Brody 1982; Wendler and Miller 2004; Miller et al. 2005). Lying is generally considered to be morally wrong, although most ethicists recognize exceptional circumstances: for example, to prevent harm to innocent persons. Moreover, in everyday life people often make deceptive statements to be kind or avoid hurting others' feelings. Can paternalistic deception be justified in medicine for the purpose of promoting a therapeutically beneficial placebo effect? In addition to violating a general moral rule prohibiting lying, deception in medicine conflicts with the contemporary understanding of the ethics of the doctor-patient relationship. Despite beneficent intent, deliberate misinformation or lack of transparency in describing placebo treatments to patients violate the principle of respect for patient autonomy and contravene the legal and ethical requirement to obtain informed consent. Physicians are obligated to provide truthful disclosure to patients about the treatment being recommended and the rationale for its selection. Patients who discover that they have been administered placebo treatments in a deceptive way are apt to feel duped, thus undermining the climate of trust that is vital to medical practice (Bok 1974).

Nevertheless, it has been argued by some commentators that the use of deception can be justified when necessary to optimally promote therapeutic benefit via the placebo effect (Boozang 2002; Kolber 2007). In view of commitments to respect patient autonomy and informed consent, however, the legitimacy of deceptive placebo treatment faces a heavy burden of proof. Certainly, this burden of proof will not be met if effective, non-deceptive ways of promoting the placebo effect can be employed. On the other hand, even if placebo treatments can be presented transparently to patients, honest disclosure may undermine placebo efficacy (Cheyne 2005). Here we face at least an apparent practical conundrum, suggesting that we may be forced to choose between truthful disclosure and taking advantage of the benefits that flow from deceptively recommended treatments aimed at promoting the placebo effect. Deception would make placebo treatments unethical; but placebo treatments without deception may not work. Is it likely that patients will obtain therapeutic benefit if they know that a treatment being prescribed lacks any inherent properties that can be effective in treating their condition and that the purpose of the treatment is to promote a placebo effect? Whether this conundrum is real or merely apparent rests on important empirical issues that we explore in the following discussion.

IS THE RITUAL OF TREATMENT NECESSARY TO OPTIMALLY PROMOTE THE PLACEBO EFFECT?

Many studies indicate that the ritual of treatment and associated patient expectations for therapeutic benefit can play a salient role in human healing. For example, it has long been known that placebo injections are more powerful than placebo pills (de Craen et al. 2000; Moerman and Jonas 2000); placebos taken four times a day are more powerful than placebos taken two times a day (de Craen et al. 1999); red and yellow tablets make better stimulants, while blue or green tablets make better tranquilizers (de Craen et al. 1996); and a validated sham acupuncture procedure had greater effects than placebo pill on self reported pain and severity of symptoms in patients with persistent arm pain (Kaptchuk et al. 2006).

Nevertheless, some commentators have argued that there is no need to resort to placebo treatments to tap the placebo effect in clinical practice (Brody 1982; Hrobjartsson 2008). Given

that the placebo effect involves therapeutic benefit that derives from the context of the clinical encounter, physicians have other potentially powerful tools at their disposal—namely, use of the clinician-patient relationship to produce positive outcomes, by means of interventions such as supportive and empathic communication with patients. Accordingly, the placebo effect can be promoted within the context of the clinical encounter without generating the ethical problems associated with the use of placebo treatments. Obviously, physicians should use their relationship with patients to promote healing, and a variety of evidence supports the therapeutic efficacy of the interpersonal dimension of the clinical encounter (Di Blasi et al. 2001; Benedetti 2002). The question remains, however, whether the use of some discrete treatment intervention—that is, the ritual of treatment—is necessary to optimally promote the placebo effect.

The potency of a treatment ritual in producing a placebo response is most clearly demonstrated in experiments comparing open versus hidden administration of analgesic medication (Colloca et al. 2004). In the open administration, patients hospitalized after surgery received an injection of analgesic drugs administered by a physician and were told that this injection contained a powerful painkiller, which should produce pain relief in a few minutes. They required a much lower dose of medication to reduce pain by 50% than those who received analgesic medication from a preprogrammed infusion machine without being told when they would be given the medication. With respect to relief of anxiety, a comparable experiment demonstrated a substantial effect of open injection of diazepam; whereas, a hidden infusion of the drug produced no symptomatic relief, suggesting that the diazepam worked entirely by means of a placebo effect. These two ways of delivering the same dose of medication with varying effects differ entirely in the patient's awareness of the treatment ritual common to clinical practice in the open administration, and its absence in the hidden administration. In a review of experiments comparing open and hidden treatment, Colloca and colleagues (2004) concluded, "although many factors and variables may contribute to the differences between the outcomes of covert and overt treatments, certainly the awareness of the treatment, the presence of the therapist, and the expectation of the outcome are likely to be very important. Because all these factors are strongly influenced by the doctor-patient interaction, the patients' knowledge about a therapy seems to be fundamental to the production of optimum therapeutic effects" (682).

The relative placebogenic power of clinician-patient interaction in ameliorating symptoms with and without a treatment ritual has not been evaluated systematically. It is reasonable to hypothesize, however, that just as open administration of analgesic drugs is more powerful than hidden administration in reducing pain, supportive clinician–patient interaction plus a treatment ritual should prove more powerful in relieving symptoms than comparable clinician–patient interaction alone. Nevertheless, there is one study in the literature that challenges this hypothesis. Thomas (1987), a British general practitioner, reported the results of an experiment in his practice involving 200 patients who visited with complaints for which no definite diagnosis could be made. He randomized them into four groups, consisting of those who received a "positive consultation" with or without treatment or a "negative consultation" with or without treatment; "In the positive consultation the patient was given a firm diagnosis and told confidently that he would be better in a few days" (1200). The negative consultation expressed uncertainty about the diagnosis and lacked assurance of benefit. The 'treatment' consisted of a prescription for pills of thiamine hydrochloride, considered a placebo. Patients were asked to complete a mailed questionnaire on how they fared 2 weeks after the consultation. Thomas found that 64% of the patients receiving a positive consultation reported that they got better after 2 weeks, compared with 39% of those who received a negative consultation (p < 0.001). There was no difference between the treated and untreated groups. Additional clinical research is needed to address this important issue.

CAN PLACEBO TREATMENTS PRODUCE CLINICALLY SIGNIFICANT BENEFIT?

Within the context of evidence-based medicine, placebo treatments can be endorsed as a legitimate option only if their efficacy is supported by scientifically sound evidence. But isn't it obvious that the response to placebos is real and powerful, as demonstrated by the outcomes of patients administered masked placebo interventions in thousands of randomized controlled trials? For many medical conditions, especially those with subjective outcomes, trial participants exhibit high rates of response to placebo, typically defined as a specified magnitude of reduction in symptoms. For example, response to drug or placebo in trials of antidepressants is defined as a 50% reduction from baseline in target symptoms as measured on a standard symptom rating scale. In the aggregate, 30% of patients with major depression respond to placebo (Walsh et al. 2002); as do 30% of migraine patients (Bendsten et al. 2003). Placebo response rates are higher in irritable bowel syndrome (43%) (Dorn et al. 2007).

From the time of Henry Beecher's classic 1955 article on the power of the placebo to the present, the placebo response has been commonly regarded as a potent therapeutic intervention, based on response rates in placebo controlled trials. However, drawing such an inference from randomized trials comparing medications or invasive interventions with placebo controls commits the logical fallacy of *post hoc ergo propter hoc* (Miller and Rosenstein 2006). Observed improvement in outcomes following administration of placebo doesn't mean that the placebo intervention caused the response. The apparent placebo response may, in fact, result from symptom fluctuation characteristic of the natural history of the disorder under investigation, including spontaneous remission, or from regression to the mean. In general, false positive errors about treatment efficacy are commonly made in medical decision-making and clinical research, by both the physician who diagnoses a patient's symptoms and patients who report symptom severity. The apparent placebo response in clinical trials also may be due to unidentified co-interventions, producing parallel effects on the observed benefit, and to the 'Hawthorne effect' that refers to the benefits arising from the fact of being under study (Colloca et al. 2008).

Just as placebos are used as controls to determine whether drugs are effective in producing clinical benefit, so determining the efficacy of placebo treatments requires comparison with a suitable control intervention. It is impossible to administer a masked intervention as a control for measuring placebo efficacy. The best possible control group consists of patients with the disorder under investigation who are randomized to receive no study treatment during the trial.

Skepticism about the efficacy of placebo interventions was produced by a landmark meta-analysis of 114 randomized controlled trials (RCTs), encompassing 8,525 participants, which included placebo and no-treatment groups in a wide range of medical conditions (Hrobjartsson and Gotzsche 2001). No effect of placebo was detected on objective outcomes. In the aggregate, there was a small, statistically significant effect of placebo on continuous, subjective outcomes—standardized mean difference of -0.36, and -0.27 for relief of pain. The authors of the meta-analysis concluded that there was no evidence of clinically significant benefit from receiving placebo interventions. Indeed, they pointed out that the modest effect of placebo on subjective outcomes may have been due to response bias, as participants in the no-treatment groups knew that they were not receiving either the study treatment or masked placebo. Based on the results of this meta-analysis, and similar results from a second meta-analysis by the same authors encompassing a larger sample of trials (Hrobjartsson and Gotzsche 2004), there appears to be no solid systematic evidence from clinical trials that placebo treatments produce clinically significant benefit.

In contrast to these meta-analytic results, numerous laboratory experiments have demonstrated consistent evidence of robust (though typically short-term) placebo effects (Benedetti 2008). These studies, designed to evaluate the placebo effect, have been able to minimize many of the methodological problems in assessing placebo efficacy encountered in the clinical trial context and have provided important and reliable evidence about the mechanisms of the placebo effect, especially in the relief of pain (Colloca and Benedetti 2005). In these experiments, placebo interventions are usually presented to human subjects deceptively as effective analgesic procedures, and responses are compared with either other subjects who do not receive placebo or with an intra-subject baseline condition. Although these experiments demonstrate that the placebo response is a real phenomenon, associated with a variety of neurobiological mechanisms across medical conditions (Benedetti 2008), they do not permit the inference that placebo treatments can produce clinically significant benefit when used in routine medical practice. Most of the placebo mechanism experiments have involved healthy volunteers, and they have measured placebo analgesia in response to pain stimuli for very short durations in the laboratory.

The placebo effect is a real neurobiological phenomenon, but can it be harnessed to promote meaningful therapeutic benefit in clinical practice by means of administering placebo treatments? Recently, a series of acupuncture trials conducted in Germany suggest solid evidence of clinically significant benefit from interventions that appear to work by virtue of the placebo effect (Haake et al. 2007; Brinkhaus et al. 2006; Linde et al. 2005; Melchart et al. 2005). This series of 3-arm trials compared acupuncture according to traditional Chinese medicine, sham acupuncture (superficial needling at non-acupuncture points) and either no-treatment (wait list) groups or those receiving usual clinical care. Conditions studied included migraine (Brinkhaus et al. 2006), tension headaches (Linde et al. 2005), chronic low back pain (Haake et al. 2007), and osteoarthritis of the knee (Melchart et al. 2005). Generally, across the various trials, there was no difference between verum and sham acupuncture, but those in both of these groups experienced substantially greater symptom improvement than no-treatment and usual care control groups. For example, in a trial of patients with chronic low back pain receiving

10 30-minute acupuncture sessions over 5 weeks (N = 1162), the response rate after 6 months was 48% in verum acupuncture and 44% in sham acupuncture, as compared with 27% in the usual care group, which received a protocol consisting of physiotherapy plus as-needed pain medication (Haake et al. 2007). Comparable results were obtained in a recent United States trial of 638 patients with chronic low back pain randomized to individualized acupuncture, standardized acupuncture, a sham acupuncture intervention without skin penetration (10 treatment sessions over 7 weeks), and usual care—after 8 weeks, 60% of the subjects reported clinically meaningful improvement on a dysfunction scale in the real and sham acupuncture groups, as compared with 39% in the usual care group (Cherkin et al. 2009).

These trials consistently demonstrated that traditional acupuncture lacks specific efficacy for the conditions investigated: that is, there is nothing specific to the needling characteristic of traditional acupuncture that contributes to therapeutic benefit. Do the trial results mean that acupuncture works by virtue of the placebo effect? This is a reasonable inference. Nevertheless, it is possible that the repetitive physical stimulus common to real and sham acupuncture was responsible for observed analgesic effects by means of some physiological mechanism (Haake et al. 2007; Cherkin et al. 2009; Liu 2009). More research will be needed to clarify the placebo response to acupuncture, but these trials at least suggest that this type of invasive but safe intervention, characterized by an elaborate treatment ritual and frequent clinician-patient interaction, may be a potent placebo treatment (Witt et al. 2005).

A recent clinical experiment involving acupuncture is noteworthy in attempting to identify components of the placebo effect and their impact on therapeutic outcomes (Kaptchuk et al. 2008). Patients with irritable bowel syndrome were randomized to two placebo acupuncture interventions that varied in the intensity and quality of communicative interaction between practitioner and patient; and both groups were compared with a waiting list group without the sham acupuncture. All patients received sham acu-

puncture during a run-in phase of a randomized trial comparing verum and sham acupuncture. Different from the German trials, this study used a validated sham acupuncture intervention consisting of a device with a retractable needle that does not penetrate the skin but retracts into the handle, creating the illusion of needling. Patients received sham acupuncture twice a week for three weeks. In the "limited" arm, communication between practitioner and patient was "business-like" and reduced to a minimum. Patients in the "augmented" arm had a 45-minute conversation relating to their condition with the practitioner at the initial visit (compared with 5 minutes in the limited arm), which was structured to be supportive and empathic and to promote positive expectations from acupuncture therapy. Patients in the augmented arm had superior outcomes of symptom relief and quality of life to those in the limited arm, which in turn had better outcomes than those in the waiting list control arm. For example, at 3 weeks 62% of the patients in the augmented group reported adequate symptom relief, as compared with 44% in the limited group and 28% in the waiting list, a difference that was sustained for the 3-week follow up.

This experiment suggests that the simulation of treatment, as reflected in the sham acupuncture intervention administered in the limited arm, by itself contributes to therapeutic benefit. When enhanced by supportive communication, the ritual of treatment produces a dramatic placebo response over a 3-week period and continued in the 3-week follow-up in a difficult-to-treat patient population.

The upshot of research to date is that we lack systematic and definitive evidence of clinically significant benefit from placebo treatments. Accordingly, more clinically relevant research is needed before placebo treatments can be recommended as evidence-based therapy, with the possible exception of acupuncture.

Our review of evidence for clinically significant benefit from placebo interventions has been based on the premise that solid evidence of benefit is an ethical requirement before placebo treatments can be legitimately recommended by physicians. Although this presumption reflects the reigning paradigm of evidence-based medicine, it might be argued that a more 'pragmatic' standard is appropriate for clinical practice. Physicians often face patients with persisting somatic complaints that are not responsive to standard medical interventions. What is wrong with recommending 'placebo treatments' known to have no risk of harm with the intent of promoting a positive placebo response, even if there is no clinical trials evidence supporting this practice? Setting aside concerns about deception, it is difficult to see any strong ethical objection. However, it clearly is preferable to base treatment recommendation on evidence of benefit. Systematic data on the conditions under which physicians actually recommend such placebo treatments, which are currently lacking, would help in clarifying the competing ethical considerations.

DO EFFECTIVE PLACEBO TREATMENTS REQUIRE DECEPTION?

A second key empirical question relating to the ethics of placebo treatments is whether their effective use requires deception of patients about the nature of the placebo intervention. Ethically problematic deception can be avoided in placebo-controlled trials, as participants are informed that they will either receive the study treatment or a placebo control designed to appear indistinguishable. Masked placebo is not an option for the administration of placebo treatments in routine clinical practice, though occasionally clinicians may employ N of 1 trials with patients alternating between active treatment and placebo under single or double-blind conditions. Moreover, the double-blind administration of placebo creates an element of uncertainty in patients, which may itself reduce the expectation of benefit from trial participation and thus diminish the prospect for a genuine placebo response (Miller and Rosenstein 2006).

Two studies shed light on the interaction between deception and therapeutic outcomes. In a study by Pollo and colleagues (2001), thoracotomized patients were treated with buprenorphine on request for 3 consecutive days, together with a basal intravenous infusion of saline solution

(Pollo et al. 2001). They were assigned to three different verbal disclosures: the first group was told nothing about any analgesic effect (natural history); the second group was told that the basal infusion was either a powerful painkiller or a placebo (classic double-blind administration), and the third group was told that the basal infusion was a potent painkiller (deceptive administration). The placebo effect of the saline basal infusion was measured by recording the doses of buprenorphine requested over the 3-day treatment. It was found that buprenorphine requests decreased in the double-blind group by 20.8% compared with natural history, and the reduction in the deceptive administration group was even greater, reaching 33.8%. These results indicated that seemingly small differences in the verbal disclosures ('It can be either placebo or painkiller. Thus we are not certain that the pain will subside' versus 'It is a painkiller. Thus pain will subside soon) produce different placebo analgesic responses, which in turn trigger a substantial change of behavior leading to a significant reduction of opioid intake. Although outside the clinical setting, Kirsch and Weixel (1988) showed that different verbal suggestions produce different outcomes. In one group, they administered regular coffee and decaffeinated coffee according to the usual double-blind design, and the subjects received the information that either the active or decaffeinated substance was being administered. In the second group decaffeinated coffee was deceptively presented as real coffee. The authors found that the placebo responses were higher following the deceptive administration than the double-blind paradigm.

These studies demonstrate that deception might not be necessary to promote a placebo response, although uncertainty relating to administration of placebo reduces placebo responses. However, they do not indicate whether placebo treatments can be administered effectively in clinical practice with honest disclosure about the intervention.

One older study in the literature provides tantalizing clues about the potential for placebo treatments to be effective in the clinical setting without deception. Park and Covi (1965) administered "open" placebo to 14 "neurotic" patients (suffering from a range of anxiety symptoms). The subjects were told that they were being given "sugar pills ... with no medication at all" (337). And the investigators communicated a positive expectation of benefit in symptom relief. All subjects reported substantial improvement in symptoms after one week of taking open placebo pills. Such a study has obvious methodological limitations in demonstrating the efficacy of placebo treatments without deception. In addition to a very small number of subjects, there was no control group. Therefore, observed responses may have been due to natural history or regression to the mean. Additionally, patients were offered pharmacologic treatment after one week of placebo, and this expectation of eventual drug therapy may have contributed to the positive response, rather than the expectation of benefit from the placebo itself. A larger and more rigorously designed clinical trial is necessary to determine whether open, inert placebo treatment can produce clinically significant benefit.

It is also noteworthy that although the aim of this study was to administer placebo with an honest disclosure, six of the 14 subjects reported that they believed that the placebo pills contained real medication. In itself, this is not evidence of deception, as the investigators did not intend to produce false beliefs in the subjects about the study intervention. Yet perhaps it still should give us some ethical pause if the efficacy of placebo treatments depends, to some extent, on patients' false beliefs.

A recent experiment by Sandler and Bodfish (2008) provides somewhat more persuasive evidence of clinically significant benefit from placebo interventions without deception. Twenty-six children age 7–15 years with attention deficit hyperactivity disorder on a stable regimen of stimulant therapy were randomized to two patterns of medication treatment and open placebo: 1) 100% of regular medication dose for 1 week, 50% medication dose for 1 week, and 50% dose plus placebo for 1 week, and 2) 100% medication dose for 1 week, 50% dose plus placebo for 1 week, and 50% medication dose. The placebo was described to both parents and children as a "dose extender" consisting of a pill with no medication in it. There was a trend for parents to perceive a worsening

of symptoms in their children when moved from the 100% dose to the 50% dose (p = 0.06), and there was no significant difference in their rating of symptom severity between the 100% dose and 50% dose plus placebo. Using the "clinical global improvement scale" clinicians judged that the children had significantly higher global improvement when receiving the 50% dose plus placebo as compared with the 50% dose alone. A real placebo effect from the use of an open "dose extender" placebo could not be conclusively demonstrated, as neither the parents nor the clinician raters were blind to the study conditions. Although the intent of the investigators was to administer placebo without any deception, the description of the placebo as a "dose extender" raises the question of whether the children or parents may have formed false beliefs or otherwise been misled about the nature of the placebo, despite being told that it contained no medication. A report of qualitative interviews with the parents and children suggest that they were not misled about the purpose or contents of the placebo, but this was not assessed systematically (Sandler and Bodfish 2008; Sandler et al. 2008).

Taken together, these experiments suggest the possibility of clinically significant benefit from placebo without deception, though questions remain about efficacy and the absence of false beliefs about open placebo. In any case, there seems to be no impossibility in principle of honest disclosure about placebo treatments. Consider, for example, the case of a physician who recommends treatment with acupuncture for a patient with chronic low back pain who has not been helped by standard medical therapy. Aware of the results of the German and United States acupuncture trials, this physician thinks that acupuncture may work as a placebogenic treatment. Can the recommendation be made without deception? The physician might provide the following disclosure to the patient:

> I recommend that you try acupuncture. Several large clinical trials have shown that traditional acupuncture is not better than a fake acupuncture treatment, but that both of these produce considerably greater symptom improvement in

patients with your condition as compared with those patients who receive no treatment or conventional medical therapy. We don't know why acupuncture works. The specific type of needling doesn't make any difference. It is likely that acupuncture works by a psychological mechanism that promotes self-healing, known as the placebo effect.

On its face, this disclosure appears honest. A patient who received this disclosure and subsequently got better after undergoing acupuncture might nonetheless develop a false belief about why it worked. This does not mean that the patient has been deceived by his physician. Whether we should have any ethical qualms about such false beliefs is a subtle, perhaps elusive, question.

CONCLUSIONS

There are two ethical requirements for the use of placebo treatments in clinical practice. First, there must be scientific evidence from well-designed randomized controlled trials in clinical settings demonstrating clinically significant benefit from a given placebo treatment as compared with a no treatment or usual care control group. Second, the disclosure to patients regarding the placebo treatment must be honest and transparent. Based on currently available evidence it is premature to judge whether placebo treatments are ethically justifiable, with the possible exception of acupuncture to relieve pain from various conditions. Before placebo treatments can legitimately become a routine part of physicians' therapeutic armamentarium, we need more clinically relevant research on the benefits resulting from placebo treatments and the possibility of recommending them without deception.

Acknowledgements

The opinions expressed are those of the author and do not necessarily reflect the position or policy of the National Institutes of Health, the Public Health Service, or the Department of Health and Human Services. Address correspondence to Franklin G. Miller, Department of Bioethics Clinical Center, National Institutes of Health, Building 10, Room 1C118, Bethesda, MD 20892–1156. E-mail: fmiller@nih.gov

---

References

Beecher, H. K. 1955. The powerful placebo. *Journal of the American Medical Association* 159: 1602–1606.

Bendsten, L, P. Mattson, J. A. Zwart, and R. G. Lipton. 2003. Placebo response in clinical randomized trials of analgesics in migraine. *Cephalalgia* 23: 487–490.

Benedetti, F. 2002.How the   doctor's words affect the patient's brain. *Evaluation & the Health Professions* 25: 369–386.

Benedetti, F. 2008. Mechanisms of placebo and placebo-related effects across diseases and treatments. *Annual Review of Pharmacology and Toxicology* 48: 33–60.

Bok, S. 1974. The ethics of giving placebos. *Scientific American* 231(5): 17–23.

Boozang, K. M. 2002. The therapeutic placebo: The case for patient deception. *Florida Law Review* 54: 687–746.

Brinkhaus, B., C. M. Witt, S. Jena, K. Linde, A. Streng, et al. 2006. Acupuncture in patients with chronic low back pain: A randomized controlled trial. *Archives of Internal Medicine* 166: 450–457.

Brody, H. 1982. The lie that heals: The ethics of giving placebos. *Annals of Internal Medicine* 97: 112–118.

Cherkin, D. C., K. J. Sherman, A. L. Avins, J. H. Erro, et al. 2009. A randomized trial comparing acupuncture, simulated acupuncture, and usual care for chronic low back pain. *Archives of Internal Medicine* 169: 858–866.

Cheyne, C. 2005. Exploiting placebo effects for therapeutic benefit. Health Care Analysis 13: 177–188.

Colloca, L., and F. Benedetti. 2005. Placebos and painkillers: Is mind as real as matter? *Nature Reviews Neuroscience* 6: 545–552.

Colloca, L., F. Benedetti, and C. A. Porro. 2008. Experimental designs and brainmapping approaches for studying the placebo analgesic effect. *European Journal of Applied Physiology* 102(4): 371–380.

Colloca, L., L. Lopiano, M. Lanotte, and F. Benedetti. 2004. Overt versus covert treatment for pain, anxiety, and Parkinson's disease. *Lancet Neurology* 3: 679–684.

de Craen, A. J., T. J. Kaptchuk, J. G. Tijssen, and J. Kleijnen. 1999. Placebos and placebo effects in medicine: Historical overview. *Journal of the Royal Society of Medicine* 92: 511–515.

de Craen, A. J., P. J. Roos, A. Leonard de Vries, and J. Kleijnen. 1996. Effect of colour of drugs: Systematic review of perceived effect of drugs and of their effectiveness. *British Medical Journal* 313: 1624–1626.

de Craen, A. J., J.G. Tijssen, J. de Gans, and J. Kleijnen. 2000. Placebo effect in the acute treatment of migraine: Subcutaneous placebos are better than oral placebos. *Journal of Neurology* 247: 183–188.

Di Blasi, Z., E. Harkness, E. Ernst, A. Georgiou, and J. Kleijnen. 2001. Influence of context effects on health outcomes: A systematic review. *Lancet* 357: 757–762.

Dorn, S. D., T. J. Kaptchuk, J. B. Park, et al. 2007. A meta-analysis of the placebo response in complementary and alternative medicine trials of irritable bowel syndrome. *Neurogastroenterology & Motility* 19: 630–637.

Grunbaum, A. 1986. The placebo concept in medicine and psychiatry. *Psychological Medicine* 16: 19–38.

Haake, M., H. H. Muller, C. Schade-Brittinger, H. D. Basler, H. Schafer, et al. 2007. German Acupuncture Trials (GERAC) for chronic low back pain: Randomized, multicenter, blinded, parallel-group trial with 3 groups. *Archives of Internal Medicine* 167: 1892–1898.

Hadler, N. M. 2008. *Worried Sick: A Prescription for Health in an Overtreated America*. Chapel Hill, NC: University of North Carolina Press.

Hrobjartsson, A. 2008. Clinical placebo interventions are unethical, unnecessary, and unprofessional. *Journal of Clinical Ethics* 19: 66–69.

Hrobjartsson, A., and P. C. Gotzsche. 2001. Is the placebo powerless? An analysis of clinical trials comparing placebo with no treatment. *New England Journal of Medicine* 344: 1594–1602.

Hrobjartsson, A., and P. C. Gotzsche. 2004. Is the placebo powerless? Update of a systematic review with 52 new randomized trials comparing placebo with no treatment. *Journal of Internal Medicine* 256: 91–100.

Hrobjartsson, A., and M. Norup. 2003. The use of placebo interventions in medical practice—a national questionnaire survey of Danish clinicians. *Evaluation & the Health Professions* 26: 153–165.

Kaptchuk, T. J., J. M. Kelley, L. A. Conboy, et al. 2008. Components of placebo effect: Randomised controlled trial in patientswith irritable bowel syndrome. *British Medical Journal* 336: 999–1003.

Kaptchuk, T. J., W. B. Stason, R. B. Davis, A. R. Legedza, R. N. Schnyer, et al. 2006. Sham device v. inert pill: Randomised controlled trial of two placebo treatments. *British Medical Journal* 332: 391–397.

Kirsch, I., and L. J. Weixel. 1988. Double-blind versus deceptive administration of a placebo. *Behavioral Neuroscience* 102: 319–323.

Kolber, A. J. 2007. A limited defense of clinical placebo deception. *Yale Law & Policy Review* 26: 75–134.

Linde, K., A. Streng, S. Jurgens, A. Hoppe, B. Brinkhaus, et al. 2005. Acupuncture for patients with migraine: A randomized controlled trial. *Journal of the American Medical Association* 293: 2118–2125.

Liu, T. 2009. Acupuncture: What underlies needle administration? *Evidence-Based Complementary and Alternative Medicine* 6(2): 185–193.

Melchart, D., A. Streng, A. Hoppe, B. Brinkhaus, C. Witt, et al. (2005) Acupuncture in patients with tension-type headache: Randomised controlled trial. *British Medical Journal* 331: 376–382.

Miller, F. G., E. J. Emanuel, D. L. Rosenstein, and S. E. Straus. 2004. Ethical issues concerning research on complementary and alternative medicine. *Journal of the American Medical Association* 291: 599–604.

Miller, F. G., and T. J. Kaptchuk. 2008. The power of context: Reconceptualizing the placebo effect. *Journal of the Royal Society of Medicine* 101: 222–225.

Miller, F. G., and D. L. Rosenstein. 2006. The nature and power of the placebo effect. *Journal of Clinical Epidemiology* 59: 331–335.

Miller, F. G., D. Wendler, and L. Swartzman. 2005. Deception in research on the placebo effect. *PLoS Medicine* 2(9): e262.

Moerman, D. E., and W. B. Jonas. 2000. Toward a research agenda on placebo. *Advances in Mind-Body Medicine* 16: 33–46.

Nitzan, U., and P. Lichtenberg. 2004. Questionnaire survey on use of placebo. *British Medical Journal* 329: 944–946.

Park, L. C., and L. Covi. 1965. Nonblind placebo trial: An exploration of neurotic patients' responses to placebo when its inert content is disclosed. *Archives of General Psychiatry* 12: 36–45.

Pollo, A., M. Amanzio, A. Arslanian, C. Casadio, G. Maggi, et al. 2001. Response expectancies in placebo analgesia and their clinical relevance. *Pain* 93: 77–84.

Sandler, A. D., and J. W. Bodfish. 2008. Open-label use of placebos in the treatment of ADHD: A pilot study. *Child: Care, Health and Development* 34: 104–110.

Sandler, A., C. Glesne, and G. Geller. 2008. Children's and parents' perspectives on open-label use of placebos in the treatment of ADHD. *Child: Care, Health and Development* 34: 111–120.

Shapiro, A. K., and E. Shapiro. 1997. The placebo: Is it much ado about nothing? In *The Placebo Effect—An Interdisciplinary Exploration*, ed. Harrington A. Cambridge, MA: Harvard University Press, 12–36.

Sherman, R., and J. Hickner. 2008. Academic physicians use placebos in clinical practice and believe in the mind-body connection. *Journal of General Internal Medicine* 23: 7–10.

Thomas, K. B. 1987. General practice consultations: Is there any point in being positive? *British Medical Journal* 294: 1200–1202.

Tilburt, J. C., E. J. Emanuel, T. J. Kaptchuk, F.A. Curlin, and F. G. Miller. 2008. Prescribing "placebo treatments": Results of a national survey of U.S. internists and rheumatologists. *British Medical Journal* 337: a1938 doi: 10.1136/bmj.a1938.

Walsh, B. T., S. N. Seidman, R. Sysko, and M. Gould. 2002. Placebo response in studies of major depression: Variable, substantial, and growing. *Journal of the American Medical Association* 287: 1840–1847.

Wendler, D., and F. G. Miller. 2004. Deception in the pursuit of science. *Archives of Internal Medicine* 164: 597–600.

Witt, C., B. Brinkhaus, S. Jena, K. Linde, A. Streng, et al. 2005. Acupuncture in patients with osteoarthritis of the knee: A randomised trial. *Lancet* 366: 136–143.

Respectful Involvement of Children in Medical Decision-Making

Nuala Kenny, Jocelyn Downie, and Christine Harrison

H is a bright, loving, 11-year-old child who has been treated for osteosarcoma. Her left arm has been amputated and she was given a course of chemotherapy. She has been cancer free for 18 months and is doing well in school. She is self-conscious about her prosthesis and sad because she had to give away her cat, Snowy, to decrease her risk of infection. Recent tests indicate that the cancer has recurred and metastasized to her lungs. Her family is devastated by this news but do not want to give up hope. However, even with aggressive treatment, H's chances for remission are less than 20%. H adamantly refuses further treatment. In the first round of treatment, she had initially acquiesced to the treatment but ultimately struggled violently when it was administered. She distrusts her healthcare providers and is angry with them and her parents. She protests, "You already made me give up Snowy and my arm. What more do you want?" Her parents insist that treatment must continue. At the request of her physician, a psychologist and psychiatrist conduct a capacity assessment. They agree that H is incapable of making treatment decisions; her understanding of death is immature and her anxiety level very high. Nursing staff are reluctant to impose treatment. In the past, H's struggling and the need to restrain her caused them serious concern.

WHAT IS RESPECTFUL INVOLVEMENT OF CHILDREN IN MEDICAL DECISIONS?

Respectful involvement of children in medical decisions requires respect for parental authority and family context as well as careful attention to the communicative and developing decisional needs and abilities of the child.

WHY IS IT IMPORTANT TO RESPECTFULLY INVOLVE CHILDREN IN MEDICAL DECISION MAKING?

Ethics

Children have traditionally been excluded from medical decision making. Inclusion was seen to be dependent upon autonomy (the capacity for self-determination) and children were considered non-autonomous. Children were seen as needing substitute decision makers, and parents

Kenny NP, Downie, J., Harrison, C. "Respectful Involvement of Children in Medical Decisions." In: Singer, P., Viens, A.M. (ed) *The Cambridge Textbook of Bioethics*. Cambridge University Press 2008. Reproduced with permission.

were generally turned to as substitutes with the right and responsibility to make medical decisions for their children.

However, ethical analysis of the involvement of children in medical decision making has evolved and at least two significant changes must be noted. Firstly, it was recognized that children from infants to teens have dramatically differing levels of capacity for decision making. Three general categories of children were described: those lacking decisional capacity, those with developing decisional capacity, and those with developed decisional capacity (American Academy of Pediatrics, 1995). The focus of respectful involvement of children in medical decisions became fixed on decisional maturity. Differing levels of inclusion in decision making, relating to these different categories of decisional capacity, came to be seen as necessary.

The North American standard for clinical decision making, for instance, evolved into parental consent/permission for the first category, the child's consent for the third category, and parental consent/permission *and* child assent for the second category (Canadian Paediatric Society and Bioethics Committee, 2004). It was claimed that assent recognizes the developing capacity of children in this second category. Assent refers to an agreement with a decision or course of action as distinct from consent, which refers to an informed and voluntary choice with respect to a decision or course of action. The capacity to assent assumes a lower standard for each of the elements of informed choice (freedom, information, and decision-making capacity) than the capacity to consent. Assent was said to demonstrate respect for the child's developing autonomy, and parental consent/permission was said to protect the child from assuming unreasonable risks (Rossi et al., 2003).

However, a second change in thinking occurred as assent has presented both practical and theoretical difficulties. Bulford (1997) has identified the lack of standards by which to judge competency and the ad hoc nature of assessment of the child's capacity for participation in the decision. Kenny and Skinner (2003) have noted that identifying the appropriate role for the child is complex. Among

other things, it requires an understanding of the neurodevelopmental capacities of children that are necessary for decision making. On a substantive level, the role of assent has become contested, as demonstrated in a special issue of the *American Journal of Bioethics* in 2003. Serious questions have been raised. Is assent required from the child? Is dissent morally binding? If so, in what way is dissent different from competent refusal? Is respectful and meaningful involvement of the child about more than decisional autonomy?

If children are to be treated with respect in medical decisions, it is imperative to have clarity regarding children's roles and to be more attentive to the developing capacities of child participants. Simpson (2003) and Baylis et al., (1999) have suggested that at least four categories of children can be described based on an understanding of the various developing capacities of the child: (i) children with no communication (neonates and young children); (ii) children with some communication but no decisional maturity (younger school-aged children); (iii) children with some communication and developing decisional authority (older school-aged children); and (iv) children with decisional maturity (i.e., equivalent to adult capacity for decisional maturity and mature and emancipated minors).

Building on this, it is argued that the appropriate involvement of the child depends upon an assessment of the child's decision-making capacity, what the child can understand, what the child can benefit from being told (even if not capable of making a decision), what the child wants to know, and what the child needs to know in order to participate appropriately (Baylis et al., 1999; Kenny and Skinner 2003).

For example, there is no role in decision making or communication (other than comforting) for an infant. A mature minor, at the other extreme, must be told everything that a competent adult would be told and has the moral authority to make the decision. A child with no decisional capacity, but good language comprehension, should be told what is going to happen to him or her. For instance, it can be morally necessary to share information even where the child has no decisional authority and it can be morally required to ask a child's opinion about various options even if the child may not yet have developed decisional authority, In other words, information sharing should be distinguished from ascribing decisional authority, and the objectives of sharing information and seeking opinions from the child can vary according to the capacities of the child.

Respectful involvement of the child, therefore, involves attention to the communicative as well as decisional needs and abilities of the child. Further, it requires careful and respectful attention to the family context of the child. It has been argued that a family-centered ethic is the best model for understanding the interdependent relationships that are at play in the clinical context. A family-centered approach considers the effects of a decision on all family members, their responsibilities toward one another, and the burdens and benefits of a decision for each member, while acknowledging the special vulnerability of the paediatric patient (Nelson and Nelson 1995; Committee on Pediatric Emergency Medicine, AAP Policy, and American Academy of Pediatrics, 2003). This approach presents special challenges for the healthcare team when there is disagreement between parent(s) and a child. Such a situation raises profound questions about the nature of the physician–patient relationship in pediatric practice. In the care of competent adults, the physician's primary relationship is with the patient. The patient's family may be involved in decision making (i.e., may participate in discussions of diagnosis, prognosis, and treatment options), but it is the patient who defines the bounds of such involvement and it is the patient who has the authority to make any and all decisions. The care of children, by comparison, involves a family-centered relationship in which the child, the parents, and the physician all have a necessary involvement. When there is disagreement between parent and child, the physician may experience some moral discomfort, feeling caught somewhat between the child and parent. The goal, however, must be to ensure the pursuit of the child's best interests and the respectful involvement of the child in the decision-making process (in a fashion appropriate to his or her capacities).

The family-centered approach can also present special challenges for the heathcare team when there is disagreement between the parent(s) and the team with respect to what is in the child's best interests. The assumption that parents best understand what is in the best interest of their child is usually sound. However, situations can arise in which the parents' distress prevents them from understanding or appropriately weighting their child's concerns and wishes. Simply complying with the parents' wishes in such cases is inadequate. Furthermore, the family-centered approach must not be taken to allow family members' interests to trump the child's interests. Rather, it must be seen as recognizing the fact that children are embedded in their families and the interests of the child can be seen as bound up with the interests of other family members. The child's interests must always be the basis for a decision to be followed by the healthcare team. This approach does not discount the parents' concerns and authority but it does recognize the child (albeit as a member of a family) as the particular patient to whom the healthcare team has a primary duty of care.

Law

Apart from exceptional circumstances (e.g., emergency), medical treatment must only be provided or withheld on the basis of a legally valid consent or refusal. To be legally valid, a consent or refusal of medical treatment must be free and informed. It must also be made by a person with appropriate authority who is deemed capable of making the treatment decision, that is, capable of understanding the nature and consequences of the recommended treatment, alternative treatments, and no treatment. If the patient is capable, then the patient has decisional authority. If the patient is a child, parents or legal guardians generally have the legal authority to act as substitute decision makers.

A child's substitute decision maker is obliged to make treatment decisions in the best interests of the child. Healthcare providers who believe that a substitute's decisions are not in the child's best interests should turn to child welfare authorities. Through child welfare legislation, the courts can ensure the appointment of a different substitute decision maker if they believe the current substitute to be acting not in accordance with the child's best interests (legislation usually provides guidance on the content of "best interests"). Courts also have the power to authorize or refuse to authorize treatment if they believe such action to be in the child's best interests. For example, courts have deemed children to be in need of protection and placed them under the care and control of child and family services and courts have themselves ordered blood transfusions in cases in which parents who are Jehovah's Witnesses refuse life-saving transfusions for their children.

Policy

Professional bodies with obligations and duties to children have formally recognized this new and emerging attention to the respectful involvement of children and youth in medical decisions. For example, the Canadian Paediatric Society policy on treatment decisions regarding infants, children, and adolescents states that "to ensure that the best decisions are made for children and adolescents, these decisions should be made jointly by members of the healthcare team, the parents of the child or adolescent, and sometimes the child or adolescent. Children and adolescents should be involved in decision-making to an increasing degree as they develop, until they are capable of making their own decisions about treatment" (Canadian Paediatric Society and Bioethics Committee, 2004, p. 99). The American Academy of Pediatrics (1995, p. 314) statement identifies the joint responsibility of physicians and parents to make decisions for very young patients in their best interest and states that "[p]arents and physicians should not exclude children and adolescents from decision-making without persuasive reasons."

Empirical Studies

There is a body of empirical research providing some information on the competence of children for assent and consent (Abramovitch et al., 1995). Miller et al. (2004) have reviewed the empirical literature focusing on the voluntariness and competence of children for medical decisions. This review identified several fundamental dilemmas underlying current approaches to children's consent, demonstrating the differences between a legal (all-or-none) and a psychological (developmental, context dependent, and interactional) perspective; differences between the clinical and research settings; and differences in studies focusing on who makes the decision in contrast to those focusing on which decision is in the child's best interest. They conclude that more research is needed in this area, with particular attention to be paid to the differences between the respectful involvement of the child in clinical and research decisions, examination of the non-cognitive aspects of children's competence, and the importance of context in the development of decisional capacity.

HOW SHOULD HEALTHCARE PROFESSIONALS RESPECTFULLY INVOLVE A CHILD IN MEDICAL DECISION MAKING IN PRACTICE?

Healthcare professionals working with children should be sensitive to the particular capacities of each child. Children are constantly developing with respect to their physical, intellectual, emotional, and personal maturity. Although developmental milestones give us a general sense of capacities, there is no bright-line of a particular age that will indicate ability to participate in independent decision making.

Where it is determined that it would not harm the child to be involved in the parental decision making and where there is sufficient language capacity to engage the child, healthcare professionals should discuss the treatment options with the child. Healthcare professionals should seek the child's opinion about the potential benefits and harms of the various options. Then, when assessing what action is in the best interests of the child, they should include a consideration of:

- the potential harm of having something done to you that you do not want done (e.g., frustration, loss of trust in healthcare providers, loss of trust in family)
- the potential harms and benefits to the child of the various options from the child's perspective as well as the perspectives of the healthcare providers and family members

• the potential harms and benefits to the child's family members and any others that the child's interests are bound up with.

Once the substitute decision maker has made the decision (likely the parents), the healthcare professionals should carefully explain to the child, at an appropriate level and with the family's assistance, what is going to happen to him or her.

THE CASE

For H, resuming aggressive treatment will have a serious negative effect on her quality of life. The chances of remission are small, yet a decision to discontinue treatment will likely result in her death. Because death is irreversible, and decisions with serious consequences require a high level of competence in decision making, the capacity required for this treatment decision is very high. It has been determined that H does not have this decisional capacity and that her parents are her substitute decision makers.

Nevertheless, H is included in discussions about the treatment options and her reasons for not wanting treatment are explored. Members of the team work hard to re-establish trust. Discussions address the hopes and fears of H and her parents, the parents' understanding of the possibility of cure, the meaning for them of the statistics provided by the physicians, as well as H's role in the decision-making process and her access to information. Members of the team include physicians, nurses, a child psychologist, a psychiatrist, a member of the clergy, a bioethicist, a social worker, and a palliative care specialist.

Discussions focus on reaching a common understanding about the goals of treatment for H. Her physician helps her to express her feelings and concerns about the likely effects of continued treatment. Consideration is given to the effects on her physical well-being, quality of life, self-esteem, and dignity of imposing treatment against her wishes. Spiritual and psychological support for H and her family is acknowledged to be an essential component of the treatment plan. Opportunities are provided for H and her family to speak to others who have had similar experiences, and staff are given the opportunity to voice their concerns.

Ultimately, a decision is made by H's parents to refuse chemotherapy and the goal of treatment shifts from "cure" to "care." H's caregivers assure her and her family that they are not "giving up" but are directing their efforts toward H's physical comfort and her spiritual and psychological needs. H returns home, supported by a community palliative care program, and is allowed to have a new kitten. She dies peacefully.

The healthcare team met after H's death to review her care. They acknowledged that some parents might have made a different decision and discussed what their plan would be should this arise in future. This would include discussions among team members and with the parents to seek consensus about the potential for benefit to the patient, ongoing communication with the parents to ensure mutual understanding of the realistic goals of treatment, and psychosocial and emotional support of the patient during his or her course of treatment. It was acknowledged that in a situation such as H's, her parents' wishes for treatment would take precedence over her dissent. The team did not agree what their approach would be in situations where treatment would not be predicted to have a chance of remission of less than 20%. Some argued that they should refuse to provide treatment in such circumstances. Others argued that, even then, the parents' decision should be respected. It was agreed that should the situation arise they would invite the hospital ethics team to assist with decision making and conflict resolution.

References

Abramovitch, R., Freedman, J.L., Henry, K., and Van Brunschot, M. (1995). Children's capacity to agree to psychological research: knowledge of risks and benefits and voluntariness. *Ethics and Behaviour* 5: 25–48.

American Academy of Pediatrics (1995). Informed consent, parental permission and assent in pediatric practice. *Pediatrics* 95: 314–17.

Baylis, F., Downie, J., and Kenny, N.P. (1999). Children and decisionmaking in health research. *IRB: Rev Hum Subject Res* 21: 5–10.

Bulford, R. (1997). Children have rights too. *BMJ* 314:1421–2.

Canadian Paediatric Society and Bioethics Committee (2004). Treatment decisions regarding infants, children and adolescents. *Paediatr Child Health* 9: 99–103.

Committee on Pediatric Emergency Medicine, AAP Policy, and American Academy of Pediatrics (2003). Consent for emergency medical services for children and adolescents. *Pediatrics* 111; 703–6.

Kenny, N.P. and Skinner, L.E. (2003). Skills for assessing the appropriate role for children in health decisions. In *Pediatric Clinical Skills*, 3rd edn, ed. R. Goldbloom. New York: Saunders, pp. 349–59.

Miller, V.A., Drotor, D., and Kodish, E. (2004). Children's competence for assent and consent: a review of empirical findings. *Ethics Behav* 14: 255–95.

Nelson, H.L., and Nelson, J.L. (1995). *The Patient in the Family: An Ethics of Medicine and Families.* New York: Routledge.

Rossi, W.C., Reynolds, W., and Nelson, R. M. (2003). Child assent and parental permission in pediatric research. *Theor Med Bioethics* 24: 131–48.

Simpson, C. (2003). Children and research participation: who makes what decisions. *Health Law Rev* 11: 20–9.

Various authors (2003). *Am J Bioethics* 3: issue 4.

CASES

AC v Manitoba (Director of Child and Family Services), 2009 SCC 30, [2009] 2 SCR 181

Summary prepared by Jacquelyn Shaw

A.C., an intelligent and mature teen-aged girl (14 years and 10 months), was admitted to hospital with serious intestinal bleeding due to her Crohn's disease. The bleeding was substantial enough to put A.C.'s health and possibly also her life in jeopardy. Her physicians determined that a blood transfusion was necessary. A.C. was a devout Jehovah's Witness, however, and she had recently signed a card stating that, in accordance with the tenets of her faith, she wished to refuse all blood transfusions, regardless of the circumstances. She verbally repeated her refusal to consent to the transfusion to her physicians. Child and Family Services subsequently took A.C. into its protection, allowing her physicians to transfuse her against her wishes in the belief that this was in her "best interests."

A.C. survived and later argued that she had been transfused against her wishes and thereby denied her rights to freedom of religion, to equal treatment compared with other patients,

to liberty, and to physical and psychological integrity.

Discussion Questions

1. Some provinces have a legislated age of consent to medical treatment, others do not. Should the patient's age be determinative in cases such as this or should the patient only have to show that she is capable of understanding and appreciating the consequences of her decision?

2. What if A.C. was an adult, her treatment refusal was not faith-based, and she simply asserted that she did not consent to a blood transfusion? Should her physicians accept her refusal, even if her decision might result in her death? Could this be considered a form of assisted suicide?

3. What if A.C. was pregnant? How, if at all, might this change your reasoning?

McInerney v MacDonald, [1992] 2 SCR 138, CanLII 57 (SCC)

Summary prepared by Victoria Apold

Margaret MacDonald was treated by various physicians over the years. Her latest physician, Dr. Elizabeth McInerney, advised her to stop taking thyroid pills that were prescribed to her by previous doctors. Mrs. MacDonald then became concerned about her preceding medical care and requested a complete copy of her medical file from Dr. McInerney.

Dr. McInerney provided Mrs. MacDonald with her own notes, memoranda, and reports she prepared herself. Dr. McInerney refused to provide copies of reports and records she received from other physicians, stating that they were the property of those physicians and it would be unethical for her to release them to Mrs. MacDonald.

_____

Reprinted by permission of the author.

Discussion Questions

1. Does the patient or the physician "own" the patient's medical records? Should a patient have an absolute right to obtain a copy of his or her complete medical record at any time?
2. Given that today's medical care is frequently provided by so many different health care providers, is it fair to expect a patient to ask each health care provider for a copy of his or her records, or should the treating physician at the time have an obligation to share all available medical records?
3. Where there are electronic medical records, who should be allowed to access them? The patient? Current health care providers? Insurers? Employers? Others?

Useful Resources

ONLINE

Canadian Medical Association (CMA) Code of Ethics

CMA policy on the rights and responsibilities of physicians and patients, including its comprehensive guide to ethical conduct and behaviour for its members.

Canadian Nurses Association Code of Ethics for Registered Nurses

This code provides guidance and education for decision-making concerning ethical matters; it also serves as a means for self-evaluation and reflection regarding ethical nursing practice.

Joint Statement on Preventing and Resolving Ethical Conflicts Involving Health Care Providers and Persons Receiving Care

"This joint statement was developed cooperatively by the Boards of Directors of the Canadian Healthcare Association, the Canadian Medical Association, the Canadian Nurses Association, and the Catholic Health Association of Canada."

Joint Statement on Resuscitative Interventions (Update 1995)

"This joint statement includes: guiding principles for health care facilities when developing cardiopulmonary-resuscitation (CPR) policy; CPR as a treatment option; competence; the treatment decision, its communication, implementation and review; and palliative care and other treatment. This joint statement was approved by the Canadian Healthcare Association, the CMA, the Canadian Nurses Association and the Catholic Health Association of Canada and was developed in cooperation with the Canadian Bar Association."

World Medical Association (WMA) Medical Ethics Manual and International Code of Medical Ethics

"Promoting the highest possible standards of medical ethics, the WMA provides ethical guidance to physicians through its Declarations, Resolutions and Statements."

READINGS

Caulfield, T. (1997). Legal aspects of the physician-patient relationship. Considerations during health care reform in Canada. *Canadian Family Physician*, 43, 2093–2095, 2098–2100.

Emmanuel, E. J., & Emmanuel, L. L. (1992). Four models of the physician-patient relationship. *Journal of the American Medical Association,* 267(16), 2221–2226.

Gabbard, G. O., & Nadelson, C. (1995). Professional boundaries in the physician-patient relationship. *Journal of the American Medical Association*, 273(18), 1445–1449.

HEALTH LAW

Norberg v Wynrib, [1992] 2 SCR 224, 1991 CanLII 14 (SCC)

Dr. Wynrib provided prescription pain killers to a patient with a known addiction to the prescribed drugs in exchange for sexual acts. The patient, Ms. Norberg, sought damages on grounds of sexual assault, negligence, breach of fiduciary duty, and breach of contract.

BR v Children's Aid Society of Metropolitan Toronto, [1995] 1 SCR 315 1995 CanLII 115 (SCC)

Physicians believed that a one-month old infant might be in need of a blood transfusion to prevent congestive heart failure and in conjunction with surgery to treat an eye condition. Her parents were Jehovah's Witnesses. They objected to blood transfusions on religious grounds and refused to give consent. The infant was temporarily placed in the care of the Children's Aid Society, who authorized the transfusions.

CanLII

CanLII is a non-profit organization managed by the Federation of Law Societies of Canada. CanLII's goal is to make Canadian law accessible for free on the Internet.

Chapter 6 AUTONOMY AND INFORMED CONSENT

INTRODUCTION

"It's my body and I get to decide what happens to it." Contemporary health care encounters are typically distinguished from those of the past by a higher level of respect for patient autonomy: patients make their own decisions about their care. However, this in itself cannot be the whole story of medical practice today. In Chapter 5 we saw that the rejection of a paternalistic approach in medicine still leaves many different types of interactions open to patients and providers. These alternatives track a variety of different accounts of autonomy, each of which has different implications for practice. This chapter begins with one such attempt to provide a conception of autonomy that goes beyond simplistic characterizations of it as self-rule or self-determination. The article reminds us, among other things, of the importance of questioning even the basic concepts and principles we use in bioethics. Given that informed consent is one of the bedrock ethical commitments of modern medical practice (and research), and the aim of informed consent is arguably to protect autonomy, it is important to begin with a clear understanding of the debates over autonomy in the bioethics literature.

In the first article, Susan Sherwin asks whether freedom from interference is enough to consider people autonomous, given that our lives are shaped in important ways by the social, institutional, and political context in which we all live. If someone has been raised in a society with sexist beauty norms, she may be inclined to pursue particular sorts of medical interventions (breast augmentation surgery, for instance) because she doesn't feel that she is living up to a certain social standard. Sherwin challenges the standard assumption that these choices are unquestionably autonomous. Sherwin argues for a relational conception of the self, and a corresponding relational account of autonomy, that more accurately capture the complicated ways in which our lives are shaped—for better and worse—by others. The relational account of autonomy she offers stands in contrast to traditional accounts that tend to focus exclusively on self-determination and freedom of choice, and which have typically characterized individuals as isolated and self-sufficient. Sherwin's account aims to be more responsive to the reality of persistent human interdependence.

The theoretical argument presented in the first article of this chapter is complemented by the second article, in which the surgeon Atul Gawande presents five cases aimed at reminding us that there may still be an important role for paternalism in health care. Drawing on his own experiences as a surgeon and as the father of a premature newborn, Gawande illustrates the many complicated ways in which paternalism still occurs—perhaps justifiably so—in contemporary medical practice. Perhaps, he suggests, patients don't want all the freedom they've been given, and perhaps we would all be better off if we recognized that. Gawande's case studies may be used as a point of departure for assessing relational autonomy and for discussions on the strengths and limitations of the general commitment to informed consent.

What implications do these insights about autonomy have for informed consent? Informed consent is thought to be necessary in medical contexts in order to adequately protect patient autonomy. It is typically characterized as consisting of five elements: competence, disclosure, understanding, voluntariness, and token consent. In the next article, Benjamin Freedman provides an analysis of informed consent that investigates the moral grounds for each of its traditional components. Freedman works reflectively between intuitions about cases and general moral principles to come up with a general moral theory of informed consent.

As noted above, competence is a necessary condition for informed consent; it is also one of the most difficult elements to define and assess. Authors of the remaining two articles take up this difficult task. Robert Pepper-Smith, William Harvey, and Michel Silberfeld define competence in terms of the practical abilities individuals employ in pursuit of their own conception of the good life. With this definition in mind, they explore the strengths and weaknesses of four different frameworks used in the evaluation of competence: psychiatric, cognitive, functional, and decision-making. They do so by developing a taxonomy of practical judgment. Mirroring the experience of making a decision, practical judgment is divided into four components: belief, deliberation and judgment, preferences, and intention. Each component bears on competence in a variety of ways, which are illustrated by a number of hypothetical cases of patients with Alzheimer's disease, psychosis, Parkinson's disease, dementia, a broken hip, bipolar disorder, and one patient with a strong desire to build a tunnel from Toronto to Montreal in order to boost the Canadian economy. Through the use of these compelling cases, Pepper-Smith and colleagues aim to clarify the strengths of their account and the inevitable challenges that arise when attempting to bring theory and practice together. They conclude the article with a short discussion of the importance of attending to the social conditions under which people are being assessed for competence. While the medical focus is often narrowly on the individual, functional supports for an individual within a particular community make a huge difference to his or her ability to achieve practical goals.

In the final article, Louis Charland provides an overview of the literature on competence, concluding that traditional accounts focus too closely on whether a person understands and appreciates the elements of a particular decision. What is lost in such accounts, according to Charland, is attention to questions about why a person wants to make a particular choice. So, in addition to asking, 'Do you understand what this decision is about?' we may want to ask 'Why do you want to choose this rather than that?' These 'why' or value questions can provide a great deal of insight into a person's competence. This in turn helps us to shape a more robust approach to informed consent, and, ultimately, to better respect patient autonomy.

A Relational Approach to Autonomy in Health Care

Susan Sherwin

Respect for patient autonomy (or self-direction) is broadly understood as recognition that patients have the authority to make decisions about their own health care. The principle that insists on this recognition is pervasive in the bioethics literature: it is a central value within virtually all the leading approaches to health care ethics, feminist and other. It is not surprising, then, that discussions of autonomy constantly emerged within our own conversations in the Network; readers will recognize that autonomy is woven throughout the book in our various approaches to the issues we take

---

Sherwin, S. (1998) "A Relational Approach to Autonomy in Health Care." In Sherwin, S. (ed.) *The Politics of Women's Health: Exploring Agency and Autonomy* (pp. 19–47). Temple University Press.

up. It is, however, an ideal that we felt deeply ambivalent about, and, therefore, we judged it to be in need of a specifically feminist analysis.

In this chapter, I propose a feminist analysis of autonomy, making vivid both our attraction to and distrust of the dominant interpretation of this concept. I begin by reviewing some of the appeal of the autonomy ideal in order to make clear why it has achieved such prominence within bioethics and feminist health care discussions. I then identify some difficulties I find with the usual interpretations of the concept, focusing especially on difficulties that arise from a specifically feminist perspective. In response to these problems, I propose an alternative conception of autonomy that I label "relational" though the terms *socially situated* or *contextualized* would describe it equally well. To avoid confusion, I explicitly distinguish my use of the term *relational* from that of some other feminist authors, such as Carol Gilligan (1982), who reserve it to refer only to the narrower set of interpersonal relations. I apply the term to the full range of influential human relations, personal and public. Oppression permeates both personal and public relationships; hence, I prefer to politicize the understanding of the term *relational* as a way of emphasizing the political dimensions of the multiple relationships that structure an individual's selfhood, rather than to reserve the term to protect a sphere of purely private relationships that may appear to be free of political influence.[1] I explain why I think the relational alternative is more successful than the familiar individualistic interpretation at addressing the concerns identified. Finally, I briefly indicate some of the implications of adopting a relational interpretation of autonomy with respect to some of the issues discussed elsewhere in this book, and I identify some of the changes that this notion of relational autonomy suggests for the delivery of health services.

THE VIRTUES OF A PRINCIPLE OF RESPECT FOR PATIENT AUTONOMY

It is not hard to explain the prominence of the principle of respect for patient autonomy within the field of health care ethics in North America:

respect for personal autonomy is a dominant value in North American culture and it plays a central role in most of our social institutions. Yet, protection of autonomy is often at particular risk in health care settings because illness, by its very nature, tends to make patients dependent on the care and good will of others; in so doing, it reduces patients' power to exercise autonomy and it also makes them vulnerable to manipulation and even to outright coercion by those who provide them with needed health services. Many patients who are either ill or at risk of becoming ill are easily frightened into overriding their own preferences and following expert advice rather than risking abandonment by their caregivers by rejecting that advice. Even when their health is not immediately threatened, patients may find themselves compelled to comply with the demands of health care providers in order to obtain access to needed services from health professionals who are, frequently, the only ones licensed to provide those services (e.g., abortion, assistance in childbirth, legitimate excuses from work, physiotherapy).[2]

Without a strong principle of respect for patient autonomy, patients are vulnerable to abuse or exploitation, when their weak and dependent position makes them easy targets to serve the interests (e.g., financial, academic, or social influence) of others. Strong moral traditions of service within medicine and other health professions have provided patients with some measure of protection against such direct harms, though abuses nonetheless occur.[3] Most common is the tendency of health care providers to assume that by virtue of their technical expertise they are better able to judge what is in the patient's best interest than is the patient. For example, physicians may make assumptions about the advantages of using fetal heart monitors when women are in labor without considering the ways in which such instruments restrict laboring-women's movement and the quality of the birthing experience from their perspective. By privileging their own types of knowledge over that of their patients (including both experiential knowledge and understanding of their own value scheme), health care providers typically ignore patients' expressed or implicit values and engage in paternalism[4] (or the overriding of patient preferences for the presumed benefit of the patient) when prescribing treatment.

Until very recently, conscientious physicians were actually trained to act paternalistically toward their patients, to treat patients according to the physician's own judgment about what would be best for their patients, with little regard for each patient's own perspectives or preferences. The problem with this arrangement, however, is that health care may involve such intimate and central aspects of a patient's life—including, for example, matters such as health, illness, reproduction, death, dying, bodily integrity, nutrition, lifestyle, self-image, disability, sexuality, and psychological well-being—that it is difficult for anyone other than the patient to make choices that will be compatible with that patient's personal value system. Indeed, making such choices is often an act of self-discovery or self-definition and as such it requires the active involvement of the patient. Whenever possible, then, these types of choices should be made by the person whose life is central to the treatment considered. The principle of respect for patient autonomy is aimed at clarifying and protecting patients' ultimate right to make up their own minds about the specific health services they receive (so long as they are competent to do so). It also helps to ensure that patients have full access to relevant information about their health status so that they can make informed choices about related aspects of their lives. For example, information about a terminal condition may affect a person's decisions to reproduce, take a leave of absence from work, seek a reconciliation from estranged friends or relatives, or revise a will.

Although theorists disagree about the precise definition of *autonomy*,[5] there are some common features to its use within bioethics. In practice, the principle of respect for patient autonomy is usually interpreted as acknowledging and protecting competent patients' authority to accept or refuse whatever specific treatments the health care providers they consult find it appropriate to offer them (an event known as informed choice). Since everyone can imagine being in the position of patient, and most can recognize the dangers of fully surrendering this authority to near strangers, it is not surprising that the principle of respect for patient autonomy is widely endorsed by nearly all who consider it. Despite different theoretical explanations, the overwhelming majority of bioethicists insist on this principle as a fundamental moral precept for health care. Support is especially strong in North America, where it fits comfortably within a general cultural milieu in which attention to the individual and protection of individual rights are granted (at least rhetorical) dominance in nearly all areas of social and political policy.[6] Both Canadian and U.S. courts have underlined the importance of protection of individual rights as a central tenet of patient–provider interactions, making it a matter of legal as well as moral concern.

Further, the principle requiring respect for patient autonomy helps to resolve problems that arise when health care providers are responsible for the care of patients who have quite different experiences, values, and world views from their own; under such circumstances, it is especially unlikely that care givers can accurately anticipate the particular needs and interests of their patients. This problem becomes acute when there are significant differences in power between patients and the health care professionals who care for them. In most cases, the relevant interactions are between patients and physicians, where, typically, patients have less social power than their physicians: doctors are well educated and they tend to be (relatively) healthy and affluent, while the patients they care for are often poor, and lacking in education and social authority. In fact, according to most of the standard dichotomies supporting dominance in our culture—gender, class, race, ability status—odds are that if there is a difference between the status of the physician and the patient, the physician is likely to fall on the dominant side of that distinction and the patient on the subordinate side. The tendency of illness to undermine patients' autonomy is especially threatening when the patients in question face other powerful barriers to the exercise of their autonomy, as do members of groups subject to systemic discrimination on the basis of gender, race, class, disability, age, sexual preference, or any other such feature. A principle insisting on protection of patient autonomy can be an important corrective to such overwhelming power imbalances.

Moreover, physician privilege and power is not the only threat to patient autonomy. Increasingly, the treatment options available to both patients and physicians are circumscribed by the policies of governments and other third-party payers. In the current economic climate, those who fund health care services are insisting on ever more stringent restrictions on access to specific treatment options; physicians find themselves asked to perform gate-keeping functions to keep costs under control. In such circumstances, where patient care may be decided by general guidelines that tend to be insensitive to the particular circumstances of specific patients, and where the financial interests of the institution being billed for the patient's care may take priority over the patient's needs or preferences, the principle of respect for patient autonomy becomes more complicated to interpret even as it takes on added importance.

The principle of respect for patient autonomy can also be seen as an attractive ideal for feminists because of its promise to protect the rights and interests of even the most socially disadvantaged patients. Feminist medical historians, anthropologists, and sociologists have documented many ways in which health care providers have repeatedly neglected and misperceived the needs and wishes of the women they treat.[7] The ideal of respect for patient autonomy seems a promising way to correct much that is objectionable in the abuses that feminist researchers have documented in the delivery of health services to women and minorities. Most feminists believe that the forces of systematic domination and oppression work together to limit the autonomy of women and members of other oppressed groups; many of their political efforts can be seen as aimed at disrupting those forces and promoting greater degrees of autonomy (often represented as personal "choice") for individuals who fall victim to oppression. For example, many feminists appeal at least implicitly to the moral norm of autonomy in seeking to increase the scope of personal control for women in all areas of their reproductive lives (especially with respect to birth control, abortion, and childbirth, often discussed under a general rubric of "reproductive freedom" or "reproductive choice").

In a world where most cultures are plagued by sexism, which is usually compounded by other deeply entrenched oppressive patterns, fundamental respect for the humanity, dignity, and autonomy of members of disadvantaged groups, though extremely fragile, seems very important and in need of strong ethical imperatives. Feminists strive to be sensitive to the ways in which gender, race, class, age, disability, sexual orientation, and marital status can undermine a patient's authority and credibility in health care contexts and most are aware of the long history of powerful medical control over women's lives. They have good reason, then, to oppose medical domination through paternalism. Promotion of patient autonomy appears to be a promising alternative.[8] Understood in its traditional sense as the alternative to heteronomy (governance by others), autonomy (self-governance) seems to be an essential feature of any feminist strategy for improving health services for women and achieving a nonoppressive society.

PROBLEMS WITH THE AUTONOMY IDEAL

Nonetheless, despite this broad consensus about the value of a principle of respect for patient autonomy in health care, there are many problems with the principle as it is usually interpreted and applied in health care ethics. As many health critics have observed, we need to question how much control individual patients really have over the determination of their treatment within the stressful world of health care services. Even a casual encounter with most modern hospitals reveals that wide agreement about the moral importance of respect for patient autonomy does not always translate into a set of practices that actually respect and foster patient autonomy in any meaningful sense. Ensuring that patients meet some measure of informed choice—or, more commonly, informed consent[9]—before receiving or declining treatment has become accepted as the most promising mechanism for insuring patient autonomy in health care settings, but, in practice, the effectiveness of the actual procedures used to obtain informed consent usually falls short of fully protecting patient autonomy. This gap is easy to understand: attention to patient autonomy can be a time-consuming business and the demands of identifying patient values and preferences are often sacrificed in the face of heavy patient loads and staff shortages. In addition, health care providers are often constrained from promoting and responding to patients' autonomy in health care because of pressures they experience to contain health care costs and to avoid making themselves liable to lawsuits. Moreover, most health care providers are generally not well trained in the communication skills necessary to ensure that patients have the requisite understanding to provide genuine informed consent. This problem is compounded within our increasingly diverse urban communities where differences in language and culture between health care providers and the patients they serve may create enormous practical barriers to informed choice.

There are yet deeper problems with the ideal of autonomy invoked in most bioethical discussions. The paradigm offered for informed consent is built on a model of articulate, intelligent patients who are accustomed to making decisions about the course of their lives and who possess the resources necessary to allow them a range of options to choose among. Decisions are constructed as a product of objective calculation on the basis of near perfect information. Clearly, not all patients meet these ideal conditions (perhaps none does), yet there are no satisfactory guidelines available about how to proceed when dealing with patients who do not fit the paradigm.

Feminist analysis reveals several problems inherent in the very construction of the concept of autonomy that is at the heart of most bioethics discussions.[10] One problem is that autonomy provisions are sometimes interpreted as functioning independently of and outweighing all other moral values. More specifically, autonomy is often understood to exist in conflict with the demands of justice because the requirements of the latter may have to be imposed on unwilling citizens. Autonomy is frequently interpreted to mean freedom from interference; this analysis can be invoked (as it frequently is) to oppose taxation as coercive and, hence, a violation of personal autonomy. But coercive measures like taxation are essential if a society wants to reduce inequity and provide the disadvantaged with access to the means (e.g., basic necessities, social respect, education, and health care) that are necessary for meaningful exercise of their autonomy. In contrast to traditional accounts of autonomy that accept and indeed presume some sort of tension between autonomy and justice, feminism encourages us to see the connections between these two central moral ideals.

In fact, autonomy language is often used to hide the workings of privilege and to mask the barriers of oppression. For example, within North America it seems that people who were raised in an atmosphere of privilege and respect come rather easily to think of themselves as independent and self-governing; it feels natural to them to conceive of themselves as autonomous. Having been taught that they need only to apply themselves in order to take advantage of the opportunities available to them, most learn to think of their successes as self-created and deserved. Such thinking encourages them to be oblivious to the barriers that oppression and disadvantage create, and it allows them to see the failures of others as evidence of the latters' unwillingness to exercise their own presumed autonomy responsibly. This individualistic approach to autonomy makes it very easy for people of privilege to remain ignorant of the social arrangements that support their own sense of independence, such as the institutions that provide them with an exceptionally good education and a relatively high degree of personal safety. Encouraged to focus on their own sense of individual accomplishment, they are inclined to blame less well-situated people for their lack of comparable success rather than to appreciate the costs of oppression. This familiar sort of thinking tends to interfere with people's ability to see the importance of supportive social conditions for fostering autonomous action. By focusing instead on the injustice that is associated with oppression, feminism helps us to recognize that autonomy is best achieved where the social conditions that support it are in place. Hence, it provides us with an alternative perspective for understanding a socially grounded notion of autonomy.

Further, the standard conception of autonomy, especially as it is invoked in bioethics, tends to place the focus of concern quite narrowly on particular decisions of individuals; that is, it is common to speak of specific health care decisions as autonomous, or, at least, of the patient as autonomous with respect to the decision at hand. Such analyses discourage attention to the context in which decisions are actually made. Patient decisions are considered to be autonomous if the patient is (1) deemed to be sufficiently competent (rational) to make the decision at issue, (2) makes a (reasonable) choice from a set of available options, (3) has adequate information and understanding about the available choices, and (4) is free from explicit coercion toward (or away from) one of those options. It is assumed that these criteria can be evaluated in any particular case, simply by looking at the state of the patient and her deliberations in isolation from the social conditions that structure her options. Yet, each of these conditions is more problematic than is generally recognized.

The competency criterion threatens to exclude people who are oppressed from the scope of autonomy provisions altogether. This is because competency is often equated with being rational,[11] yet the rationality of women and members of other oppressed groups is frequently denied. In fact, as Genevieve Lloyd (1984) has shown, the very concept of rationality has been constructed in opposition to the traits that are stereotypically assigned to women (e.g., by requiring that agents demonstrate objectivity and emotional distance),[12] with the result that women are often seen as simply incapable of rationality.[13] Similar problems arise with respect to stereotypical assumptions about members of racial minorities, indigenous peoples, persons with disabilities, welfare recipients, people from developing countries, those who are nonliterate, and so on. Minimally, then, health care providers must become sensitive to the ways in which oppressive stereotypes can undermine their ability to recognize some sorts of patients as being rational or competent.

Consider, also, the second condition, which has to do with making a (reasonable) choice from the set of available options. Here, the difficulty is that the set of available options is constructed in ways that may already seriously limit the patient's autonomy by prematurely excluding options the patient might have preferred. There is a whole series of complex decisions that together shape the set of options that health care providers are able to offer their patients: these can involve such factors as the forces that structure research programs, the types of results that journals are willing to publish, curriculum priorities in medical and other professional schools, and funding policies within the health care system.[14] While all patients will face limited choices by virtue of these sorts of institutional policy decisions, the consequences are especially significant for members of oppressed groups because they tend to be underrepresented on the bodies that make these earlier decisions, and therefore their interests are less likely to be reflected in each of the background decisions that are made. In general, the sorts of institutional decisions in question tend to reflect the biases of discriminatory values and practices.[15] Hence, the outcomes of these multiple earlier decisions can have a significant impact on an oppressed patient's ultimate autonomy by disproportionately and unfairly restricting the choices available to her. Nevertheless, such background conditions are seldom visible within discussions of patient autonomy in bioethics.

The third condition is also problematic in that the information made available to patients is, inevitably, the information that has been deemed worthy of study and that is considered relevant by the health care providers involved. Again, research, publication, and education policies largely determine what sorts of data are collected and, significantly, what questions are neglected; systemic bias unquestionably influences these policies. Further, the very large gap in life experience between physicians, who are, by virtue of their professional status, relatively privileged members of society, and some of their seriously disadvantaged patients makes the likelihood of the former anticipating the specific information needs of the latter questionable. While an open consent process will help reduce this gap by providing patients with the opportunity to raise questions, patients often feel too intimidated to ask or even formulate questions, especially when they feel socially and intellectually inferior to their physicians and when the physicians project an image of being busy with more important demands. Often, one needs some information in order to know what further questions to ask, and large gaps in perspective between patients and their health care providers may result in a breakdown in communication because of false assumptions by either participant.

The fourth condition, the one that demands freedom from coercion in exercising choice, is extremely difficult to evaluate when the individual in question is oppressed. The task becomes even trickier if the choice is in a sphere that is tied to her oppression. The condition of being oppressed can be so fundamentally restrictive that it is distorting to describe as autonomous some specific choices made under such conditions. For example, many women believe they have no real choice but to seek expensive, risky cosmetic surgery because they accurately perceive that their opportunities for success in work or love depend on their more closely approximating some externally defined standard of beauty. Similar sorts of questions arise with respect to some women's choice of dangerous, unproven experiments in new reproductive tech-

nologies because continued childlessness can be expected to have devastating consequences for their lives. In other cases, women sometimes choose to have abortions because they fear that giving birth will involve them in unwanted and lifelong relationships with abusive partners. Some women have little access to contraceptives and find themselves choosing sterilization as the most effective way of resisting immediate demands of their partners even if they might want more children in the future. Or, some women seek out prenatal diagnosis and selective abortion of cherished fetuses because they realize that they cannot afford to raise a child born with a serious disability, though they would value such a child themselves. Many middle-class Western women choose hormone replacement therapy at menopause because they recognize that their social and economic lives may be threatened if they appear to be aging too quickly. When a woman's sense of herself and her range of opportunities have been oppressively constructed in ways that (seem to) leave her little choice but to pursue all available options in the pursuit of beauty or childbearing or when she is raised in a culture that ties her own sense of herself to external norms of physical appearance or fulfillment associated with childbearing or, conversely, when having a(nother) child will impose unjust and intolerable costs on her, it does not seem sufficient to restrict our analysis to the degree of autonomy associated with her immediate decision about a particular treatment offered. We need a way of acknowledging how oppressive circumstances can interfere with autonomy, but this is not easily captured in traditional accounts.

Finally, there are good reasons to be wary of the ways in which the appearance of choice is used to mask the normalizing powers of medicine and other health-related institutions. As Michel Foucault (1979, 1980) suggests, in modern societies the illusion of choice can be part of the mechanism for controlling behavior. Indeed, it is possible that bioethical efforts to guarantee the exercise of individual informed choice may actually make the exercise of medical authority even more powerful and effective than it would be under more traditionally paternalistic models. In practice, the ideal of informed choice amounts to assuring patients of the opportunity to consent to one of a limited list of relatively similar, medically encouraged procedures. Thus, informed consent procedures aimed simply at protecting autonomy in the narrow sense of specific choice among preselected options may ultimately serve to secure the compliance of docile patients who operate under the illusion of autonomy by virtue of being invited to consent to procedures they are socially encouraged to choose. Unless we find a way of identifying a deeper sense of autonomy than that associated with the expression of individual preference in selecting among a limited set of similar options, we run the risk of struggling to protect not patient autonomy but the very mechanisms that insure compliant medical consumers, preoccupied with the task of selecting among a narrow range of treatments.

FOCUS ON THE INDIVIDUAL

A striking feature of most bioethical discussions about patient autonomy is their exclusive focus on individual patients; this pattern mirrors medicine's consistent tendency to approach illness as primarily a problem of particular patients.[16] Similar problems are associated with each discipline. Within the medical tradition, suffering is located and addressed in the individuals who experience it rather than in the social arrangements that may be responsible for causing the problem. Instead of exploring the cultural context that tolerates and even supports practices such as war, pollution, sexual violence, and systemic unemployment—practices that contribute to much of the illness that occupies modern medicine—physicians generally respond to the symptoms troubling particular patients in isolation from the context that produces these conditions. Apart from population-based epidemiological studies (which, typically, restrict their focus to a narrow range of patterns of illness and often exclude or distort important social dimensions), medicine is primarily oriented toward dealing with individuals who have become ill (or pregnant, [in]fertile, or menopausal). This orientation directs the vast majority of research money and expertise toward the things that can be done to change the individual, but it often ignores key elements at the source of the problems.

For example, physicians tend to respond to infertility either by trivializing the problem and telling women to go home and "relax," or by prescribing hormonal and surgical treatment of particular women, rather than by demanding that research and public health efforts be aimed at preventing pelvic inflammatory disease, which causes many cases of infertility, or by encouraging wide public debate (or private reflections) on the powerful social pressures to reproduce that are directed at women. In similar fashion, the mainstream scientific and medical communities respond to the growth of breast cancer rates by promoting individual responsibility for self-examination and by searching for the gene(s) that makes some women particularly susceptible to the disease; when it is found in a patient, the principal medical therapy available is to perform "prophylactic" double mastectomies. Few physicians demand examination of the potential contributory role played by the use of pesticides or chlorine, or the practice of feeding artificial hormones to agricultural animals. Or they deal with dramatically increased skin cancer rates by promoting the personal use of sunscreens while resigning themselves to the continued depletion of the ozone layer. In another area, health care professionals generally deal with the devastating effects of domestic violence by patching up its victims, providing them with medications to relieve depression and advice to move out of their homes, and devising pathological names for victims who stay in violent relationships ("battered woman syndrome" and "self-defeating personality disorder"), but few actively challenge the sexism that accepts male violence as a "natural" response to frustration and fears of abandonment.[17]

Some qualifications are in order. Clearly, these are crude and imprecise generalizations. They describe a general orientation of current health practices, but they certainly do not capture the work of all those involved in medical research and practice. Fortunately, there are practitioners and researchers engaged in the very sorts of investigation I call for, but they are exceptional, not typical. Moreover, I do not want to imply that medicine should simply abandon its concern with treating disease in individuals. I understand that prevention strategies will not eliminate all illness and I believe that personalized health care must continue to be made available to those who become ill. Further, I want to be clear that my critique does not imply that physicians or other direct care providers are necessarily the ones who ought to be assuming the task of identifying the social and environmental causes of disease. Health care training, and especially the training of physicians, is directed at developing the requisite skills for the extremely important work of caring for individuals who become ill. The responsibility for investigating the social causes of illness and for changing hazardous conditions is a social one that is probably best met by those who undertake different sorts of training and study. The problem is that medicine, despite the limits of its expertise and focus, is the primary agent of health care activity in our society and physicians are granted significant social authority to be the arbiters of health policy. Hence, when medicine makes the treatment of individuals its primary focus, we must understand that important gaps are created in our society's ability to understand and promote good health.

In parallel fashion, autonomy-focused bioethics concentrates its practitioners' attention on the preferences of particular patients, and it is, thereby, complicit in the individualistic orientation of medicine. It asks health care providers to ensure that individual patients have the information they need to make rational decisions about their health care, yet it does not ask the necessary questions about the circumstances in which such decisions are made. The emphasis most bioethicists place on traditional, individualistic understandings of autonomy reinforces the tendency of health care providers and ethicists to

neglect exploration of the deep social causes and conditions that contribute to health and illness. Moreover, it encourages patients to see their own health care decisions in isolation from those of anyone else, thereby increasing their sense of vulnerability and dependence on medical authority.

The narrow individual focus that characterizes the central traditions within both medicine and bioethics obscures our need to consider questions of power, dominance, and privilege in our interpretations and responses to illness and other health-related matters as well as in our interpretations of the ideal of autonomy. These ways of structuring thought and practice make it difficult to see the political dimensions of illness, and, in a parallel way, they obscure the political dimensions of the conventional criteria for autonomous deliberation. As a result, they interfere with our ability to identify and pursue more effective health practices while helping to foster a social environment that ignores and tolerates oppression. In both cases, a broader political perspective is necessary if we are to avoid the problems created by restricting our focus to individuals apart from their location.

Feminism offers just such a broader perspective. In contrast to the standard approaches in bioethics, feminism raises questions about the social basis for decisions about health and health care at all levels. Here, as elsewhere, feminists are inclined to ask whose interests are served and whose are harmed by the traditional ways of structuring thought and practice. By asking these questions, we are able to see how assumptions of individual-based medicine help to preserve the social and political status quo. For example, the current taxonomy in Canada designates certain sorts of conditions (e.g., infertility, cancer, heart disease, anxiety) as appropriate for medical intervention, and it provides grounds for ensuring that such needs are met. At the same time, it views other sorts of conditions (e.g., malnutrition, fear of assault, low self-esteem) as falling beyond the purview of the health care system and, therefore, as ineligible to draw on the considerable resources allocated to the delivery of health services.[18] In this way, individualistic assumptions support a system that provides expert care for many of the health complaints of those with greatest financial privilege while dismissing as outside the scope of health care many of the sources of illness that primarily affect the disadvantaged. A more social vision of health would require us to investigate ways in which nonmedical strategies, such as improving social and material conditions for disadvantaged groups, can affect the health status of different segments of the community.[19]

None of the concerns I have identified argues against maintaining a strong commitment to autonomy in bioethical deliberations. In fact, I have no wish to abandon this ideal (just as I have no desire to abandon patient-centered medical care). I still believe that a principle of respect for patient autonomy is an important element of good patient care. Moreover, I believe that appeal to a principle of respect for autonomy can be an important instrument in challenging oppression and it can actually serve as the basis for many of the feminist criticisms I present with respect to our current health care system.[20]

What these criticisms do suggest, however, is that we must pursue a more careful and politically sensitive interpretation of the range of possible restrictions on autonomy than is found in most of the nonfeminist bioethics literature. We need to be able to look at specific decisions as well as the context that influences and sometimes limits such decisions. Many of the troublesome examples I review above are entirely compatible with traditional conceptions of autonomy, even though the patients in question may be facing unjust barriers to care or may be acting in response to oppressive circumstances; traditional conceptions are inadequate to the extent that they make invisible the oppression that structures such decisions. By focusing only on the moment of medical decision making, traditional views fail to examine how specific decisions are embedded within a complex set of relations and policies that constrain (or, ideally, promote) an individual's ability to exercise autonomy with respect to any particular choice.

To understand this puzzle it is necessary to distinguish between agency and autonomy. To exercise agency, one need only exercise reasonable choice.[21] The women who choose some of the controversial practices discussed (e.g., abortion to avoid contact with an abusive partner, cosmetic surgery to conform to artificial norms of beauty, use of dangerous forms of reproductive technology) are exercising agency; clearly they are making choices, and, often, those choices are rational under the circumstances.[22] They also meet the demands of conventional notions of autonomy that ask only that anyone contemplating such procedures be competent, or capable of choosing (wisely), have available information current practice deems relevant, and be free of direct coercion. But insofar as their behavior accepts and adapts to oppression, describing it as autonomous seems inadequate. Together, the habits of equating agency (the making of a choice) with autonomy (self-governance) and accepting as given the prevailing social arrangements have the effect of helping to perpetuate oppression: when we limit our analysis to the quality of an individual's choice under existing conditions (or when we fail to inquire why some people do not even seek health services), we ignore the significance of oppressive conditions. Minimally, autonomous persons should be able to resist oppression—not just act in compliance with it—and be able to refuse the choices oppression seems to make nearly irresistible. Ideally, they should be able to escape from the structures of oppression altogether and create new options that are not defined by these structures either positively or negatively.

In order to ensure that we recognize and address the restrictions that oppression places on people's health choices, then, we need a wider notion of autonomy that will allow us to distinguish genuinely autonomous behavior from acts of merely rational agency. This conception must provide room to challenge the quality of an agent's specific decision-making ability and the social norms that encourage agents to participate in practices that may be partially constitutive of their oppression.[23] A richer, more politically sensitive standard of autonomy should make visible the impact of oppression on a person's choices as well as on her very ability to exercise autonomy fully. Such a conception has the advantage of allowing us to avoid the trap of focusing on the supposed flaws of the individual who is choosing under oppressive circumstances (e.g., by dismissing her choices as "false consciousness"), for it is able to recognize that such choices can be reasonable for the agent. Instead, it directs our attention to the conditions that shape the agent's choice and it makes those conditions the basis of critical analysis.

The problems that I identify with the conventional interpretation of patient autonomy reveal a need to expand our understanding of the types of forces that interfere with a patient's autonomy. On nonfeminist accounts, these are irrationality, failure to recognize that a choice is called for, lack of necessary information, and coercion (including psychological compulsion). Since each of these conditions must be reinterpreted to allow for the ways in which oppression may be operating, we must add to this list recognition of the costs and effects of oppression and of the particular ways in which oppression is manifested. But we must do more than simply modify our interpretation of the four criteria reviewed above. We also need an understanding of the ways in which a person can be encouraged to develop (or discouraged from developing) the ability to exercise autonomy. For this task, we need to consider the presence or absence of meaningful opportunities to build the skills required to be able to exercise autonomy well (Meyers 1989), including the existence of appropriate material and social conditions. In addition, our account should reflect the fact that many decision makers, especially women, place the interests of others at the center of their deliberations. Such an analysis will allow us to ensure that autonomy standards reflect not only the quality of reasoning displayed by a patient at the moment of medical decision making but also the circumstances that surround this decision making.

A RELATIONAL ALTERNATIVE

A major reason for many of the problems identified with the autonomy ideal is that the term is commonly understood to represent freedom of action for agents who are paradigmatically regarded as independent, self-interested, and self-sufficient. As such, it is part of a larger North American cultural ideal of competitive individualism in which every citizen is to be left "free" to negotiate "his" way through the complex interactions of social, economic, and political life.[24] The feminist literature is filled with criticism of such models of agency and autonomy: for example, many feminists object that this ideal appeals to a model of personhood that is distorting because, in fact, no one is fully independent. As well, they observe that this model is exclusionary because those who are most obviously dependent on others (e.g., because of disability or financial need) seem to be disqualified from consideration in ways that others are not. Many feminists object that the view of individuals as isolated social units is not only false but impoverished: much of who we are and what we value is rooted in our relationships and affinities with others. Also, many feminists take issue with the common assumption that agents are single-mindedly self-interested, when so much of our experience is devoted to building or maintaining personal relationships and communities.[25]

If we are to effectively address these concerns, we need to move away from the familiar Western understanding of autonomy as self-defining, self-interested, and self-protecting, as if the self were simply some special kind of property to be preserved.[26] Under most popular interpretations, the structure of the autonomy–heteronomy framework (governance by self or by others) is predicated on a certain view of persons and society in which the individual is thought to be somehow separate from and to exist independently of the larger society; each person's major concern is to be protected from the demands and encroachment of others. This sort of conception fails to account for the complexity of the relations that exist between persons and their culture. It idealizes decisions that are free from outside influence without acknowledging that all persons are, to a significant degree, socially constructed, that their identities, values, concepts, and perceptions are, in large measure, products of their social environment.

Since notions of the self are at the heart of autonomy discussions, alternative interpretations of autonomy must begin with an alternative conception of the self. Curiously, despite its focus on individuals, standard interpretations of autonomy have tended to think of selves as generic rather than distinctive beings. In the traditional view, individuals tend to be treated as interchangeable in that no attention is paid to the details of personal experience. Hence, there is no space within standard conceptions to accommodate important differences among agents, especially the effects that oppression (or social privilege) has on a person's ability to exercise autonomy. In order to capture these kinds of social concerns, some feminists have proposed turning to a relational conception of personhood that recognizes the importance of social forces in shaping each person's identity, development, and aspirations.[27] Following this suggestion, I now explore a relational interpretation of autonomy that is built around a relational conception of the self that is explicitly feminist in its conception.

Under relational theory, selfhood is seen as an ongoing process, rather than as something static or fixed. Relational selves are inherently social beings that are significantly shaped and modified within a web of interconnected (and sometimes conflicting) relationships. Individuals engage in the activities that are constitutive of identity and autonomy (e.g., defining, questioning, revising, and pursuing projects) within a configuration of relationships, both interpersonal and political. By including attention to political relationships of power and powerlessness, this interpretation of relational theory provides room to recognize how the forces of oppression can interfere with an individual's ability to exercise autonomy by undermining

her sense of herself as an autonomous agent and by depriving her of opportunities to exercise autonomy. Thus, it is able to provide us with insight into why it is that oppressed people often seem less autonomous than others even when offered a comparable range of choices. Under a relational view, autonomy is best understood to be a capacity or skill that is developed (and constrained) by social circumstances. It is exercised within relationships and social structures that jointly help to shape the individual while also affecting others' responses to her efforts at autonomy.[28]

Diana Meyers (1989) has developed one such theory of personal autonomy. She argues that autonomy involves a particular competency that requires the development of specific skills. As such, it can be either enhanced or diminished by the sort of socialization the agent experiences. Meyers shows how the specific gender socialization most (Western) women undergo trains them in social docility and rewards them for defining their interests in terms of others, thereby robbing them of the opportunity to develop the essential capacity of self-direction. Such training relegates most women to a category she labels "minimally autonomous" (as distinct from her more desirable categories of medially autonomous and fully autonomous). Relational theory allows us to appreciate how each relationship a person participates in plays a role in fostering or inhibiting that individual's capacity for autonomous action by encouraging or restricting her opportunities to understand herself as an autonomous agent and to practice exercising the requisite skills. Such a conception makes clear the importance of discovering the ways in which oppression often reduces a person's ability to develop and exercise the skills that are necessary for achieving a reasonable degree of autonomy.

For instance, relational theory allows us to see the damaging effects on autonomy of internalized oppression. Feminists have long understood that one of the most insidious features of oppression is its tendency to become internalized in the minds of its victims. This is because internalized oppression diminishes the capacity of its victims to develop self-respect, and, as several feminists have argued, reduced (or compromised) self-respect undermines autonomy by undermining the individual's sense of herself as capable of making independent judgments (Meyers 1989; Dillon 1992; Benson 1991, 1994). Moreover, as Susan Babbitt (1993, 1996) has argued, these oppression-induced barriers to autonomy cannot necessarily be rectified simply by providing those affected with more information or by removing explicit coercive forces (as the traditional view assumes). When the messages of reduced self-worth are internalized, agents tend to lose the ability even to know their own objective interests. According to Babbitt, in such cases transformative experiences can be far more important to autonomy than access to alternative information. Feminist theory suggests, then, that women and members of other oppressed groups can be helped to increase their autonomy skills by being offered more opportunities to exercise those skills and a supportive climate for practicing them (Meyers 1989), by being provided with the opportunity to develop stronger senses of self-esteem (Benson 1994; Dillon 1992; Meyers 1989), by having the opportunity for transformative experiences that make visible the forces of oppression (Babbitt 1993, 1996), and by having experiences of making choices that are not influenced by the wishes of those who dominate them (Babbitt 1993, 1996).

Autonomy requires more than the effective exercise of personal resources and skills, however; generally, it also demands that appropriate structural conditions be met. Relational theory reminds us that material restrictions, including very restricted economic resources, on-going fear of assault, and lack of educational opportunity (i.e., the sorts of circumstances that are often part of the condition of being oppressed), constitute real limitations on the options available to the agent. Moreover, it helps us to see how socially constructed stereotypes can reduce both society's and the agent's sense of that person's ability to act autonomously. Relational

theory allows us to recognize how such diminished expectations readily become translated into diminished capacities.

The relational interpretation I favor is feminist in that it takes into account the impact of social and political structures, especially sexism and other forms of oppression, on the lives and opportunities of individuals. It acknowledges that the presence or absence of a degree of autonomy is not just a matter of being offered a choice. It also requires that the person have had the opportunity to develop the skills necessary for making the type of choice in question, the experience of being respected in her decisions, and encouragement to reflect on her own values. The society, not just the agent, is subject to critical scrutiny under the rubric of relational autonomy.

It is important, however, to avoid an account that denies any scope for autonomy on the part of those who are oppressed. Such a conclusion would be dangerous, since the widespread perception of limited autonomy can easily become a self-fulfilling prophecy. Moreover, such a conclusion would be false. Many members of oppressed groups do manage to develop autonomy skills and, thus, are able to act autonomously in a wide variety of situations, though the particular demands of acting autonomously under oppression are easily overlooked (Benson 1991). Some feminists, such as bell hooks (1990) and Sarah Hoagland (1992), have observed that the marginality associated with being oppressed can sometimes provide people with better opportunities than are available to more well-situated citizens for questioning social norms and devising their own patterns of resistance to social convention. Because those who are especially marginalized (e.g., those who are multiply oppressed or who are "deviant" with respect to important social norms) may have no significant social privilege to lose, they are, sometimes, freer than others to demand changes in the status quo. They may be far more likely to engage in resistance to the norms of oppression than are those who derive some personal benefits from oppressive structures (e.g., middle-class, able-bodied, married women).

Still, we must not make the mistake of romanticizing the opportunities available to the oppressed. An adequate conception of autonomy should afford individuals more than the opportunity to resist oppression; it should also ensure that they have opportunities to actively shape their world. A relational conception of autonomy seems better suited than the traditional models to handle the complexities of such paradoxes because it encourages us to attend to the complex ways in which the detailed circumstances of an individual's social and political circumstances can affect her ability to act in different kinds of contexts.

When relational autonomy reveals the disadvantage associated with oppression in terms of autonomy, the response should not be that others are thereby licensed to make decisions for those who are oppressed; this response would only increase their powerlessness. Rather, it demands attention to ways in which oppressed people can be helped to develop the requisite autonomy skills. The best way of course to help oppressed people to develop autonomy skills is to remove the conditions of their oppression. Short of that, long-term social projects can help to provide educational opportunities to counter the psychological burdens of oppression. In the short term, it may be necessary to spend more time than usual in supporting patients in the deliberative process of decision making and providing them with access to relevant political as well as medical information when they contemplate controversial procedures (e.g., information about the social dimensions of hormone replacement therapy).

Relational autonomy is not only about changing the individual, however. It also demands attention to ways in which the range of choices before those who belong to oppressed groups can be modified to include more nonoppressive options, that is, options that will not further entrench their existing oppression (as often happens, for example, when women choose cosmetic surgery or the use of many reproductive technologies). Whereas in traditional autonomy theory only the mode and quality of specific decisions are evaluated, feminist relational autonomy regards the range and nature of available and acceptable options as being at least as important as the quality of specific decision making. Only when we understand the ways in which oppression can infect the background or baseline conditions under which choices are to be made will we be able to modify those conditions and work toward the possibility of greater autonomy by promoting nonoppressive alternatives.

As in health matters, it is important in relational discussions not to lose sight of the need to continue to maintain some focus on the individual. Relational autonomy redefines autonomy as the social project it is, but it does not deny that autonomy ultimately resides in individuals. Our attention to social and political contexts helps deepen and enrich the narrow and impoverished view of autonomy available under individualistic conceptions, but it does not support wholesale neglect of the needs and interests of individuals in favor of broader social and political interests. Rather, it can be seen as democratizing access to autonomy by helping to identify and remove the effects of barriers to autonomy that are created by oppression. A relational approach can help to move autonomy from the largely exclusive preserve of the socially privileged and see that it is combined with a commitment to social justice in order to ensure that oppression is not allowed to continue simply because its victims have been deprived of the resources necessary to exercise the autonomy required to challenge it.

Acknowledgements

This chapter has evolved over the course of the Network interactions and has benefited enormously from Network discussions. I am grateful to all Network members for careful readings of many earlier drafts and stimulating comments. In addition to input from Network members, I have also benefited from the generous attention paid by Keith Burgess-Jackson, Sue Campbell, Richmond Campbell, Carmel Forde, Jody Graham, Carl Matheson, Barbara Secker, and Eldon Soifer.

Notes

1. Some Network members prefer the terms, "contextual" or "situated" as a way of avoiding all confusion with those feminists who reserve the term "relational" to refer exclusively to interpersonal relations. I feel that this usage perpetuates the misleading sense that interpersonal relations are themselves "apolitical." I have, therefore, chosen to insist on a thoroughly political reading of the term "relational" that applies to both interpersonal and more public sorts of relations.

2. While questions of patient autonomy arise in interactions with all health care providers, North American health care delivery is largely structured around provision of medical services; moreover, physicians control most of the decision making that determines provision of health care services. Hence, much of the subsequent discussion focuses explicitly on patient autonomy in relation to physician authority, even though many of the concerns raised also extend to other (nonmedical) types of health care practice.

3. The most vivid examples appear in the distressing history of medical research with human subjects. See, for example, Katz 1972.

4. I deliberately retain the gendered term in this particular instance since it accurately reflects the connection to the traditional gendered role of patriarchal father who presumes authority to make decisions on behalf of all other family members. Traditional stereotypes of mothering and gender-neutral parenting do not retain this hierarchical flavor.

5. For a review of most of the common interpretations, see Dworkin 1988.

6. Interest in respect for patient autonomy is hardly unique to North America, however. See note 20.

7. See, for example, Corea 1985; Ehrenreich and English 1979; Fisher 1986; Perales and Young 1988; and White 1990. This is not a straightforward history of constant abuse or one-sided power, however; as Wendy Mitchinson documents in Chapter 6, the relationship between women and their doctors has long been complex and ambiguous.

8. At the very least, we need a more complex analysis of the options for decision making than is provided by the familiar dichotomous structure of patient autonomy versus medical paternalism. See Mahowald 1993 for development of the idea of maternalism as an alternative that is aimed at capturing both these aspects of medical responsibility; see also Sherwin 1992 for a brief proposal of "amicalism."

9. *Informed choice* suggests a wider scope for patient autonomy than *informed consent* in that it includes the possibility of patients' initiating treatment suggestions, where *informed consent* implies that the role of the patient is merely to consent to the treatment proposed by the physician; further, *informed choice* makes more explicit that patients ought also to be free to refuse recommended treatments as well as to accept them.

10. Many of these concerns are not exclusive to feminists; several have also been raised by other sorts of critics. I call them feminist because I came to these concerns through a feminist analysis that attends to the role in society of systems of dominance and oppression, especially those connected with gender.

11. This reduction may be a result of a tendency to collapse the ideal of personal autonomy central to bioethics discussions with the concept of moral autonomy developed by Immanuel Kant.

12. It is often taken as a truism in our culture that emotional involvement constitutes irrationality, that emotions are direct threats to rationality. It is hard to see, however, how decisions about important life decisions are improved if they are made without any emotional attachment to the outcomes.

13. Susan Babbitt (1996) argues that the traditional conception of rationality is defined in terms of propositional understanding in ways that obscure the experiences and needs of oppressed people.

14. For example, research priorities have led to the situation where birth control pills are available only for women and this increases the pressure on women seeking temporary protection against pregnancy to take the pill even when it endangers their health.

15. See Chapter 10.

16. I focus primarily on medicine since it is the dominant health profession and is responsible for organization of most health services in developed countries. Most health professions involve a similar bias toward treatment of individuals, though some (e.g., social work) pride themselves on attending to social structures as well as individual need, and most health professions, including medicine, include subspecialties concerned with matters of public health.

17. See Chapter 9.

18. Because health care is a provincial responsibility, there are differences in the precise services offered from province to province and from one

administration to the next within provinces. The examples here are broad generalizations.

19. Such considerations do play a role in health care planning at a governmental level where the focus shifts from medical interventions to the idea of *health determinants*, but here, too, there is excessive attention paid to what the individual can and should be doing ("healthism") and insufficient concern about promoting egalitarian social conditions. See Chapters 3 and 4.

20. When I read an early version of this section of the paper to the Second World Congress of the International Association of Bioethics in Buenos Aires, Argentina, in November 1994, I was struck by how passionately committed local feminists were to retaining a version of the respect for autonomy principle. They felt that most women in their country had very little authority over decisions about their health care, and so they were struggling to reverse a strongly paternalistic bias on the part of physicians by appeal to the principle of respect for autonomy. While they acknowledged that this principle was not as well-entrenched in their society as it is in North America, they considered it very important to their own feminist health agenda. They see respect for patient autonomy as having profoundly liberatory potential in their own society; this perspective provides clear reason not to dismiss this principle lightly, flawed though it may be.

21. The language of agency and autonomy is quite varied within feminist (and other) discourse. For example, the term *agency* is used throughout the collection *Provoking Agents: Gender and Agency in Theory and Practice* (Gardiner 1995) in ways that sometimes appear to overlap with my usage of *relational autonomy*. Susan Babbitt (1996), on the other hand, seems to use the two terms in ways analogous to the use here.

22. The notion of agency is itself highly contested within current feminist theory. Postmodern accounts seem to deny the possibility of subjectivity in any familiar sense; since agency is traditionally assigned to a single subject, once the subject is eliminated, the possibility of agency seems to disappear as well. I do not address this complex theoretical issue here but continue to rely on common sense understandings of both subjectivity and agency. Readers interested in understanding the feminist debates around agency may consult Gardiner 1995.

23. In addition, we need the conceptual space to be able to acknowledge that restrictive definitions of

health sometimes preempt autonomy analysis by limiting the opportunity of some people even to enter the relatively well-funded health care system for assistance with problems (e.g., poverty) that affect their health.

24. The agent imagined in such cases is always stereotypically masculine.

25. Feminist discussion of these and other critiques can be found in Gilligan 1982; Baier 1985; Code 1991; and Held 1993.

26. See Nedelsky 1989 for discussion of this view and its limitations.

27. For example, Baier 1985; Code 1991; and Held 1993.

28. An alternative feminist conception of a relational view of autonomy is provided by Anne Donchin (1998). I see her account as complementary to, not competitive with, this one.

References

Babbitt, Susan. 1993. "Feminism and Objective Interests." In *Feminist Epistemologies*, eds. Linda Alcoff and Elizabeth Potter. New York: Routledge.

———. 1996. *Impossible Dreams: Rationality, Integrity, and Moral Imagination*. Boulder, Colo.: Westview Press.

Baier, Annette. 1985b. "What Do Women Want in a Moral Theory?" *Nous* 19(1): 53–63.

Benson, Paul. 1991. "Autonomy and Oppressive Socialization." *Social Theory and Practice* 17(3): 385–408.

———. 1994. "Free Agency and Self-Worth." *Journal of Philosophy* 91(12): 650–68.

Code, Lorraine. 1991. *What Can She Know? Feminist Theory and the Construction of Knowledge*. Ithaca, N.Y.: Cornell University Press.

Corea, Gena. 1985. *The Hidden Malpractice: How American Medicine Mistreats Women*. New York: Harper Colophon Books.

Dillon, Robin. 1992. "Toward a Feminist Conception of Self-Respect." *Hypatia* 7(1): 52–69.

Donchin, Anne. 1998. "Understanding Autonomy Relationally: Toward a Reconfiguration of Bioethical Principles." *Journal of Medicine and Philosophy* 23.

Dworkin, Gerald. 1988. *The Theory and Practice of Autonomy*. Cambridge: Cambridge University Press.

Ehrenreich, Barbara, and Deirdre English. 1972. *Witches, Midwives, and Nurses: A History of Women Healers*. Glass Mountain Pamphlet, no. 1, Old Westbury, N.Y.: The Feminist Press.

Fisher, Sue. 1986. *In the Patient's Best Interests: Women and the Politics of Medical Decisions.* New Brunswick, N.J.: Rutgers University Press.

Foucault, Michel. 1979. *Discipline and Punish.* New York: Vintage.

———. 1980. *Power/Knowledge.* Ed. Colin Gordon. Brighton, Eng.: Harvester

Gardiner, Judith Kegan. 1995. *Provoking Agents: Gender and Agency in Theory and Practice.* Chicago: University of Illinois Press.

Gilligan, Carol. 1982. *In a Different Voice: Psychological Theory and Women's Moral Development.* Cambridge, Mass.: Harvard University Press.

Held, Virginia. 1993. *Feminist Morality: Transforming Culture, Society, and Politics.* Chicago: University of Chicago Press.

Hoagland, Sarah Lucia. 1992. "Lesbian Ethics and Female Agency." In *Explorations in Feminist Ethics: Theory and Practice,* ed. Susan Browning Cole and Susan Coultrap-McQuin. Bloomington: Indiana University Press.

hooks, bell. 1990. *Yearning: Race, Gender, and Cultural Politics.* Toronto: Between the Lines.

Katz, Jay, ed. 1972. *Experimentation with Human Beings: The Authority of the Investigator, Subject, Professions, and State in the Human Experimentation Process.* New York: Russell Sage Foundation.

Lloyd, Genevieve. 1984. *The Man of Reason: "Male" and "Female" in Western Philosophy.* Minneapolis: University of Minnesota Press.

Mahowald, Mary Briody. 1993. *Women and Children in Health Care: An Unequal Majority.* New York: Oxford University Press.

Meyers, Diana T. 1989. *Self, Society, and Personal Choice.* New York: Columbia University Press.

Nedelsky, Jennifer. 1989. "Reconceiving Autonomy." *Yale Journal of Law and Feminism* 1(1): 7–36.

Perales, Cesar A., and Lauren S. Young, eds. 1988. *Too Little, Too Late: Dealing with the Health Needs of Women in Poverty.* New York: Harrington Park Press.

Sherwin, Susan. 1992. *No Longer Patient: Feminist Ethics and Health Care.* Philadelphia: Temple University Press.

White, Evelyn C., ed. 1990. *The Black Women's Health Book: Speaking for Ourselves.* Seattle, Wash.: Seal Press.

Whose Body Is It, Anyway?

Atul Gawande

The first time I saw the patient it was the day before his surgery, and I thought he might be dead. Joseph Lazaroff, as I'll call him, lay in bed, his eyes closed, a sheet pulled up over his thin, birdlike chest. When people are asleep—or even when they are anesthetized and not breathing by themselves—it does not occur to you to question whether they are alive. They exude life as if it were heat. It's visible in the tone of an arm muscle, the supple curve of their lips, the flush of their skin. But as I bent forward to tap Lazaroff on the shoulder I found myself stopping short with that instinctive apprehension of touching the dead. His color was all wrong—pallid, fading. His cheeks, eyes, and temples were sunken, and his skin was stretched over his face like a mask. Strangest of all, his head was suspended two inches above his pillow, as if rigor mortis had set in.

"Mr. Lazaroff?" I called out, and his eyes opened. He looked at me without interest, silent and motionless.

I was in my first year of surgical residency and was working on the neurosurgery team at the time. Lazaroff had a cancer that had spread throughout his body, and he had been scheduled for surgery to excise a tumor from his spine. The senior resident had sent me to "consent" him —that is, to get Lazaroff's signature giving final permission for the operation. No problem, I had said. But now, looking at this frail, withered man, I had to wonder if we were right to operate on him.

His patient chart told the story. Eight months earlier, he had seen his doctor about a backache. The doctor initially found nothing suspicious, but three months later the pain had worsened and he ordered a scan. It revealed extensive cancer—multiple tumors in Lazaroff's liver, bowel, and up and down his spine. A biopsy revealed it was an untreatable cancer.

Lazaroff was only in his early sixties, a longtime city administrator who had a touch of diabetes, the occasional angina, and the hardened manner of a man who had lost his wife a few years earlier and learned to live alone. His condition deteriorated rapidly. In a matter of months, he lost more than fifty pounds. As the tumors in his abdomen grew, his belly, scrotum, and legs filled up with fluid. The pain and debility eventually made it impossible for him to keep working. His thirty-something son moved in to care for him. Lazaroff went on around-the-clock morphine to control his pain. His doctors told him that he might have only weeks to live. Lazaroff wasn't ready to hear it, though. He still talked about the day he'd go back to work.

Then he took several bad falls; his legs had become unaccountably weak. He also became incontinent. He went back to his oncologist. A scan showed that a metastasis was compressing his thoracic spinal cord. The oncologist admitted him to the hospital and tried a round of radiation, but it had no effect. Indeed, he became unable to move his right leg; his lower body was becoming paralyzed.

He had two options left. He could undergo spinal surgery. It wouldn't cure him—surgery or not, he had at the most a few months left—but it offered a last-ditch chance of halting the progression of spinal-cord damage and possibly restoring some strength to his legs and sphincters. The risks, however, were severe. We'd have to go in through his chest and collapse his lung just to get at his spine. He'd face a long, difficult, and painful recovery. And given his frail condition—not to mention the previous history of heart disease—his chances of surviving the procedure and getting back home were slim.

The alternative was to do nothing. He'd go home and continue with hospice care, which would keep him comfortable and help him maintain a measure of control over his life. The immobility and incontinence would certainly worsen. But it was his best chance of dying peacefully, in his own bed, and being able to say good-bye to his loved ones.

The decision was Lazaroff's.

That, in itself, is a remarkable fact. Little more than a decade ago, doctors made the decisions; patients did what they were told. Doctors did not consult patients about their desires and priorities, and routinely withheld information—sometimes crucial information, such as what drugs they were on, what treatments they were being given, and what their diagnosis was. Patients were even forbidden to look at their own medical records: it wasn't their property, doctors said. They were regarded as children: too fragile and simple-minded to handle the truth, let alone make decisions. And they suffered for it. People were put on machines, given drugs, and subjected to operations they would not have chosen. And they missed out on treatments that they might have preferred.

My father recounts that, through the 1970s and much of the 1980s, when men came to see him seeking vasectomies, it was accepted that he would judge whether the surgery was not only medically appropriate but also personally appropriate for them. He routinely refused to do the operation if the men were unmarried, married but without children, or "too young." In retrospect, he's not sure he did right by all these patients, and, he says, he'd never do things this way today. In fact, he can't even think of a patient in the last few years whom he has turned down for a vasectomy.

One of the reasons for this dramatic shift in how decisions are made in medicine was a 1984 book, *The Silent World of Doctor and Patient,* by a Yale doctor and ethicist named Jay Katz. It was a devastating critique of traditional medical decision making, and it had wide influence. In the book, Katz argued that medical decisions could and should be made by the patients involved. And he made his case using the stories of actual patients.

One was that of "Iphigenia Jones," a twenty-one-year-old woman who was found to have a malignancy in one of her breasts. Then, as now, she had two options: mastectomy (which would mean removing the breast and the lymph nodes of the nearby axilla) or radiation with minimal surgery (removing just the lump and the lymph nodes). Survival rates were equal, although in a spared breast the tumor can recur and ultimately make mastectomy necessary. This surgeon preferred doing mastectomies, and that's what he told her he'd do. In the days leading up to the operation, however, the surgeon developed misgivings about removing the breast of someone that young. So the night before the operation he did an unusual thing: he discussed the treatment options with her and let her choose. She chose the breast-preserving treatment.

Sometime later, both patient and surgeon appeared on a panel discussing treatment options for breast cancer. Their story drew a heated response. Surgeons almost uniformly attacked the idea that patients should be allowed to choose. As one surgeon asked, "If doctors have such trouble deciding which treatment is best, how can patients decide?" But, as Katz wrote, the decision involved not technical but personal issues: Which was more important to Iphigenia—the preservation of her breast or the security of living without a significant chance that the lump would grow back? No doctor was the authority on these matters. Only Iphigenia was. Yet in such situations doctors did step in, often not even asking about a patient's concerns, and made their own decisions—decisions perhaps influenced by money, professional bias (for example, surgeons tend to favor surgery), and personal idiosyncrasy.

Eventually, medical schools came around to Katz's position. By the time I attended, in the early 1990s, we were taught to see patients as autonomous decision makers. "You work for

them," I was often reminded. There are still many old-school doctors who try to dictate from on high, but they are finding that patients won't put up with that anymore. Most doctors, taking seriously the idea that patients should control their own fates, lay out the options and the risks involved. A few even refuse to make recommendations, for fear of improperly influencing patients. Patients ask questions, look up information on the Internet, seek second opinions. And they decide.

In practice, however, matters aren't so straightforward. Patients, it turns out, make bad decisions, too. Sometimes, of course, the difference between one option and another isn't especially significant. But when you see your patient making a grave mistake, should you simply do what the patient wants? The current medical orthodoxy says yes. After all, whose body is it, anyway?

Lazaroff wanted surgery. The oncologist was dubious about the choice, but she called in a neurosurgeon. The neurosurgeon, a trim man in his forties with a stellar reputation and a fondness for bow ties, saw Lazaroff and his son that afternoon. He warned them at length about how terrible the risks were and how limited the potential benefit. Sometimes, he told me later, patients just don't seem to hear the dangers, and in those cases he tends to be especially explicit about them—getting stuck on a ventilator because of poor lung function, having a stroke, dying. But Lazaroff wasn't to be dissuaded. The surgeon put him on the schedule.

"Mr. Lazaroff, I'm a surgical resident, and I'm here to talk to you about your surgery tomorrow," I said. "You're going to be having a thoracic spine corpectomy and fusion." He looked at me blankly. "This means that we will be removing the tumor compressing your spine," I said. His expression did not change. "The hope is that it will keep your paralysis from worsening."

"I'm not paralyzed," he said at last. "The surgery is so I won't become paralyzed."

I quickly retreated. "I'm sorry—I meant, keep you from becoming paralyzed." Perhaps this was just semantics—he could still move his left leg some. "I just need you to sign a permission form so you can have the surgery tomorrow."

The "informed-consent form" is a relatively recent development. It lists as many complications as we doctors can think of—everything from a mild allergic reaction to death—and, in signing it, you indicate that you have accepted these risks. It has the mark of lawyerdom and bureaucracy, and I doubt that patients feel any better informed after reading it. It does, however, provide an occasion to review the risks involved.

The neurosurgeon had already gone over them in detail. So I hit the highlights. "We ask for your signature so we're sure you understand the risks," I said. "Although you're having this done to preserve your abilities, the operation could fail or leave you paralyzed." I tried to sound firm without being harsh. "You could have a stroke or a heart attack or could even die." I held the form and a pen out to him.

"No one said I could die from this," he said, tremulously. "It's my last hope. Are you saying I'm going to die?"

I froze, not knowing quite what to say. Just then, Lazaroff's son, whom I'll call David, arrived, with his wrinkled clothes, scraggly beard, and slight paunch. The father's mood changed abruptly, and I remembered from notes in the medical chart that David had recently raised the question with him of whether heroic measures were still appropriate. "Don't you give up on me," Lazaroff now rasped at his son. "You give me every chance I've got." He snatched the form and the pen from my hand. We stood, chastised and silent, as Lazaroff made a slow, illegible scrawl near the line for his signature.

Outside the room, David told me that he wasn't sure this was the right move. His mother had spent a long time in intensive care on a ventilator before dying of emphysema, and since then his father had often said that he did not want anything like that to happen to him. But now he was adamant about doing "everything." David did not dare argue with him.

Lazaroff had his surgery the next day. Once under anesthesia, he was rolled onto his left side. A thoracic surgeon made a long incision, opening into the chest cavity from the front around to the back along the eighth rib, slipped in a rib spreader, cranked it open, and then fixed in place a retractor to hold the deflated lung out of the way. You could see right down into the back of the chest to the spinal column. A fleshy, tennis ball-size mass enveloped the tenth vertebra. The neurosurgeon took over and meticulously dissected around and under the tumor. It took a couple of hours, but eventually the tumor was attached only where it invaded the bony vertebral body. He then used a rongeur—a rigid, jawed instrument—to take small, painstaking bites in the vertebral body, like a beaver gnawing slowly through a tree trunk, ultimately removing the vertebra and, with it, the mass. To rebuild the spine, he filled the space left behind with a doughy plug of methacrylate, an acrylic cement, and let it slowly harden in place. He slipped a probe in behind the new artificial vertebra. There was plenty of space. It had taken more than four hours, but the pressure on the spinal cord was gone. The thoracic surgeon closed Lazaroff's chest, leaving a rubber chest tube jutting out to reinflate his lung, and he was wheeled into intensive care.

The operation was a technical success. Lazaroff's lungs wouldn't recover, however, and we struggled to get him off the ventilator. Over the next few days, they gradually became stiff and fibrotic, requiring higher ventilator pressures. We tried to keep him under sedation, but he frequently broke through and woke up wild-eyed and thrashing. David kept a despondent bedside vigil. Successive chest X rays showed worsening lung damage. Small blood clots lodged in Lazaroff's lungs, and we put him on a blood thinner to prevent more clots from forming. Then some slow bleeding started—we weren't sure from where—and we had to give him blood transfusions almost daily. After a week, he began spiking fevers, but we couldn't find where the infection was. On the ninth day after the operation, the high ventilator pressures blew small holes in his lungs. We had to cut into his chest and insert an extra tube to keep his lungs from collapsing. The effort and expense it took to keep him going were enormous, the results dispiriting. It became apparent that our efforts were futile. It was exactly the way Lazaroff hadn't wanted to die—strapped down and sedated, tubes in every natural orifice and in several new ones, and on a ventilator. On the fourteenth day, David told the neurosurgeon that we should stop.

The neurosurgeon came to me with the news. I went to Lazaroff's ICU room, one of eight bays arrayed in a semicircle around a nursing station, each with a tile floor, a window, and a sliding glass door that closed it off from the noise but not from the eyes of the nurses. A nurse and I slipped in. I checked to make sure that Lazaroff's morphine drip was turned up high. Taking my place at the bedside, I leaned close to him and, in case he could hear me, told him I was going to take the breathing tube out of his mouth. I snipped the ties securing the tube and deflated the balloon cuff holding it in his trachea. Then I pulled the tube out. He coughed a couple of times, opened his eyes briefly, and then closed them. The nurse suctioned out phlegm from his mouth. I turned the ventilator off, and suddenly the room was quiet except for the sound of his labored, gasping breaths. We watched as he tired out. His breathing slowed down until he took only occasional, agonal breaths, and then he stopped. I put my stethoscope on his chest and listened to his heart fade away. Thirteen minutes after I took him off the ventilator, I told the nurse to record that Joseph Lazaroff had died.

Lazaroff, I thought, chose badly. Not, however, because he died so violently and appallingly. Good decisions can have bad results (sometimes people must take terrible chances), and bad decisions can have good results ("Better lucky than good," surgeons like to say). I thought Lazaroff chose badly because his choice ran against his deepest interests—interests not as I or anyone else conceived them, but as he conceived them. Above all, it was clear that he wanted to live. He would take any risk—even death—to live. But, as we explained to him, life was not what we had to offer. We could offer only a chance of preserving minimal lower-body function for his brief remaining time—at a cost of

severe violence to him and against extreme odds of a miserable death. But he did not hear us: in staving off paralysis, he seemed to believe that he might stave off death. There are people who will look clear-eyed at such odds and take their chances with surgery. But, knowing how much Lazaroff had dreaded dying the way his wife had, I do not believe he was one of them.

Could it have been a mistake, then, even to have told him about the surgical option? Our contemporary medical credo has made us exquisitely attuned to the requirements of patient autonomy. But there are still times—and they are more frequent than we readily admit—when a doctor has to steer patients to do what's right for themselves.

This is a controversial suggestion. People are rightly suspicious of those claiming to know better than they do what's best for them. But a good physician cannot simply stand aside when patients make bad or self-defeating decisions—decisions that go against their deepest goals.

I remember a case from my first weeks of internship. I was on the general surgical service, and among the patients I was responsible for was a woman in her fifties—I'll call her Mrs. McLaughlin—who had had a big abdominal operation just two days before. An incision ran the entire length of her belly. Fluids and pain medication dripped through an intravenous line into her arm. She was recovering according to schedule, but she wouldn't get out of bed. I explained why it was essential for her to get up and around: it cuts the risk of pneumonia, clot formation in leg veins, and other detrimental effects. She wasn't swayed. She was tired, she said, and didn't feel up to it. Did she understand that she was risking serious problems? Yes, she said. Just leave me be.

During rounds that afternoon, the chief resident asked me if the patient had gotten out of bed. Well, no, I said—she had refused. That's no excuse, the chief said, and she marched me back to Mrs. McLaughlin's room. The chief sat down on the edge of the bed and, as friendly as a country pastor, said, "Hi, how're you doing," made some small talk, took Mrs. McLaughlin by the hand, and then said, "It's time to get out of bed now." And I watched Mrs. McLaughlin get up without a moment's hesitation, shuffle over to a chair, plop herself down, and say, "You know, that wasn't so bad after all."

I had come into residency to learn how to be a surgeon. I had thought that meant simply learning the repertoire of moves and techniques involved in doing an operation or making a diagnosis. In fact, there was also the new and delicate matter of talking patients through their decisions—something that sometimes entailed its own repertoire of moves and techniques.

Suppose you're a doctor. You're in an examination room of your clinic—one of those cramped spaces with fluorescent lights, a Matisse poster on the wall, a box of latex gloves on the counter, and a cold, padded patient table as centerpiece—seeing a female patient in her forties. She's a mother of two and a partner in a downtown law firm. Despite the circumstances, and the flimsy paper gown she's in, she manages to maintain her composure. You feel no mass or abnormality in her breasts. She had a mammogram before seeing you, and now you review the radiologist's report, which reads, "There is a faint group of punctate, clustered calcifications in the upper outer quadrant of the left breast that were not clearly present on the prior examination. Biopsy must be considered to exclude the possibility of malignancy." Translation: worrisome features have appeared; they could mean breast cancer.

You tell her the news. Given the findings, you say, you think she ought to have a biopsy. She groans, and then stiffens. "Every time I see one of you people, you find something you want biopsied," she says. Three times in the past five years, her annual mammogram has revealed an area of "suspicious" calcifications. Three times a surgeon has taken her to the operating room and removed the tissue in question. And three times, under the pathologist's microscope, it has proved to be benign. "You just don't know when enough is enough," she says. "Whatever these specks are that keep turning up, they've proved to be normal." She pauses, and decides. "I'm not

getting another goddam biopsy," she says, and she stands up to get dressed.

Do you let her go? It's not an unreasonable thing to do. She's an adult, after all. And a biopsy is not a small thing. Scattered across her left breast are the raised scars—one almost three inches long. Enough tissue has already been taken out that the left breast is distinctly smaller than the right one. And, yes, there are doctors who biopsy too much, who take out breast tissue on the most equivocal of findings. Patients are often right to push for explanations and second opinions.

Still, these calcifications are not equivocal findings. They commonly do indicate cancer—even if they don't always—and typically at an early and treatable stage. Now, if having control over one's life is to mean anything, people have to be permitted to make their own mistakes. But when the stakes are this high, and a bad choice may be irreversible, doctors are reluctant to sit back. This is when they tend to push.

So push. Your patient is getting ready to walk out the door. You could stop her in her tracks and tell her she's making a big mistake. Give her a heavy speech about cancer. Point out the fallacy in supposing that three negative biopsies proves that the fourth one will be negative as well. And in all likelihood you'll lose her. The aim isn't to show her how wrong she is. The aim is to give her the chance to change her own mind.

Here's what I've seen good doctors do. They don't jump right in. They step out for a minute and give the woman time to get dressed. They take her down to the office to sit and talk, where it's more congenial and less antiseptic—with comfortable chairs instead of a hard table, a throw rug instead of linoleum. And, often, they don't stand or assume the throne behind the big oak desk but pull up a chair and sit with her. As one surgical professor told me, when you sit close by, on the same level as your patients, you're no longer the rushed, bossy doctor with no time to talk; patients feel less imposed upon and more inclined to consider that you may both be on the same side of the issue at hand.

Even at this point, many doctors won't fuss or debate. Instead, some have what can seem like strange, almost formulaic conversations with the patient, repeating, virtually word for word, what she tells them. "I see your point," they might say. "Every time you come in, we find something to biopsy. The specks keep coming up normal, but we never stop biopsying." Beyond this, many doctors say almost nothing until they're asked to. Whether one calls this a ruse or just being open to their patients, it works, oddly enough, nine times out of ten. People feel heard and like they have had an opportunity to express their beliefs and concerns. At that point, they may finally begin to ask questions, voice doubts, even work through the logic themselves. And once they do, they tend to come around.

A few still resist, though, and when doctors really think someone is endangering himself or herself, other tactics are not beyond the pale. They may enlist reinforcements. "Should we call the radiologist and see what he really thinks?" they might ask, or "Your family's out in the waiting room. Why don't we ask them to come in?" They might give the patient time "to think it over," knowing that people often waver and change their minds. Sometimes they resort to subtler dynamics. I once saw a doctor, faced with a heart disease patient who wouldn't consider quitting smoking, simply fall silent, letting the complete extent of his disappointment show. The seconds tocked by until a full minute had passed. Before a thoughtful, concerned, and, yes, sometimes crafty doctor, few patients will not eventually "choose" what the doctor recommends.

But it's misleading to view all this simply as the art of doctorly manipulation: when you see patients cede authority to the doctor, something else may be going on. The new orthodoxy about patient autonomy has a hard time acknowledging an awkward truth: patients frequently don't want the freedom that we've given them. That is, they're glad to have their autonomy respected, but the exercise of that autonomy means being able to relinquish it. Thus, it turns out that patients commonly prefer to have others make their medical decisions. One study found that although 64 percent of the general public thought they'd want to select their own treatment if they developed cancer, only 12 percent of newly diagnosed cancer patients actually did want to do so.

This dynamic is something I only came to understand recently. My youngest child, Hunter, was born five weeks early, weighing barely four pounds, and when she was eleven days old she stopped breathing. She had been home a week and doing well. That morning, however, she seemed irritable and fussy, and her nose ran. Thirty minutes after her feeding, her respiration became rapid, and she began making little grunting noises with each breath. Suddenly, Hunter stopped breathing. My wife, panicked, leaped up and shook Hunter awake, and the baby started breathing again. We rushed her to the hospital.

Fifteen minutes later, we were in a large, bright, emergency department examination room. With an oxygen mask on, Hunter didn't quite stabilize—she was still taking over sixty breaths a minute and expending all her energy to do it—but she regained normal oxygen levels in her blood and held her own. The doctors weren't sure what the cause of her trouble was. It could have been a heart defect, a bacterial infection, a virus. They took X rays, blood, and urine, did an electrocardiogram, and tapped her spinal fluid. They suspected—correctly, as it turned out—that the problem was an ordinary respiratory virus that her lungs were too little and immature to handle. But the results from the cultures wouldn't be back for a couple of days. They admitted her to the intensive care unit. That night, she began to tire out. She had several spells of apnea—periods of up to sixty seconds in which she stopped breathing, her heartbeat slowed, and she became pale and ominously still—but each time she came back, all by herself.

A decision needed to be made. Should she be intubated and put on a ventilator? Or should the doctors wait to see if she could recover without it? There were risks either way. If the team didn't intubate her now, under controlled circumstances, and she "crashed"—maybe the next time she would not wake up from an apneic spell—they would have to perform an emergency intubation, a tricky thing to do in a child so small. Delays could occur, the breathing tube could go down the wrong pipe, the doctors could inadvertently traumatize the airway and cause it to shut down, and then she might suffer brain damage or even die from lack of oxygen. The likelihood of such a disaster was slim but real. I myself had seen it happen. On the other hand, you don't want to put someone on a ventilator if you don't have to, least of all a small child. Serious and detrimental effects, such as pneumonia or the sort of lung blowout that Lazaroff experienced, happen frequently. And, as people who have been hooked up to one of these contraptions will tell you, the machine shoots air into and out of you with terrifying, uncomfortable force; your mouth becomes sore; your lips crack. Sedation is given, but the drugs bring complications, too.

So who should have made the choice? In many ways, I was the ideal candidate to decide what was best. I was the father, so I cared more than any hospital staffer ever could about which risks were taken. And I was a doctor, so I understood the issues involved. I also knew how often problems like miscommunication, overwork, and plain hubris could lead physicians to make bad choices.

And yet when the team of doctors came to talk to me about whether to intubate Hunter, I wanted them to decide—doctors I had never met before. The ethicist Jay Katz and others have disparaged this kind of desire as "childlike regression." But that judgment seems heartless to me. The uncertainties were savage, and I could not bear the possibility of making the wrong call. Even if I made what I was sure was the right choice for her, I could not live with the guilt if something went wrong. Some believe that patients should be pushed to take responsibility for decisions. But that would have seemed equally like a kind of harsh paternalism in itself. I needed Hunter's physicians to bear

the responsibility: they could live with the consequences, good or bad.

I let the doctors make the call, and they did so on the spot. They would keep Hunter off the ventilator, they told me. And, with that, the bleary-eyed, stethoscope-collared pack shuffled onward to their next patient. Still, there was the nagging question: if I wanted the best decision for Hunter, was relinquishing my hard-won autonomy really the right thing to do? Carl Schneider, a professor of law and medicine at the University of Michigan, recently published a book called *The Practice of Autonomy,* in which he sorted through a welter of studies and data on medical decision making, even undertaking a systematic analysis of patients' memoirs. He found that the ill were often in a poor position to make good choices: they were frequently exhausted, irritable, shattered, or despondent. Often, they were just trying to get through their immediate pain, nausea, and fatigue; they could hardly think about major decisions. This rang true to me. I wasn't even the patient, and all I could do was sit and watch Hunter, worry, or distract myself with busywork. I did not have the concentration or the energy to weigh the treatment options properly.

Schneider found that physicians, being less emotionally engaged, are able to reason through the uncertainties without the distortions of fear and attachment. They work in a scientific culture that disciplines the way they make decisions. They have the benefit of "group rationality"—norms based on scholarly literature and refined practice. And they have the key relevant experience. Even though I am a doctor, I did not have the experience that Hunter's doctors had with her specific condition.

In the end, Hunter managed to stay off the ventilator, although she had a slow and sometimes scary recovery. At one point, less than twenty-four hours after the doctors had transferred her to a regular floor, her condition deteriorated and they had to rush her back to the ICU. She spent ten days in intensive care and two weeks in the hospital. But she went home in fine shape.

Just as there is an art to being a doctor, there is an art to being a patient. You must choose wisely when to submit and when to assert yourself. Even when patients decide not to decide, they should still question their physicians and insist on explanations. I may have let Hunter's doctors take control, but I pressed them for a clear plan in the event that she should crash. Later, I worried that they were being too slow to feed her—she wasn't given anything to eat for more than a week, and I pestered them with questions as to why. When they took her off the oxygen monitor on her eleventh day in the hospital, I got nervous. What harm was there in keeping it on, I asked. I'm sure I was obstinate, even wrongheaded, at times. You do the best you can, taking the measure of your doctors and nurses and your own situation, trying to be neither too passive nor too pushy for your own good.

But the conundrum remains: if both doctors and patients are fallible, who should decide? We want a rule. And so we've decided that patients should be the ultimate arbiter. But such a hard-and-fast rule seems ill-suited both to a caring relationship between doctor and patient and to the reality of medical care, where a hundred decisions have to be made quickly. A mother is in labor: should the doctor give hormones to stimulate stronger contractions? Should he or she break the bag of water? Should an epidural anesthetic be given? If so, at what point in labor? Are antibiotics needed? How often should the mother's blood pressure be checked? Should the doctor use forceps? Should the doctor perform an episiotomy? If things don't progress quickly, should the doctor perform a cesarean section? The doctor should not make all these decisions, and neither should the patient. Something must be worked out between them, one on one—a personal modus operandi.

Where many ethicists go wrong is in promoting patient autonomy as a kind of ultimate value in medicine rather than recognizing it as one value among others. Schneider found that what patients want most from doctors isn't

autonomy per se; it's competence and kindness. Now, kindness will often involve respecting patients' autonomy, assuring that they have control over vital decisions. But it may also mean taking on burdensome decisions when patients don't want to make them, or guiding patients in the right direction when they do. Even when patients do want to make their own decisions, there are times when the compassionate thing to do is to press hard: to steer them to accept an operation or treatment that they fear, or forgo one that they'd pinned their hopes on. Many ethicists find this line of reasoning disturbing, and medicine will continue to struggle with how patients and doctors ought to make decisions. But, as the field grows ever more complex and technological, the real task isn't to banish paternalism; the real task is to preserve kindness.

One more case, again from my internship year. The patient—I'll call him Mr. Howe—was in his late thirties, stout, bald, and with a muted, awkward manner. I wanted to turn the sound up when he spoke, and pictured him as someone who worked alone, perhaps as an accountant or a computer programmer. He was in the hospital following an operation for a badly infected gallbladder. Whenever I saw him, he wore the sad look of someone caged, and he asked no questions. He could not wait to leave the hospital.

Late Saturday afternoon, maybe three days after his surgery, his nurse paged me. He had spiked a high fever and become short of breath. He didn't look well, she said.

I found him sweating profusely, his face flushed, eyes wide. He was sitting bent forward, propped up on his thick arms, panting. He had an oxygen mask on, and, even with the flow turned up to the maximum, the pulse-oximeter readings showed barely adequate oxygen levels in his blood. His heart was racing at well over a hundred beats a minute, and his blood pressure was much too low.

His wife, a small, thin, pale woman with lank black hair, stood to the side, rocking on her feet and hugging herself. I examined Mr. Howe, drew blood for tests and cultures, and asked the nurse to give him a bolus of intravenous fluid, trying to appear as confident as I could. Then I went out into the hall and paged K., one of the chief residents, for help.

When she called back, I filled her in on the details. I think he's septic, I said. Sometimes a bacterial infection gets into the bloodstream and triggers a massive, system-wide response: high fevers and dilation of the body's peripheral blood vessels, causing the skin to flush, the blood pressure to drop, and the heart to speed up. After abdominal surgery, a common cause of this is an infection of the surgical wound. But his incision was not red or hot or tender, and he had no pain in his belly. His lungs, however, had sounded like a washing machine when I listened with my stethoscope. Perhaps a pneumonia had started this disaster.

K. came right over. She was just past thirty, almost six feet tall, with short blond hair, athletic, exhaustingly energetic, and relentlessly can-do. She took one look at Howe and then murmured to the nurse to keep an intubation kit available at the bedside. I had started antibiotics, and the fluids had improved his blood pressure a bit, but he was still on maximal oxygen and working hard to maintain his breathing. She went over to him, put a hand on his shoulder, and asked how he was doing. It took a moment before he managed to reply. "Fine," he said—a silly answer to a silly question, but a conversation starter. She explained the situation: the sepsis, the likely pneumonia, and the probability that he would get worse before he got better. The antibiotics would fix the problem, but not instantly, she said, and he was tiring out quickly. To get him through it, she would need to put him to sleep, intubate him, and place him on a breathing machine.

"No," he gasped, and sat straight up. "Don't... put me ... on a ... machine."

It would not be for long, she said. Maybe a couple of days. We'd give him sedatives so he'd be as comfortable as possible the whole time. And—she wanted to be sure he understood—without the ventilator he would die.

He shook his head. "No ... machine!"

He was, we believed, making a bad decision—out of fear, maybe incomprehension. With antibiotics and some high-tech support, we had every reason to believe, he'd recover fully. Howe had a lot to live for—he was young and otherwise healthy, and he had a wife and a child. Apparently, he thought so, too, for he had cared enough about his well-being to accept the initial operation. If not for the terror of the moment, we thought, he would have accepted the treatment. Could we be certain we were right? No, but if we were right could we really just let him die?

K. looked over at Howe's wife, who was stricken with fear and, in an effort to enlist her in the cause, asked what she thought her husband should do. She burst into tears. "I don't know, I don't know," she cried. "Can't you save him?" She couldn't take it anymore, and left the room. For the next few minutes, K. kept trying to persuade Howe. When it was clear that she was making no headway, she left to phone his attending surgeon at home, and then returned to the bedside. Soon Howe did tire out. He leaned back in his bed, pale, sweaty strands of hair sticking to his pate, oxygen levels dropping on the monitor. He closed his eyes, and he gradually fell into unconsciousness.

That was when K. went into action. She lowered the head of Howe's bed until he lay flat. She had a nurse draw up a tranquilizing agent and administer it in his IV. She pressed a bag mask to his face and squeezed breaths of oxygen down into his lungs. Then I handed her the intubation equipment, and she slipped a long, clear plastic breathing tube down into his trachea on the first try. We wheeled Howe in his bed to the elevator and took him down a few floors to the intensive care unit.

Later, I found his wife and explained that he was now on a ventilator in the ICU. She said nothing and went to see him.

Over the next twenty-four hours, his lungs improved markedly. We lightened up on the sedation and let him take over breathing from the machine. He woke up and opened his eyes, the breathing tube sticking out of his mouth. He did not struggle.

"I'm going to take this tube out of your mouth now, OK?" I said. He nodded. I cut the ties and deflated the balloon cuff holding the tube in place. Then I pulled it out, and he coughed violently a few times. "You had pneumonia," I told him, "but you're doing just fine now."

I stood there silent and anxious for a moment, waiting to see what he would say. He swallowed hard, wincing from the soreness. Then he looked at me, and, in a hoarse but steady voice, he said, "Thank you."

A Moral Theory of Informed Consent

Benjamin Freedman

Most medical codes of ethics, and most physicians, agree that the physician ought to obtain the "free and informed consent" of his subject or patient before attempting any serious medical procedure, experimental or therapeutic in nature. They agree, moreover, that a proxy consent ought to be obtained on behalf of the incompetent subject. And informed consent is seen as not merely a legal requirement, and not merely a formality: it is a substantial requirement of morality.

Acceptance of this doctrine, however, requires the solution of a number of problems. How much information need be imparted? At what age is a person mature enough to consent on his own behalf? Can prisoners give a "free and informed consent" to be experimented upon? Lurking behind these and similar questions there are more fundamental difficulties. What are the functions of consent for the competent and the incompetent? What is the sense in which the patient/subject must be "free," "informed," and "competent?" It is by way of an approach to these latter questions that I shall attempt to respond to the more specific questions.[1]

I. CONSENT AND THE COMPETENT

The negative aspects of the doctrine of informed consent have ordinarily been the focus of attention; difficulties in obtaining the informed consent of the subject/patient render the ethics of experimentation and therapeutic measures questionable. Our common view of informed consent is that, when at all relevant, it represents a minimum condition which ethics imposes upon the physician. It is seen as a necessary condition for medical manipulation, but hardly as a sufficient condition.

The reasons why this is so—why it is not sufficient that an experimenter, for instance, have received informed consent from his subject before proceeding—are quite obvious. The scarcity of medical resources (which includes a scarcity of qualified physician-investigators) forbids us from wasting time upon poorly-designed experiments, or upon experiments which merely replicate well-established conclusions. There seems to be, as well, a limit to the dangers which we (ordinarily) allow subjects to face. We do not, as a matter of policy, think it wise to allow would-be suicides to accomplish their end with the aid of a scientific investigator. Many other reasons could be given for the proposition that a person does not have a right to be experimented upon, even when he has given valid consent to the procedure.

The Right to Consent

But there does seem to exist a positive right of informed consent, which exists in both therapeutic

"A Moral Theory of Informed Consent," *Hastings Center Report* 5, no. 4 (1975): 32–39. Reproduced by permission © The Hastings Center.

and experimental settings. A person who has the capacity to give valid consent, and who has in fact consented to the procedure in question, has a right to have that fact recognized by us. We all have a duty to recognize a valid consent when confronted with it.

From whence derives this right? It arises from the right which each of us possesses to be treated as a person, and in the duty which all of us have, to have respect for persons, to treat a person as such, and not as an object. For this entails that our capacities for personhood ought to be recognized by all—these capacities including the capacity for rational decision, and for action consequent upon rational decision. Perhaps the worst which we may do to a man is to deny him his humanity, for example, by classifying him as mentally incompetent when he is, in fact, sane. It is a terrible thing to be hated or persecuted; it is far worse to be ignored, to be notified that you "don't count."

If an individual is capable of and has given valid consent, I would argue that he has a right, as against the world but more particularly as against his physician, to have it recognized that valid consent has been given. (The same applies, of course, with still greater force, with regard to *refusals* to consent to medical procedures.) The limited force of this claim must be emphasized: it does not entail a right to be treated, or to be experimented upon. It is a most innocuous right, one which most of us would have little hesitation about granting.

It is, therefore, curious that the literature on informed consent has failed to recognize this right—has, in fact, tacitly denied this right, at least as regards experimentation. In writings on informed consent it seems to have been assumed that if, under certain conditions, it is *doubtful* that valid consent to an experiment has been granted, it is best to "play it safe" ethically. In cases of doubt, we prefer not to take chances: in this case, we will not take a chance upon violating the canons of ethics by experimenting without being certain that the subject has validly consented to the experiment. Since we do not at present know whether a prisoner can give a valid consent, let us not take chances: we call for a moratorium on prison experimentation. Since we do not know at what age a person has the capacity to give a valid consent, we avoid the problem by setting the age of majority at a point where it is beyond doubt that maturity has been attained. If we must err, we shall ensure that we err in being overly ethical.

The establishment of the innocuous right to have valid consent recognized as such eliminates this expedient. Other writers have conceptualized the conflict as one between a right and, at best, a mere liberty. From the patient's point of view, he has a right to have his health protected by the physician, and a mere liberty to be experimented upon. From the physician-investigator's point of view, he has a duty to protect the subject's health, and a mere liberty to experiment upon the subject (contingent, of course, upon obtaining the subject's consent). A recognition of the claims of personhood and autonomy, however, reveals this to be a conflict between rights and duties. The physician-investigator has a duty to recognize consent when validly offered. When the consent is of doubtful validity, therefore, the physician experiences a conflict between two duties. He will not be ethically well-protected by choosing not to experiment, for there exists the possibility—which, as cases are multiplied, becomes a probability—that he is violating a duty in so choosing. Problems in informed consent present us with a dilemma. It is no longer the case that the burden of proof devolves upon the would-be experimenter. The would-be abstainer-from-experiments may have to prove his case as well.

These considerations give us a new point of departure in investigating problems of informed consent. They show us that there is no "fail-safe" procedure which we can fall back upon in cases of doubt. Rather, what is required is an exhaustive examination of each case and issue, to see whether or not a valid consent has in fact been obtained....

The Requirement of Information

The most common locution for the requirement which I am discussing is "informed consent"—we require "informed consent" to protect a doctor from legal liability resultant from his therapeutic endeavors, or to ensure the "ethicacy" of an experiment. But I believe "informed consent" to be a serious misnomer for what we do, in fact, want medical practice to conform to.

No lengthy rehearsal of the absurdities consequent upon taking the term "informed consent" at face value is necessary. The claim has been made, and repeated with approval, that "fully informed consent" is a goal which we can never achieve, but toward which we must strive. In order to ensure that fully informed consent has been given, it has seriously been suggested that only medical students or graduate students in the life sciences ought to be accepted as subjects for experimentation. *Reductio ad absurdum* examples of "fully informed consent" have been elaborated, in forms which list all the minutiae of the proposed medical procedure, together with all of its conceivable sequelae. With such a view of "informed consent" and its requirements, it is not surprising to find doctors who claim that since they cannot fully inform patients, they will tell them nothing, but instead will personally assume the responsibility for assuring the subject's safety.

In truth, a *reductio ad absurdum* of this view of "informed consent" need not be constructed; it serves as its own *reductio ad absurdum*. For there is no end to "fully informing" patients. When the doctor wishes to insert a catheter, must he commend to the subject's attention a textbook of anatomy? Although this, of course, would not suffice: he must ensure that the patient understand the text as well. Must he tell the patient the story of Dr. X, that bogey of first-year medical students, who, in a state of inebriation, inserted ("by mistake") his pen-refill instead of the catheter? With, of course, the assurance that *this* physician never gets drunk ("Well, rarely, anyway.") Must the patient be informed of the chemical formula of the catheter? Its melting point?

The basic mistake which is committed by those who harp upon the difficulties in obtaining informed consent (and by critics of the doctrine) is in believing that we can talk about information in the abstract, without reference to any human

purpose. It is very likely impossible to talk about "information" in this way; but impossible or not, when we do in fact talk about, or request, information, we do not mean "information in the abstract." If I ask someone to "tell me about those clouds" he will, ordinarily, know what I mean; and he will answer me, in the spirit in which he was asked, by virtue of his professional expertise as an artist, meteorologist, astronomer, soothsayer, or what-have-you. The meteorologist will not object that he cannot tell you the optical refraction index of the clouds, and therefore that he cannot "fully answer" your question. He knows that you are asking him with a given end in mind, and that much information about the cloud is irrelevant *relative to that purpose.*

That this "abstract information" requirement is not in question in obtaining valid consent is hardly an original point, but it is worth repeating. One of the leading court opinions on human experimentation puts it like this: "… the patient's interest in information does not extend to a lengthy polysyllabic discourse on all possible complications. A mini-course in medical science is not required…."[2]

The proper question to ask, then, is not "What information must be given?" That would be premature: we must first know for what purpose information is needed. *Why* must the patient be informed? Put that way, the answer is immediately forthcoming. The patient must be informed so that he will know what he is getting into, what he may expect from the procedure, what his likely alternatives are—in short, what the procedure (and forbearance from it) will mean, so that a responsible decision on the matter may be made. This is the legal stance, as well as, I think, a "common sensical" stance; as Alexander Capron writes, the information component in valid consent derives in law from the recognition that information is "necessary to make meaningful the power to decide."[3] The proper test of whether a given piece of information needs to be given is, then, whether the physician, knowing what he does about the patient/subject, feels that that patient/subject would want to know this before making up his mind. Outré, improbable consequences would not ordinarily, therefore, be relevant information. Exceptionally, they will be: for example, when there is a small risk of impotence consequent upon the procedure which the physician proposes to perform upon a man with a great stake in his sexual prowess. This is only sensible.

Our main conclusion, then is that valid consent entails only the imparting of that information which the patient/subject requires in order to make a responsible decision. This entails, I think, the possibility of a valid yet ignorant consent.

Consider, first, the therapeutic context. It is, I believe, not unusual for a patient to give his doctor *carte blanche* to perform any medical procedure which the physician deems proper in order to effect a cure. He is telling the doctor to act as his agent in choosing which procedure to follow. This decision is neither unwise nor (in any serious sense) an abdication of responsibility and an unwarranted burden upon the physician. We each of us choose to delegate our power of choice in this way in dealing with our auto mechanic or stockbroker.

It may be harder to accept an ignorant consent as valid in the purely experimental context. I think, however, that much of this difficulty is due to our paucity of imagination, our failure to imagine circumstances in which a person might choose to proceed in this way. We might approach such a case, for example, by imagining a Quaker who chooses to serve society by acting as a research subject, but who has a morbid fear of knives and pointed instruments. The Quaker might say to the physician-investigator that he wants to serve science but is afraid that his phobia would overcome his better judgment. He might consequently request that any experiment which would involve use of scalpels, hypodermic needles, and such, be performed without informing him: while, say, he is asleep or unconscious. He might further ask the doctor not to proceed should the experiment involve considerable risk. In such a case, or one similar, we would find an instance of a valid yet ignorant consent to experimentation.

The ostensible differences between the therapeutic and experimental contexts may be resolved into two components: in the therapeutic context it is supposed that the physician knows what the sequelae to treatment will be, which information, by definition, is not available in the experimental situation; and in the therapeutic context the doctor may be said to be seeking his patient's good, in contrast to the experimental context where some other good is being sought. On the basis of these differences it may be claimed that a valid yet ignorant consent is enough permission for therapy, but not for experimentation.

Closer examination, however, reveals that these differences do not necessarily obtain. First, because I believe it would be granted that a valid yet ignorant consent can be given in the "therapeutic-experimental" situation, where a new drug or procedure is being attempted to aid the patient (in the absence of any traditional available therapy). In the therapeutic-experimental situation, as in the purely experimental situation, the sequelae are not known (although of course in both cases some definite result is expected or anticipated). If a valid yet ignorant consent is acceptable in the one, therefore, it must be acceptable in the other.

Secondly, because it is patently not the case that we can expect there to be no good accruing to the subject of an experiment by reason of his participation. There are, commonly, financial and other "tangible" benefits forthcoming (laboratory training, and so on). And it must ... be said that the pleasures of altruism are not negligible. The proposed differences between experimentation and therapy do not stand up, and so we must say that if a valid yet ignorant consent is acceptable in the one it must be acceptable in the other. It must be remembered that this statement only concerns itself with one part of the consent doctrine, which is, itself, only one of the requirements which the ethical experiment must satisfy....

Our conclusion, then, is that the informing of the patient/subject is not a fundamental requirement of valid consent. It is, rather, derivative from the requirement that the consent be the expression of a responsible choice. The two requirements which I do see as fundamental in this doctrine are that the choice be responsible and that it be voluntary.

The Requirement of Responsibility

What is meant by saying that the choice must be "responsible?" Does this entail that the physician may at any time override a patient's judgment on the basis that, in the physician's view, the patient has not chosen responsibly? Surely not; to adopt such a criterion would defeat the purpose embodied in the doctrine of consent. It would mean that a person's exercise of autonomy is always subject to review.

Still, some such requirement would appear to be necessary. A small child can certainly make choices.[4] Small children can also be intelligent enough to understand the necessary information. Yet surely we would not want to say that a small child can give valid consent to a serious medical procedure.[5] The reason for this is that the child cannot choose *responsibly.*

We are faced with a dilemma. On the one hand, it appears that we must require that the choice be responsible. To require only that the choice be free would yield counter-intuitive results. On the other hand, if we do require that the choice made be a responsible one, we seem to presuppose some body which shall judge the reasonableness of choices; this represents a paternalism which is antithetical to the doctrine of consent. An elderly patient chooses to forgo further life-saving measures. How are we to judge whether or not this choice is a responsible one?

The path between the horns of this dilemma involves saying that the "responsibility" which we require is to be predicated not on the nature of the particular choice, but on the nature of the patient/subject. What we need to know is whether *he* is a responsible man ("in general," so to speak), not whether the choice which has been made is responsible. In this way, we avoid the danger of upholding as "responsible" only those choices which we ourselves feel are good choices. We can and do admit into the community of responsible persons individuals who make choices with which we do not agree.

In this sense, responsibility is a dispositional characteristic. To say that someone is a responsible individual means that he makes choices, typically, on the basis of reasons, arguments, or beliefs—and that he remains open to the claims of reason, so that further rational argument might lead him to change his mind. It is to say that a person is capable of making and carrying through a life-plan—that he is prepared to act on the basis of his choices. It is to say that a person is capable of living with his life-plan; he can live with the consequences of his choices, he *takes responsibility* for his choices.[6] Of course, none of these are absolutes: all responsible people are at times pigheaded, at times short-sighted, at times flighty. That is to say, all responsible men at times act irresponsibly. Should the lack of responsibility persist, of course, to an extreme degree, we may say that the person has left the community of responsible folk.

Voluntarism and Reward

The other requirement of valid consent is that it be given voluntarily. The choice which the consent expresses must be freely made.

We all know some conditions which, if satisfied, make us say that a consent has been given involuntarily. The case which immediately springs to mind occurs when an individual succumbs under a threat: we call this duress or coercion. But the threat need not be overt; and perhaps there need not be a threat at all to render consent involuntary.

Hence, the major problem currently engendered by the requirement of voluntariness. It is typified by the prisoner who "volunteers" for an experiment in the hope or expectation of a reward: significantly higher wages, an opportunity for job training, better health care while involved in the experiment, a favorable report to his parole board. Is the consent which the prisoner offers a voluntary consent? The problem may be stated more generally thus: At what point does reward render consent involuntary?

The problem of reward is particularly difficult, since it involves questions of degree. Is a prisoner's consent involuntary if the reward for his participation in the experiment is a three-month reduction of sentence? Is it relevant here that the prisoner is serving a twenty-year sentence, rather than a one-to-five-year sentence? Does a possible increase in wages from twenty-five cents per hour to one dollar per hour constitute duress? Should we consider the percentage increase, or the increase in absolute value, or the increase in actual value which the seventy-five-cent disparity represents in the prison environment?

To some, of course, questions like these have little meaning. They have little meaning to those who are indifferent to the demands of justice and autonomy which the consent doctrine represents, to those who are willing to buy guinea pigs, rather than to reward human beings. And they have little meaning for those who are convinced that prisoners are inherently unfree, and who thus would call for a total cessation of prison experimentation. Each of these positions denies, in an *a priori* fashion, freedom to prisoners; each must be rejected. A recognition of the fact that decisions about consent may be over- as well as under-protective forces us to deal with this sort of question, complex though it may be.

As is so often the case, posing the question in a different way may facilitate response. We have been considering the question of how much reward nullifies the validity of consent, how much reward renders the subject unfree. But is it in fact the case that *reward* is the disruptive factor here?

This problem may be clarified by the following examples. Imagine an upper-middle-class individual, who can provide for his family all of their needs and most of the amenities of civilized life. Let us say that this person is offered one hundred dollars to cross the street—if you like, make it one thousand or ten thousand dollars? He chooses to cross the street. Is his choice *involuntary*? Despite the substantial reward, I think most of us would agree that the consent was freely offered (and would that we should have such problems!).

Consider a person who deeply wants to be an astronaut. He is told that as part of the program he must participate in experiments to determine resistance to high-G conditions. Is his consent to this invalid, involuntary? I think not. We would say, this is part of his job; he should have expected it; and if he can't stand the heat, he should get out of the kitchen. In this vein, consider Evel Knievel, a financially prosperous man, who is offered millions of dollars to perform daredevil stunts. His choice may be bizarre, even crazy: but has his reward rendered it unfree?

Finally, consider a man who is informed by his doctor that he will most likely die unless he has open-heart surgery. His "reward" for consenting is his life; the penalty for not consenting is death. Does this mean this man cannot give the doctor valid consent—morally valid consent—to proceed?

There are two distinctions which, I think, go a long way towards dispelling these problems. First, I think it must be granted that natural contingencies ("acts of God," things which come to pass naturally, those contingencies which we cannot hold anyone responsible for) do not render a person unfree, nor do they render unfree the choices which a person makes in light of those contingencies.[7]

That natural contingencies do not render a man unfree is a point which is apt to be forgotten in the present context. I am not—in the morally relevant sense—lacking in freedom because I cannot, unaided, fly through the air, or live on grass. Nor am I unfree because my heart is about to give out. Nor am I unfree when, recognizing that my heart may give out, I choose to undergo surgery. I may, of course, be so crazed by knowing that I am near death's door that I am in a state of general impotence, and hence must have the choice made for me; but general incompetence is not in question here. The distinction between choices forced by man, and choices forced by nature, is, then, of importance.

The second distinction is between those pressures which are, and those which are not, in Daube's words, "consonant with the dignity and responsibility of free life."[8] I would explain this as follows: there are certain basic freedoms and rights which we possess which *entitle* us (morally) to certain things (or states of affairs). We would all, no doubt, draw up different lists of these rights and freedoms; but included in them would be safety of person, freedom of conscience and religion, a right to a certain level of education, and, for some of us, a right to some level of health care. When the "reward" is such as only to give us the necessary conditions of these rights and freedoms—when all that the reward does is to bring us up to a level of living to which we are entitled, and of which we have been deprived by man—then the "reward," I think, constitutes duress. A reward which accrues to one who has achieved this level, or who can easily achieve it (other than by taking the reward option), and which hence serves only to grant us "luxury" items, does not constitute duress, and hence does not render choice unfree, no matter how great this reward may be.

The rewards above the moral subsistence level are true rewards. In contrast, we may say (with some touch of metaphor) that the "rewards" which only bring us up to the level to which we were in any event entitled are properly viewed as functioning as *threats:* "Do this, or stay where you are:"—when you should not have been "where you are" in the first place.

The astronaut, Evel Knievel, and the upper-middle-class street-crosser are being granted "luxury" items, and hence are capable of giving free consent. But consider a man who will not be admitted to the hospital for treatment unless he agrees to be a subject in an experiment (unrelated to his treatment). Those who feel, as I do, that we are, here and now, morally entitled to medical treatment would agree, I trust, that this illegitimate option coerces the man into agreeing. Or consider a man who has religious scruples against donating blood, who takes his daughter to a hospital for treatment. He is told that the doctors will not treat her unless the family donates a certain amount of blood. His freedom has been nullified; his "consent" to donating blood is morally invalid. Similarly, the college student whose grade is contingent upon his participation in the instructor's psychological experiments is not validly consenting to serve. He is entitled to have his grade based upon his classroom work.

It yet remains to apply this distinction to our original problem, prison experimentation. The application will not be attempted here, for we would first need to be clear in our minds what rights and freedoms a prisoner is entitled to. I would not hesitate to say, though, that when a situation is created whereby a prisoner can only receive decent health care by participating in an experiment, he is being coerced into that experiment. I would have little hesitation in claiming that if subjecting himself to experimentation is the only way in which a prisoner could learn a trade which maybe used "outside," then that prisoner is being coerced, his consent is not free. When we take into account the condition of our society, these would seem to be reasonable entitlements for the prisoner. Other rewards—for example, higher pay—may or may not constitute rewards above the moral subsistence level; if they are, then consent in light of these rewards could be freely offered. Perhaps too much has been said already; judgments like these must be made in an individualized fashion, one which is sensitive to the realities of prison life.

II. CONSENT AND THE INCOMPETENT

In this section will be discussed, first, the question of how the age of majority and minority with reference to valid consent ought to be set; and secondly, the problems associated with the concept of proxy consent.

The Age of Consent

It has been argued that the requirements for obtaining valid consent are that the patient/subject must have consented freely and that he must be a responsible individual. The requirement of voluntariness does not raise any novel problems when applied to minors. Rather, what we usually have in mind when restricting the power of the minor to consent is that he is not, in the sense required, a responsible individual.

I have claimed that to be a responsible individual one must be capable of rationally adopting, following through, and accepting the consequences of a life-plan. The age, therefore, at which society indicates a presumption that individuals can satisfy these conditions can be said to be the age at which society ought to grant the right to give valid consent to serious medical procedures. The examples which spring to mind are the age of conscription and the age of marriageability. At these ages society has indicated that one is capable of acting, in a complex society, as an individual.

This is not an argument like that which says "If you are old enough to fight, then you are old enough to vote." The requirements necessary for being a soldier may be wholly unrelated to the requirements necessary before the franchise may be properly exercised. In contrast, the responsibility which we assume to be possessed by those capable of soldiering and contracting marriage is the same responsibility which is required to make consent valid: the ability to work through and with a life-plan....

But the setting of an age of consent indicates only a presumption and nothing more. The fact that someone has passed the age of consent is not conclusive proof that he is responsible (in the sense required); the fact that someone is below the age of consent is not conclusive proof of irresponsibility. The presumption may be defeated in either direction.

It is clear, for example, that an adult is not, *ipso facto,* responsible. The adult may be insane.

It is equally clear that a minor need not be irresponsible. People mature at different rates. If evidence of responsibility may be supplied on behalf of one below the age of consent, the presumption of irresponsibility should be defeated. The sort of evidence which would be necessary is that which indicates that the person can work through a life-plan. It may be said that this notion is being approached by the law in the special provisions sometimes made for the "emancipated minor." Marriage or economic self-sufficiency are among the common requirements for being considered an emancipated minor. One of the special prerogatives of the emancipated minor is that he may consent on his own behalf to medical care. I would argue that this should be extended to cover participation in experimentation as well.

Proxy Consent

Proxy consent is consent given on behalf of an individual who is himself incapable of granting consent. The major category of those who require proxy consent are minors, but proxy consent may need to be obtained for the insane or the unconscious as well. My comments will nevertheless be restricted to the case of minors, leaving the other cases to be dealt with by implication. In minors, proxy consent is ordinarily granted by the child's parent or guardian; exceptionally, it may be given by another close relative or by an individual appointed by the court for the specific purpose of granting consent to some procedure.

I have argued that the function of informed consent is to respect the autonomy and dignity of the individual. This cannot be the function of proxy consent. The minor patient/subject cannot fully express autonomy and dignity through choices. It may be said that the function of proxy consent is to protect the right of the parents to raise their child as they see fit, to do with the child as they like. But the child is not the property of the parents; parents do not have an absolute right of disposal over the child. In law we recognize constraints upon the parental power, and common morality affirms the justice in this. What then is the function of proxy consent?

I think it would be best to turn this question on its head. By virtue of what right which the child possesses do we require the granting of proxy consent before a medical procedure may be initiated? What *could* be the source of such an obligation? We ordinarily recognize that there is only one fundamental right possessed by minors, a right to be protected and aided in development. "... A child, unlike an adult, has a right 'not to liberty but to custody.'"[9] All other rights which a child possesses, all other duties which we have towards children, are derivative from this single right, and are void when inconsistent with it. Broadly speaking, in consequence of this right, we must do what we may to promote the welfare of the child; we must abstain from doing what will injure the child, physically or otherwise; and, as far as this right goes, we are at liberty to deal with the child in ways which neither help nor hurt.

That proxy consent is ordinarily to be obtained from the parent or guardian of the child is understandable. We feel that the parent has the best interests of the child at heart, and knows how best to seek the child's welfare. It also follows from this right, however, that, when the parent does not have the best interests of the child in mind, the power of proxy consent should be transferred to another. It is on such a basis that society feels justified in removing a child from his parent's custody, and in appointing another to act *in parens patriae*. If this system is to be effective, society must, by and large, act on the basis of shared common views about what the welfare of the child consists of. We cannot allow anything which a parent considers to be a benefit to the child—being boiled in oil to save his eternal soul—to count as action in the child's best interests. This does not preclude a certain amount of leeway in a liberal society as to permitted views of welfare: if most feel that it is better, when the money is available, to send the child to a private school, we yet will not fault an affluent parent who decides to send his child to a public school.

The consequences of these propositions for cases when proxy consent is being sought for the purpose of giving therapy to a child accord well with the way the law handles this subject. The problem situation which arises concerns parents who, because of religious scruples, refuse to consent to needed medical treatment for their child. Jehovah's Witnesses, for example, who believe that blood transfusions are forbidden by the law of God, will not consent on behalf of their child to blood transfusions. Society feels that the benefit of the child is to be found in allowing the procedure. Because of this, the hospital will often turn to a judge, who appoints someone to act *in parens patriae* for the purpose of consenting to the specific procedure....

Proxy consent to experimentation on children is a more complicated matter. In law, there are two kinds of intervention in the person of another which are actionable in the absence of consent: those interventions where harm does,

and where harm does not, result. The latter are termed "wrongful" or "harmful touchings" (though no harm has occurred). In other words, the mere *doing* of something to a person without his consent is, in itself, an actionable wrong.

We may say that, corresponding to this division, there are two sorts of experiments: those which do, and those which do not, injure the subject appreciably. Beecher has noted, for example, that "Many thousands of psychomotor tests and sociological studies have been carried out in children during the child's development and have revealed much information of value.... Sound nutritional studies without risk have been carried out. So have certain blood studies."[10] It must be added that many studies of value cannot, due to metabolic and other differences, be carried out in adults with results which will be valid for children.

It is clear, on the basis of the principle of benefit, that proxy consent to dangerous or harmful experiments on children cannot be valid. What about those experiments which carry no appreciable risk—the "wrongful touchings" sort? In an adult, it would seem, the right to autonomy, the right "to be let alone," is sufficient basis for the action of wrongful touching. But the child does not have a right to autonomy, except insofar as some measure of autonomy is necessary to promote the child's development and well-being.

Harmless experiments on children, therefore, which satisfy the other canons of medical ethics—good design, well-trained experimenters, and so forth—could be performed. Parents would not be derelict in their duty should they consent, on behalf of their child, to experiments of this sort. Participation in these experiments [does] not infringe the child's right to welfare, unless they would result in a *harmful* (and not just any) restriction of autonomy.

As I see it, the fundamental problem with those who would forbid *all* experimentation upon children[11] is that they confuse consent in adults with proxy consent for children. These two are fundamentally different requirements. Children are not small adults; our relations with children must not be made to approach as nearly as possible to our relations with adults. There are things which you ought to grant to children which need not be granted to adults: if a child is thirsty you provide him with drink. And there are things which may licitly be done to children which could not be done with adults: if my parents annoy me I may not send them to their room. A child is (morally) a different sort of thing than is an adult; we must adjust our relations with them according to their claims upon us.

CONCLUSION

This paper represents an attempt to formulate what I call a "moral theory" of the requirement of consent to serious medical procedures. The method used involves an interplay between cases and principles, such that each influences the other. Well-established moral intuitions about cases suggested some principles and called for the rejection of others. These principles in turn, once established, enabled the clarification of a proper approach to other, borderline cases.

Under the influence of situation ethics, much of the work on medical ethics has stressed the respects in which cases differ. This has resulted in the development of an *ad hoc* literature on cases which pose difficulty for the doctrine of informed consent. As the cases accumulated the doctrine began to seem more and more amorphous.

In contrast, this paper has sought to unify the doctrine of consent. Principles which are developed through considering the problems raised by prison experimentation in turn suggested solutions to other situations; rather than stressing the differences between the experimental and the therapeutic contexts, their similarities were emphasized. There is, I think, a need for such efforts at unification, as there is a need for a literature which is committed to the unique aspects of different cases.

Acknowledgements

The research for this paper was begun during an internship at the Institute of Society, Ethics and the Life Sciences in the month of June, 1973. I gratefully acknowledge the help of Drs. Daniel Callahan, Marc Lappé, Peter Steinfels, and Robert Veatch, of the Institute, who helped make my internship profitable and enjoyable. My wife Barbara read the manuscript and suggested a number of needed changes.

Notes

1. For examples of a similar method applied to different problems, see Thomas I. Emerson, *Toward A General Theory of the First Amendent* (New York: Vintage Books, 1967).
2. *Cobbs* v. *Grant,* 502 P. 2d 1, 11.
3. Alexander M. Caron, "Legal Rights and Moral Rights," in Hilton, et al., eds., *Ethical Issues in Human Genetics* (Plenum Press, 1978), 228.
4. The counter-suggestion may be made that children cannot *really* make choices. This would, I think, put too great a weight upon the requirement of voluntarism. We would be recruiting the concepts of choice and volition to do a job which they have not been designed for.
5. I am speaking of course in the moral, not the legal, context. It may be that in an emergency a child may, in the absence of his parents, give legally valid consent.
6. This gives us the link between "responsible" in the dispositional sense explained here, and "responsible" in the blame-sense of the word ("I'll hold you responsible for that.").
7. The *caveat* must be added: natural contingencies do not have, as their *sole* result, the rendering of a person unfree, in the sense which vitiates consent: a man's brain tumor can make the man an idiot, schizophrenia can make a man insane, but these do not so much affect a person's volition as they do disturb his entire psychic structure.
8. David Daube, quoted in Henry K. Beecher, *Research and the Individual: Human Studies* (Boston: Little, Brown, 1970), p. 146.
9. *In re Gault.* 387 U.S. 1 (1967).
10. Beecher, p. 67.
11. See, for example, Paul Ramsey, "Consent as a Canon of Loyalty With Special Reference to Children in Medical Investigations," in *The Patient as Person* (New Haven: Yale University Press, 1970).

Competency and Practical Judgment

Robert Pepper-Smith, William R.C. Harvey, and M. Silberfeld

1. INTRODUCTION

Many recognize that the notion of competency remains confused and open to capricious interpretation and application.[1] Yet a determination of incompetence, however subjective and idiosyncratic, may lead to the removal of fundamental rights and freedoms. If a psychiatric outpatient is found financially incompetent, control of her finances may revert to the Public Trustee. If an individual is found incompetent to make medical decisions, his course of treatment may be decided by a close relative, or, in the last instance, by the Public Guardian.

At least four different frameworks—psychiatric, cognitive, functional and decision-making—are used in the evaluation of competence, all of which remain more or less unrelated. The purpose of this paper is to develop an alternate conceptual framework for the determination of competence, which we refer to as a taxonomy of practical judgment. The taxonomy shows when each of the traditional frameworks mentioned above may or may not be useful in a determination of competence.

2. AN OVERVIEW OF VARIOUS FEATURES OF "COMPETENCE"

In this section, through a review of the everyday notion of competence and of medico-legal features of competence, we sketch out a definition of competence. We then turn to an evaluation of the traditional frameworks used in a determination of competence.

2.1. The Everyday Notion of Competence

In the everyday sense, competency refers to a level of skill. Saying that "X" is a competent doctor means that he has shown expertise and skill in practice. However, not just any level of skill is sufficient for competency. The competent physician has skills which meet norms set by the profession itself. In everyday terms, "competency" is an evaluative notion related to practical skills.

Finally the term can be a bit pejorative. The competent doctor may be an "average" physician. Competency need not denote an extraordinary level of expertise, but something shading toward the run-of-the-mill.

2.2. Competency in the Medical Setting

Patient competency has a restricted meaning, based upon the patient's role in her own treatment. The everyday notion of competency emphasizes practical skills measured against some community or professional norm. In medical treatment the role of the patient requires skills of judgment. To question a patient's competence is to question her ability to make treatment *decisions*.[2] We discuss these skills below, in the section on practical judgment.

Further, "competence" means exercising certain practical skills so as to meet some standard. Just as the competent physician has skills that meet or exceed standards set by the College of Physicians, so the competent patient must have practical skills that meet some standard or norm. The standard served by the patient's practical skills are her own autonomous goals in life. A medical decision may profoundly affect the course of a patient's life. The skills that she brings to bear in making such a decision aim to realize, in a concrete manner, her own preferences and values. The practical skills of competence serve the value of autonomy. Autonomy—directing one's life as one

With kind permission from Springer Science + Business Media: *Theoretical Medicine and Bioethics* 17(2), "Competency and Practical Judgment" by Robert Pepper-Smith, William R. C. Harvey and M. Silberfeld, pp. 135–150. © 1996.

chooses[3]—is not only an ideal but a practice that requires certain mundane practical skills.

2.3. Legal Notions of Competence

Legal notions of competence highlight two aspects of competence which are also present in the everyday and medical setting. First, the law explicitly links competence to responsibility. In civil law, for instance, competency refers to the ability to understand the nature and effects of a transaction. Individuals are competent to enter into a specific contract if they understand the nature and effects of the contract. They can be held responsible for obligations they incur under the contract. On the other hand, if it can be shown that one of the parties did not understand the nature and effects of the contract at the time of signing, her responsibility is vitiated.[4]

Further, the law recognizes that if an adult is unable to competently manage her own interests, another—including the state—may have, out of beneficence, an obligation to manage her interests on her behalf. Traditionally the law in Western society has restricted the scope of its involvement in these matters to financial management. Recently personal care matters have fallen under its purview, including medical decision-making. If an individual is no longer able to responsibly manage her finances, another may have the obligation to assume control of her finances, to protect her interests as well as those of her dependents and heirs.

In sum, we define competency as the exercise of practical skills that meet (and are evaluated according to) some norm. Patient or client competency refers to practical skills that maintain or further the individual's own preferences and goals in life. These skills serve the value of autonomy. Only through the exercise of these skills are individuals able to realize an autonomous life.

In the following section we review and criticize four standard frameworks for the evaluation of competence. In the fourth section we show how a systematic categorization of the practical skills of competence—which we refer to as a taxonomy of practical judgment—can be used to show when each of the disparate frameworks

may or may not be useful in the evaluation of specific competencies.

3. FOUR STANDARDS FOR THE EVALUATION OF COMPETENCE

> Competency has not been well defined in law: no court decision has yet produced a specific definition, no formal guidelines exist, and no detailed and standardized assessment information is required to reach a conclusion of mental incapacity.[5]

There is no one widely recognized framework for the assessment of competence. Depending on the professionals involved, the setting and the particular competence in question, one or more of the following frameworks may be used to determine the relevant parameters of an assessment.

3.1. Psychiatric Status

Competency determinations in the recent past were marked by their simplicity: one was either sane and responsible or mentally ill and incompetent, to manage one's estate, for example, or to vote.[6] The current literature no longer tends to equate mental illness with incompetency.[7] In part this is due to the recognition that competency does not refer to global capacity but to the ability to perform a specific task or set of tasks.[8] One may no longer be competent to instruct counsel but still competent to change one's Will. Such task-specific notions of competency relate well to the observation that mental illness may [affect] decision-making in certain areas while not in others, or not at all.[9] For instance, an individual suffering from paranoid ideation may still be competent to consent to medical treatment, insofar as his paranoia does not extend to his physician or affect his understanding of his medical condition and the proposed treatment.

In sum, though psychiatric status may bear upon specific competencies, the relation is at best indirect. There is no easy link between a psychiatric diagnosis and a determination of incompetence.

3.2. Cognitive Status

Cognitive status refers to such factors as attention and memory as measured, say, by the MSE (Mental Status Examination). These factors may figure prominently in a competency determination. A psychiatrist may, for instance, justify a finding of financial incompetency by citing test results which show impaired short-term memory and partial disorientation to time and place. Poor short-term memory may suggest, for instance, that the individual will be unable to recall if and when bills have been paid.

Poor memory, however, does not necessarily affect one's ability to make a choice or to state a preference. For instance, an individual who can no longer remember the contents of her Will may recognize the contents as reflecting her wishes upon reading the Will and may show consistency of preference and reasonableness in accounting for her beneficiaries. Her inability to recall the contents of her Will has no significant effect upon her testamentary capacity. An individual who is disoriented to time and place may nevertheless retain the ability to clearly articulate his financial preferences.

Though such factors as impaired memory and recall or disorientation may bear upon one's ability to make sound judgments, they do not do so necessarily.[10]

3.3. Functional Ability

Functional ability refers to the individual's ability to act upon his or her decision. Functional ability is a key consideration in discharge planning. For instance, an elderly woman who is about to be discharged home may be asked to undergo an in-hospital kitchen assessment. The purpose of such an assessment may be to determine whether she is able to cook safely for herself at home. Here competency criteria typically swing towards assessments of risk and safety in light of certain actions of the patient.[11]

Such assessments may give an inaccurate picture of the patient's competence to live at home on at least two grounds. First, they may fail to take into account the patient's own reasons and motivations which lie behind the action. That is, they may fail to take into account her directive capacity. For instance, during one assessment with which we are familiar, the patient neglected to turn off a stove burner. The assessor (an occupational therapist) concluded that she was at great risk of starting a fire in her own home, and therefore unable (incompetent) to live at home. However later, when asked why she had left the burner on, the patient replied that she thought the assessor would turn it off.

Second, functional assessments may fail to take into account that the ability to act effectively often depends on the familiarity of one's surroundings. An elderly patient who can find her way around her own kitchen with ease may find the unfamiliar outlay of the hospital kitchen confusing and upsetting, especially if she knows that she is being "tested", and that the results of the tests will be used to determine whether she ought to be allowed to go home.

3.4. Decision-making Ability

This dimension of competency has received the greatest attention within the specific sphere of consent to, or the refusal of, medical treatment. Most of the medical and bioethical literature on competency confines discussion of the topic to this particular context. An assessment of the competence of a treatment decision may focus either on the process of decision-making (How did the patient come to make this particular decision?) or the outcome (Is the decision itself a "reasonable" one?). Such factors as the patient's understanding of the treatment proposed and the patient's appreciation of the consequences of consenting to or declining the treatment may figure heavily in this sort of competency determination.[12]

In the medical setting competency criteria vary between the minimal "evincing a choice" to a demonstrated appreciation of the risks and benefits attendant upon the choice. Justification for the choice of particular criteria is either not given or seen to be a matter of policy.[13]

In sum, there are at least four different approaches (psychiatric, cognitive, functional and decision-making) to the assessment of competency, each with its own inherent limitations. In the following section we develop a systematic categorization of the practical skills involved in "competence". This categorization, which we refer to as a taxonomy of practical judgment, allows us to begin to critically coordinate the four frameworks, showing when they may or may not be useful in the assessment of a particular competence.

4. COMPETENCE AND PRACTICAL JUDGMENT

In section 2, we mentioned that competence has to do with a demonstrated level of skill measured against some norm. The competent physician is skilful (though not necessarily *extraordinarily* skilful) at her work. The level of skill required, the level of "competent medical practice", is determined by the medical profession as a community.

In section 2 we also stated one underlying supposition of this paper. In speaking of patient or client competence, we are speaking of the individual's ability to maintain, in a practical manner, her values and fulfil her interests. Her "skills" of competence are the skills involved in making practical decisions which affect the course of her life and in acting upon these decisions. The standards against which these skills ought to be evaluated are the patient's own core preferences and values. Broadly speaking, the incompetent physician is one whose level of skilful practice falls below the standards set by her profession. The incompetent patient is one whose decisions (or lack of a decision) frustrate *her own* autonomously held preferences and values.

In addition, we indicated that autonomy, in the functional sense, is about determining the course of one's own life. It involves making practical decisions in real situations, decisions about the sort of life one would like to lead, and with whom. The skills of *practical judgment* serve the value of autonomy. These are the skills that individuals are called on to exercise when they make medical or legal decision affecting their own lives. By "practical judgment" we mean reasoning in the service of action. Individuals use practical judgment to determine *what to do* in concrete circumstances, in light of the things they care about.[14]

Practical judgment can be divided into four related components: belief, deliberation and judgment, preferences, and intention.[15] This categorization readily accords with the experience of making a practical decision. For instance, consider an individual who has suffered a brain injury during a car accident and who, after a long period of cognitive rehabilitation, wishes to regain control of his finances. First, he will have to formulate *accurate beliefs* about his financial circumstances and about his financial abilities: "My assets and income are such, my expenses are such. I'm still having difficulty with calculations, so I may need the assistance of an accountant," etc. Second, he must have the *ability to deliberate* about the concrete options that are available to him and to make choices based on his *preferences and values*. Finally, in order to effectively manage his finances on his own, his *intentions* must generally accord with his decisions. For instance, if he decides he needs the assistance of an accountant, but is unable to formulate the intention to seek one out, then his prudential decision may come to nothing.

4.1. Belief

To demonstrate how each of the four components of practical reason (the formulation of relevant beliefs, deliberation, preferences and values, intention) may bear upon competence in a variety of ways, we give a detailed, case-based exposition of the category of "belief". We conclude this section with brief examples of how the three remaining components of practical judgment may be relevant to a competency determination.

At least four categories of belief may be relevant to a competency determination: (1) none, (2) irrational, (3) incomplete and (4) fluctuating.

4.2. No Beliefs

The patient who has advanced Alzheimer disease may no longer have the ability to formulate any beliefs about his medical care or the proper disposition of his estate. It follows that he is incapable of making decisions in these matters. The neurological basis for the formulation of belief has been irreversibly eroded.

Sometimes it is difficult to determine whether the patient is unable to formulate relevant beliefs or whether he is incapable of communicating them. While on holidays in Florida, Mr. H., a 65-year-old business entrepreneur, suffered a stroke which resulted in marked aphasia and paralysis of the right hand. He could no longer write and verbal expression was limited to a few short expressions: "Yes, but …" "You see …" "No". Mr. H. had several business transactions outstanding. He indicated to his physician his wish to discuss his finances. When presented with contrary propositions written on cards, e.g. "I am able to manage my finances", "I am unable to manage my finances", the physician established Mr. H's belief that he was incapable of managing his finances and that the Public Trustee was the best person to do so for him (over his wife and lawyer). By choosing between contrary propositions, Mr. H. was able to consistently indicate his beliefs. In this instance the assessment of competency (to appoint financial committee) turned on the physician's ability to find an effective way of communicating with the patient, rather than upon the patient's ability to verbally express his beliefs. Had the physician relied on a standard cognitive instrument in his assessment of competency (such as the MSE), Mr. H. would have probably appeared financially incompetent. These tests tend to rely on communicative ability.[16]

4.3. Irrational Beliefs

The psychotic patient who holds the unassailable belief that his medication is poison and therefore refuses it, or the testator who cuts her caring husband out of her Will with the claim that he is literally the devil, may find the competency of their decisions challenged on the basis that they are drawn from irrational beliefs.[17] An irrational belief is one which does not accord with reality and which is held despite overwhelming and ready evidence to the contrary. In this regard it

is important to distinguish between false beliefs and irrational beliefs. An individual who holds false beliefs about the nature of his illness is not necessarily incompetent to make decisions about his course of treatment: presumably, if properly informed, he will come to see the true nature of his illness. However, if he persists in his beliefs despite the information with which he has been presented, then his beliefs may appear not only false but irrational.

"Having no relevant beliefs" and "having irrational beliefs" show, in a concrete manner, how practical judgment may be linked to the value of autonomy. Practical judgment involves reasoning about what to do in light of one's preferences and values and in light of one's circumstances. Competent practical judgment serves the value of autonomy in that a truly autonomous life requires the exercise of such practical skills. Returning to our examples, we can see why "having no ability to formulate relevant beliefs" may lead almost automatically to a determination, say, of testamentary incapacity. Without the ability to formulate specific, relevant beliefs, the individual cannot possibly direct the course of his life. He is no longer oriented to his circumstances and cannot choose a course of action that reflects his own values.

An individual who reasons from irrational beliefs occasioned by a psychotic illness has also at least partially lost the direction of his life. His decisions and actions are guided by persistent beliefs that do not accord with reality, beliefs that he would reject, were he not ill.

Now, too, we can begin to see when a psychiatric diagnosis may be useful in a competency determination. A diagnosis of paranoia, for instance, is not conclusive for a determination of incompetence. It must be shown that the illness is actually affecting the individual's ability to make the decision at hand, say, through a distortion of relevant belief.

4.4. An Incomplete Set of Relevant Beliefs

Mrs. W. has a lengthy history of Parkinson's disease. Recently she has begun to suffer from periodic hallucinations and delusions, perhaps resulting from the medication used to control the symptoms of her disease. When lucid, she shows an active interest in her treatment. Recently the illness has affected Mrs. W's ability to keep in mind the intricacies of her treatment. She is no longer able to formulate and keep in mind a complete set of specific beliefs related to the nature and purpose of her various medications. Still, with her daughter's assistance, she is able to maintain directive control over her treatment. Her daughter monitors changes in dosage, and assists her mother with decisions related to major changes in treatment. Thus incompleteness of belief does not necessarily affect Mrs. W.'s ability to maintain directive control over her treatment.

In contrast, incompleteness of belief does prevent Mr. P. from choosing an attorney. Mr. P. is suffering from an advanced progressive dementia, probably Pick's disease. In the early stages of his illness, Mr. P. quit his work, began to neglect his personal care and spent recklessly. As a result, his spouse Mrs. P. made informal arrangements which prevent Mr. P. from writing cheques or making major purchases. She gives him an allowance which he spends on cigarettes and in the Italian cafes of the city. During an assessment of his ability to appoint a power of attorney (sought by Mrs. P.) Mr. P. showed that his general beliefs about his assets and own abilities were accurate. He states that he owned three properties and that he needed help in their management. However, he was unable to formulate a belief as to who might serve as his attorney. On this he remained persistently silent, even when presented with viable options. Mr. P. was found incompetent to appoint a Power of Attorney, in part because incompleteness of belief went to the heart of the requisite skills. A key consideration in the appointment of an attorney is the ability to form beliefs about suitable candidates.

Incompleteness of belief may or may not provide sufficient reason for a determination of incompetence. According to the decision (or set of decisions at hand), certain beliefs may be more central than others which are nevertheless relevant. For instance, beliefs about one's own surgical abilities may be largely irrelevant to one's decision to undergo surgery. The ability to formulate relevant beliefs about one's own financial abilities, however, may play a key role in determining one's ability to assign a Power of Attorney.

4.5. Fluctuating Belief

Related difficulties arise with fluctuating belief. With regard to a certain category of decisions, fluctuating belief need not result in incompetence. We refer to these as temporally discreet decisions, like making changes to a Will or deciding whether or not to accept a specific course of medical treatment. Consider Mrs. L. who, in the advanced stages of a dementing illness, wishes to alter the contents of her Will. Several of her beneficiaries have failed to remain in contact with her since the original Will was drafted in 1980. Her lawyer notes down her suggestions, but out of concern for her forgetfulness and fluctuating lucidity (Mrs. L. is most confused in the morning, better toward evening), the lawyer decides to have her testamentary capacity assessed. Towards evening, we discover that Mrs. L. is unable to recall the contents of her Will, but recognizes her Will and its contents when it is presented to her. Moreover, having the document in hand, which acts as a kind of memorative cue, provides the occasion for her to indicate her new preferences: "I haven't seen Mr. D. in years. He doesn't deserve $5000, give it to my grandchildren," etc. By reviewing the document with her on several evenings, the interviewers establish the consistency and reasonableness of her preferences.

There are periods during the day when Mrs. L. is too disoriented to undertake such a task, and without the document before her she is unable to recount her beliefs about who should benefit and why. Still, because having testamentary capacity is only necessary at the time when one executes a Will, fluctuating ability does not prevent Mrs. L. from making competent changes. One has only to choose the right time of day and to provide mnemonic cues. Once these helped her to orient herself to the contents of her estate and her beneficiaries, Mrs. L. was able to make decisions which consistently reflected her preferences.

The key here is the temporal discreteness of the set of decisions Mrs. L. must make and account for, in order to demonstrate her testamentary capacity. It is enough that she showed ability in this regard at the time of execution of the new Will. In other instances, where competency refers to some sort of *ongoing ability,* fluctuating belief may severely compromise that ability. Mr. S. is a 78-year-old retired artist who recognizes that his short-term memory is beginning to fail. He misplaces bills and forgets to cash pension cheques, which are left to accumulate in a dresser drawer. His niece Ms. B. offers to help with bill payments and bank deposits. They consult a lawyer who advises Mr. S. to assign his niece a power of attorney specific to everyday financial transactions. Bills and cheques continue to arrive at Mr. S.'s house, where Ms. B. collects them bi-weekly.

Mr. S.'s short-term memory continues to deteriorate. The family physician arranges for a psycho-geriatric assessment. Diagnosis is of a major depression, for which Mr. S. receives treatment as an outpatient. During this time he begins to call Ms. B. in a panic late at night, demanding to know what she has done with his pension cheques. At first she patiently explains that she has deposited them in his bank account, according to his instructions. Relieved, he apologizes. However the calls persist. In the end Ms. B. refuses to continue acting as Mr. S's attorney. In this instance fluctuating belief makes it impossible for Mr. S. to maintain an effective working relationship with his attorney. He regularly forgets what she is doing for him and panics. He cannot effectively direct her. Because he can no longer manage his everyday finances on his own, and because he can no longer maintain directive control over his estate, Mr. P. is found financially incompetent.

The above phenomenological exploration of one category of the taxonomy of practical judgment—belief—begins to highlight the specific applicability of each of the four traditional frameworks for the evaluation of competence. A diagnosis of paranoia, for instance, may be applicable when it is shown that the illness occasions irrational beliefs. However, these must be irrational beliefs that result in a decision or

course of action which, however valid, the individual would recognize as not her own, were she well. Reliance on instruments for the assessment of cognitive ability or decision-making ability may fail to take into account the question as to whether an incomplete set of beliefs or fluctuating belief go to the heart of the competence in question.

To conclude this section, we now introduce the three remaining components of the taxonomy: decision-making, preferences and values, and intention. Each of these could be given the same detailed exposition that we have devoted to "belief". For instance, an individual may be unable to formulate intentions with regard to seeking medical treatment, though he has *decided* to do so. Alternatively, his intentions may fluctuate dramatically from day to day. A complete exposition of the taxonomy, however, would result in a paper of unacceptable length. Instead, we give brief case examples that illustrate the importance of the three remaining components of practical judgment.

4.6. Decision-making Ability

Mrs. K., a 75-year-old widow, is in hospital for treatment of a broken hip resulting from a fall. She has two sons, Don and Phil. Two years ago, she assigned her eldest son Don a Durable Power of Attorney. Since then Phil has frequently accused Don of neglecting their mother. For instance, he claims that Don should have used some of Mrs. K.'s savings to hire a homemaker to assist her, and that, had he done so, she wouldn't have fallen at home. Don claims that his mother cannot afford such an expense. Now that she is ready to be discharged from hospital, Mrs. K. is presented with two options. Don wants her to move in with him and his family. Phil has arranged for her to move into a nursing home where he feels she will receive good care. When she speaks with Don, she agrees to his proposal; when she speaks to Phil, she agrees with him. When the discharge planner sees her alone to ask her what she really wants, she lowers her head and is unable to answer. Despite several attempts, the discharge planner receives no response from her as to her preference. Mrs. K is equally attached to her sons and is emotionally devastated by the conflict between them. Her inability to make a choice is not related to her having certain cognitive deficits. Rather her ability to choose has been overwhelmed by family conflicts.

4.7. Preferences and Values

Mr. C. is an elderly individual who has a long history of bipolar affective disorder which has resulted in several hospitalizations. Recently, after spending recklessly during a manic phase of his illness, Mr. C. arranged for his sister to assume informal control of his finances. Mr. C.'s financial decisions fluctuate according to mood swings associated with his illness. Still, he is able to protect himself from reckless spending during manic phases through informal arrangements with his sister. His illness does not affect his instrumental ability to make financial decisions—he is still able to make specific, effective decisions about how and where to spend his money. However, the illness temporarily distorts the preferences or values that guide his decisions. The issue here is not one of "cognitive deficits" but of the distortion of fundamental preferences and values, a facet in his life that Mr. C. is able to recognize and counter.

4.8. Intention

During an evaluation of his financial competency, Mr. W. indicates to his psychiatrist that he has decided to build a tunnel from Toronto to Montreal. He claims that such a tunnel will bolster the Canadian economy, that it will serve as a good bomb shelter and that he has more than enough funds to complete the project. The psychiatrist finds him financially incompetent and control of his finances reverts to the Public Trustee. Still, though Mr. W. may have actually decided to build such a tunnel, perhaps he had no intention of actually carrying out the plan. The decision itself may have posed no threat to his finances, which he had managed well hitherto. His character might provide an appropriate context for interpreting such pronouncements: does he have, for instance, a tendency to dream up quixotic plans without acting on them?

5. SOME NORMATIVE CONSIDERATIONS UNDERLYING THE TAXONOMY

To this juncture, our analysis of "competence" refers entirely to practical abilities possessed by individuals. Competence, however, is not only related to intrinsic abilities. It is also related to resources available in the community. These points figure in the discussion below.

5.1. The Normative Weighting of "Relevant Belief" and "Irrational Belief"

Mrs. G., an elderly widow who has lived on her own for a number of years, is hospitalized for treatment of a fractured hip resulting from a fall at home. In-hospital rehabilitation has restored some of her functional ability, but she shows some cognitive impairment. Moreover, an occupational therapy assessment has documented she is unable to get to the toilet or cook without assistance. Mrs. G. cannot afford live-in help. In effect, like many elderly women in Canada, she is impoverished:[18] she has no savings, has lived in government housing for a number of years and gets by on a meagre pension.

Out of concern that Mrs. G. may be at considerable risk at home, of falling while bathing, or of setting a fire while attempting to cook, the physician recommends that she consider placement in a nursing home. Mrs. G. denies that the OT assessment had demonstrated serious risk and demands to go home. In her opinion, the risks mentioned are not of overriding importance. Both the physician and the occupational therapist feel that Mrs. G.'s decision is irrational. She persistently denies the seriousness of the risks she will face. On these grounds they decide to question her competency to choose her place of residence.[19]

Application of the taxonomy outlined above may justify the team's conclusion. Mrs. G.'s persistent, unshakeable belief that the risks attendant upon her decision to go home are insignificant appears irrational. She persists in believing something despite overwhelming and ready evidence to the contrary. Irrational beliefs are obviously compromising her ability to make a competent decision about where she will live.

What counts as "relevant" or as a "relevant belief," however, depends upon what we are concerned with. The team is concerned with risk and safety. They begin with the normative presumption that the patient ought to want to avoid risks to her physical health.[20] As a result, Mrs. G.'s persistent denial of the risk appears "irrational". Still, the affective tie of "being at home" might be given its due in relation to the team's preoccupation with risk. For many elderly, "home" is a sustaining place where habits and abilities are vitally maintained. Mrs. G. may have an unarticulated sense that the loss of her home through removal to an unfamiliar environment is more of a threat to her integrity than the risks with which the team is preoccupied.[21]

The latter remark indicates another shortcoming of the taxonomy, indeed of most assessment procedures or instruments. So much depends upon articulated belief. Say that Mrs. G. evaluates the risks of being at home as insignificant *in relation to* an inchoate sense that being at home is really what matters to her. If she is able to articulate this for herself and explain it to the team, her evaluation of the risks may appear more reasonable. If she is unable to articulate her beliefs in this regard, even to herself, the team's evaluation may hold sway.

The conflict is significant. Those who designate that beliefs about risk to physical health are of overriding importance are also those who perform the competency assessment. If Mrs. G. is found incompetent, she may lose her right to choose her place of residence.

5.2. Competency and the Allocation of Resources

> Decisions about the distribution of resources and risks reflect both prevailing values and power structures. In a society where power relations are unequal it is inevitable that risks are ... unfairly distributed.[22]

So far we have indicated some of the abilities the individual must have in order to demonstrate her competency, abilities related to the formulation and maintenance of belief. Competency, however, is not only related to intrinsic ability but also to functional supports available in the community. The risks that Mrs. G. is being asked to appreciate have to do with her impoverished circumstances. If she could afford live-in help, or if long-term, around-the-clock community services were in place, the risks that worry the team would no longer exist. As a result the perceived justification for questioning her competence (to decide her place of residence) would disappear.

The taxonomy has nothing to say about the circumstances within which an individual may find her competence questioned. Usually we do not question the competence of another adult to make personal care decisions. This is in line with the law's presumption that individuals are competent to care for themselves, unless something happens to indicate otherwise, some failure or other. But such failures may equally suggest questions related to the fair distribution of social resources. In the case under discussion, poverty and its attendant risks may lead to the questioning of the patient's competence to decide her place of residence, simply because she wants to go home. Her impoverishment, when linked to the team's concern with physical safety, leads to a questioning of the "competence" of her decision.

Acknowledgements

The authors gratefully acknowledge the financial support of the Social Sciences and Humanities Research Council of Canada. We would also like to thank the three reviewers of the manuscript for their incisive comments, patience and encouragement.

Notes

1. Working Group on Legal Issues. Legal Issues in the Care of Mentally Impaired Elderly Persons: Competence, Surrogate Management and the Protection of Rights. *Canada's Mental Health* 1978;26:6–11. See also Culver C, Gert B. The inadequacy of incompetence. *The Milbank Quarterly* 1990;68:619–643.

2. Freedman B. Competence, marginal or otherwise. *International Journal of Law and Psychiatry* 1981;4:53–72. See also Applebaum P, Grisso T. Assessing patients' capacity to consent to treatment. *N Engl J Med* 1988;319:1635–1638.

3. Dworkin, G. *The Theory and Practice of Autonomy*. Cambridge: Cambridge University Press, 1989.

4. The competent patient, too, is responsible for his decisions. However, one major difference between the two contexts is that in medicine the decision primarily affects the patient, whereas in law the decision, say, to contract, primarily affects both parties to the contract.

5. Working Group on Legal Issues: 7.

6. Alexander G. Legal perspectives: Issues of competency. In: Lesnoff-Caravaglia G, ed. *Values, Ethics and Aging*. New York: Human Sciences Press, 1985: 62–78.

7. Macklin R. Philosophical conceptions of rationality and psychiatric notions of competency. *Synthese* 1983;57:205–224.

8. Meyers D. Personal autonomy and the paradox of feminine socialization. *The Journal of Philosophy* 1987;84:619–628. See also Buchanan A, Brock R. Deciding for others. *The Milbank Quarterly* Suppl. 2 1986;64:17–94.

9. Macklin: 210–224.

10. Tancredi L. The mental status examination. *Generations* 1987;11:24–31.

11. Zuckerman C. Conclusions and guidelines for practice. *Gerontologist* 1987;27:67–73.

12. Ontario's *Mental Health Act,* R. S, O., 1980.

13. Freedman: 65–72.

14. Robins M. Practical reasoning, commitment, and rational action. *The American Philosophical Quarterly* 1984;21:55–68.

15. Aristotle (Apostle H. trans.). *Nicomachean Ethics*. Grinnell: The Peripatetic Press, 1975. See also Audi R. Intending, intentional action and desire. In: Marks J, ed. *The Ways of Desire*. Chicago: Precedent Publishing, 1986: 17–37.

16. All scenarios in this article are compiled from a number of cases at the Competency Clinic, Baycrest Centre for Geriatric Care.

17. Culver and Gert argue that one may be justified in overruling an irrational decision made by a competent patient. Their claim, however, depends upon a sharp distinction between rationality and competence. They define competence as, "… the understanding and appreciation of information given during a properly conducted consent process." But "understanding" and "appreciation" depend on the ability to formulate relevant, rational beliefs. Thus a notion of rationality is already implicit in their definition of competence. Culver C, Gert B: 621–627.

18. Chappell N. Social policy and the elderly. In: Marshall V, ed. *Aging in Canada: Social Perspectives*. Don Mills: Fitzhenry and Whiteside, 1980: 35–42. See also Gutman, G. The elderly at home and in retirement housing. Ibid: 189–190.

19. Pepper-Smith R, Harvey W. Competency assessments in discharge planning and the question of intergenerational justice. *Westminster Affairs* 1990;3:3–5.

20. This presumption is reinforced by a legal obligation to discharge the patient to a "safe" environment.

21. Langer E. The illusion of incompetence. In: Perlmuter LC, Monty RM, eds. *Choice and Perceived Control*. Hillsdale: Lawrence Elbaum Associates, 1979: 301–313.

22. Brearly C. *Risk and Social Work*. London: Routledge and Kegan Paul, 1982: 51.

Mental Competence and Value:
The Problem of Normativity in the
Assessment of Decision-Making Capacity

Louis C. Charland

THE DUAL NATURE OF COMPETENCE

The right of an individual to make his or her own medical treatment decisions goes to the heart of what it means to be an autonomous individual. However, there exist circumstances where that right needs to be curtailed. This can occur when an individual is deemed mentally incompetent to make his or her own decisions. Children below a certain age are usually considered incompetent,

Charland, L.C., "Mental Competence and Value: The Problem of Normativity in the Assessment of Decision-Making Capacity" from *Psychiatry, Psychology and the Law* 8(2), pp. 135–145, © 2001 Taylor & Francis. Reprinted by permission.

as are individuals subject to medical or psychiatric conditions that compromise decision-making capacity. Judgments regarding mental competence are often based on special operationalised standards developed to assess it. This article is about the nature of those standards, why they must incorporate elements of value and rationality, and how to reconcile this normative dimension of competence with the requirement that assessments of competence be sufficiently objective. The problem is not only theoretical, but also practical. For in the end, when competence is assessed, either individual freedom is protected or it is violated. You cannot get much more practical about the ethics of autonomy than that.

It is reasonable to require that standards designed to assess competence be objective. Similar tests should yield similar judgments in like cases. The standards employed should be sufficiently objective to be replicable in a manner that yields consistent results across like cases. Anything less would be unjust to those whose competence is at issue. The problem is that objectivity of this sort is both difficult to formulate theoretically and difficult to realise practically. Aside from the fact that existing laws relating to competence vary across jurisdictions, which implies that general criteria must be flexible, there is the deeper problem of how to formulate objective standards for something that is inherently normative. Not surprisingly, standards for competence tend to be extremely open-ended. They tend also to vacillate between specifying what competence is and prescribing what it should be. This is not surprising, since competence is neither pure description nor pure evaluation. It is rather a mixture of both. As one commentator explains: "a psychiatrist may give expert testimony, in his capacity as a trained observer, about a person's competence seen as a factual matter, and the judge may or may not give this testimony practical effect in deciding how we ought to treat that person."[1] Thus in the former case the issue is whether the individual is competent, while in the latter it is whether the individual *should* be considered competent. The dual nature of the concept of competence raises special problems for the requirement that assessments of competence be objective.

One approach to the problem of objectivity is essentially to try to define it away. The strategy is to limit assessment to so-called cognitive capacities and mechanisms alone; for example, the ability to store and retrieve information, to process information, and to appropriately identify what count as the relevant pieces of information. Very basically, the capacities involved are memory, reasoning, and understanding. Many accounts of competence also mention the notion of appreciation. Appreciation consists in an individual's ability to apply his or her current understanding of a given medical condition and its treatment options to him- or herself. It is one thing to understand what schizophrenia is, but quite another to recognise that this information applies to you.

Most existing tests for competence are designed to assess abilities such as those mentioned above. The fact that these abilities are characterised as cognitive is usually deemed essential to the objectivity of the proposed operationalised standards for assessing them. Defining competence in exclusively cognitive terms thus provides a strategy for addressing the problem of objectivity. So defined, competence has little or nothing to do with value. That makes it easier to view it as an objective commodity. Whether or not such a vision is ethically desirable, it is in any case empirically inadequate. The reason is that decision-making capacity is inextricably normative. There is no such thing as mental competence without value, and normative considerations associated with value cannot be eliminated from the assessment of decision-making capacity. Moreover, the manner in which values figure in competence is not gratuitous. Simply having values is not enough. A certain kind of rationality is also required.

There are a few important precedents that address the relationship between mental competence and value.[2] They are largely the work of philosophers, and two have had an impact far beyond the confines of what is normally considered the province of philosophy. One is referred to in a major legal case.[3] The other is now a matter of United States government policy.[4] Sadly, both initiatives have gone largely unnoticed in academic philosophical circles. It is time to introduce these developments in the philosophy of mental competence to a wider audience.

Unfortunately, the philosophical literature on competence is riddled with problems. Its diverse strands form a tangled web of mutually incompatible terms and distinctions combined in arguments that regularly miss their targets. Introducing two distinctions will help to make some exegetical sense of this terrain. The first distinction is between putative decisions and actual decisions. A putative decision is one that is currently being entertained but has not yet been made. An actual decision is one that is no longer being entertained but has been made. The second distinction is between internal as opposed to external rationality. External rationality has to do with the outcome of actual decisions. Internal rationality has to do with the coherence of putative decisions within a set of values and beliefs.

The assessment of decision-making capacity is normative because value and rationality are involved. Specifically, mental competence is normative because it involves assessing the internal rationality of a putative decision against a background set of values and beliefs. Therefore, the idea that competence can be entirely objective is misguided, and the attempt to downplay or ignore the role of value in competence is wrongheaded. So is the strategy of restricting competence and its standards to what is purely cognitive and mechanistic. None of this means giving up on objectivity entirely. As is common in this area, objectivity is provided by insisting on rigorous operationalised measures for all standards and tests. Together with third-party consensus and agreement, this is about as much as can be reasonably expected in this domain.

RECOGNISABLE REASONS

In a landmark publication, the philosopher Benjamin Freedman states that competence requires alluding to "an individual's own value system."[5] Making value a component of competence invites the question of whether rationality might also play a role in competence. Freedman

explicitly links value and rationality. He alludes to both in his discussion of recognisable reasons, his proposed criterion for competency.

Along with many others, Freedman believes that understanding and appreciation are necessary for competence. However, according to him they are not sufficient. In this respect he departs from established tradition. According to Freedman, in order to be deemed competent, an individual must not only understand and appreciate the nature and consequences of the decision at hand, the individual must also be able to provide recognisable reasons for it.[6] Freedman initially flirts with the idea of calling those reasons "rational," but eventually opts for the less redundant formulation that they be termed "recognisable." He does so partly in order to accommodate the fact that an assessor can recognise the legitimacy of a subject's reasons for a decision without having to share or agree with those beliefs.

Recognisable reasons take the form of arguments. Thus for a reason to be recognisable, "it must contain acceptable premises and a conclusion related to those premises."[7] The obvious objection to this proposal, which Freedman anticipates, is that it risks being overly paternalistic: anybody whose reasons you do not deem recognisable will on those grounds be deemed incompetent by you. To remedy the problem, Freedman qualifies what counts as a recognisable reason. He writes: "Since we wish to give latitude to an individual's own value system, one which we do not necessarily share, it is not required that the conclusion 'follow' from the premises."[8] The point is that reasons do not have to logically *entail* the decision they are reasons for in order to be considered recognisable. It is sufficient that they be capable of providing a strong justification for that decision.

In order to be considered recognisable, reasons must at least be relevant to the decision they are reasons for. But relevant in what light? No doubt, reasons are considered relevant to a decision partly according to the values and standards of those assessing competence. However, more importantly, the reasons must also be relevant in light of the individual's own value system. Conflict between the two standards is of course possible. What is unclear is how to resolve it, and in whose favor. On this point Freedman is almost entirely silent. All we are told is that an individual's reasons can be deemed recognisable by others who do not necessarily share that person's values. This, it seems reasonable, is what it means to give "latitude" to an individual's own value system. The proposal is admittedly vague. But it is at least capable of satisfying an important kind of legal consideration. For example, blood transfusions are contrary to the religious value system held by adherents of the Jehovah's Witness faith. Nevertheless, in some jurisdictions the courts have recognised the right of Jehovah's Witnesses to make such choices, even if they result in death.[9] The religious reasons for such refusals were deemed sufficiently strong to count as recognisable reasons even though the presiding judge was not a Jehovah's Witness and probably did not share or agree with that value system.

There are two other features of Freedman's account that are worth noting here. First, he claims that it is process-centered. By this he means that it is concerned with what "goes into the decision, not merely with the result."[10] Second, he claims it involves a reversal of the traditional roles ascribed to information and competence. He writes:

> Traditionally, it was thought that the ascertainment of competence was an issue which needed to be decided prior to the transmittal of information. To the contrary, I believe that information is prior to competence, in that competence includes, but extends beyond, that the person involved be able to allow the informing process to enter into his decision-making in a substantial way. He must be capable of utilizing the information provided in formulating his reasons ... [C]ompetence is primarily concerned with the manner in which the person uses the information.[11]

Both of these points are worth pondering. Consider first the claim that competence is process-centered.[12] The idea is that the actual consequences of a decision should not be a factor in assessing competence. It is not necessary for the decision to have been made and for its consequences to have been assessed in order to determine whether or not the individual is competent to make that decision. Dealing with the putative decision, one that remains to be made but has not yet been made, is sufficient. Here it is important to keep in mind that an assessment of competence is required in order to determine whether a person is even capable of making a decision. Competence needs to be assessed before a decision is made. Obviously, then, the actual decision a person actually makes cannot be what is assessed for competence.

Competence then has to do with our capacity to make decisions and that is independent of the consequences of the actual decisions we make. Now in evaluating the consequences of a decision we may wish to inquire into its rationality. But the term is ambiguous. On the one hand, there is a sense in which the rationality of a decision can be assessed before it is made. On the other hand, there is a sense in which the rationality of a decision can be assessed only after it has been made. In assessing the rationality of an actual decision, we often want to look at its consequences. Call this "the external sense of 'rationality'." Rationality in that sense requires appealing to what goes on outside the mind, so to speak. It requires looking beyond the internal mental processes involved in reasoning to the actual external consequences of decisions once they have been made.

According to Freedman, it is possible to assess the rationality of a putative decision without looking at its actual consequences or results. Yet he also wants to maintain that rationality somehow is a component of competence and he does refer to rationality in his account of recognisable reasons. Call this "the internal sense of 'rationality'." Internal rationality has to do with whether the putative decision an individual is entertaining coheres with his or her system of values in a manner that satisfies the recognisable reasons criterion. Note that while this conception of competence refers to the content of the putative decision involved, the assessment of competence is restricted to the internal processes that underlie decision-making and does not require reference to the external consequences of that decision. As indicated in the passage quoted above, the recognisable reasons model requires alluding to the content of decisions. Competence then cannot be assessed without alluding to content in that sense. The requirement is sensible, since it would appear to be impossible to assess the reasons for a decision without knowing what that decision is about. There are, however, some who seem committed to denying this, as we shall see in the following section.

To sum up, Freedman's recognisable reasons account of competence is as interesting as it is cryptic. Nevertheless his strategy is clear. First, assessing competence requires inquiring into an individual's ability to make a putative decision by getting him or her to provide reasons for that decision. Those reasons are specified in the form of an argument with premises and conclusion. Second, assessing the internal rationality of a putative decision requires that we interpret that decision and the reasons for it against the background of the individual's own values and not simply our own. Third, competence is a matter of process. Fourth, competence does not require alluding to the consequences of the actual decision that is made, nor does it require an evaluation of its external rationality. All that is required for competence is internal rationality.

AN ENDURING SET OF VALUES

In a classic discussion on the topic of competence, Alan Buchanan and Dan Brock say quite a bit more about the place of value in mental competence than does Freedman. While Freedman talks of a system of values, Buchanan and Brock refer instead to "a *set of values* or *conception of what is good.*"[13] Elsewhere they speak of "relatively stable values or a conception of the good life."[14] At times they also speak of an individual's "underlying and enduring values."[15] One virtue of their account is that it is far more explicit than Freedman's about

how value fits into competence. To see this, we need first to review their overall account of competence.

According to Buchanan and Brock, competence is a threshold concept. Either you are competent or you are not. Like virtually everyone else working in the area, they also maintain that competence is decision-relative. Thus "a person may be competent to make a particular decision at a particular time, under certain circumstances, but incompetent to make another decision or even the same decision, under different conditions."[16] Buchanan and Brock's theory of competence has three components: (1) understanding and communication; (2) reasoning and deliberation; (3) a set of values or conception of the good. Understanding is said to consist in part of basic conceptual, linguistic and cognitive abilities. It requires "the capacities to receive, process, and make available for use the information relevant to particular decisions."[17] As the following passage states, it also involves the notion of appreciation.

> Understanding is not merely a formal or abstract process, but also requires the ability to appreciate the nature and meaning of potential alternatives—what it would be like and "feel" like to be in possible future states and to undergo various experiences—and to integrate this appreciation into one's decision making."[18]

The capacity for appreciation is one reason why competence requires value. For otherwise how could an individual evaluate the nature and personal meaning of the alternatives he or she faces? You cannot rank and weigh alternatives unless you have a set of values. Here then is one reason why a set of values is required for competence.

For much the same reasons, values are also required for reasoning and deliberation. These capacities "require the capacity to draw inferences about the consequences of making a certain choice and to compare alternative outcomes based on how they further one's good or promote one's ends."[19] Of course, those two subcomponents also rely on understanding and the information it provides. Buchanan and Brock say they require "applying the decision-maker's values."[20] This is because in order to deliberate and reason about alternatives we need some way to rank and attach weights to those alternatives. Without values, that task is impossible. Therefore, on the whole, competence requires a set of values or a conception of the good. This is necessary "in order to be able to evaluate particular outcomes as benefits or harms, goods or evils, and to assign different relative weight or importance to them."[21]

Buchanan and Brock are careful to qualify the sense in which competence requires values. They note:

> [S]ufficient internal consistency and stability over time in the values relative to a particular decision are needed to yield and enable pursuit of a decision outcome; for example, a depressed patient subject to frequent mood changes may repeatedly consent to electroconvulsive treatment, but then change his or her mind before treatment is carried out.[22]

The point is that "sufficient value stability is needed to permit, at the very least, a decision that can be stated and adhered to over the course of its discussion, initiation, and implementation."[23] This is not meant to deny the fact that personal values change and evolve over time, or that people undergo radical changes in some of their most cherished desires and preferences. Neither does it rule out the fact that individuals may be ambivalent about which values they hold. No doubt, there will always be difficult cases and that is something this account needs to deal with. Changes in values in radical end-of-life circumstances are likely to be one problem area. Mental disorders of certain kinds are another. Nevertheless, the fact remains that in many less complex circumstances the requirement that an individual's values be minimally consistent and relatively stable is reasonable. So "competence does not require a fully consistent set of goals, much less a detailed 'lifeplan' to cover all contingencies."[24] All that is required are that

the values in question be relatively stable and minimally consistent.

Like Freedman, Buchanan and Brock want to give latitude to an individual's own values when assessing competence. They also grant that conflicts can arise between an individual's stated values and the values of those appointed to assess their competence. For example, people can sometimes entertain decisions that appear contrary to their own self-interests and which, if enacted, would compromise their well-being. In such cases, it is important to weigh the need to protect an individual's well-being against his or her right to self-determination. Among the difficulties is the risk of setting too high a standard for competence and ruling persons incompetent who ought not to be declared so. There is also the risk of setting too low a standard of competence and thereby failing to protect individual well-being. In the end, the challenge is to avoid succumbing to either of these two errors.[25] This sort of balancing act is impossible without some appeal to value. On the one hand, there are the values of the individual whose competence is being assessed. And, on the other hand, there are the values of those assessing competence.

It should be evident by now that there are important parallels between Buchanan and Brock, and Freedman on the place of value in competence. The parallels in the case of rationality are not as clear and there the exegetical situation is more complicated. Buchanan and Brock argue that so-called outcome accounts of competence need to be rejected. They characterise those as ones that "look solely to the content or outcome of the decision—for example, the standard that the choice be a reasonable one, or be what other reasonable or rational persons would chose."[26] On the face of it, this would appear to be tantamount to a rejection of Freedman's model, since it appeals both to the content of decisions and to what counts as recognisable reasons for those decisions. The problem is that Buchanan and Brock appear to have conflated the notions of content and outcome. They also appear to have conflated external and internal rationality. Yet, like Freedman, they also claim to be committed to an account of competence given in terms of process. To sort things out, we look first at the alleged disagreement over content.

PROBLEMS WITH CONTENT

We have seen that according to Freedman assessing competence requires alluding to the content of the putative decision involved. This is because competence is a matter of how an individual uses information and this is impossible to determine without adverting to what the decision is about. Like Freedman, Buchanan and Brock want to embrace a process account of competence. However, because of the stand they take on the issue of content, their account appears to be incompatible with Freedman's. Thus, in stating the overall aim of their project they say their intention is "to focus primarily on the process of reasoning, not on the content of the decision itself."[27] I believe that Buchanan and Brock are mistaken in thinking they need to reject the notion of content entirely: their account requires a notion of content for just the same reasons as Freedman's. If this is right, then there is more consensus in the literature on competence than even its proponents seem to have realised. However, in order to set the record straight we will have to introduce two additional players, Charles Culver and Bernard Gert.

Recall the fact that Freedman rejects the idea that the actual results of decisions should play a role in determining competence. A version of that condition is the view that someone is competent to consent to something if in consenting he or she achieves a reasonable outcome.[28] On their side, Culver and Gert also reject the idea that the results or outcomes of decisions should be determining factors in competence. As we saw, so do Buchanan and Brock. So everyone seems to be in agreement. Unfortunately, in rejecting the outcome of a decision as an operative factor in competence, Culver and Gert also introduce complications that confuse the overall picture of how decisional content works its way into a process account of competence.

Culver and Gert propose the concept of a kind of decision, which they sharply distinguish from an actual decision.[29] According to them,

competence has to do with the former and not the latter. They propose the following definition of competence:

> [A] patient is competent to decide whether to consent or refuse treatment if she adequately understands and appreciates the information given to her during a properly conducted consent process. This definition of competence does not include within it any reference to whether the patient *decided* to consent to or refuse, nor does it indicate whether the patient's consent or refusal seems, on either subjective or objective grounds, to be wise or foolish, rational or irrational, impulsive or deliberate.[30]

In other words, competence is "determined by the ability of the patient to understand and appreciate all of the relevant information, but independent of the actual decision the patient makes."[31] It is a matter of an individual's "ability to carry out certain mental tasks."[32]

It is now possible to say why Buchanan and Brock do not need to abandon the notion of content in espousing a process account of competence and why, like Freedman, they need a notion of content to ground their account of competence. The reason for the trouble is that they fail to distinguish a putative decision from an actual one. A putative decision is one you are entertaining and deliberating about but have not yet made. An actual decision is one you have made. A putative decision cannot have an *actual* outcome or result, only an actual decision can. However, a putative decision can have an *expected* outcome or result.[33] But in order for this to be the case, the putative decision must have a content in this sense: a semantic interpretation that specifies what the decision is about. The content of a decision in this semantic sense is distinct from its outcome. Therefore, Buchanan and Brock are mistaken to conflate the two. They are also mistaken that a process account of competence can do without alluding to the semantic content of decisions. It follows that in so far as competence is meant to be process-centered and requires content, there are no incompatibilities between the account provided by Buchanan and Brock and the account provided by Freedman.

Where does this leave Culver and Gert? They agree that only an actual decision can have an outcome or result. They also agree with the others that the actual results or outcomes of decisions should not play a role in competence. On the matter of content, however, the situation is more problematic. In fact, they never mention content. Their focus is the notion of a kind of decision as opposed to a particular individual decision.[34] They depart from tradition in selecting a different unit of analysis for the theory of competence. Unfortunately, their alternative does not appear to be satisfactory.

KINDS OF DECISIONS

Culver and Gert provide the following characterisation of what it means to speak of a kind of decision:

> [T]wo decisions are of the same kind with regard to competence when a person who understands and appreciates the pertinent information relevant to deciding in one way—for example, consenting to a treatment—also understands and appreciates the pertinent information relevant to deciding in the other—refusing the very same treatment … [I]f we accept that a patient is competent to make a kind of decision—for example, he is competent to consent to a treatment in specific circumstances—then we must accept that he is competent to refuse the very same treatment in these same circumstances.[35]

No argument is given in favor of this characterisation. The authors simply assert that it is common to many standard accounts. Maybe so, but which ones? It is certainly inconsistent with at least the accounts of Buchanan and Brock, and Freedman. For according to them, competence is decision-relative in quite a strict sense. Recall that "a person may be competent to make a particular decision at a particular time, under

certain circumstances, but incompetent to make another decision or even the same decision, under different conditions."[36] Decision relativity is incompatible with Culver and Gert's notion of a kind of decision. Since decision relativity is apparently here to stay, it is the notion of a kind of decision that will have to be abandoned.

First, note that what is involved in decision relativity is a particular instance of a decision, not a general kind of decision. Second, simply to assert that consent and refusal are the same kind of decision seems to beg the question whether they should be treated as such. In fact, Buchanan and Brock explicitly distinguish the two. They argue that "consent to a low-risk life-saving procedure by an otherwise healthy individual should require only a minimal level of competence, but refusal of that same procedure by such an individual should require the highest level of competence."[37] What varies here is not simply the level of competence required, with the kind decision remaining unchanged. Indeed, the reason the level of competence must vary is that the two decisions and their associated conditions are not the same. They are in fact two different particular decisions, not one general kind of decision. Thus, to declare a *priori* that the conditions for treatment and refusal decisions are the same is to beg the issue at hand. Considered individually, such decisions commonly have different conditions associated with them. Therefore, to focus on kinds of decisions as opposed to individual particular decisions as Culver and Gert suggest is not only incompatible with the spirit of a decision-relative account of competence, it also begs the issue at hand. Consent and refusal are not the same kind of decision. The reason is that they have different expected consequences and associated risks and benefits. This is sufficient to count them as different decisions.

A related problem with the notion of a kind of decision proposed by Culver and Gert is that it is semantically empty. As we have seen, when you deliberate or reason about an individual particular decision there needs to be something you are deliberating about, a specified semantic content. However, Culver and Gert never mention content. In their discussion they are concerned with the case where an individual is being asked to consent to or to refuse treatment. But if the unit of analysis being assessed is a kind of decision, then what is being assessed is this general kind of decision to consent to or to refuse that kind of treatment, not a particular decision to choose or refuse a particular treatment. Decisions of the latter sort are concrete enough. But ones of the former sort appear strangely empty. They do not have a specific semantic content. How then can competence be assessed? The answer is, it cannot. If Culver and Gert are right, then the basic unit of analysis in a competency assessment really turns out to be a sort of abstract place-holder without any specified semantic content. What after all is the semantic content of a kind of decision? What is such a decision about? Suppose a treatment X is involved. Then what is at issue in competency assessment on Culver and Gert's account is this: deciding to consent-to-or-refuse X. But the true object of a competency determination is more fine-grained and concrete than this. It is a particular decision to do a particular thing at a given time. I see no alternative but to conclude that the notion of a kind of decision proposed by Culver and Gert is inadequate as a unit of analysis for the purposes of assessing competence.[38]

A ROLE FOR RATIONALITY

By now it should be clear that there is no incompatibility between endorsing a process account of competence and espousing a notion of decisional content. It should also be clear that a process account of competence requires an appeal to value. In this section, we look more closely at how a process account of competence can incorporate rationality.

To start, it is worth pointing out that Culver and Gert explicitly argue that the assessment of competence should not rest on the rationality of an individual's decision. This is obviously incompatible with the thesis that internal rationality is a condition of competence. The problem is easily resolved. Very simply, Culver and Gert conflate internal and external rationality. They consider all rationality to be external, a feature of actual decisions. Because they do not distinguish actual from putative decisions, it is impossible for them to countenance the possibility that rationality might be a component of competence in the internal sense suggested by Buchanan and Brock, and Freedman. They are right that rationality in the external sense should not be considered a condition of competence, but they are wrong that rationality in the internal sense is not important.

Freedman explicitly endorses an internal account of rationality to complement his process account of competence. So do Buchanan and Brock, once the confusion between decisional content and outcomes is resolved. In the following passage they appear to endorse a version of the recognisable reasons model:

> A crude but perhaps helpful way of characterising the proper aim of the evaluator of the competence of a seemingly harmful or bad patient choice is to think of him or her addressing the patient in this fashion: 'Help me try to understand and make sense of your choice. Help me to see whether your choice is reasonable, not in the sense that it is what I or most people would choose, but that it is reasonable for you in light of your underlying and enduring aims and values.' This is the proper focus of a process account of competence.[39]

So according to Buchanan and Brock, competence involves appealing to the reasonableness of the putative choice in question. Like Freedman, they believe that this determination is internal to the reasoning process. It is now time to try to look more closely at internal rationality and its role in the recognisable reasons account of competence. A putative decision is rational in the internal sense if: (a) it coheres with an individual's enduring aims and values; (b) it is justified in light of those values and their associated beliefs; and (c) the proposed justification is deemed appropriate by the third party responsible for assessing competence. Again, the reasons offered do not have to entail the proposed decision. It is sufficient that they be recognised as an appropriate justification for selecting that option by the assessors. The reasons do not even have to be true, nor do the assessors have to believe they are true. All that is required is that the individual in question believes them to be true.

Consider again the example of the Jehovah's Witnesses and blood transfusions. A Jehovah's Witness's putative decision to refuse a life-saving transfusion may appear unreasonable when assessed against the general public's values and beliefs regarding the preservation of life. But the system of values that define the Jehovah's Witness faith constitutes a strong justification for that decision, one that is recognisable to a suitably disposed third party, and one that coheres with the overall set of values and beliefs associated with that faith. If, as some legal precedents suggest we must, we opt to give latitude to a Jehovah's Witness's value system in assessing his or her competence to make treatment decisions, then it is possible to count those decisions as competent even though they may ensue in death. The Jehovah's Witness's reasons for refusing transfusions are recognisable even to those who might not share them. They are rational in light of, and internal to, the Jehovah's Witness faith. That does not mean that assessments of competence must necessarily collapse into subjectivity. It is not too hard to imagine satisfactory objective means of determining whether a Jehovah's Witness's decision to refuse a transfusion is made in conformity with his or her religious principles and with a basically sound mind. The Jehovah's Witness who refuses a transfusion on the grounds that he or she is Jesus Christ is just as incompetent to make that decision as a severely schizophrenic patient who says the same thing.

ASKING "WHY?"

It is time to leave the realm of philosophical theory and to turn to more practical matters. Having articulated the case for including considerations of value in the assessment of mental competence, we are left with the challenge of how to devise operationalised measures which do that.

The traditional approach to competence requires understanding and appreciation. However, if the arguments provided here are correct, then this is not enough. In order to judge competence we need to know more than simply the fact that a patient understands and appreciates the nature of a putative decision. Those conditions only capture a person's abilities to comprehend what the relevant facts of a situation are. If value is going to count as a component of competence we also need to know why a person proposes to choose as they do. This is because it is primarily values that define goals and aspirations and, thereby, direct conduct.

In determining whether an individual understands and appreciates the nature of a certain decisional task we normally ask questions such as: "Do you understand what this decision is about?" "Do you appreciate what will happen if you choose this rather than that?"[40] Such "What?" questions deal with facts. Answers to them are assessed by determining whether the person involved can demonstrate that he or she has those facts right. Let us grant that all of this is more or less amenable to objective scrutiny. "Why?" questions are a different matter. They are also notoriously absent from competency assessment tools, probably because of their association with questions of value and rationality. "Why?" questions delve into a person's reasons for wanting to choose as he or she does, and that often involves inquiring into that person's values. Assessing the answers to "Why?" questions is likely to be more complicated than assessing the answers to "What?" questions. At the very least, the criteria are going to be different.

The recognisable reasons criterion requires that we ask "Why?" To see the point of that condition imagine the following situation. Patient X understands what is involved in the putative decision to do Y. Patient X also appreciates what it means to opt in favor of the putative decision to do Y. Therefore, so far as understanding and appreciation are concerned, patient X is competent. But now imagine that when asked why she wants to opt to do Y, patient X says "I am inclined to choose Y because I am Jesus Christ!" Is patient X competent? Not likely. Is she incompetent? Perhaps. But there are at least grounds for overriding the usual presumption of competence and inquiring into this individual's competence. The point is that without asking this last question one would probably never come to that inquiry. For it is perfectly conceivable that someone might satisfy the understanding and appreciation conditions and yet at the same time choose to do Y for irrational reasons. It is worth noting that the rare instances when "Why?" questions are employed in assessments of competence; it is not specifically to inquire into the grounds for competence. It is rather to screen out impediments to competence such as pathological extremes of affect, psychosis and the like. However, "Why?" questions do much more. They not only help isolate factors outside competence that may impede or compromise it, they also capture factors that are constitutive of competence, namely, reasons. Thus, "Why?" questions are the clinical key to reasons.

To sum up, considerations of value could probably be incorporated into assessments of competence employing specially tailored "Why?" questions. Such reason-seeking probes should be accompanied by carefully defined operationalised criteria for evaluating what counts as the coherence of a putative decision with an individual's overall set of values, and what counts as a recognisable reason. This is obviously more a strategy than a solution. But it is a start.

CONCLUSION

The aim of this discussion has been to try and clarify the place of value and rationality in the theory and assessment of mental competence. With a few interpretive adjustments, it is possible to make a convincing case for the thesis that there is a lot more consensus in the literature on this topic than might at first appear to be the case. In particular, there is agreement that assessments of competence cannot be carried out independently of certain considerations of value and rationality. This poses problems for the requirement that assessments of competence be objective. Buchanan and Brock say that competence is not something that can be determined scientifically.[41] They are right about this, but that does not mean giving up entirely on objectivity, as they also seem to suggest.

Third party agreement is probably the best and only way to address the requirements of objectivity involved in the assessment of decision-making capacity. This might seem unsatisfactory to those versed in the philosophical intricacies of the problem of objectivity. However, keep in mind that in addition to being objective to some degree, operationalised criteria for assessing competence must also be sufficiently general and flexible to apply across different jurisdictions (such as different states or provinces in the case of some federations). Precision of a certain sort is therefore not desirable. It is also unrealistic. After all, the purpose of philosophical inquiry here is to facilitate problem-solving in a practical domain, not to paralyse it by setting impossible goals and standards. The onus is on those who desire more objectivity in that domain to specify how it might be attained in a manner that meets the practical exigencies of the task.

Notes

1. Freedman, B (1981), Competence, Marginal and Otherwise, *International Journal of Law and Psychiatry* 4, 53–72: p. 55.
2. For an account of the evaluative contribution of emotion to competence see Charland, LC (1999). Appreciation and Emotion: Theoretical Reflections on the MacArthur Treatment Competence Study, *Kennedy Institute Journal of Ethics* 8(4), 359–377; and Charland, LC (1998), Is Mr. Spock Mentally Competent: Competence to Consent and Emotion, *Philosophy, Psychiatry, Psychology* 5(1), 67–95.
3. Freedman's recognisable reasons criterion is referred to in *US v Charters,* F 2d, No. 86–5568, United States Court of Appeals Fourth Circuit, Sept. 18, 1988 *per* Murnaghan Circuit Judge.
4. Both Buchanan and Brock were consulting members of the President's Commission for the Study of Ethical Problems in Biomedical and Behavioral Research and co-authors of its report, *The President's Commission for the Study of Ethical Problems in Medicine and Biomedical and Behavioral Research.* (1982) Making Health Care Decisions, Vol 1 Washington: US Government Printing Office). In that document "a set of enduring values" is listed as a condition of competence.
5. Freedman, *op cit*, p. 61.

6. For an intriguing view of competence that incorporates elements of responsibility in addition to value and rationality see: Elliott, C (1991), Competence as Accountability, *Journal of Clinical Ethics* 2(3), 167–171. Elliott argues that competence should be construed as accountability.
7. Freedman, *op cit*, p. 61.
8. *Ibid*, p. 61.
9. In Canadian law there is the case of *Mallete v Shulman* (1990) 72 OR (2d) 417 (CA).
10. Freedman, *op cit*, p. 61.
11. *Ibid*, p. 62.
12. A similar point is made in: Buchanan, AE, and Brock, DW (1989), *Deciding for Others: The Ethics of Surrogate Decision Making*. Cambridge, Cambridge University Press. The details differ somewhat from Freedman's account.
13. Buchanan and Brock, *op cit*, p. 25.
14. *Ibid*, p. 84.
15. *Ibid*, p. 32.
16. *Ibid*, p. 18.
17. *Ibid*, p. 24.
18. *Ibid*, p. 24.
19. *Ibid*, p. 25.
20. *Ibid*, p. 25.
21. *Ibid*, p. 25
22. *Ibid*, p. 25.
23. *Ibid*, p. 25.
24. *Ibid*, p. 25.
25. *Ibid*, pp. 40–1.
26. *Ibid*, p. 49.
27. *Ibid*, p. 84.
28. Freedman, *op cit*, p. 59; see also: Roth, LH, Meisel, A, Litz, W (1977), Test of Competency to Consent, *American Journal of Psychiatry* 134, 279–284.
29. Culver and Gert (1990), The Inadequacy of Competence. *Millbank Quarterly*, pp. 620, 629, respectively.
30. *Ibid*, p. 621; emphasis added.
31. *Ibid*, p. 634; emphasis added.
32. *Ibid*, p. 621.
33. See, for example, Buchanan and Brock, *op cit*, p. 85.
34. Culver and Gert, *op cit*, pp. 619–620; see also Buchanan and Brock, *op cit*, p. 65.
35. Culver and Gert, *op cit*, p. 620.
36. Buchanan and Brock, *op cit*, p. 18.
37. *Ibid*, p. 52.
38. See Cale, Gita S (1999), Risk-Related Standards of Competence, *Bioethics 13(2)*. 131–148, for a recent discussion of the problem of asymmetry in the area of competence.
39. *Ibid*, p. 56.
40. There are a number of interesting "Why?" questions in Paul Appelbaum and Tom Grisso's MacCAT-T assessment tool. The manual and assessment tool are contained in an appendix to T, Grisso and Appelbaum, PA (1998), *The Assessment of Decision-Making Capacity: A Guide for Physicians and Other Health Professionals*. Oxford: Oxford University Press.
41. Buchanan and Brock, p. 47.

CASES

Reibl v Hughes, [1980] 2 SCR 880, 1980 CanLII 23 (SCC)

Summary prepared by Matthew Herder

Mr. Reibl, a 44-year-old Hungarian immigrant, elected to undergo an internal carotid endarterectomy to remove an occlusion in an artery near his brain that was preventing a significant amount of blood flow through the artery. The operation was performed competently by Dr. Hughes, a fully qualified neurosurgeon. However, following the procedure, Mr. Reibl suffered a massive stroke, resulting in the paralysis of his entire right side. He also became impotent. Mr. Reibl claimed that

Reprinted by permission of the author.

he had not been told of the serious risks of the surgery (e.g., stroke) and that, had he been told, he would not have consented to the surgery (particularly because the risk of stroke associated with not having the surgery was not imminent and because he was only one-and-a-half years away from being eligible for pension benefits from his employer). He sued Dr. Hughes in battery and negligence, arguing that he had not given a valid informed consent.

Discussion Questions

1. What standard of disclosure is necessary in order to ensure informed consent to medical treatment?

2. What level of understanding is required in order to ensure informed consent to medical treatment?

3. Given that disclosing every possible risk of medical interventions, however remote and unlikely, would be incredibly time-consuming (and perhaps impossible for some interventions given uncertainty in the current state of knowledge) what reasonable limits on disclosure might be necessary in the health care context?

Starson v Swayze, 2003 SCC 32, [2003] 1 SCR 722

Summary prepared by Sheila Wildeman

Mr. Starson, an unusually gifted thinker in the area of theoretical physics, was involuntarily committed to a psychiatric hospital in 1999 by disposition of the Ontario Review Board, following a criminal court finding that he was not criminally responsible for two counts of uttering death threats. Mr. Starson had a history of psychiatric admissions reaching back to 1985. His most consistent diagnosis was bipolar disorder.

Once in hospital, Mr. Starson refused prescribed medications (neuroleptic medication, mood stabilizers, anti-anxiety medication, and anti-Parkinsonian medication), consenting to psychotherapy only. While Mr. Starson refused to accept any psychiatric diagnosis, there was sufficient evidence (from Mr. Starson and in letters from third parties) that he "clearly recognized" that he had "mental problems" and also recognized that his "perception of reality" differed from that of others. His physicians found him to be incapable of refusing treatment. He challenged this finding before the Ontario Consent and Capacity Board.

Discussion Questions

1. The right to refuse medical treatment is thought to be justified by a general commitment to respect for personal autonomy. How might commitment to a non-traditional account of autonomy, for instance relational autonomy, change our understanding of the right to refuse medical treatment (if at all)?

2. What level of competence is required for informed refusal of medical treatment? Is this different from the level of competence required for informed consent to medical treatment?

3. Health care systems are always in some danger of going too far in 'normalizing' individuals with idiosyncratic or unorthodox beliefs or lifestyles, even when those individuals are not harming others. How can health care systems be designed so that individuals are protected against this tendency?

Reprinted by permission of the author.

Useful Resources

READINGS

Berg, J. W., Appelbaum, P. S., Lidz, C. W., & Parker, L. S. (Eds.). (2001). *Informed consent: Legal theory and clinical practice* (2nd ed.). New York, NY: Oxford University Press.

Faden, R. R., Beauchamp, T. L., King, N. M. P. (Eds.). (1986). *A history and theory of informed consent.* New York, NY: Oxford University Press.

Freedman, B. (1981). Competence, marginal and otherwise: Concepts and ethics. *International Journal of Law and Psychiatry, 4*(1–2), 53–61, 64–66.

Kukla, R. (2005). Conscientious autonomy: Displacing decisions in health care. *Hastings Center Report, 35,* 34–44.

Manson, N., & O'Neill, O. (2007). *Rethinking informed consent in bioethics.* Cambridge, MA: Cambridge University Press.

Miller, F. G., & Wertheimer, A. (Eds.). (2010). *The ethics of consent: Theory and practice.* New York, NY: Oxford University Press.

Misak, C. (2005). ICU psychosis and patient autonomy: Some thoughts from the inside. *Journal of Medicine and Philosophy, 30,* 411–430.

HEALTH LAW

Malette v Shulman (1987), 72 OR (2d) 417 (CA)

Georgette Malette, a Jehovah's Witness, was seriously injured in a car accident. Dr. Shulman determined that a blood transfusion was necessary to save her life. He administered the treatment even though he knew, on the basis of a card Ms. Malette carried and discussions with her daughter, that she rejected blood transfusions for religious reasons.

Arndt v Smith, [1997] 2 SCR 539, 1997 CanLII 360 (SCC)

Ms. Arndt contracted chickenpox during the 12th week of her pregnancy, as a result of which her daughter was injured. Ms. Arndt sued her physician Dr. Smith for the costs associated with raising her daughter. She claimed that she would have aborted her fetus if she hadn't been reassured by her physician that the risks of fetal injury were very small.

CanLII

CanLII is a non-profit organization managed by the Federation of Law Societies of Canada. CanLII's goal is to make Canadian law accessible for free on the Internet.

Chapter 7 **CLINICAL RESEARCH**

INTRODUCTION

Experimentation on human subjects has always been controversial, since it frequently involves risks to individual subjects for the benefit of others (in the medical context, the benefits often accrue to future patients). What, then, makes clinical research ethical? A popular response—informed consent—is surely part of the answer. But it is not the whole answer, since we can easily imagine trivial, poorly designed or extremely risky trials that might be unethical even if there were people willing to consent to participation. For a clinical trial to be ethical, it must, among other things, attempt to answer an important clinical question, enroll participants as required by the hypothesis under investigation (not merely for reasons of convenience or habit), have a favourable (or at least proportionate) risk–benefit ratio, and ensure respect for research participants. The articles in this chapter highlight some of the specific ethical problems that arise when attempting to sort through the details of the requirements outlined above.

Before we can assess the ethics of clinical research, we need to understand the distinction between research and practice (after all, if there was no difference, we wouldn't need to pay any special attention to research ethics. We could just apply lessons from clinical practice.). Franklin Miller and Howard Brody offer a critique of the longstanding bioethical commitment to clinical equipoise as a pre-condition for research. Clinical equipoise exists when there is genuine uncertainty within the medical community over which treatment option is best for some condition. Miller and Brody suggest that the longstanding problem of therapeutic misconception in clinical research—the conflation of research and practice—can be corrected and eliminated by properly distinguishing research from practice. They offer

an argument in support of a clear distinction, and suggest that this eliminates any need for a concept of equipoise.

Jonathan Kimmelman challenges Miller and Brody's attempt to draw a sharp distinction between research and practice, and argues that an understanding of the ways in which research and practice are interrelated has implications for the way in which trials are presented to prospective participants. If there is no clear research-practice distinction, researchers aren't off the hook for providing therapeutic benefit where possible, and this in turns means there will be more reason to try to design studies that are maximally beneficial for participants.

Challenges in assessing the social benefit of clinical trials often arise in the context of research conducted in developing countries (which is often sponsored by governments and industries from more developed countries). The proposed (though ultimately abandoned) Surfaxin trial in Bolivia provides a case study from which to analyze these issues. The case description is followed by two analyses: one, by Robert Temple, defends the use of placebo controls in the proposed Surfaxin study on the grounds that such trials are best positioned to answer questions of genuine clinical importance for members of the local community. The other, by Peter Lurie and Sidney Wolfe, argues that the trial was unjustified because it proposed to treat Bolivian patients worse than patients from developed countries. Current trends indicate that medical research is increasingly shifting to sites in developing countries, so there is a pressing need for resolution of the questions raised by this case—particularly on the question of whether there should be global or local standards of care for research participants in control groups.

In the next article Gopal Sreenivasan raises concerns about the informed consent requirement for clinical research. In particular, he focuses on problems with comprehension or understanding. He points out that while bioethicists seem to suggest that prospective research participants must fully understand a trial in order to give informed consent to participate, this position is in tension with recent empirical literature that suggests most research participants fail to understand common features of clinical trials such as randomization and blinding. If bioethicists were to enforce the requirement that participants understand most or all elements of the trials they enter, clinical research would grind to a halt. Sreenivasan explores what ought to be done in light of this tension between theory and practice.

One of the requirements of ethical medical research that has received only scattered attention over the years is that of fair participant selection. In the early 1990s feminist bioethicists drew attention to problems with inclusion/exclusion criteria for clinical trials. At the time, a glaring problem was the exclusion of women from clinical trials. Recent empirical evidence suggests that, after a great deal of activism and governmental intervention, women are now well represented in clinical trials. However, Anne Lyerly, Margaret Little, and Ruth Faden draw our attention to one sub-group still vastly underrepresented in clinical trials: pregnant women. Lyerly, Little, and Faden offer four arguments for fair representation of pregnant women in clinical trials: the research is needed to find effective treatments for women during pregnancy, without such research we cannot protect fetal safety, reluctance to prescribe potentially beneficial medications to pregnant women can be harmful, and it is only fair that pregnant women have access to the benefits of research participation.

In the final article of this chapter, we broaden our perspective and consider some of the practical challenges shaping contemporary clinical research. Steven Lewis and colleagues outline some of the incentives created by industry funding of clinical research, including pressures to suppress negative results and ask only commercially profitable questions. They ask whether the universities pursuing closer ties to industry have exercised due diligence in protecting the university's fundamental commitment to the pursuit of truth. The integrity of the research enterprise depends on the ability of researchers and research institutions to negotiate competing demands without compromising important goals.

A Critique of Clinical Equipoise: Therapeutic Misconception in the Ethics of Clinical Trials

Franklin G. Miller and Howard Brody

The Hypericum Depression Trial Study Group published in 2002 the results of a randomized trial comparing hypericum (St. John's Wort), sertraline (Zoloft), and placebo in the treatment of major depression.[1] In the study, funded by the National Institutes of Health, 340 subjects from twelve participating centers were randomized to three trial arms for an eight-week period, with careful monitoring to assure that patients who worsened significantly or who became suicidal were removed from the study and received adequate treatment. Neither hypericum nor sertraline was found to be superior to placebo on the primary outcome

Miller, F. & Brody, H. (2003) "A Critique of Clinical Equipoise: Therapeutic Misconception in the Ethics of Clinical Trials." *Hastings Center Report* 33(3): pp. 19–28.

measures. The authors noted, "From a methodological point of view, this study can be considered an example of the importance of including inactive and active comparators in trials testing the possible antidepressant effects of medications. In fact, without a placebo, hypericum could easily have been considered as effective as sertraline."[2]

What can we conclude about the ethics of this trial? One dominant viewpoint in research ethics would have prohibited the study. On this viewpoint, a randomized trial is ethical only in circumstances of "clinical equipoise"—a genuine uncertainty within the medical community as to whether (in this case) any of the three treatment arms are superior to the other two. No such uncertainty exists. Approximately twenty-five clinically available antidepressants, including sertraline, have been shown to be superior to placebo.[3] Moreover, the majority opinion within psychiatry probably holds that sertraline is definitely superior to hypericum for major depression, even if hypericum has potential for the treatment of mild to moderate depression. But another widespread viewpoint would hold that the trial was ethically sound. Depressed individuals widely use hypericum, a "natural" agent, despite the lack of proven efficacy. Accordingly, a rigorous evaluation offered scientific, clinical, and social value. According to the report of trial results, the study was approved by institutional review boards (IRBs) at twelve sites and subjects provided written informed consent.

But if clinical equipoise is a basic requirement for ethical research, how could all these review boards be blind to the unethical nature of this trial? And how could two such radically divergent viewpoints exist, without research ethics being widely regarded as in a state of crisis?

THERAPEUTIC MISCONCEPTIONS

The prevailing ethical perspective on clinical trials holds that physician-investigators can discharge their "therapeutic obligation" to patients in the context of randomized clinical trials (RCTs) as long as treatments being tested scientifically satisfy clinical equipoise. We contend that this ethical perspective is fundamentally flawed. An ethical framework that provides normative guidance about a practice should accurately characterize the practice. The prevailing ethical perspective fails this test: All sound ethical thinking about clinical research, and the regulatory framework for review of protocols for clinical investigation, depends on a basic distinction between research and therapy. But the claims in the prevailing ethical perspective on clinical trials conflate research and therapy. These claims are that the ethics of the physician-patient relationship must govern RCTs, that physicians who conduct these trials have a "therapeutic obligation" to patients enrolled in them, and that RCTs must be compatible with some form of equipoise.

Certainly, investigators and ethicists recognize that clinical trials are scientific experiments, which differ from standard medical care. They also recognize that they are subject to regulatory requirements which do not apply to routine medical practice. However, the prevailing ethical framework views clinical trials through a therapeutic lens. The mainstream ethical approach to clinical trials attempts to have it both ways: to view the clinical trial as a scientific experiment, aimed at producing knowledge that can help improve the care of future patients, and as treatment conducted by physicians who retain fidelity to the principles of therapeutic beneficence and therapeutic non-maleficence that govern the ethics of clinical medicine. The doctrine of clinical equipoise has emerged as the bridge between medical care and scientific experimentation, allegedly making it possible to conduct RCTs without sacrificing the therapeutic obligation of physicians to provide treatment according to a scientifically validated standard of care. This constitutes a "therapeutic misconception" concerning the ethics of clinical trials, analogous to the tendency of patient volunteers to confuse treatment in the context of RCTs with routine medical care.[4] As Paul

Appelbaum has recently observed, "In fact, this confusion between the ethics of research and of ordinary clinical care appears rampant in the world of clinical trials."[5]

The therapeutic misconception in the ethics of clinical trials is reflected in the language commonly used within the clinical research enterprise. Clinical trials are often described as "therapeutic research," and investigators are regarded as having a "therapeutic intent." Research participants who are being studied because they have a medical condition under investigation are referred to as "patients," and investigators as "physicians" or "doctors," without qualification.

To demonstrate our contention about the mainstream approach to the ethics of clinical trials, we will offer an intellectual reconstruction of some of the history of research ethics since the 1970s. This history is characterized by incoherence resulting from commitment to two incompatible positions, each approaching research ethics in a fundamentally different way. The therapeutic misconception about the ethics of clinical trials has emerged from the "similarity position," which argues that ultimately, the ethics of clinical trials rest on the same moral considerations that underlie the ethics of therapeutic medicine. The "difference position" argues that the ethics of clinical trials must start with the realization that medical research and medical treatment are two distinct forms of activity, governed by different ethical principles.

The reigning ethical paradigm for clinical trials has coexisted with clinical trials practice that departs from its guidance. Clinical equipoise, the cornerstone of the similarity position, rules out placebo-controlled trials whenever there is a proven effective treatment for the disorder under investigation.[6] However, IRBs have routinely approved such placebo-controlled trials. These two anomalies—unappreciated theoretical incoherence and conflict between the theoretical paradigm and the practice of ethical review of clinical trials—call for critical examination of the similarity position and the doctrine of clinical equipoise.

THE DISTINCTION BETWEEN RESEARCH AND THERAPY

In 1979, Robert Levine summarized "the most important achievements of the National Commission" for the Protection of Human Subjects of Biomedical and Behavioral Research in "correcting the conceptual and semantic errors that had undermined virtually all previous attempts to develop rational public policy on research involving human subjects."[7] Two portions of Levine's summary capture the essential ingredients of the difference position: recognizing the distinction between research and therapy and, accordingly, abandoning the distinction between therapeutic and nontherapeutic research.

Clinical research shares with medical care the fact that both are performed by physicians in clinical settings, and both often use similar diagnostic and treatment interventions. When the commission began its work, physicians commonly regarded clinical research and medical therapy as inextricably connected. One authority quoted by Levine claimed that "Every time a physician administers a drug to a patient, he is in a sense performing an experiment." But the commission recognized the importance of determining the boundaries between routine medical practice and research. For Levine, the commission's conceptual breakthrough came with the realization that the physicians of the day were thinking about clinical research in the wrong way, and that the boundary between research and therapy was clear rather than fuzzy. The commission came to hold that clinical research is fundamentally different from medical practice.[8]

Clinical medicine aims at providing optimal medical care for individual patients. Ethically, it is governed by the principles of therapeutic beneficence and therapeutic nonmaleficence. Therapeutic beneficence directs physicians to practice medicine with primary fidelity to promoting the health of particular patients. According to therapeutic nonmaleficence, the risks of medical care to which a patient is exposed are to be justified by the prospect of compensating medical benefits for that patient. The physician uses scientific knowledge to care for the patient and engages in therapeutic experimentation with the aim only of finding optimal treatment. It is not part of the role of the physician in providing medical care to develop scientific knowledge that can help future patients.

Clinical research, in contrast, is not a therapeutic activity devoted to the personal care of patients. It is designed for answering a scientific question, with the aim of producing "generalizable knowledge." The investigator seeks to learn about disease and its treatment in *groups* of patients, with the ultimate aim of improving medical care. Scientific interest in any particular patient concerns what can be learned that is applicable to other patients. In view of the nature and purpose of clinical research, the principles of beneficence and nonmaleficence applicable to clinical research lack the therapeutic meaning that guides their application to medical care. Clinical research is dedicated primarily to promoting the medical good of future patients by means of scientific knowledge derived from experimentation with current research participants—a frankly utilitarian purpose.

A major reason for distinguishing research from therapy is to underscore that clinical research has an inherent potential for exploiting research participants.[9] Exploitation also may occur in clinical medicine—venal physicians sometimes perform medically unnecessary procedures for the sake of profit, for example. Yet when physicians of integrity practice medicine, physicians' and patients' interests converge. The patient desires to regain or maintain health or to relieve suffering; the physician is dedicated to providing the medical help that the patient needs.

In clinical research, by contrast, the interests of investigators and patient volunteers are likely to diverge, even when the investigator acts with complete integrity. Patient volunteers, especially in clinical trials, typically seek therapeutic benefit, though they also may be motivated by altruism.[10] Investigators are interested primarily in developing scientific knowledge about groups of patients. Regardless of investigators' motivations, patient volunteers are at risk of having

their well-being compromised in the course of scientific investigation. Clinical research involves an inherent tension between pursuing rigorous science and protecting research participants from harm.[11]

Historically, the ethical distinction between research and therapy emerged out of concern about exploitive abuses of patients in clinical research. Reflection on this dark history gave rise to a major development in the ethics of clinical research: the requirement for independent, prospective review and approval of research protocols.[12] Prior independent review was considered necessary for clinical research because of the divergence between the interests of the investigator and the research participant. Self-regulation by physician-investigators could not be trusted in the research context to the same extent that self-regulation by physicians was appropriate in the therapeutic context. The basic rationale for prospective, independent research review depends on the distinction between research and therapy.

The point of distinguishing research and therapy is not to make an invidious comparison, implying that clinical trials are more risky or ethically problematic than routine clinical practice. Indeed, there is some evidence that patients receive more favorable medical outcomes in many clinical trials,[13] and clinical medicine is certainly rife with ethical problems. Further, since research is more carefully regulated than medical practice, it is quite likely that fewer ethical violations occur in research. To say that two activities are ethically different is not to say that either is inherently better than the other.

ABANDONING THE DISTINCTION

The distinction between research and therapy is most likely to be obfuscated in the context of clinical trials, which test the safety or efficacy of investigational and standard treatments. Since patients may derive medical benefit from trial participation, especially in phase III RCTs (the final stage of testing, which many investigational drugs never even reach), clinical trials are often characterized as "therapeutic research."

Nonetheless, the process of treatment in RCTs differs radically from routine clinical practice.[14] Consider the contrast between the hypericum-sertraline trial and routine medical care for depression. If a physician treated 340 patients for major depression, she would not decide which drug to administer by flipping a coin. If the physician elected to use sertraline, she would judge each case individually to determine dose, when to change the dose, and whether to prescribe a second antidepressant or recommend other treatment. We would expect to find considerable variation in the treatment administered to those 340 patients after eight weeks or so. From the vantage point of therapy, this is what it means to provide care to patients.

From the vantage point of research, such variation would wreak havoc on experimental design and the validity and generalizability of findings. So when patients are randomized to one or another experimental drug, and are treated according to relatively inflexible protocols, the activity is very different from therapeutic medicine.

In many other ways, too, routine aspects of research deviate from what would be required by the duties of therapeutic beneficence and nonmaleficence. Volunteer patients and physician investigators are often ignorant of assignment to the experimental or control treatment, which may be a placebo. Trials often include interventions such as blood draws, lumbar punctures, radiation imaging, or biopsies that measure trial outcomes but in no way benefit participants. RCTs often contain a drug "washout" phase before randomization to avoid confounding the evaluation of the investigational treatment with the effects of medication that patients were receiving prior to the trial. These various features of research design promote scientific validity; they carry risks to participants without the prospect of compensating therapeutic benefit.

For these reasons, Levine argued that the second major contribution of the commission was to abandon the "illogical" distinction between therapeutic and nontherapeutic research, which previous policymakers thought was essential to the proper regulation of research

and the protection of human subjects.[15] Because research and therapy are distinct activities, and the ethics of therapeutic medicine therefore cannot be automatically extended to guide research, it is mistaken to label research as "therapeutic" or "nontherapeutic," as if that made any fundamental ethical difference. Many research trials consist of a complex mix of therapeutic and nontherapeutic elements— the placebo-controlled trial being only one obvious example—such that labeling the trial as a whole as "therapeutic" or "nontherapeutic" is misleading. In addition, the therapeutic-nontherapeutic distinction diverts attention from key ethical issues. Consider a nontherapeutic trial in which one interviews subjects and takes saliva samples, and a therapeutic trial in which one is testing a new cancer drug that has some promise for creating remission, but also has potentially life-threatening toxicity. Is the latter trial less in need of stringent regulatory oversight because it is "therapeutic"? Or does the therapeutic-nontherapeutic distinction distract the observer from those aspects of the trials that assume far greater moral weight, such as the level of risks and the potential vulnerability of subjects?

Once one understands the distinction between research and therapy, one realizes that "therapeutic" research is still research, and that the ethical rules appropriate to it are those appropriate for clinical research generally. Even though the patient may derive benefit from treatment being evaluated, the basic goal of the activity is not personal therapy, but rather the acquisition of generally applicable scientific knowledge. The basic goal and nature of the activity determines the ethical standards that ought to apply.

Writing in 1993, Jay Katz affirmed the vital importance of the distinction between research and therapy and deplored its blurring in practice: "The astronomical increase in clinical research has, in practice, not led to a clear demarcation between therapy and research, bioethical theories notwithstanding. This vital distinction remains blurred when physician-investigators view subjects as patients, and then believe that patients' interests and not science's are being served by participation in randomized clinical trials that are so commonly conducted in today's world."[16] One of the reasons investigators (and bioethicists) have failed to appreciate the distinction between research and therapy is that the similarity position has conceived the ethics of clinical trials within the context of the physician–patient relationship.

CHARLES FRIED AND THE SIMILARITY POSITION

In 1974, Fried published *Medical Experimentation: Personal Integrity and Social Policy,* which launched the similarity position within bioethics.[17] Fried assumed that answers to ethical dilemmas in research would have to be found within the ethics of therapeutic medicine. He defended fidelity to the interests of the individual patient against a model in which "medicine is to be viewed as caring for populations."[18] What made the RCT ethically suspect was that it seemed to him a prime example of population-focused—rather than individualized—and utilitarian medicine.

Fried devoted most of his book to defending patients' "rights in personal care."[19] Returning to medical research, he took issue with trials in which patients were randomized to receive either the experimental intervention or standard care. Fried coined the term "equipoise" to describe the ethically necessary condition for conducting an RCT: physician-investigators must be indifferent to the therapeutic value of the experimental and control treatments evaluated in the trial. The basic idea of equipoise had previously been articulated by Bradford Hill, a pioneer in the development of RCTs.[20] But what Fried objected to primarily in RCTs was not randomization per se, but the fact that no informed consent had been obtained. Fried saw the threat of "care for groups" (instead of "care for individuals") as residing primarily in the idea that it was legitimate to enroll subjects in an RCT without explicit, informed consent because the results of the trial would provide new medical knowledge that would improve the lot of future patients.[21] Because Fried was concerned chiefly about informed consent, an essential ingredient of both medical research and therapeutic medicine, he saw no problem in applying the ethics of medical therapy to medical research.

In the 1970s, the "respect for patient autonomy" movement was gaining steam as a replacement for the old Hippocratic ethic of paternalistic beneficence. Since both Fried and the National Commission seemed on the surface to be championing patient autonomy, it was easy to miss the point that they were proposing two fundamentally different strategies for approaching the ethics of clinical trials. Put another way, so long as the bioethics debate of the moment has to do with whether research ethics requires all competent subjects to give fully informed consent, any fundamental divergence between the similarity and the difference positions is likely to be obscured.

THE EMERGENCE OF CLINICAL EQUIPOISE

During the 1980s, philosophers interested in research ethics recognized a tension between the obligation of physicians to offer optimal care to their patients ("the therapeutic obligation") and the provision of medical treatment in the context of clinical trials. Don Marquis addressed this problem in a 1983 essay, "Leaving Therapy to Chance."[22] The title is significant, suggesting that the RCT is a form of therapy rather than an ethically distinct activity. Marquis began his essay, "Consider this dilemma: according to an argument that is hard to refute, the procedure for conducting randomized clinical trials of anticancer drugs is incompatible with the ethics of the physician–patient relationship. If this problem is to be resolved, then either a key procedure for achieving scientific knowledge in medicine must be given up or unethical behavior by physicians must be tolerated."[23] In framing this "RCT dilemma," Marquis assumed that the appropriate ethic for clinical trials was that of the (therapeutic) physician–patient relationship.

Fred Gifford, following the lead of Marquis, examined the RCT dilemma in greater depth: "The central dilemma concerning randomized clinical trials (RCTs) arises out of some simple facts about causal methodology (RCTs are the best way to generate the reliable causal knowledge necessary for optimally informed action) and a *prima facie* plausible principle concerning how physicians should treat their patients (always do what it is most reasonable to believe will be best for the patient)."[24] Neither Marquis nor Gifford found what they regarded as a satisfactory solution, and neither considered the possibility that the difference position could dismiss the "RCT dilemma" as misguided to begin with.

In a landmark 1987 article, Benjamin Freedman offered a solution to the RCT dilemma that gained widespread acceptance within bioethics. He argued that the tension between ethically legitimate scientific experimentation and the therapeutic obligation of physicians could be overcome by the principle of "clinical equipoise."[25] Freedman agreed with Fried and Marquis that ethical clinical trials had to be compatible with therapeutic beneficence and nonmaleficence. But he argued that Fried's formulation of equipoise was too constraining. Freedman called Fried's original concept "theoretical equipoise" (sometimes called "individual equipoise") and contrasted it with his favored concept of "clinical equipoise" (sometimes called "collective equipoise"). In the latter sense of equipoise, any individual investigator or physician might have reasons to believe that one arm of the RCT offers a therapeutic benefit over the other arm, but the medical profession as a whole remains divided. According to Freedman, an RCT is ethical so long as the professional community has not yet reached a consensus, which recognizes that "medicine is social rather than individual in nature."[26] When, and only when, clinical equipoise is satisfied will patients enrolled in a clinical trial be assured that they will not be randomized to treatment known to be inferior. Freedman thus asserted in a later article that clinical equipoise is "grounded in the normative nature of clinical practice, the view that

a patient is ethically entitled to expect treatment from his or her physician—an entitlement that cannot be sacrificed to scientific curiosity."[27]

The bioethics community perceived Freedman's concept of clinical equipoise as both a theoretical and a practical advance. Theoretically, it appeared to offer a more intellectually compelling argument than Fried's initial formulation. Practically, it would permit useful RCTs that would otherwise be ethically proscribed to go forward. Since it appeared to solve the RCT dilemma by accommodating the conduct of clinical trials with the therapeutic obligation of physicians to offer optimal medical care, clinical equipoise gained wide currency as a fundamental concept of the ethics of clinical trials.[28] The persuasive way in which Freedman fortified the similarity position diverted attention from the fact that clinical equipoise collapsed the distinction between research and therapy.

The similarity position and clinical equipoise have been popular not only among bioethicists, but also among investigators. We speculate that this ethical perspective helps to address investigators' psychological needs. Physician-investigators, after all, went to medical school, not investigator school. To think of research with patients outside the ethical framework of the physician–patient relationship, as the difference position requires, may be difficult and threatening to them. Clinical equipoise offers a formula that seems to allow them to mix both physician and investigator roles—even if the psychological comfort is purchased at the price of ethical obfuscation.

The anomaly therefore exists that much of today's bioethical thinking accepts clinical equipoise as an outgrowth of the similarity position, while the Federal regulations grew out of the work of the National Commission, which largely endorsed the difference position. One would imagine that sooner or later proponents of clinical equipoise would realize the need to defend this doctrine from the charge that it conflates the ethics of clinical trials with the ethics of medical care. But this is precisely what has not yet happened.

THE CASE OF PLACEBO-CONTROLLED TRIALS

Although the similarity position, bolstered by clinical equipoise, became the reigning paradigm in the ethics of clinical trials, its dominion over practice was limited. This divorce between theory and practice has been particularly pronounced in the case of placebo-controlled trials. Freedman and his colleagues argued that the use of placebo controls is unethical whenever proven effective treatment exists for the medical condition under investigation in a clinical trial because those randomized to placebo would receive treatment known to be inferior.[29]

Despite the clear implications of clinical equipoise for the ethics of placebo-controlled trials, numerous trials, such as the hypericum-sertraline trial, continued to use placebo controls despite proven effective treatment. Placebo controls have typically been used in trials of new treatments for a wide range of chronic conditions—including mood and anxiety disorders, asthma, stable angina, hypertension, and migraine headaches—all of which can be treated with medication of proven efficacy.

There are two explanations for this incoherence between theory and practice. First, the FDA has encouraged the use of placebo controls in trials concerning these and other chronic conditions.[30] Active-controlled trials designed to test the equivalence of the experimental treatment with a standard treatment suffer from serious methodological limitations. Whenever active-controlled trials show no statistically significant difference between the investigational treatment and an active comparator, two conclusions are possible. Either both were effective in the trial sample of patients, or neither was effective. Without the use of a placebo control, such trials lack internal validity. Accordingly, the FDA has insisted that pharmaceutical companies use placebo controls in trials of new treatments for conditions characterized by fluctuating symptoms and high rates of placebo response.[31] Second, the U.S. federal regulations governing human subjects research do not provide any explicit guidance on the use of placebo controls.[32] IRBs have been free to approve such placebo-controlled trials, provided that they meet regulatory requirements for a favorable risk-benefit ratio, including the potential value of knowledge to be gained and informed consent.

For the most part, this lack of fit between theory and practice received little critical attention until the publication in 1994 of an article in the *New England Journal of Medicine* entitled "The Continuing Unethical Use of Placebo Controls."[33] Kenneth Rothman and Karin Michels castigated the practice of placebo-controlled trials in the face of proven effective treatment and the role of the FDA in encouraging these trials. They cited the Declaration of Helsinki, which relies heavily on the similarity position, as prohibiting this widespread "unethical" practice.

Their article stimulated a lively debate over the ethics of placebo-controlled trials. Freedman and his colleagues attacked "the placebo orthodoxy" in a two-part article that challenged the scientific value of placebo-controlled trials and reiterated that they are unethical when proven effective treatments exist because they contravene clinical equipoise.[34] Other commentators, writing in leading medical journals, defended more or less extensive use of placebo-controlled trials on methodological and ethical grounds.[35] Without directly challenging the doctrine of clinical equipoise, they implied that clinical equipoise provides erroneous ethical guidance for placebo-controlled trials. Accordingly, the debate over placebo-controlled trials jeopardizes the reigning ethical paradigm of the similarity position and clinical equipoise.

CRITIQUE OF THE SIMILARITY POSITION AND CLINICAL EQUIPOISE

Our reconstruction of the recent history of the ethics of clinical trials has traced the emergence and dominance of the similarity position. This history also reveals cracks in the foundation of this ethical paradigm. Simultaneous endorsement of the difference position, reflected in the federal regulatory system and the Belmont Report, and the similarity position, which invokes the doctrine of clinical equipoise, has left the ethics of clinical trials in a state of incoherence. Although this incoherence has not received critical attention, it becomes apparent once the assumptions underlying the similarity position and clinical equipoise are challenged. In addition, the divorce between research ethics theory and clinical trials practice in the case of placebo-controlled trials suggests that a critique of the similarity position and clinical equipoise is overdue.

We contend that clinical equipoise is fundamentally mistaken because "the RCT dilemma," for which it was proposed as a solution, is false. Clinical equipoise and all other forms of equipoise make sense as a normative requirement for clinical trials only on the assumption that investigators have a therapeutic obligation to the research participants. The "therapeutic obligation" of investigators, forming one horn of the RCT dilemma, constitutes a therapeutic misconception about the ethics of clinical trials. The presumption that RCTs must be compatible with the ethics of the physician–patient relationship assumes erroneously that the RCT is a form of therapy, thus inappropriately applying the principles of therapeutic beneficence and nonmaleficence that govern clinical medicine to the fundamentally different practice of clinical research. It is impossible to maintain fidelity to doing what is best medically for patients in the context of RCTs because these are not designed for, and may conflict with, personalized care. Although ethically appealing, the project of bridging the gap between therapy and research via the doctrine of clinical equipoise is doomed to fail.

The insight that the RCT contravenes the ethics of the physician–patient relationship led Samuel Hellman and Debra Hellman to argue that the RCT is unethical and that other methods of evaluating treatments should be employed.[36] This stance, however, would deprive patients and society of the benefits that flow from rigorous scientific evaluation of experimental and standard treatments. The more reasonable conclusion is that RCTs should be governed by ethical norms appropriate to clinical research, which are distinct from therapeutic beneficence and therapeutic nonmaleficence.

Clinical equipoise is neither necessary nor sufficient for ethically justifiable RCTs. The use of placebo controls when proven effective treatment exists violates clinical equipoise; however, when methodologically indicated, their use is no different in principle from any research intervention that poses risks to subjects without the prospect of benefiting them.[37] In many cases, the risks of withholding effective treatment are excessive, and the use of placebo controls would thus be unethical. Nevertheless, it is the unacceptable level of risk, not the violation of investigators' alleged "therapeutic obligation," that makes these trials unethical. In other cases, including the hypericum-sertraline trial, use of placebo controls when proven effective treatment exists is ethically justifiable.

By conflating the ethics of clinical trials with the ethics of therapeutic medicine, proponents of the similarity position may also contribute to the lack of adequate informed consent. If investigators view the ethics of clinical trials through a therapeutic lens, they may explicitly or implicitly foster the therapeutic misconception among research participants—that is, the tendency of participants in trials to confuse clinical trials with medical care. Research participants need to know that the overall activity is aimed not at their own ultimate benefit, but at discovering new knowledge to help future patients. If they think that clinical trial participation is a form of therapy, then they cannot give informed consent. Moreover, unlike the therapeutic context, the patient-subject cannot delegate the decision to the physician-researcher. In the therapeutic setting, a patient can decide to trust the physician to choose the best treatment because the physician has the patient's best interests at heart. The investigator has the interests of future patients at heart, and so cannot decide for the subject whether or not to participate in the research. To be trustworthy, investigators must themselves understand clearly the ways in which clinical research differs from clinical practice and convey this forthrightly to potential research subjects.

It is worth pondering, however, the practical consequences that might ensue if physicians, investigators, patients, and ethicists understood clinical trials without distortion by therapeutic misconceptions. Would recruitment of participants for valuable clinical trials become substantially more difficult, slowing progress in medical care? The fact that clinical trials are no longer seen as a mode of therapy leaves unchanged the real prospect of therapeutic benefits offered to patients from trial participation, including the opportunity to receive promising investigational agents, ancillary medical care, expert diagnostic evaluations, and education about their disorder. Nonetheless, some patients might be less inclined to participate in clinical trials when they appreciate the differences between these scientific experiments and medical care.

To attract enough subjects, researchers might have to pay people for their participation, as researchers in industry-sponsored clinical trials already do with increasing frequency. Payments would add to the cost of conducting clinical trials, but it might help prevent the therapeutic misconception among trial participants.[38] To be paid signifies that the trial participant is not merely a patient seeking therapy. If additional expenditure is necessary to motivate clinical trial participation, then this is a price worth paying for enhanced professional integrity and informed consent.

AN ALTERNATIVE ETHICAL FRAMEWORK

In view of the theoretical and practical problems associated with the similarity position and its logical offspring, clinical equipoise, an alternative framework for the ethics of clinical trials is needed. The most promising recent treatment of research ethics has been developed by Ezekiel Emanuel, David Wendler, and Christine Grady.[39] They propose seven ethical requirements for all clinical research: (1) scientific or social value; (2) scientific validity; (3) fair subject selection; (4) favorable risk-benefit ratio; (5) independent review; (6) informed consent; and (7) respect for enrolled research participants. This framework is built on the difference between research and therapy and on the core value of *protecting research participants from exploitation.*

Yet even this formulation of an ethical framework appropriate to clinical research testifies to the hold of the similarity position. The authors endorse clinical equipoise, claiming it is implied by the requirements of value, validity, and risk-benefit ratio. We contend, by contrast, that the endorsement of clinical equipoise renders incoherent any account that arises from the difference position. The most important next step for research ethics is to develop this "non-exploitation" framework systematically in a way that avoids any conflation of clinical research with medical care.

Those who agree that physician-investigators who conduct clinical trials are not governed by therapeutic beneficence still might argue that clinical equipoise provides important methodological guidance for justifying clinical trials. Freedman and his colleagues have argued that clinical equipoise is both an ethical and a scientific principle: "That principle can be put into normative or scientific language. As a normative matter, it defines ethical trial design as prohibiting any compromise of a patient's right to medical treatment by enrolling in a study. The same concern is often stated scientifically when we assert that a study must start with an honest null hypothesis, genuine medical uncertainty concerning the relative merits of the various treatment arms included in the trial's design."[40] Nevertheless, whatever is valid methodologically in clinical equipoise—the honest null hypothesis—can be stated more clearly and without confusion with the therapeutic obligation, by appeal to the requirement of scientific value: no research participants should be exposed to the risks of valueless research. Clinical trials must be designed to answer valuable scientific questions. If the answer is already known or the question is trivial, then there is no honest null hypothesis, and a clinical trial should not be conducted. But this is logically independent of whether all the patients enrolled in the trial would receive medical treatment that is believed by the expert medical community to be at least as good as the standard of care.

This alternative framework provides accurate ethical guidance concerning clinical research without presuming that the ethics of therapeutic medicine should govern clinical trials. We illustrate this by applying the seven ethical requirements to the example of the hypericum-sertraline trial.

Scientific or social value and scientific validity.

The study has social value owing to the widespread use of herbal remedies. Since the efficacy of hypericum in treating depression (especially major depression) was uncertain, there was an honest null hypothesis that hypericum would be no better than placebo. It would have been unreasonable to design the trial as an active-controlled superiority trial, since it is highly unlikely that hypericum could be shown to be more effective than sertraline. An active-controlled equivalence trial would lack "assay sensitivity" because the finding that the reduction in symptoms of depression experienced by those trial participants receiving hypericum was not significantly different for those receiving sertraline would not validly support the inference that hypericum was effective.[41] It would remain possible that neither treatment was effective in the study sample—as was in fact shown. The study, therefore, was properly designed as a three-arm placebo-controlled trial.

Fair subject selection.

There is no evidence to suggest that particularly vulnerable patients were recruited inappropriately for this study, which included a sample representative of depressed patients.

Favorable risk–benefit ratio.

Risk–benefit assessment of research protocols ultimately comes down to a matter of judgment. With respect to the use of the placebo control—the aspect of the trial that violated clinical equipoise—the risks to participants from an eight-week trial, with careful exclusionary criteria and monitoring, were not excessive and were justifiable by the anticipated value of the knowledge to be gained from the research. Hence, the placebo component of the study had a favorable risk–benefit ratio. Eliminating the placebo would have made the risk-benefit ratio unfavorable by virtue of undermining the scientific validity of the research.

Independent review, informed consent, and respect for enrolled research participants.

The report of the study asserted that IRB approval was obtained at all sites and that all subjects gave informed consent. In addition, the described procedures for monitoring subjects for possible risk of harm indicated an acceptable level of respect.

In sum, this study was ethically justifiable despite violating clinical equipoise; moreover, had it been designed in accordance with clinical equipoise, it would have been methodologically deficient and therefore ethically questionable.

Charles Weijer, a leading advocate of clinical equipoise and the similarity position, has recently claimed that "Placebo-controlled trials in the context of serious illnesses such as depression or schizophrenia are ethically egregious precisely because no competent physician would fail to offer therapy to a patient with the condition."[42] Although we agree that depression is a serious illness, the hypericum-sertraline trial demonstrates that there is nothing "ethically egregious" about the use of placebo controls in trials of treatment for depression, as long as the ethical requirements for clinical research are satisfied. Whether or not one agrees that, all things considered, the placebo control was ethical in this trial, the ethical justification of placebo controls has nothing to do with the therapeutic practice of competent physicians. In any case, the alternative ethical framework with its seven requirements provides adequate guidance for clinical trials without appeal to the incoherent doctrine of clinical equipoise and without conflating the ethics of research with the ethics of therapy.

Notes

1. Hypericum Depression Trial Study Group, "Effect of *Hypericum Perforatum* (St John's Wort) in Major Depressive Disorder: a Randomized Controlled Trial," *JAMA* 287 (2002):1807–1814.
2. Ibid., 1813.

3. S.M. Stahl, *Essential Psychopharmacology of Depression and Bipolar Disorder* (New York: Cambridge University Press, 2000).

4. P.S. Appelbaum, L.H. Roth, C.W. Lidz, P. Benson, and W. Winslade, "False Hopes and Best Data: Consent to Research and the Therapeutic Misconception," *Hastings Center Report* 17, no. 2 (1987):20–24.

5. P.S. Appelbaum, "Clarifying the Ethics of Clinical Research: a Path Toward Avoiding the Therapeutic Misconception," *American Journal of Bioethics* 2, no. 2 (2002):22.

6. B. Freedman, "Placebo-Controlled Trials and the Logic of Clinical Purpose," *IRB* 12, no. 6 (1990):1–6.

7. R.J. Levine, "Clarifying the Concepts of Research Ethics," *Hastings Center Report* 9, no. 3 (1979):21–26.

8. National Commission for the Protection of Human Subjects of Biomedical and Behavioral Research, *The Belmont Report* (Washington, D.C.: U.S. Government Printing Office, 1979), p. 3.

9. E.J. Emanuel, D.Wendler, and C. Grady, "What Makes Clinical Research Ethical?" *JAMA* 283 (2000):2701–2711.

10. J. Sugarman, N.E. Kass, S.N. Goodman, P. Perentesis, P. Fernandes, and R.R. Faden, "What Patients Say About Medical Research," *IRB* 20, no. 4 (1998):1–7.

11. F.G. Miller, D.L. Rosenstein, and E.G. DeRenzo, "Professional Integrity in Clinical Research," *JAMA* 280 (1998):1449–54.

12. R.R. Faden and T.L. Beauchamp, *A History and Theory of Informed Consent* (New York: Oxford University Press, 1986):200–232.

13. D.A. Braunholtz, S.J.L. Edwards, and R.J. Lilford, "Are Randomized Clinical Trials Good For Us (in the Short term)? Evidence for a 'Trial Effect,'" *Journal of Clinical Epidemiology* 54 (2001):217–224.

14. J.W. Berg, P.S. Appelbaum, C.W. Lidz, and L.S. Parker, *Informed Consent: Legal Theory and Clinical Practice,* 2nd edition (New York: Oxford University Press, 2001):280–283.

15. R.J. Levine, *Ethics and Regulation of Clinical Research,* 2nd ed. (New Haven: Yale University Press, 1986):8–10.

16. J. Katz, "'Ethics and clinical research' revisited: a tribute to Henry K. Beecher," *Hastings Center Report* 23, no. 5 (1993):36.

17. C. Fried, *Medical Experimentation: Personal Integrity and Social Policy* (New York: American Elsevier, 1974).

18. Ibid., 5.

19. Ibid., 94.

20. A.B. Hill, "Medical ethics and controlled trials," *British Medical Journal* 1 (1963):1043–1049.

21. C. Fried, *Medical Experimentation: Personal Integrity and Social Policy* (New York: American Elsevier, 1974): 8.

22. D. Marquis, "Leaving therapy to chance," *Hastings Center Report* 13, no. 4 (1983):40–47.

23. Ibid., 40.

24. F. Gifford, "The Conflict Between Randomized Clinical Trials and the Therapeutic Obligation," *Journal of Medicine and Philosophy* 11 (1986):347–366.

25. B. Freedman, "Equipoise and the Ethics of Clinical Research," *NEJM* 317 (1987):141–145.

26. Ibid., 144.

27. B. Freedman, "Placebo-Controlled Trials and the Logic of Scientific Purpose," *IRB* 12, no. 6 (1990):5.

28. T.L. Beauchamp, and J.F. Childress, *Principles of Biomedical Ethics* 5th edition (New York: Oxford University Press, 2001):323–327.

29. B. Freedman, K.C. Glass, and C. Weijer, "Placebo Orthodoxy in Clinical Research. II: Ethical, Legal and Regulatory Myths," *Journal of Law, Medicine & Ethics* 24 (1996):252–259.

30. R. Temple and S. E. Ellenberg, "Placebo-Controlled Trials and Active-Control Trials in the Evaluation of New Treatments: Part 1: Ethical and Scientific Issues," *Annals of Internal Medicine* 133 (2000):455–63.

31. T.P. Laughren, "The Scientific and Ethical Basis for Placebo-Controlled Trials in Depression and Schizophrenia: an FDA Perspective," *European Psychiatry* 16 (2001):418–423.

32. Department of Health and Human Services. Protection of Human Subjects. Code of Federal Regulations. 45CFR46, 1991.

33. K.J. Rothman and K.B. Michels, "The Continuing Unethical Use of Placebo Controls," *NEJM* 331 (1994):394–8.

34. See B. Freedman, K.C. Glass, and C.Weijer, "Placebo Orthodoxy in Clinical Research. I: Empirical and Methodological Myths," *Journal of Law, Medicine & Ethics* 24 (1996):243–51; and B. Freedman, K.C. Glass, and C.Weijer, "Placebo Orthodoxy in Clinical Research. II: Ethical, Legal and Regulatory Myths," *Journal of Law, Medicine & Ethics* 24 (1996):252–259.

35. R. Temple and S.E. Ellenberg, "Placebo-Controlled Trials and Active-Control Trials in the Evaluation of New Treatments: Part 1: Ethical and Scientific Issues," *Annals of Internal Medicine* 133 (2000):455–63; E.J. Emanuel

and F.G. Miller, "The Ethics of Placebo-Controlled Trials-a Middle Ground," *NEJM* 345 (2001):915–919.

36. S. Hellman and D.S. Hellman, "Of Mice But Not Men: Problems of the Randomized Controlled Trial," *NEJM* 324 (1991):1585–1589.

37. F.G. Miller and H. Brody, "What Makes Placebo-Controlled Trials Unethical?" *American Journal of Bioethics* 2, no. 2 (2002):3–9.

38. N. Dickert and C. Grady, "What's the Price of a Research Subject? Approaches to Payment for Research Participation," *New England Journal of Medicine* 341 (1999): 198–203.

39. See E.J. Emanuel, D. Wendler, and C. Grady, "What Makes Clinical Research Ethical?" *JAMA* 283 (2000):2701–2711.

40. B. Freedman, K.C. Glass, and C.Weijer, "Placebo Orthodoxy in Clinical Research. II: Ethical, Legal and Regulatory Myths," *Journal of Law, Medicine & Ethics* 24 (1996):253.

41. R. Temple and S.E. Ellenberg, "Placebo-Controlled Trials and Active-Control Trials in the Evaluation of New Treatments: Part 1: Ethical and Scientific Issues," *Annals of Internal Medicine* 133 (2000):455–63.

42. C. Weijer, "When Argument Fails," *American Journal of Bioethics* 2, no. 2 (2002): 10.

The Therapeutic Misconception at 25: Treatment, Research, and Confusion

Jonathan Kimmelman

"Therapeutic misconception" has been misconstrued, and some of the newer, mistaken interpretations are troublesome. They exaggerate the distinction between research and treatment, revealing problems in the foundations of research ethics and possibly weakening informed consent.

Years ago, a friend of mine who sits on an institutional review board was diagnosed with cancer. When her oncologist invited her to participate in a randomized controlled trial studying two approved therapies, she enrolled. She is well versed in the research ethics literature, and she knows what ethicists mean by "therapeutic misconception"—namely (and roughly), the phenomenon of conflating research and therapy. She also knew—although she was somewhat troubled by the fact—that participation in the study required her to forgo a treatment that she would have preferred to receive simultaneously. And years later, she knows that the study failed to demonstrate the superiority of the arm to which she was assigned. Yet if you ask her whether she was receiving treatment for her cancer while on protocol, she will unhesitatingly answer in the affirmative.

In the past half decade, this view has suffered a bruising, partly because of the ever-broadening interpretation of the concept of "therapeutic misconception." This expansion has largely been salutary for the ethics of clinical trials. Fields like gene transfer have long been faulted for inflating medical benefits and exploiting therapeutic misconceptions; that researchers running gene transfer protocols have responded to the phenomenon, and informed consent guidelines have changed, is evidence that the concept has stimulated important reflection.[1]

Kimmelman, J., "The Therapeutic Misconception at 25: Treatment, Research, and Confusion", *Hastings Center Report*, pp. 36–42. Published by the Hastings Center © 2007. Reprinted by permission.

However, like "paradigm," "empowerment," and "social capital," the concept of therapeutic misconception is showing signs of wear typical of concepts that are developed in one context and generalized to others. Some flawed interpretations are merely annoying. But others are more worrying because they reveal unrest about one of research ethics' foundational issues: how to demarcate the boundary between research and care.

This year marks the twenty-fifth anniversary of the seminal article that first introduced the "therapeutic misconception." In what follows, I describe the therapeutic misconception's evolution and argue that recent interpretations of the concept might weaken aspects of informed consent and exaggerate the distinction between therapy and treatment, thereby eroding human protections.

THE RISE OF THE THERAPEUTIC MISCONCEPTION

The problem of therapeutic misconception was first articulated by Paul Appelbaum and colleagues in 1982 and introduced to the wider bioethical community in 1987 (I will call the idea as presented in the 1987 publication simply the "original formulation").[2] In studies of psychiatric drugs, Appelbaum and colleagues noticed that research subjects frequently misinterpreted the risks and benefits of participation because they failed to appreciate how various research procedures interfered with their care. For example, after being told that investigators would randomize participants to a placebo arm, prospective subjects continued to believe that the investigator would assign them to whichever arm best suited their medical needs. "To maintain a therapeutic misconception," wrote Appelbaum et al., "is to deny the possibility that there may be major disadvantages to participating in clinical research that stem from the nature of the research process itself."[3]

Although the term was used sporadically throughout the early 1990s, it lay more or less dormant until a revival in 2000, when its meaning, and influence, significantly expanded.

The reasons for this sudden expansion are not clearly attributable to any single factor, but do present an interesting sociological question. The original formulation had discussed only randomized controlled trials; now the phenomenon was generalized to phase I oncology and other kinds of studies. The term's uptake is evident from its widening clientele, which now includes nurses, sociologists, neuroscientists, and clinical investigators.[4] But some ways of expanding the original formulation raise problems: these concern the concept's definition, its object, and consequences.

DEFINING THERAPEUTIC MISCONCEPTION

The original formulation, quoted above, centered on the failure of subjects to appreciate that research imposes practices on investigators that conflict with conventional ways of practicing medicine. Many who later adopted the term have strayed to a definition along the following lines: "the mistaken belief held by many research subjects that research projects will directly benefit them."[5] More recent writings also imply that patients who join trials in order to obtain medical benefits are enrolling "under the influence."[6] The influence has seemed clearest when patients join trials that are still in early phases, where the primary goal is to gauge an experimental agent's toxicity.

Should anticipation of benefit or misestimation of risk and benefit be considered a component of the therapeutic misconception? Appelbaum and his collaborators allowed that a failure to appreciate restrictions imposed on care by protocol design—the core element of therapeutic misconception—might lead to a misestimation of risk and benefit. A subject might overestimate a trial's benefits because she does not understand that she will be randomized to a placebo, for example. But in this formulation, the benefit overestimation is an outcome of the therapeutic misconception, rather than the misconception itself. As noted by Horng and Grady, this distinction seems important for conceptual clarity: for one thing, subjects can overestimate a trial's medical benefits while fully understanding how research procedures might interfere with typical care.[7] Second, patients—and, for that matter, clinicians—frequently have unrealistic expectations about benefits in clinical care settings. In fact, some commentators warn that overestimating the benefits of standard care can lead patients to decline participation in trials that offer better prospects of benefit.[8] Thus, overestimation of benefits usually has little to do with distinguishing care and research.

Incorporating benefit misestimation into therapeutic misconception may obscure problems with informed consent.[9] But another reason to be wary of considering benefit misestimation "misconceived" is that it may overextend the informed consent process. The idea that subjects misconceive trials because they overestimate benefits or underestimate risks implies that some perceptions of risk and benefit are "correct" and others are "incorrect," and that ethicists and clinicians are well positioned (or at least better positioned) for deciding which perceptions are appropriate. I do not wish to categorically dismiss this view. Nevertheless, studies repeatedly demonstrate that risk and benefit perceptions are influenced by the perceiver's values, culture, and worldviews.[10] Although we can and should develop mechanisms for dispelling the most extreme misestimations, applying the concept of therapeutic misconception to rectify the perception of benefits transforms it from a tool for correcting falsehoods (such as that randomization is compatible with individualized assignment) to one that potentially antagonizes the research subject's worldviews.

THE OBJECT: WHAT IS BEING MISCONCEIVED?

Another way that the conceptual territory of the therapeutic misconception has widened concerns its object. Consider the wording of Appelbaum's 1987 description of a subject-patient: "this man ... has interpreted, even distorted, the information he received to maintain the view ... that every aspect of the research project to which a patient consents is designed to benefit the subject directly. This belief ... we call the therapeutic misconception."[11] In the original formulation, the misconception centered on confusion about procedures *within* a protocol. Randomization is one such procedure. More recent work has broadened the object of confusion to trials, classes of trials, and clinical research in general.

This broadening from confusion within a protocol to confusion *about* protocols is reflected in the way some commentators use the concept of therapeutic misconception to pry apart the boundaries of clinical care and research. Again, consider the original formulation's careful description of the difference between research and care: "[the] methods of science *inhibit* the application of personal care" (emphasis added). This leaves the door open a crack for some trials to perform therapeutic functions. Franklin Miller and various collaborators use therapeutic misconception to shut that door. In their interpretation, research and care become "fundamentally different activities" that are "governed by different ethical principles."[12] In research, as opposed to clinical practice, the interests of clinical investigators and subjects are likely to diverge. Whereas clinical care mandates that physicians provide "optimal medical care for individual patients," the obligations of researchers to their subjects consist only of protecting research participants from exploitation. In defining the differences between care and research so starkly, direct medical benefit in all clinical trials becomes "incidental."[13]

Is so sharp a distinction warranted? Clinical practitioners, too, can harbor interests that legitimately compete with their therapeutic obligations. In medical training, for example, a clinician's responsibilities as an educator can compete with optimizing the care of individual patients.[14] Similarly, competing interests are introduced when a practitioner transplants an organ donated by a healthy person, thereby exposing that person to significant risks for the benefit of somebody else, and when a practitioner withholds antibiotics in elderly, terminal patients because of concerns about the spread of antibiotic resistance.[15] Triage is another scenario in which decisions about whether and when to treat a given patient are made with respect to the needs and interests of others. So while it is true that physicians generally owe their primary obligation to patients in their care, this obligation, as the fourth edition of the American College of Physicians ethics manual states, "has its limits."[16]

It is also true that clinical research activities are sometimes conducted in circumstances where the investigator maintains a therapeutic alliance with the subject. Surgical research, for example, frequently mingles individualized care and investigation. Alternative medicine and psychotherapeutic interventions are two other clinical activities in which the contrast between clinical care and research is often less striking. In all three, the failure to customize care would abrogate the study's validity, since customization is central to each. Novel medical devices, which involve variation and rapid technological modification, are also often best evaluated in trials that bring research activities and clinical care into much greater proximity than could be supported by a sharp distinction between care and research.[17] Clinical research in all four of these areas tends to employ "pragmatic trial designs," which are aimed at testing interventions as they will actually be applied, instead of the traditional approach sometimes known as explanatory design.[18]

One of the most common tropes in the therapeutic misconception literature is the notion that research and care have different primary aims— that the primary purpose of research is knowledge, whereas medical practice is primarily aimed at clinical care. Presumably, a secondary goal of the former might be care. The question then becomes, To what degree should we let secondary goals shape the primary agenda, and under what circumstances? If my primary goal in a shopping run is to pick up bread, and my secondary goal to buy cheese, the secondary goal may constrain my choice of baker, and consequently my choice of bread. Similarly, secondary

therapeutic goals can and should influence the investigator's choice of research design.

A doctrinaire distinction between research and care undermines trial design reforms aimed at enhancing subject welfare. In phase I oncology trials—often thought to represent an extreme of nontherapeutic research—these reforms include customizing dosing, maximizing the number of subjects receiving levels of test drugs that are anticipated to be therapeutic, or allowing subjects to select their dose level.[19]

In deciding whether ethicists should separate the ethics of care and research, perhaps one question that needs to be asked is, Whose interests would best be served? According to Miller and Rosenstein, investigators who regard trials as therapy may "find it easy to tolerate or rationalize research activities that may compromise the subjects' well being,"[20] This concern seems important, but the alternative they propose sounds even riskier. Encouraging clinicians to check their therapeutic impulses at the door whenever they walk into a research clinic attenuates their ethical obligations. The therapeutic misconception, which was originally intended to strengthen the responsibilities of investigators to research subjects, flirts with excusing physicians from ethical commitments. Perhaps evidence could be marshaled in support of Miller's view: investigators who harbor therapeutic intentions when conducting trials might conduct shabbier informed consent and expose their volunteers to greater risks. Absent such evidence, though, this interpretation of the therapeutic misconception seems to weaken protections.

THE CONSEQUENCES: WHY WORRY?

A third dimension in which the concept of therapeutic misconception has been expanded concerns its consequences. In the original formulation, Appelbaum and colleagues articulated two ethical concerns about studies that are misconceived by subjects: exploitation and validity of informed consent. Later commentators have added several other ethical concerns: diminished study value (because the misconception inhibits compliance with research activities), validity (because the misconception produces a large placebo effect or interferes with the use of procedures like placebo controls), and professional integrity (because the misconception leads investigators to have incoherent beliefs about medical practice).[21]

Some of these additions require qualification. For example, therapeutic misconceptions need not always antagonize validity, and in some circumstances they may actually enhance it. Drug trials, like any scientific model, attempt to emulate conditions under which the experimental agent will ultimately be applied. Since validated drugs are typically administered in therapeutic settings, therapeutic expectations may be acceptable—indeed the *absence* of therapeutic expectations may arguably lessen the external validity of trials.[22]

The charge that the therapeutic misconception undermines professional integrity also seems questionable. Some commentators suggest that physicians who harbor therapeutic intentions in clinical research lack coherent professional self-understanding.[23] But the remedy—encouraging physicians to suppress their therapeutic self-understanding when they participate in clinical research—may be more incoherent. Years of training and practice have acculturated physicians to regard themselves as healers.

Finally, the central charge that the therapeutic misconception invalidates informed consent needs further elaboration. Some think that it can have "tolerable" ethical consequences.[24] In addition, despite many empirical studies of the therapeutic misconception, there is little evidence that it leads people to make erroneous decisions. It would be helpful to know, for example, whether the therapeutic misconception is important in a potential subject's consent decision. Perhaps the therapeutic misconception often represents a pathway through which more deep-seated factors, like poor comprehension or emotional turmoil, can interfere with informed consent. If so, studies indicating that low educational attainment, impaired social functioning, and emotional problems correlate significantly with the therapeutic misconception (defined as research-treatment confusion) raise the possibility that the therapeutic misconception may be only a marker, not a cause, of "uninformed" consent.[25] Of course, in the absence of information showing otherwise, it would be prudent to assume that the therapeutic misconception is determinative in informed consent, but the issue deserves examination (and the growing use of empirical methodologies to study the therapeutic misconception provides reason to expect that these questions will soon have answers).

TOWARD A MORE NUANCED UNDERSTANDING OF THE RESEARCH-TREATMENT BOUNDARY

One alternative way of viewing the relationship between research and care borrows from a notion developed by historians and sociologists of technology. They reject the view that technologies have (or should have) solitary, obvious applications. They argue instead that users understand them in many different ways, just as citizens do laws.[26] And as with interpretations of laws, understandings of technology have a tendency to feed back on and reshape the technology. Since clinical trials are a type of technology, their form and application can be modified by different interests. As long as activists, patients, ethicists, and others encourage investigators to implement trials that serve the multiple interests of present and future subjects, "research" and "care" need not be a dichotomy.

If that's right, then the concept of therapeutic misconception seems flawed if it categorically labels as mistaken those subjects who enter trials seeking or expecting medical benefits, reproaches investigators and ethicists who regard trial participation as serving therapeutic ends, or reifies the distinction between care and research. Ethicists who use the therapeutic misconception in this way seem to be suggesting that study design reforms should not aim to improve the therapeutic value of trials (thus advancing the interests of research subjects).

They seem to dismiss the convictions of those clinical investigators who embrace their commitment to promote their subjects' best interests. They also seem to denigrate the worldviews on which an optimistic subject's benefit assessments are built and to reject legitimate reasons subjects with refractory diseases might have for participating in research.

A better, more defensible option might be to refocus attention on situations where a subject's expectations and goals for care cannot be achieved within the parameters of a study's design. Consider the following examples.

- Some gene transfer studies administer a vector into one tumor in order to compare its growth with that of uninjected tumors. The subject who enters such a trial intending to receive curative care may have misconceived the trial, since such a study design is incompatible with cure.
- Some subjects with untreatable illnesses enter randomized controlled trials in order to gain access to an unapproved drug that they believe will benefit them. These subjects are not necessarily misconceiving research. They are, however, if they fail to appreciate that the investigator has no intention of ensuring that the subject receives the unapproved drug.
- A person with a chronic, incurable disease might enter a trial in hopes of building a long-term therapeutic alliance with a clinical investigator. That decision is mistaken if, upon the trial's completion, the investigator has no intention of continuing to follow the subject.

To head off such clearly problematic "strong" therapeutic misconceptions, investigators might invite subjects to describe their objectives in entering a trial and then disabuse them of expectations incompatible with trial design. If empirical studies show that subjects frequently fail to appreciate how trial design can interfere with their own therapeutic objectives, then this sort of intervention is warranted. One way of handling it would be to include an addendum to consent documents that itemizes the practices or constraints (such as randomization, blinding, subtherapeutic dosing, nonclinically indicated testing, or trial closure) that are at odds with the way care is typically provided.

At the same time, there is something to be said for the more generalized version of the therapeutic misconception, which is grounded in the notion that, from the standpoint of persons who design or conduct them, clinical trials and clinical care have different primary objectives. First, the research-treatment distinction obviously has repercussions for IRB review and the stringency of informed consent. It also often has implications for insurance reimbursement and research funding.

Second, recognizing the primacy of knowledge creation in research (again, from the standpoint of investigators) has important implications for justice. For instance, various policy documents require that trials conducted in the developing world be responsive to the health needs of the communities from which subjects are drawn. Conflating the primary objectives of research and care would relieve investigators of the obligation to demonstrate responsiveness, if they could claim that a trial offered sufficient direct benefits to participating subjects. Third, the distinction is relevant to the obligations that derive from respect for persons. I have suggested that in many research contexts, subjects may reasonably define their primary objectives upon entering a trial as therapeutic. Nevertheless, when subjects consent to a trial, they volunteer to endure burdens that will advance interests external to their own.

It seems appropriate, therefore, to recognize the existence of a "weaker" version of the therapeutic misconception in which research subjects—or, for that matter, investigators and ethicists—fail to appreciate or understand that trial participation advances ends other than care. Empirical studies clearly document that this weaker therapeutic misconception is not uncommon among ill subjects.[27] In some circumstances, appreciation of a study's scientific objectives, or even *that* a study has scientific objectives, may affect the subject's decision, her comfort level, or her experience with research participation. However, the consequences of this weaker misconception are less severe: unlike a strong therapeutic misconception, the weaker misconception does not threaten to directly frustrate a subject's therapeutic goals on entering a trial. Also, as previously noted, research is not the only circumstance where accepted clinical practice advances other interests. Nevertheless, the weaker misconception is clearly undesirable; whether in the context of medical education, HMO clinics, or research, patients should be informed about the existence and role of external interests in influencing their care.

Two important criticisms might be leveled against the foregoing arguments. First, some might hold that drawing attention to the malleability of the research-treatment distinction or suggesting that subjects can legitimately harbor therapeutic motivations when entering a trial invites practices that have been rightly criticized. It may encourage clinicians to "rationalize research activities that may compromise the subjects' well-being" or use referrals to phase I oncology studies to "avoid the … uncomfortable discussions that loom when therapeutic options are exhausted."[28] But the sin in both cases is a failure of self-awareness and honesty. Nothing in what I have argued excuses a clinical investigator who misrepresents a trial's benefits or denies the existence and influence of external interests in clinical research.

Second, why all the fuss over an intellectual construct? How can misconstruing the research-treatment distinction possibly harm human subjects? The answer is that the therapeutic misconception purports to diagnose an ethical problem. As in medicine, diagnoses help determine a course of action, and a wrong or invalid diagnosis can lead to interventions that, despite good intentions, divert attention from the major problems—or worse, jeopardize a patient's welfare. I've tried to enumerate some of the ways that misunderstanding the research-treatment distinction can subvert the interests of research subjects.

In the original formulation, Appelbaum and collaborators emphasized the tenaciousness of the therapeutic misconception among some subjects. Although investigators should do all they can to dispel this misconception, it will often persist. Nevertheless, the insight that the therapeutic misconception is not always gravely problematic suggests another way of reducing the moral fallout from research-treatment confusion. Researchers should try to design studies so that the therapeutic misconception will have limited ethical consequences. This is a reason for requiring that a trial be conducted only when the experimental regimen is in clinical equipoise with standard practice. It is also a reason for designing studies that maximize the therapeutic benefits for enrolled subjects.

We should be particularly cautious about research circumstances in which the stronger and more ethically problematic therapeutic misconception can flourish. These circumstances might include trials involving riskier designs or interventions, and trials in which grandiose claims are made about the social or medical value of a particular research undertaking or research design. Greater caution in these circumstances would help ensure that the concept of the therapeutic misconception continues to serve as it was originally intended: to protect persons rendered weak and dependent by their illnesses.

Acknowledgements

Without wishing to suggest their endorsement of my positions, I thank Kathy Glass, Alberto Cambrosio, Stan Shapiro, and several anonymous reviewers for comments on a previous draft. This work was funded by the Canadian Institutes of Health Research.

Notes

1. L.M. Arkin et al., "Confronting the Issues of Therapeutic Misconception, Enrollment Decisions, and Personal Motives in Genetic Medicine-Based Clinical Research Studies for Fatal Disorders," *Human Gene Therapy* 16 (2005): 1028–36; Office of Biotechnology Activities, National Institutes of

Health, "NIH Guidance on Informed Consent for Gene Transfer Research," at http://www4.od.nih.gov/oba/ rac/ic/.

2. P.S. Appelbaum, L.H. Roth, and C. Lidz, "The Therapeutic Misconception: Informed Consent in Psychiatric Research," *International Journal of Law and Psychiatry* 5 (1982): 319–29; P.S. Appelbaum et al., "False Hopes and Best Data: Consent to Research and the Therapeutic Misconception," *Hastings Center Report* 17, no. 2 (1987): 20–24.

3. Appelbaum et al., "False Hopes and Best Data," 20.

4. E.E. Steinke, "Research Ethics, Informed Consent, and Participant Recruitment," *Clinical Nurse Specialist* 18 (2004): 88–95; R.C. Fox and J.P. Swazey, "'He Knows That Machine Is His Mortality'': Old and New Social and Cultural Patterns in the Clinical Trial of the AbioCor Artificial Heart," *Perspectives in Biology and Medicine* 47 (2004): 74–99; G.J. Boer and H. Widmer, "Clinical Neurotransplantation: Core Assessment Protocol Rather Than Sham Surgery as Control," *Brain Research Bulletin* 58 (2002): 547–53; Arkin, "Confronting the Issues of Therapeutic Misconception."

5. M. Hochhauser, "'Therapeutic Misconception' and 'Recruiting Doublespeak' in the Informed Consent Process," *IRB: Ethics & Human Research* 24 (2002): 11–12; M.A. Williams and C. Haywood, "Critical Care Research on Patients with Advance Directives or Do-Not-Resuscitate Status: Ethical Challenges for Clinician-Investigators," *Critical Care Medicine* 31 (2003): S167–71.

6. R. Dresser, "The Ubiquity and Utility of the Therapeutic Misconception," *Social Philosophy & Policy* 19, no. 2 (2002): 271–94; G.E. Henderson et al., "Therapeutic Misconception in Early Phase Gene Transfer Trials," *Social Science & Medicine* 62 (2006): 239–53.

7. S. Horng and C. Grady, "Misunderstanding in Clinical Research: Distinguishing Therapeutic Misconception, Therapeutic Misconception, and Therapeutic Optimism," *IRB: Ethics & Human Research* 25 (2003): 11–16.

8. J.M. Sheldon, J.H. Fetting, and L.A. Siminoff, "Offering the Option of Randomized Clinical Trials to Cancer Patients Who Overestimate Their Prognoses with Standard Therapies," *Cancer Investigation* 11 (1993): 57–62.

9. K.P. Weinfurt et al., "Patient Expectations of Benefit from Phase 1 Clinical Trials: Linguistic Considerations in Diagnosing a Therapeutic Misconception," *Theoretical Medicine* 24 (2003): 329–44.

10. P. Slovic, "Trust, Emotion, Sex, Politics, and Science: Surveying the Risk-Assessment Battlefield," *Risk Analysis* 19 (1999): 689–701; M. Douglas and A. Wildavsky, *Risk and Culture: An Essay on the Selection of Technological and Environmental Dangers* (Berkeley: University of California Press, 1982).

11. Appelbaum et al., "False Hopes and Best Data," 20.

12. The first clause is from F.G. Miller and H. Brody. "Reply," *Hastings Center Report* 33, no. 5 (2003): 6–7; the second is from F.G. Miller and H. Brody, "A Critique of Clinical Equipoise: Therapeutic Misconception in the Ethics of Clinical Trials," *Hastings Center Report* 33, no. 3 (2003): 19–28, at 20.

13. H. Brody and F.G. Miller, "The Clinician-Investigator: Unavoidable but Manageable Tension," *Kennedy Institute of Ethics Journal* 13 (2003): 329–46, at 334.

14. A.J. Raja and A.V. Levin, "Challenges of Teaching Surgery': Ethical Framework," *World Journal of Surgery* 27 (2003): 948–51; A. Gawande, *Complications: A Surgeon's Notes on an Imperfect Science* (New York: Henry Holt and Company, 2002), 24.

15. E.L Marcus, M. Clarfield, and A.E. Moses, "Ethical Issues Relating to the Use of Antimicrobial Therapy in Older Adults," *Clinical Infectious Diseases* 33 (2001): 1697–1705.

16. American College of Physicians, "Ethics Manual: Fourth Edition," *Annals of Internal Medicine* 128 (1998): 576–94.

17. R.J. Lilford et al., "Trials and Fast Changing Technologies: The Case for Tracker Studies," *British Medical Journal* 320 (2000): 43–46.

18. S.R. Tunis, D.B. Stryer, and C.M. Clancy, "Practical Clinical Trials: Increasing the Value of Clinical Research for Decision Making in Clinical and Health Policy," *Journal of the American Medical Association* 290 (2003): 1624–32: H. MacPherson, "Pragmatic Clinical Trials," *Complementary Therapies in Medicine* 12 (2004): 136–40.

19. E.A. Eisenhauer et al., "Phase I Clinical Trial Design in Cancer Drug Development," *Journal of Clinical Oncology* 18 (2000): 684–92; J.S. Babb and A. Rogatko, "Patient Specific Dosing in a Cancer Phase 1 Clinical Trial,' *Statistics in Medicine* 20 (2001): 2079–90: C.K. Daugherty et al., "Study of Cohort-Specific Consent and Patient Control in Phase 1 Cancer Trials," *Journal of Clinical Oncology* 16, no. 7 (1998); 2305–2312.

20. F.G. Miller and D.L. Rosenstein, "The Therapeutic Orientation to Clinical Trials," *New England Journal of Medicine* 348 (2003): 1383–86.

21. N.M.P King, "Accident and Desire: Inadvertent Germline Effects in Clinical Research," *Hastings Center Report* 33, no. 2 (2003): 23–30; J. Kimmelman. "Recent Developments in Gene Transfer: Risk and Ethics," *British Medical Journal* 330 (2005): 79–82; Miller and Rosenstein, "The Therapeutic Orientation."

22. MacPherson. "Pragmatic Clinical Trials."

23. Miller and Rosenstein, "The Therapeutic Orientation."

24. Horng and Grady, "Misunderstanding in Clinical Research."

25. Henderson et al., "Therapeutic Misconception in Early Phase Gene Transfer Trials"; Appelbaum, Roth, and Lidz, "The Therapeutic Misconception: Informed Consent in Psychiatric Research."

26. T. Pinch and W. Bijker, "The Social Construction of Facts and Artifacts," in *The Social Construction of Technological Systems*, ed. W. Bijker, T. Hughes, and T. Pinch (Cambridge, Mass.: MIT Press. 1987), 17–50.

27. S. Joffe et al., "Quality of Informed Consent in Cancer Clinical Trials: A Cross-Sectional Survey," *Lancet* 358 (2001): 1772–77; Henderson et al., "Therapeutic Misconception in Early Phase Gene Transfer Trials."

28. The first comes from Miller and Rosenstein, "The Therapeutic Orientation," and the second from M. Miller, "Phase 1 Cancer Trials: A Collusion of Misunderstanding," *Hastings Center Report* 30, no. 4 (2000): 34–42.

Pharmaceutical Research in Developing Countries: Testing a New Surfactant in Bolivia

James V. Lavery, Christine Grady, Elizabeth R. Wahl, and Ezekiel E. Emanuel

BACKGROUND ON BOLIVIA

Located in central South America, Bolivia is...one of the least developed countries in South America. About two-thirds of the population lives below the poverty line, many as subsistence farmers.

Consistent with income disparities, 21% of the population is undernourished and 15% lack access to improved water sources. Nonetheless, life expectancy in Bolivia has increased from 46.7 years in 1975 to 63.9 years in 2005. Infant and child mortality rates have also improved dramatically over the last 30 years, yet infant mortality remains relatively high at 53 per 1,000 live births and mortality rate for children under 5 is now 66 per 1,000 children.... Health care spending is approximately US$180 per capita (in purchasing power parity).

. . .

RESPIRATORY DISTRESS SYNDROME AND SURFACTANTS

Respiratory distress syndrome, or RDS, is a common and potentially fatal disease in premature infants that is caused by insufficient surfactant in the lungs. Surfactant is a protein that reduces alveolar surface tension, enabling proper lung inflation and aeration. In most full-term infants, surfactant ensures soft and pliable lungs that stretch and contract with each breath. Premature infants have underdeveloped lungs

Ethical Issues in International Biomedical Research: A Casebook, edited by James V. Lavery et al (2007) Chp. "Commentaries on Pharmaceutical Research in Developing Countries" by Temple, Lurie, & Wolfie pp. 151–170. By permission of Oxford University Press.

with insufficient surfactant and consequently their lungs are stiff and do not inflate as easily. As a result premature infants are more likely to have RDS.

RDS in infants is ideally treated by general supportive care, including intravenous fluids and mechanical ventilation and the administration of surfactant. The use of surfactant replacement therapy as the standard treatment for RDS in the Western world has produced a 34% reduction in neonatal mortality in randomized trials.[1]...

Surfactant therapy has been approved for use in Latin America, but its high cost, about US$1,100–2,400 per child, precludes it as a viable option for most infants in Latin America, where per capita annual health spending ranges from US$60–225. In Bolivia, Ecuador, and Peru, where only a privileged minority has access to surfactant therapies and adequate prenatal monitoring, RDS continues to be responsible for at least 30% of neonatal deaths.

. . .

Of the current available surfactants, Exosurf is synthetic, and Infasurf, Survanta, and Curosurf are animal-derived (pig lung and cow lung respectively). All are administered in the neonatal period through the endotracheal tube while the infant is receiving mechanical ventilation.

THE STUDY

In 2000, Discovery Labs, a private U.S. drug company, proposed a phase 3 study to demonstrate the efficacy of a new synthetic surfactant called Surfaxin for the treatment of RDS in premature infants. The drug company deliberated with the Food and Drug Administration about an acceptable study design. Although a superiority trial designed to demonstrate the superiority of Surfaxin to Exosurf might have been accepted by the FDA as evidence of Surfaxin's effectiveness, the sponsor did not think it could succeed with such a trial. Based on its experience with

previous surfactant studies, the FDA concluded that a noninferiority trial of Surfaxin against Survanta could not yield data that would support the approval of Surfaxin. Despite the clear overall evidence of the effectiveness of surfactants, data on the performance of various clinical measures used in effectiveness studies of each individual surfactant has been inconsistent in studies of the prevention and treatment of RDS. This made it very difficult to identify a credible "noninferiority margin"[2] for surfactant drugs in...comparison trials with other surfactants.

After some deliberation, a multicenter, double-blinded, randomized, two-arm, placebo-controlled trial was proposed to be conducted in Bolivia, and three other Latin American countries. The study population was to be 650 premature infants with RDS. The hospitals chosen for participation in the study generally did not have surfactant available for the treatment of RDS. The sponsor proposed to provide endotracheal tubes, ventilators, and antibiotics for all study participants. The proposal also included sending a team of American neonatologists to supervise the study and help train local health care personnel.

In participating research centers, parents of infants showing symptoms of RDS would be asked to give consent for their infants to participate in the study. With consent, a health care provider would intubate the infants with an endotracheal tube, and either give air suffused with Surfaxin or air without any drug. Endpoints for the proposed study were all-cause mortality by day 28, and mortality due to RDS.

. . .

The principal target market for the drug was the United States and Europe, and the sponsor had no specific plans for marketing Surfaxin in Latin America. However, the sponsor engaged in some preliminary discussions with the participating hospitals making Surfaxin available to them at reduced cost if it proved to be efficacious in the trial. No firm agreement was reached in these negotiations.

THE ETHICAL ISSUES

Surfactants have been used for more than a decade in the treatment of respiratory distress syndrome in infants. Placebo-controlled surfactant trials for premature infants with RDS would currently be considered unethical in the United States and other developed countries because surfactant treatment is widely available and known to improve survival compared to mechanical ventilation alone; a placebo-controlled trial would require withholding life saving treatment that is available to those who can afford it.

Even though financial constraints prevent the Bolivian hospitals from routinely providing surfactant treatment for RDS, the hospitals were of sufficient quality to support and run the ICU facilities promised by the sponsor in return for participation. In the study, although half the infants with RDS would not receive surfactant, they would not be denied a treatment that they otherwise would have received because of economic limits. The ventilator support that both the Surfaxin and "placebo" patients would receive in the proposed study was known to improve survival more effectively than treatments generally available to both groups prior to the initiation of the study. Although offering a higher standard of care than many Bolivian infants would have received, the level of care provided in the control arm—ventilation without a surfactant—would most likely not have been permitted in the United States and other developed countries.

Were the researchers in the Surfaxin trial obligated to use the same surfactant therapies in the control group in Bolivia that would have been required in any developed country? Was it ethical to provide medical care that although better than what the patients normally received was not better than the worldwide best standard of care? Did this study violate the Declaration of Helsinki which states:

> The benefits, risks, burdens and effectiveness of a new method should be tested against those of the best current prophylactic, diagnostic, and therapeutic methods. This does not exclude the use of placebo, or no treatment, in studies where no proven prophylactic, diagnostic or therapeutic method exists.[3]

If the study was ultimately approved, what information should the Bolivian parents receive? Should they be informed that although this study did not include them, several other surfactants were available for those who could afford them?

Notes

1. Soll RF. Synthetic Surfactant for Respiratory Distress Syndrome in Prenatal Infants (Cochrane Review). In The Cochrane Library, issue 4. Oxford: Update Software; 2000.
2. International Conference on Harmonization: Choice of control group in clinical trials. *Federal Register,* 2001;66:24390 24391.
3. World Medical Association Declaration of Helsinki: ethical principles for medical research involving human subjects. Principle #29. Adopted by the 52nd World Medical Assembly, Edinburgh, 2000. Available at http://www.wma.net/e/policy/b3.htm. Accessed Sept. 3, 2006.

Commentary: Benefit to Trial Participants or Benefit to the Community? How Far Should the Surfaxin Trial Investigators' and Sponsors' Obligations Extend?

Robert J. Temple

The Surfaxin case presents a perfect example of the problem of deciding what constitutes "available" therapy for a population in a trial involving a serious disease. Despite some degree of discussion following the 2000 revision of the Declaration of Helsinki, it is widely accepted,[1-4] and clearly stated in guideline E10 of the International Conference on Harmonization (ICH), Choice of Control Group and Related Issues in Clinical Trials,[2] that patients can be invited to participate in a placebo-controlled trial, even if there is existing available effective treatment, if they will not be harmed, that is, suffer death, irreversible morbidity, or perhaps very severe discomfort, by the delay or denial of the treatment. In contrast, and not at all debated, patients cannot be randomized to a placebo treatment when available therapy for that patient population, given as it would be used in the study, is known to prevent death or irreversible morbidity.[1,2]

The ICH E–10 guideline does not consider, however, what "available therapy" means in a clinical-trial context in a country in which limited economic resources means that there will be limited medical services. Other documents have considered this question, but not always persuasively, often using the evocative language of social justice at the expense of rational consideration of the real interests of potential participants in the trial.

. . .

It is…important to know that were an active-control trial considered interpretable, it almost surely would be conducted in the United States or another developed country. Given the decreased assurance of the applicability of results of a Latin American trial to the U.S. population there is reason to believe an active control trial would not be done in Bolivia. Therefore, under these circumstances, there would be no trial of any kind of a surfactant in Latin America. Consequently, babies born with RDS in Bolivia would not have received either ventilator support or surfactant. Forcing an active control study might have resulted in more than the 17 deaths from RDS in Bolivia that the advocates of an active-control trial claim a placebo-controlled design would produce.

There is no question that conducting a placebo-controlled trial that denies trial subjects effective therapy widely used in other countries, when the beneficiary of the trial is a developed nation and is not the country where the trial is to be conducted, is unsettling. Nonetheless, it is worth asking the basis for insisting that people in a clinical study are entitled to treatment not available to others in their own country and worth exploring the full consequences of not permitting such a trial. There are at least two aspects of this question that need to be explored.

People in the Trial versus the Community as a Whole

One discomfort expressed about trials in developing countries relates to whether the trial serves the needs of the community where the study takes place or serves only the needs of a commercial sponsor. Indeed, the 2000 Declaration of Helsinki (paragraph 19) and guideline 10 of the 2002 CIOMS guideline[5] state that any trial in a developing country must in some way serve the needs of that country. Although the sponsor of the Surfaxin trial will make the drug available to the participating community at reduced cost, this will not affect Bolivia as a whole, and the purpose of the trial is primarily to market the drug in developed countries.

The critical question, however, is whether a trial must indeed serve the community in which it is conducted or whether it is sufficient to be a desirable trial for the people who participate in it. In other clinical research situations, we appear to act as if the most important ethical consideration is the interest of the people in the trial. For instance, we are not allowed to increase risks to those who participate in research because the results would be more generalizable to other people.

Although it is recognized that individuals can behave altruistically, contributing time and possible discomfort to the cause of advancing scientific knowledge, it is generally agreed that it would not be ethical to put people at real avoidable risk compared to their prior status even for a considerable benefit to the community. No one, for example, thinks it would be reasonable or ethical to study nerve agent antidotes in humans given harmful doses of such agents even though the public benefit might be very great. The FDA promulgated the "animal rule"[6] to allow reliance on animal studies as evidence of effectiveness for such antidotes because it considered human studies "infeasible." In brief, it seems clear that ethical principles demand that the focus of trials must be on the people in them, not the communities from which they are drawn.

One must then ask why, if everyone in a trial is better off because of participation, and no one is denied anything otherwise available to them, the trial is not ethically acceptable. In the Surfaxin case, all participants would receive ventilator support, a higher level of care than would otherwise be available, a clear and almost surely life-saving benefit for some infants, but only half would randomly receive the surfactant, which would be very likely to provide additional life-saving benefit.

It is hard to see why a rational patient would not prefer study participation to nonparticipation and, indeed, local authorities were enthusiastic about the trial. If the focus is on trial participants, it seems clear that they receive an advantage by participating in the trial. By analogy with the principle that you should not harm patients for the good of the community, failure to help the community is not a reason not to help the people in the trial. It is also very clear what the consequences of failing to do the studies would be. The infant lives that would have been saved by improved care in all patients and treatment with surfactant in 50% of patients will not be saved. Although there can be no doubt that all patients would prefer to receive active treatment, in an active control trial. But as we have seen, if such a trial were thought to be informative, it would be conducted in the United States, not in Latin America, and patients in Bolivia would receive no benefit.

Is the Placebo-Controlled Trial "Exploitative"?

Once again, the answer depends on whether the focus is on study participants or the whole community. Plainly the proposal makes use of the severe wealth and health care inequalities that exist among countries and regions in the world. These differences are distressing, but there is no easy or rapid way to eliminate them. Importantly, the drug company did not create or foster these inequalities. Furthermore, the world makes use of such inequalities in other ways, accepting goods made at the low prices made possible by cheaper labor, with appropriate debate about how much advantage should be taken of this, but little real debate about the overall situation. It thus appears that not all use of inequalities is "exploitative." There is, for example, a real difference between paying people in a developing country to participate in a study of a substance too toxic to be acceptable in the United States, or one that has had no animal studies to assess its toxicity—a risk that could not be imposed on U.S. citizens—and studying a probably useful treatment in a developing country, but not giving an active drug to everyone. In the first case, people may be worse off than they were before the study and would accept this possible deterioration because they are poor. In the second case, they would be accepting a random possibility of gain with no risk of potential worsening of their state.

While paying poor people to risk their health may be exploitative, offering a benefit to all—although some would benefit more than others—does not seem exploitative, even if it makes use of the fact of their poor medical care.

SUMMARY AND CONCLUSIONS

It is clear that the fact of disparate access to health care is troubling to everyone and there have been discussions of developed countries' responsibilities with respect to treatment of AIDS, malaria, diarrhea, and many other illnesses that devastate developing countries. The argument that a placebo-controlled surfactant trial is ethical in a country that is not able to provide surfactant treatment for its citizens is in no way related to the question of whether we should be doing more to change the underlying inequality of the situation; it says only that while that situation obtains, a trial that makes everyone better off is ethical.

Notes

1. Temple R, Ellenberg SS. Placebo controlled trials and active control trials in the evaluation of new treatments. Part I: Ethical and scientific issues. *Annals of Internal Medicine*. 2000;133:455–463.
2. International Conference on Harmonization: Choice of control group in clinical trials. Federal Register. 2001;66:24390–24391.
3. Lewis JA, Jonsson B, Krentz G, Sampaio C, van Zwieten-Boot B. Placebo-controlled trials and the Declaration of Helsinki. *Lancet*. 2002;359:1337–1340.
4. Emanuel EJ, Wendler D, Grady C. What makes research ethical? *JAMA*. 2000, 283:2701–2711.
5. Council for International Organizations of Medical Sciences (CIOMS). International ethical guidelines for biomedical research involving human subjects. Geneva: CIOMS;2002.
6. U.S. Food and Drug Administration "Animal Rule" (21 C.F.R. 314.600).

Commentary: The Developing World as the "Answer" to the Dreams of Pharmaceutical Companies: The Surfaxin Story

Peter Lurie and Sidney M. Wolfe

A recent trend in biomedical research is to conduct research in developing countries, rather than just in industrialized ones. The number of new foreign investigators in the U.S. Food and Drug Administration's (FDA) database grew from 988 in the 1990–1992 period to 5,380 in the 1996–1998 period.[1] If the result were therapies for or knowledge relevant to developing country scourges such as malaria or onchocerciasis, this would clearly be a step in the right direction, particularly because pharmaceutical companies have essentially turned a blind eye to the needs of developing-country residents with limited purchasing power. But if the result were a series of research studies with little prospect of generating direct benefit to the local communities, both during the trial and after, we would risk a transformation of contemporary research culture into one with strong echoes of colonialism.

In 1997, we criticized a series of 15 planned clinical trials in Africa and Thailand, including 9 conducted or funded by the U.S. government, in which researchers gave HIV-positive pregnant women in the control arms placebos or drugs not proven to be effective, rather than the proven-effective drug AZT.[2] The trials attempted to identify affordable drug regimens for developing countries to prevent the transmission of HIV from mother to infant. We argued that researchers, particularly those running multimillion dollar trials, are obligated to provide the best scientifically proven intervention—independent of the economic status of the volunteers and regardless of where the study is conducted. In the perinatal trials specifically, we argued that, rather than comparing the less-expensive regimens to unproven regimens or placebo, as the 15 trials planned to do, the less-expensive regimens could have been compared to the proven-effective more-expensive regimens. Such an approach was taken in a sixteenth trial,[3] and, despite the absence of a placebo group, its results left little doubt as to the effectiveness of several less-expensive regimens, while providing additional information comparing their efficacy.

While we never disputed that the researchers in the government-funded perinatal trials actually intended to aid people in developing countries (although we rejected their methods), we always understood that the more worrisome prospect was pharmaceutical company-funded studies in developing countries in which lower ethical standards would be adopted in the pursuit of profit. In the proposed placebo-controlled trial of Surfaxin, a synthetic surfactant for the treatment of neonatal Respiratory Distress Syndrome (RDS), we encountered exactly that situation. The primary concern of Discovery Laboratories, the manufacturer of Surfaxin, appears to have been to conduct a trial with its preferred design in Latin America and then to obtain approval in industrialized countries, where they are likely to reap by far their greatest sales. At the time of the proposed study, pharmaceutical sales in Latin America represented a mere 7% of international pharmaceutical sales, compared with 40% in North America and 27% in Europe.[4]

In an unequivocal demonstration of the double standard represented by the proposed research, Discovery Laboratories planned to conduct a study in Europe in which Surfaxin would be compared to an already FDA-approved surfactant drug. As the internal FDA documents on which we based our exposé of this trial correctly stated, "Conduct of a placebo controlled surfactant trial for premature infants with RDS is considered unethical in the USA." These documents were made available to hundreds of FDA employees in conjunction with an internal FDA Scientific Rounds on January 24, 2001, and were subsequently made public by us in a letter to Health and Human Services Secretary Tommy Thompson seeking that the placebo-controlled study not be allowed to proceed. The meeting had the extraordinarily inappropriate but revealing title "Use of Placebo-Controls in Life Threatening Diseases: Is the Developing World the Answer?"

Clear Evidence that Surfactant Saves Newborn Lives Available at the Time of Study Design

The basic ethical principle of equipoise requires that, among the community of knowledgeable researchers, there be genuine uncertainty as to a study's likely outcome.[5] In the Surfaxin case, the data documenting the efficacy of previously approved surfactants were overwhelming: there were literally dozens of clinical trials, including many with placebo, that together had demonstrated the effectiveness of both synthetic (like Surfaxin) and natural surfactants before the

Surfaxin study was proposed. For this reason, surfactant was described in an article in the *New England Journal of Medicine* as long ago as 1993 as "without doubt the most thoroughly studied new therapy in neonatal care" and as "a major advance in neonatal care."[6] ...

The Cochrane Collaboration had conducted a meta-analysis of six placebo-controlled studies of synthetic surfactant in the treatment of RDS in premature infants and concluded that the use of synthetic surfactant for the treatment of RDS "has been demonstrated to improve clinical outcome."[7] In a section of the review entitled "Implications for research," the reviewer stated unequivocally: "Further placebo controlled trials of synthetic surfactant are no longer warranted." ...

This strong scientific grounding has two consequences: first, it made it very likely that Surfaxin would prove more effective than placebo and, second, it made the withholding of known-effective drugs from any comparison arm all the more unconscionable. The FDA estimated the neonatal mortality rate among premature infants in the potential host countries to be at least 30%. If half of the infant deaths were due to RDS (this was the case in the U.S. in the pre-surfactant era),[8] the provision of placebo (instead of another surfactant) to the 325 infants in the control group would have resulted in the preventable deaths of 17 infants.

Historical Trends in the Design of Surfactant Clinical Trials

At the time of the Surfaxin controversy, we examined all 5 Cochrane reviews of surfactant efficacy in the treatment of RDS as well as a book chapter published by the Cochrane review author.[9] We also included 3 additional clinical trials[10–12] that could be identified through PubMed.

A total of 42 randomized trials of surfactant for the treatment of RDS had been published; 22 of these (52%) utilized placebos. Between 1985, when the first placebo-controlled trial appeared, and 1990, a total of 15 placebo-controlled (and no active-controlled) trials were published. Between 1991, when the first active-controlled trial was published, and 1995, both active- and placebo-controlled trials were published, though the former predominated (16/19 trials). From 1996 onward, there were a total of 8 active-controlled trials and not a single placebo-controlled trial. Clearly, the trend in surfactant clinical trials for RDS has been toward active-controlled trials. The proposed Surfaxin study would therefore have been a landmark of unethical behavior— a turning to the developing world to conduct studies that the FDA acknowledged could never occur in the United States. In so doing, the study would have turned back the ethical clock by at least 5 years for developing-country studies, while industrialized-country studies (including the European Surfaxin trial) used active controls.

Alternatives to Placebo-Controlled Trials

Neither federal laws nor FDA regulations actually require placebo-controlled trials for drug approval. Rather, the regulations require "adequate and well-controlled studies," and list 5 types of acceptable studies: (1) randomized, placebo-controlled trials; (2) dose response studies; (3) active-controlled studies; (4) no treatment, concurrent-controlled studies; and (5) historical controls.[13] Indeed, in some divisions of the FDA, active-controlled trials are commonly used as the basis for drug approval. The field of oncology has for years eschewed pure placebo controls in trials of treatments of cancers for which effective therapy exists. Similarly, drugs for the treatment of pelvic inflammatory disease, bacterial pneumonia, and most other bacterial infections would never be tested against a placebo.

In fact, the FDA has accepted active-controlled trials in the past to support approval of a surfactant. In the FDA-approved label for Infasurf (a natural surfactant), the only 2 clinical trials mentioned are active-controlled trials.[14] Both the treatment and prophylaxis indications were supported by trials comparing Infasurf to Exosurf (a synthetic surfactant). The trials were conducted between 1991 and 1993.

Active-controlled trials may be divided into 2 categories: superiority trials (in which the object is to demonstrate that the new therapy is superior to existing therapy) and noninferiority trials (in which the goal is to prove that the new therapy is not inferior to existing therapies by a prespecified amount). In the Surfaxin case, the FDA raised questions about a noninferiority trial because previous studies were said to have given inconsistent results. However, we have shown above that the results of previous placebo-controlled studies of synthetic surfactant in the treatment of RDS were remarkably consistent. Statistical significance has not generally been a problem for these extremely effective interventions, as long as the study is adequately powered. As noted, the FDA can assure that this occurs. It is noteworthy that the planned study in Europe was a noninferiority trial.

An alternative would be a superiority study, the basis of approval for Infasurf. The FDA documents state that a superiority study in an industrialized country was not considered feasible by the sponsor due to enrollment difficulties and unspecified "ethics." While these "ethical" concerns in industrialized countries, whatever they were, seemed to resonate with the sponsors, providing second-rate treatment to desperately ill infants in developing countries simply because they were poor apparently did not.

According to the FDA documents, "The sponsor has not yet provided justification for why they haven't planned a superiority trial versus Exosurf in *underdeveloped* Latin American countries" (emphasis in original). Even if one accepted (which we do not) that a noninferiority trial was not feasible, one is left wondering why the FDA did not force the company to conduct a superiority trial as Infasurf had been approved on that basis. Perhaps the company was concerned that Surfaxin would prove no more effective and perhaps less effective than another surfactant, a marketing problem for the company. (As the FDA explained in the documents we obtained, "a superiority trial versus an approved therapy presents a clinical efficacy hurdle that the sponsor deems too high for this drug.")

While this altitude may be understandable from a corporate perspective, the FDA is not charged with promoting corporate interests. If an active-controlled trial is the ethical approach from a patient-protection perspective and provides the most useful data (the clinically relevant question is how Surfaxin compares to already-approved surfactants, not whether it is better than nothing), the FDA should have insisted upon such a design. Instead the FDA has been the leading intellectual force behind attacks on the usefulness of active-controlled trials.[15-20]

Another reason to avoid a superiority trial may be the FDA's claim that a superiority study against Exosurf would take longer to conduct for statistical reasons due to larger sample-size requirements. Of course, this is only due if one expects there to be only a small advantage for the new treatment; clearly superior new therapies can be proved superior with studies that are not very different in size from placebo-controlled studies.[21] Every patent-protected day a drug is on the market is a day of increased profit for the company. But with four surfactants already on the U.S. market and the patients at the participating centers in the four Latin American countries currently receiving none of them, even though some of them were approved locally, why is speed a factor for either U.S. or developing-country patients?

Intra-Trial Issues

We do not raise any objection to the use of placebos per se. Placebos are acceptable when no proven therapy exists or when the condition being treated is mild or self-limited, such as common headache or seasonal allergy. But they are considered inappropriate in industrialized countries when the best available science has identified a treatment that may reduce or prevent serious harm, improve health, or prolong life. A therapy proven to reduce neonatal mortality by 34% in placebo-controlled trials certainly meets that criterion. In order to justify the withholding of effective therapy in a developing country, therefore, the researchers had to rely on an economic argument: because the other surfactants were unavailable to the potential patients in the developing countries due to cost, the researchers were under no obligation to provide them no matter how strong the science supporting them. This has come to be known as the "standard of care argument." This term, borrowed inappropriately from malpractice jurisprudence (in which physicians can be found liable for damages if they fail to provide the "standard of care" offered by others in their communities), seeks to sugarcoat the ethical sleight of hand that is in operation....

London has distinguished between what he terms the de facto and de jure standards of care.[22] The de facto standard is defined as being set by "the actual medical practices of that community." In contrast, the de jure standard is determined by "the judgment of experts in the medical community as to which diagnostic and therapeutic practices have proven most effective against the illness in question." In part because it has a basis in the rigors of science, not the vagaries of the world economic order, we endorse the de jure approach.

The de facto standard of care argument has two important consequences for the Surfaxin trial. First, it essentially lays waste to the bedrock ethical principle of equipoise. Due to the large number of previously positive phase 3 trials of similar products as well as phase 1/2 studies and animal studies of Surfaxin presumably in the company's possession, there is little question that Surfaxin will prove superior to placebo. There is, however, genuine doubt as to whether Surfaxin will be as efficacious as the already approved surfactants. This is the ideal situation for an active-controlled trial.

Second, the de facto standard of care argument endorses the notion that researchers' responsibilities are determined in part by nonclinical factors external to the trial. This is completely inconsistent with the Hippocratic oath in which physicians undertake to "look upon [God's] offspring in the same footing as my own brothers." As physician scientists, the only reasonable standard for defining an acceptable control arm is scientific. Patients should not be treated inferiorly because of an accident of birth, residence, or global economic conditions. The laudable work of physicians in bringing

anti-HIV treatments to poor countries bears witness to researchers' potential as opinion leaders, influencing the quality of health care delivered in the countries in which they are working, rather than relegating themselves to the status of bystanders who exploit adverse economic circumstances to conduct a study designed primarily to benefit corporate interests. As medical historian Rothman has observed, "As soon as [researchers] attempt to take advantage of the social predicament in which the subjects are found, they become accomplices to the problem, not observers of it. For usually the investigators have the ability to alter the social deprivation of their particular subjects."[23]

The researcher's obligation to provide interventions to their study participants is not one without limits. We do not suggest that tuberculosis researchers who recognize cases of depression among their patients are obligated to treat those patients' depression themselves. For conditions not being studied but encountered during the course of the study, referral for appropriate care is reasonable, wherever the study is conducted. Nor do we suggest that unreasonable infrastructure building be undertaken before a study can commence. As we have stated previously,[24] a study of the treatment of hypertension in the developing world would not require the construction of a coronary care unit in case the patients develop complications of hypertension. However, reasonable expenditures for care related to the condition under study are, in our view, ethically required when the researchers continue to examine the patients prospectively. The Surfaxin researchers could easily provide an active control drug, particularly since they were planning to go to the effort and expense of upgrading intensive care units so that they could conduct their study.

There are often massive economically based differences in the quality of care provided within a country, even within industrialized countries; these are susceptible to exploitation by any researcher brandishing the de facto standard of care argument. Under such circumstances there is no national standard of care at all: there are those who receive scientifically proven care and those who do not. In the countries where the trial would have taken place (Bolivia, Ecuador, Peru, and Mexico were candidates), surfactants were being used in some hospitals, but, according to the FDA documents, "surfactants are completely unavailable to infants at many other hospitals, secondary to rationing or economic limitations." It is in these latter hospitals that the studies were planned. The researchers thus had to tread a narrow line: they had to identify a target population within a country that was (1) poor enough to not be receiving surfactant; (2) not so well off as to have an expectation of receiving the drug; and (3) receiving care in a facility sophisticated enough to be upgraded to study requirements.

By definition, the proposed trial would have required at least a certain level of infrastructure, because both the placebo and Surfaxin patients would have had endotracheal tubes and would probably have been on ventilators. The logistical feasibility of providing Surfaxin (and thus an active control ding) during the study was therefore not in question, since it would simply have been squirted down the endotracheal tube. Such studies have budgets in the hundreds of thousands, if not millions, of dollars. The physician-investigators who conducted the study would clearly have been making the choice not to provide this lifesaving therapy for some patients, even as they had before them infants suffering from a frequently fatal disease. This represents a very fundamental undermining of the doctor-patient relationship.

Post-Trial Issues

A central tenet of research in developing countries is that the subject of the research must be relevant to the host country's needs.[25] While RDS is certainly an important problem in many developing countries, the notion that the lack of surfactant, which can only be delivered in sophisticated settings, is an important priority in such countries is absurd, particularly after the previous surfactants had been approved and had proved unaffordable in the proposed host countries. In the more likely event that the study pro-duced findings that were beneficial to patients in wealthier countries but the drug was not widely available in the countries in which it was tested, an additional dimension of unethical behavior would have been added.

The investigators claimed that they would provide benefits to the hospital by training neonatologists and providing the drug to those hospitals after the trial. In other words, they were willing to aid these countries in several different ways—just not the most straightforward way, which would have been to treat the control group. Although that would have spared many infants' lives, it would preclude the company from conducting the study the way it wished. This is the very definition of conflict of interest.

Efforts to improve health care infrastructure are hard to oppose; the problem is that the benefits accrue to people outside the trial, while the actual volunteers may not benefit from these infrastructural improvements. In some cases, subjects may actually be denied care as a quid pro quo for others to receive the infrastructural improvements. The Declaration of Helsinki is clear that the researcher's most fundamental ethical responsibility is to his or her patients: "In medical research on human subjects, considerations related to the well-being of the human subject should take precedence over the interests of science and society."[26]

Absent a clear agreement on paper to make the drug available to the general community after the trial (a "prior agreement"[27]), post-trial availability promises may prove empty. Once the trial has been conducted, developing countries have little leverage to insist upon such availability. Prior agreements must specify, to the extent possible, to whom the drug will be made available, at what cost, and for how long. To our knowledge, the offer from Discovery Laboratories included none of these details.

Some may argue that if the company were not permitted to conduct the study with a placebo, it would instead do an active-controlled trial in an industrialized country, denying the developing country the benefits of the research project. In the first place, this would be an acknowledgment that the company never had any interest in the health needs of the developing country, which is, as we noted above, the most basic prerequisite for any developing country research.[25] It would also dispense with the claim, often heard in the defense of these sorts of unethical developing-country studies, that the research was a product of due collaboration between the sponsor and the host country. Obviously, the fact that Discovery had not even decided in which country the research would occur undermines that argument.

We believe that ethical standards have unique value as a statement of the equality of all persons[28] and are therefore themselves important to maintain; they should not be sacrificed to this kind of coercion. In their absence, exploitative studies are sure to proliferate, to the detriment of developing country-health. The long-term health of people in developing countries will be better served by standards that protect all patients in all studies and set a higher standard for acceptable medical care than by accepting occasional exploitative studies that do not provide full benefit to all subjects. (In the Surfaxin case, the threat proved empty; after the placebo-controlled study was canceled, the company converted, without apparent incident, to an active-controlled trial at 49 sites in the developing world and elsewhere.[29])

Procedural Safeguards Do Not Guarantee Ethical Trial Designs

When challenged, researchers commonly seek to justify research by claiming that participants are protected by informed consent....

There is strong evidence of a lack of informed consent in research conducted in developing countries.[30] An adequate informed consent process in a placebo-controlled Surfaxin study would have to make reference, at a minimum, to the 22 placebo-controlled studies collectively showing the known effectiveness of other surfactants in the treatment of RDS in newborns and would have to explain why these drugs were not being provided to the infants in the present study. It would also have to explain that there have been 20 active-controlled trials and that

because the study could not be conducted with a placebo in an industrialized country, it was being conducted in a developing one instead. Even so, the desperate parents of these infants are likely to give consent for the trial, for at least they have a 50% chance of receiving the surfactant treatment. No doubt they would be at least as likely to sign up if they knew they had a 100% chance of receiving an active treatment, as previous research has shown.[31]

. . .

SUMMARY AND CONCLUSIONS

The ethical obligation of the researcher is to obtain needed scientific information in the manner most protective of the health of his or her study participants. Given the proven, life-saving effectiveness of other surfactants, a placebo-controlled trial could not satisfy this requirement, and an active-controlled trial was mandatory. Contrary to the FDA's assertions, we believe that a noninferiority trial was indeed feasible from a statistical point of view. Even if one hypothetically conceded that this was not so, the manufacturer was still left with an ethical option: a superiority trial, the basis for the approval of a previous surfactant. Clearly, the company was opposed to this option, leaving unresolved the question of why the FDA did not insist upon the ethical design, even though, as the gateway to the world's most lucrative pharmaceutical market, it holds enormous sway over the industry. But, even if one rejected both active-controlled designs, one would still have to resort to the de facto standard of care argument to justify the withholding of effective therapy from poor patients.

The Surfaxin trial is one of the best examples to date of the race to the ethical bottom that the de facto standard of care argument ensures. Unable to conduct a placebo-controlled study in an industrialized country, or even in the wealthier parts of these developing countries, the researchers hit upon the idea of experimenting on the poorest of the poor, even as they proposed an active-controlled trial in Europe. Such behavior might be expected from a profit-driven drug company. However, it has become clear that the FDA played a central role in supporting this study design.[32] The FDA's role is to prevent such unethical behavior, not to give it the agency's stamp of approval.

Postscript

On April 14, 2004, Discovery Laboratories announced that it had filed a New Drug Application seeking FDA approval for Surfaxin for RDS in premature infants, citing the favorable results from two clinical trials.[33] In the European noninferiority study, Surfaxin proved statistically equivalent to Curosurf, another surfactant.[34] Despite the company's protestations, the second trial was redesigned as a superiority study and implemented in 49 centers, including some in developing countries. In a paper presented at a pediatric conference, the company reported that Surfaxin was more efficacious than Exosurf at preventing the development of RDS at 24 hours (39% vs. 47%) and RDS-related death by 14 days (4.7% vs. 9.6%).[29]

Notes

1. Office of the Inspector General. Recruiting human subjects: pressures in industry-sponsored clinical research. Washington, D.C: Department of Health and Human Services, June 2000.

2. Lurie P, Wolfe SM. Unethical trials of interventions to reduce perinatal transmission of the human immunodeficiency virus in developing countries. *N Engl J Med.* 1997;337:853–856.

3. Lallemant M, Jourdain G, Le Coeur S et al. A trial of shortened zidovudine regimens to prevent mother-to-child transmission of human immunodeficiency virus type 1. *N Engl J Med.* 2000;343:982–991.

4. IMS. World-wide Pharmaceutical Market 1999. Available at: http://www.ims global.com/insight/world_in_brief/review99/year.htm. Accessed March 15, 2006.

5. Freedman B. Equipoise and the ethics of clinical research. *N Engl J Med.* 1987;317:141–145.

6. Jobe AH. Pulmonary surfactant therapy. *N Engl J Med.* 1993;328:861–868.

7. Soll RF. Synthetic surfactant for respiratory distress syndrome in preterm infants (Cochrane Review). In: *The Cochrane Library,* issue 4. Oxford: Update Software;2000.

8. Behrman RE, Kliegman RM, Nelson WE, Vaughan VC, eds. *Nelson Textbook of Pediatrics*, 14th ed. W. B. Saunders Company; Philadelphia, 1992;463.

9. Soll RF, McQueen MC. Respiratory distress syndrome: In: Sinclair JC, Bracken MB, eds. *Effective Care of the Newborn Infant.* Oxford: Oxford University Press 1992;325–358.

10. Ainsworth SB, Beresford MW, Milligan DW, Shaw NJ, Matthews JN, Fenton AC. Pumactant and poractant alfa for treatment of respiratory distress syndrome in neonates born at 25–29 weeks' gestation: a randomised trial, *Lancet.* 2000;355:1387–1392.

11. da Costa DE, Pai MG, Al Khusaiby SM. Comparative trial of artificial and natural surfactants in the treatment of respiratory distress syndrome of prematurity: experiences in a developing country. *Pediatiic Pulmonology.* 1999, 27:312–317.

12. Kattwinkel J, Bloom BT, Delmore P el al. High-versus low-threshold surfactant retreatment for neonatal respiratory distress syndrome. *Pediatrics.* 2000; 106:282–288.

13. 21 CFR 314.126(b)(2) (1991).

14. *Physicians Desk Reference.* Medical Economics. Montvale, NJ, 2001.

15. Temple RJ. When are clinical trials of a given agent vs. placebo no longer appropriate or feasible? *Controlled Clinical Trials* 1997;18:613–620.

16. Temple RJ. Special study designs: early escape, enrichment, studies in nonresponders. *Communications in Statistics* 1994;23:499–531.

17. Temple RJ. Problems in interpreting active control equivalence trials. *Accountability in Research.* 1996;4:267–275.

18. Temple R. Difficulties in evaluating positive control trials. Proceedings of the American Statistical Association, Biopharmaceutical Section. 1983:1–7.

19. Temple R, Ellenberg SS. Placebo-controlled trials and active-control trials in the evaluation of new treatments, Part 1: ethical and scientific issues. *Ann Intern Med.* 2000;133:455–463.

20. Ellenberg S.S, Temple R. Placebo-controlled trials and active-control trials in the evaluation of new treatments, Part 2: practical issues and specific cases. *Ann Intern Med.* 2000;133:464–470.

21. Freedman B, Weijer C, Glass KC. Placebo orthodoxy in clinical research. I. Empirical and methodological myths. *Journal of Law, Medicine and Ethics.* 1996;24:243–251.

22. London AJ. The ambiguity and the exigency: clarifying "standard of care" arguments in international research. *Journal of Medicine and Philosophy.* 2000;25:379–397.

23. Rothman DJ. Were Tuskegee and Willowbrook "studies in nature"? *Hastings Center Report.* 1982;12:5–7.

24. Lurie P, Wolfe SM. Unethical trials of interventions to reduce perinatal transmission of the human immunodeficiency virus in developing countries. *N Engl J Med.* 1997;337:853–856.

25. Shapiro HT, Meslin EM. Ethical issues in the design and conduct of clinical trials in developing countries. *N Engl J Med.* 2001;345:139–142.

26. World Medical Association Declaration of Helsinki: ethical principles for medical research involving human subjects. Adopted by the 18th World Medical Assembly, Helsinki, 1964, and revised by the 29th World Medical Assembly, Tokyo, 1975; the 35th World Medical Assembly, Venice, 1983, the 41st World Medical Assembly, Hong Kong, 1989, the 48th World Medical Assembly, Somerset West, 1996; and the 52nd World Medical Assembly, Edinburgh, 2000.

27. Glanatz. LH, Annas GJ, Grodin MA, Mariner WR. Research in developing countries: taking "benefit" seriously. *Hastings Center Report.* 1998;28:38–42.

28. United Nations. Universal Declaration of Human Rights. 1948. Available at: http:// www.un.org/ Overview/rights.html. Accessed August 21, 2006.

29. Moya F, Gadzinowski J, Bancalari E et al. Superiority of a novel surfactant, Surfaxin (Lucinactant), over Exosurf in preventing respiratory distress syndrome in very preterm infants: a pivotal, multinational, randomized trial (Abstract 2643). Presented at: Pediatric Academic Societies Meeting; May 2, 2004; San Francisco, Calif.

30. Karim QA, Karim SSA, Coovadia HM, Susser M. Informed consent for HIV testing in a South African hospital: is it truly informed and truly voluntary? *Am J Public Health.* 1998;88. 637–640.

31. Welton AJ, Vickers MR, Cooper JA, Meade TW, Marteau TM. Is recruitment more difficult with a placebo arm in randomised controlled trials? a quasirandomised, interview based study. *Br Med J.* I999;318:1114–1117.

32. Temple explains ethical issues in Latin American placebo trial. Camp Hill, Pa.: Ferdic, Incorporated, FDA Webview, March 2, 2001.

33. Available at: http://www.discoverylabs.com/ 2004pt/041404_PR.pdf. Accessed August 21, 2006.

34. Sinha S, Lacaze-Masmonteil T, Valls i Soler A et al. Randomized, controlled trial of a new generation surfactant, Surfaxin (Lucinactant), versus Curosurf (Poractant Alfa) for the prevention and treatment of RDS in very preterm infants (Abstract 2644). Presented at: Pediatric Academic Societies Meeting; May 2, 2004, San Francisco, Calif.

Does Informed Consent to Research Require Comprehension?

Gopal Sreenivasan

The doctrine of informed consent is a cornerstone of ethical medicine, both in clinical and in research settings.[1–9] It consists of two parts: a duty to obtain the voluntary agreement of patients or trial participants before treatment or enrolment; and a duty to disclose adequate information to the patient or participant before seeking this agreement.[1] The two parts evolved separately.[1–3] Indeed, the first is centuries old,[10] whereas the second is a relatively recent development.[11] Yet, according to the standard view of informed consent, they are best understood, morally, as closely integrated parts of a single requirement.[3–7] This interpretation has an ethically weighty implication; that the validity of an individual's consent depends on him or her actually comprehending the information disclosed.[3–7] To remove doubt, comprehension or understanding is often listed in addition to disclosure, voluntary participation, and competence as an explicit requirement of informed consent.[3–7]

Although the issue of whether disclosure actually results in comprehension is not irrelevant, the standard view of informed consent is mistaken. Obviously, the point of disclosing information is to impart a certain grasp of the procedure or protocol in question. An aspiration to produce adequate comprehension is therefore inseparable from the requirement of disclosure. It does not follow, however, that success in producing comprehension is likewise required. The standard view confuses an ethical aspiration with a minimum ethical standard.

Another defect of the standard view is that the physician shoulders the entire responsibility for achieving comprehension in the patient—an unwitting irony from the advocates of individual autonomy. Physicians and investigators should take reasonable steps to ensure that the information they disclose has been adequately understood. But if adequate comprehension is strictly required and reasonable steps fail to produce it, the physician or investigator must keep on taking further steps until it is achieved—even when the failure is on the part of an otherwise competent patient or participant. In a shared relationship, successful communication is normally a shared responsibility. Why should the physician-patient relationship be an exception?

The most serious defect of the standard view of informed consent, however, is that it threatens to bring enrolment in many ethical clinical trials to a near standstill.

CONSENT TO RESEARCH AND THERAPEUTIC MISCONCEPTION

To simplify matters, consider informed consent specifically in clinical research. US regulations require that disclosure to prospective research participants includes certain basic elements, such as the risks and benefits of the research, available alternatives to study participation, and the fact that participants have the right to withdraw from the trial at any time.[12] Can the consent of participants who do not adequately comprehend this

standard disclosure be morally valid? To address this issue in isolation, imagine that consent is voluntary and that participants are all competent to consent—ie, they have the ability to comprehend, even if they fail to comprehend on a given occasion.

My argument begins from the "therapeutic misconception"[13–16]—a tendency to mistake the nature of clinical research and to confuse its aims with those of clinical care. Appelbaum and colleagues[13] reported widespread failure among participants in psychiatric research to appreciate the significance of randomisation, non-individualised treatment, placebo controls, and double-blinding. As a result of these mistakes, an individual might overestimate the therapeutic benefit of participating in research. Appelbaum and colleagues concluded: "research subjects systematically misinterpret the risk/benefit ratio of participating in research because they fail to understand the underlying scientific methodology."[13] Other researchers have reported similar findings in various populations of research participants.[17] Joffe and colleagues[18] reported "major deficiencies" among cancer trial participants in their comprehension of the nonstandard character of their treatment, the risks of their participation, the unproven nature of their treatment, and the uncertainty of benefit to themselves.

If comprehension is a necessary condition of valid consent, as the standard view maintains, then consent given by participants with a therapeutic misconception is invalid. Proponents of the standard view sometimes distinguish between full comprehension and adequate or substantial comprehension,[3,4] meaning that the less rigorous standard is acceptable. But this approach does not avoid the conclusion that consent is invalid, since the risks and benefits of study participation are a central part of the standard disclosure procedure. Since the risk-benefit ratio seems to be profoundly misunderstood by many participants,[13,18] these participants clearly fail the requirement of even adequate comprehension.

This line of reasoning entails that any clinical trial in which participants with a therapeutic misconception are enrolled is unethical. For informed consent remains a fundamental ethical requirement of research;[5-9] and the consent given by such participants has been deemed invalid. The standard view of informed consent therefore burdens researchers with a commitment not to enrol anyone with a therapeutic misconception. But if the therapeutic misconception is widespread, enrolment in many clinical trials should then be brought to a near standstill, which seems unacceptable.

For example, imagine a clinical trial that satisfies the applicable local regulations and otherwise conforms to the ethical requirements described by Emanuel and colleagues.[9] Two of their requirements, in particular, should be considered: a favourable risk-benefit ratio and independent review. Imagine, then, that the hypothetical trial has passed institutional review board assessment and has been independently assessed as having a favourable risk-benefit ratio. Furthermore, suppose that the trial is not a phase I or other study in which benefit to society in knowledge gained is required to render the risk-benefit ratio favourable—ie, that the risk-benefit ratio is favourable, even when direct benefit to the participant is the only benefit taken into account.

Such a trial has a good claim to being ethical. I submit that this claim is not undermined if researchers enrol participants with a therapeutic misconception. After all, their misconception does not actually change the trial's risk-directbenefit ratio. The ratio is, in fact, favourable, even though it is not as favourable as some participants believe. Moreover, provided they are otherwise competent, agreed voluntarily, and received the standard disclosure, their consent is perfectly valid. Yet the standard view of informed consent requires them to be excluded from the trial.

THREE OBJECTIONS

Proponents of the standard view of informed consent might retort that reducing enrolments is a price worth paying to uphold ethical standards.

I will discuss three arguments that they might offer to defend their viewpoint.

Protection

First, it might be argued that treating adequate comprehension as a precondition of valid consent protects prospective participants, especially those who do not want to participate in research. No-one would dispute that protection of participants is the lodestar of research ethics. But it is not necessary to insist on comprehension to achieve a high level of protection. Individuals are already protected in two critical ways. First, and foremost, there is the requirement that an institutional review board establish that the clinical trial's risk-benefit ratio is favourable. It is a mistake to prefer an individual participant's judgment to careful institutional review board assessment as the first line of defence.[19] Second, individuals always retain the right not to enrol in a trial or to withdraw from it, even if it has been passed by an institutional review board. Even without comprehension, individuals are always free to choose not to participate in research.

Privileged Authority

Second, some may contend that institutional review boards are inadequate judges of a trial's risk-benefit ratio for a particular individual. Judgments of this kind lack final moral force until confirmed by the individual, since individuals are privileged authorities on their own interests. At least since the publication of John Stuart Mill's *On Liberty* (1859),[20] this conception has been a sacred liberal dogma. However, we should distinguish two versions of this dogma.

In one version, an individual's view of his or her own interests is infallible. Unfortunately, this version is untenable.[21-23] Consider a man who wants to drink the glass in front of him, but does not know that it contains poison. No-one believes that the man's "thinking it so" makes drinking the glass in his interest. Now, consider a man with a seriously infected tooth and an irrational fear of the dentist. Again, no-one believes that his "thinking it not so" prevents going to the dentist from being in the man's interest.

In a second version, two facts are combined with empirical generalisations.[21] First, what is objectively in a person's interest varies from individual to individual. This fact is reason to privilege an individual's view of his or her own interests because individuals are generally more familiar than anyone else with the details of their own situation. Second, weighing risks and benefits against each other is inherently difficult. This fact supports the same privilege because individuals also generally have the greatest motivation to weigh correctly in their own case.

These empirical generalisations are highly plausible, and may be invoked to question an institutional review board's expertise in assessing the risk-benefit ratio for a particular individual. However, the second version of the liberal dogma is fully accommodated by giving individuals the right to second-guess the institutional review board's assessment of the ratio in their own case; a right that individuals hold anyway, irrespective of the standard view of informed consent. Furthermore, this version of the argument holds only up to a point. It says that individuals are generally better judges of their own interests, not that they are infallible. But a therapeutic misconception is precisely a case of misunderstanding the risk-benefit ratio—a case, that is, in which the individual's fallible judgment about what serves his or her interest has failed. Clearly, in these cases, the claim to privileged authority does not hold.

Playing It Safe

Finally, proponents of the standard view might argue that comprehension should be required if only as a safety precaution. What harm can there be in an extra safeguard? The cost of playing it safe would be a commitment to exclude participants with a therapeutic misconception from clinical trials. To act on this commitment would bring many otherwise ethical trials to a near standstill, with a concomitant loss of scientific and medical progress. If researchers baulk at actually excluding such participants, while condemning their enrolment as unethical, they will fail to practise what they preach and thereby fall

into hypocrisy. It is difficult to see how a superfluous safeguard could be worth this moral cost.

AN ALTERNATIVE VIEW OF INFORMED CONSENT

What alternative is there to the standard view of informed consent? The duty of disclosure and the duty to obtain a prospective participant's consent should be treated as largely independent ethical requirements. The duty to obtain consent is a duty to respect an individual's right not to participate in research. This right protects an individual's ordinary interest in liberty, well described by the US Judge Benjamin Cardozo: "every human being of adult years and sound mind has a right to determine what shall be done with his body."[24] Within prescribed limits, the exercise of this right depends on nothing other than an individual's election; there is no basis for making its validity contingent on comprehending a trial's risk-benefit ratio. Would an ignorant decision not to participate in research be invalid? Obviously not. So why should there be an asymmetry? The natural answer is that it exists to protect participants, but this does not stand up. If reliable independent judgment of a trial's risk-direct benefit ratio is favourable, an individual's ignorant decision to participate should not be treated any differently from an ignorant decision not to participate.

Strictly speaking, consent cannot be entirely ignorant. The very act of consent arguably entails a bare minimum of comprehension. Participants must comprehend both what it means to consent and a basic description of what they will undergo—injections, for example. However, this minimal comprehension is fully consistent with a therapeutic misconception, since it includes nothing about risks or benefits or the difference between research and clinical care.

The standard disclosure thus goes well beyond what consent itself requires. But it does not thereby lose its moral basis. Various reasons to require greater disclosure remain in force. First, most people want the relevant information to be disclosed to them, quite apart from how it relates to their decision-making process.[25] Furthermore, wider disclosure is vital to maintain trust in the researcher-participant relationship. Finally, it would obviously make for better decisions if participants did comprehend the information disclosed. All these factors are also reasons to assign investigators some share of responsibility for producing comprehension of the standard disclosure.

What are the reasonable steps investigators must take to ensure such comprehension? Plainly, these steps include using clear, non-technical language, at an appropriate reading level, in the prospective participant's mother tongue; providing opportunities to ask questions throughout the trial; and using short consent forms. Would it be reasonable to require further steps? This question remains open. The crucial point is that some limit must be drawn— the minimum standard cannot simply be whatever it takes to produce comprehension. To see the need for a limit is already to reject the standard view of informed consent.

The most important advantage of the alternative view of informed consent is relief from the pressure on researchers to lapse into hypocrisy; pressure that results from confusion of an ethical aspiration with a minimum standard. Investigators should aspire to dispel the therapeutic misconception. But failure to satisfy this aspiration does not itself invalidate an individual's consent. Once comprehension of the standard disclosure is no longer treated as a minimum standard, researchers will not have to choose between assigning it no ethical importance and excluding participants who fail to achieve it from otherwise ethical clinical trials.

Acknowledgements

I am grateful to Frank Miller, Ezekiel Emanuel, Donna Chen, and Dan Brock for helpful comments. There was no funding source for this article.

Notes

1. Berg JW, Appelbaum PS, Lidz CW, Parker LS. Informed consent: legal theory and clinical practice, 2nd edn. New York: Oxford University Press, 2001.

2. Katz J. The silent world of doctor and patient. New York: Fress Press, 1984.

3. Faden RR, Beauchamp TL. A history and theory of informed consent. New York: Oxford University Press, 1986.

4. Beauchamp TL, Childress JF. Principles of biomedical ethics, 5th edn. New York: Oxford University Press, 2001: 77–93.

5. National Commission for the Protection of Human Subjects of Biomedical and Behavioral Research. The Belmont report. Washington: US Government Printing Office, 1979.

6. Levine RJ. Ethics and regulation of clinical research, 2nd edn. New Haven: Yale University Press, 1988: 95–153.

7. Nuremberg Military Tribunal. The Nuremberg Code. *JAMA* 1996; 276: 1691.

8. World Medical Association. Declaration of Helsinki: ethical principles for medical research involving human subjects. *JAMA* 2000; 284: 3044.

9. Emanuel EJ, Wendler D, Grady C. What makes clinical research ethical? *JAMA* 2000; 283: 2701–11.

10. English legal case. Slater v Baker and Stapleton. 95 Eng Rep 860 (KB 1767).

11. US legal case. Salgo v Leland Stanford Jr Univ Bd of Trustees. 317 P2d 170 (Cal Ct App 1957).

12. US Federal Government. General requirements for informed consent. Code of Federal Regulations. 45 CFR 46.116. (http://frwebgate2.access.gpo.gov, accessed Dec 1, 2003).

13. Appelbaum PS, Roth LH, Lidz CW, Benson P, Winslade W. False hopes and best data: consent to research and the therapeutic misconception. *Hastings Cent Rep* 1987; 17: 20–24.

14. Appelbaum PS, Roth LH, Lidz C. The therapeutic misconception: informed consent in psychiatric research. *Int J Law Psychiatry* 1982; 5: 319–29.

15. Benson PR, Roth LH, Winslade WJ. Informed consent in psychiatric research: preliminary findings from an ongoing investigation. *Soc Sci Med* 1985; 20: 1331–41.

16. Lidz CW, Appelbaum PS. The therapeutic misconception: problems and solutions. *Med Care* 2002; 40 (suppl): V55–63.

17. Sugarman J, McCrory DC, Powell D, et al. Empirical research on informed consent: an annotated bibliography. *Hastings Cent Rep* 1999; 29 (suppl): S1–42.

18. Joffe S, Cook EF, Cleary PD, Clark JW, Weeks JC. Quality of informed consent in cancer clinical trials: a cross-sectional survey. *Lancet* 2001; 358: 1772–77.

19. Truog RD, Robinson W, Randolph A, Morris A. Is informed consent always necessary for randomized, controlled trials? *N Engl J Med* 1999; 340: 806.

20. Mill JS. On liberty. Indianapolis: Hackett Publishing Company, 1978.

21. Brock DW. Informed consent. In: Life and death. New York: Cambridge University Press, 1993: 21–54.

22. Griffin J. Well-being. Chapter 1. New York: Oxford University Press, 1986.

23. Geuss R. The idea of a critical theory. Chapter 2. New York: Cambridge University Press, 1981.

24. US legal case. Schloendorff v Society of New York Hospital. 105 NE 92 (NY 1914).

25. Schneider CE. The practice of autonomy. New York: Oxford University Press, 1998.

The Second Wave: Toward Responsible Inclusion of Pregnant Women in Research

Anne Drapkin Lyerly, Margaret Olivia Little, and Ruth Faden

INTRODUCTION

In the 1990s, prominent reports emerged indicating that women were underrepresented in biomedical research. By now, the findings are well-known: many significant studies on aging and heart disease were performed without adequate representation of women, and the health concerns of women were frequently under-investigated (General Accounting Office 1992; Merton 1996). Also well-known by now is the progress made following the establishment in the United States of the Women's Health Initiative at the National Institutes of Health (NIH) and the passage of the NIH Revitalization Act of 1993, with provisions that each NIH-funded study include representative samples of subpopulations unless their exclusion can be justified on a basis other than cost. More than a decade later, though some disparities have persisted (Chronic Disease Prevention and Control Research Center at Baylor College of Medicine and Intercultural Cancer Council 2008), women now make up the majority of participants in clinical research (General Accounting Office 2001).

Although progress was made on the inclusion of non-pregnant women in research, thoughtful discussion of how to reason about the inclusion of pregnant women in clinical research lags far behind. Despite a 1994 Institute of Medicine report recommending that pregnant women be "presumed eligible for participation in clinical studies" (Mastroianni, Faden, and Federman 1994), many researchers and institutional review boards (IRBs) continue to regard pregnancy as a near-automatic cause for exclusion, regardless of the costs of exclusion or the magnitude or likelihood of the risks of participation.

This reticence brings with it a profound cost. Of the more than four million women giving birth in the United States every year (Martin et al. 2007), many face medical conditions during their pregnancies that require clinical treatment, but they lack adequate data to inform their care. Indeed, chronic diseases during pregnancy are common: chronic hypertension and diabetes each complicate nearly 4 percent or 40,000 pregnancies each year (Martin et al. 2007); an estimated 500,000 pregnant women experience psychiatric illness (American College of Obstetricians and Gynecologists 2007); cancer, autoimmune disease, and a plethora of other conditions commonly occur with pregnancy

Lyerly, A.D., Little, M.O., and Faden, R. (2008) "The Second Wave: Toward Responsible Inclusion of Pregnant Women in Research." *International Journal of Feminist Approaches to Bioethics* 1(2): pp. 5–22. Published by Indiana University Press. Reprinted by permission.

and often require treatment. Further, gestation engenders a host of pregnancy-specific conditions that range from difficult (extreme nausea and vomiting) to disabling (sciatic nerve compression) to life-threatening for the woman or her fetus (preeclampsia). Pregnancy is not a prophylaxis against medical illness.

Yet only a dozen medications are approved by the United States Food and Drug Administration (FDA) for use during pregnancy. All of them are medications for gestation- or birth-related issues, such as regional anesthesia, nausea and vomiting, the prevention of congenital malformation, and the induction or delay of labor (Haire 2001). Any medication used to *treat illness* during pregnancy— be it hypertension, diabetes, depression, or cancer—is used without approval from the FDA, often leaving doctors and patients alike worried whenever they face decisions about using medication during pregnancy. Pregnancy, it turns out, is an "off label" condition.

In contemplating treatment of these conditions, an overarching concern, for providers and women alike, is of course the safety of medication for the fetus. Medications can cross the placenta and irreversibly affect fetal growth, structure, and function. Newer research has shown how environmental, nutritional, and other health factors during pregnancy can have an impact on an offspring's gene expression (Jirtle 2008). These potentially profound implications ground the reluctance in the research community to include pregnant women in clinical investigations.

Unfortunately, this conservative stance turns out to enhance neither fetal nor maternal safety. Certainly, guidelines for research in pregnancy must include careful and responsible criteria for protections. Consideration of fetal well-being will, in any framework, constitute a crucial component in shaping criteria for inclusion; further, as in any research involving a party whose capacity for consent is limited or absent, such as children, inclusion will require extra layers of protection and scrutiny of the risks, benefits, and alternatives. But currently, there are few oppor-

tunities for such a framework to be applied. With pregnant women effectively deemed untouchable in the research community, obstetricians care for their patients without meaningful data regarding the safety and efficacy of most of the medications used in pregnancy.

In what follows, we review the price of turning a blind eye to pregnancy in research and research ethics. We describe both the knowledge gaps around the use of medication during pregnancy and their costs, highlighting four reasons why ethically we are obliged to confront the challenges of including pregnant women in clinical research studies: the need for effective treatment for women during pregnancy, considerations of fetal safety, the harm from reticence to prescribe potentially beneficial medication, and the broader issues of justice and access to the benefits of research participation.

THE COSTS OF EXCLUSION

Effective Medical Treatment for Women during Pregnancy

The first reason to confront the challenges of including pregnant women in research is a simple one: women need effective treatment during pregnancy. Without adequate research on how drugs are metabolized during pregnancy, we have very little evidence on how to treat illnesses when they occur in the pregnant body.

Pregnancy extends and alters the impact of sex differences on absorption, distribution, metabolism, and excretion of drugs—often times in ways that are both dramatic and difficult to predict. Pregnancy-related changes in the gastrointestinal tract, the cardiovascular system, the kidneys, and other organs may profoundly alter the ways that drugs are processed by the body (pharmacokinetics) or the ways that drugs act on the body (pharmacodynamics) (Mattison and Zajicek 2006). For instance, a 30–40 percent increase in blood flow through the kidneys means that some medications are cleared at much higher rates during pregnancy (Mattison and Zajicek 2006). Increases in blood volume, decreases in gastric emptying time, changes in the concentrations of sex hormones, alterations in liver enzymes, the presence (to say the least) of a fetal-placental unit, can all alter the activity of a drug. In the end, the pregnant body processes and eliminates drugs in ways that may differ both surprisingly and substantially from the non-pregnant body processing the same substance.

Indeed, evidence suggests that pregnancy often acts as a significant wild card in clinical management. In a 1999 review of the literature reporting pharmacokinetic differences between pregnant and non-pregnant women, the sixty-one studies reporting on pharmacokinetics during pregnancy revealed little or no consistency of results in studies during pregnancy, even for the same class of drugs or the same drug (Little 1999). Sometimes the pharmacokinetic parameters increase, sometimes they decrease, and sometimes they stay the same, suggesting that intuition and even clinical experience may not be trustworthy.

Opportunistic studies of drug metabolism and activity during pregnancy corroborate. In 2003, the Obstetric-Fetal Pharmacology Research Unit (OPRU) Network was founded through the United States National Institutes of Health to identify, characterize, and study drugs of therapeutic value in normal and abnormal pregnancies (Zajicek and Giacoia 2007). Initial studies generated findings that are of concern. For instance, pharmacokinetic measurements on a pregnant woman receiving chemotherapy during pregnancy revealed that the drug was so quickly and thoroughly metabolized and excreted by her pregnant body that the drug never approached a therapeutic range, despite the fact that she and her fetus were exposed to its toxicities.[1]

Of potentially even broader applicability are the implications of knowledge regarding amoxicillin pharmacokinetics during pregnancy. Given heightened concern about bioterrorism, the American College of Obstetricians and Gynecologists (ACOG) recommended using amoxicillin for post-exposure prophylaxis in pregnant women in the setting of penicillin-sensitive bacteria (American College

of Obstetricians and Gynecologists 2002). Yet a 2007 OPRU study revealed that concentrations of amoxicillin adequate to prevent anthrax may be unachievable during pregnancy due to altered kidney function and that amoxicillin ultimately may not be an appropriate antibiotic for post-anthrax exposure prophylaxis (Andrew et al. 2007).

With regard to dosing medications, our best predictions can be disastrously wrong. But predictions are largely all that physicians and policymakers have for making decisions. The same 1999 review that highlighted the variability in pharmacokinetic parameters also highlighted standardized pharmacokinetic studies as a major area of need (Little 1999). Of more than one thousand articles published on pregnancy pharmacokinetics, only sixty-one reported relevant pharmacokinetic data, and only two synthesized data into guidelines for clinical care. When physicians prescribe medications during pregnancy, they do so in the absence of data regarding the dosage required to achieve the desired therapeutic result.

As often is said in research ethics, there is no one-size-fits-all research subject. Children are not just small adults; women are not just men with a bit less on-average muscle. Developmental stage and gender make a difference in how drugs act in the body and how the body acts on drugs (Mattison and Zajicek 2006). So, too, with gestation—a pregnant woman is not just a woman with a bigger belly. The maternal-fetal-placental system brings its own pharmacokinetics and dynamics. If we are to treat pregnant women's illnesses effectively— something crucial to the health of *both* pregnant women and that of the children they may bear—we must study medications in pregnant women.

Fetal Safety

The second reason to address the challenges of including pregnant women in research is the very same reason that is given for excluding them— fetal safety. Given their medical needs, pregnant women *do* use medications during pregnancy. The average woman receives 1.3 prescriptions per obstetric visit (Lee et al. 2006), and two-thirds of women use four to five medications during pregnancy and labor (National Institute of Child Health and Human Development 2003). More than 40 percent of pregnant women use drugs classified as C or D by the U.S. FDA risk classification.[2] Further, given that almost half of pregnancies are unintended (Finer and Henshaw 2006), exposure to a fetus can occur when a woman taking medication unexpectedly becomes pregnant. Without information on the fetal safety of these medications, we are left with the variable predictive value of animal studies (Brent 2004), considerable anxiety, and a paucity of data with which to reason about the trade-offs that mark decisions about the use of medication in—or continuation of—pregnancy.

Indeed, a 2002 review of fetal risk associated with all 468 of the medications approved in the United States for use in humans between 1980 and 2000 revealed just how little we know (Lo and Friedman 2002). Only 6.4 percent were recognized as safe in pregnancy (in that their teratogenic risk was considered as "none, minimal or unlikely"); and 2.5 percent were associated with some risk, ranging from small or moderate (fetal growth restriction with cyclophosphamide chemotherapy, goiter with amiodarone) to high (severe limb abnormalities with thalidomide). This leaves us without any substantive guidance regarding the risk to the fetus of more than 91 percent of the drugs on the market. Worse, this percentage has shifted very little over the last two decades. More than 80 percent of drugs are classified as "undetermined" with respect to fetal risk, whether approved 15–20 years ago (96%), 10–14 years ago (83%), 5–9 years ago (88%), or 0–4 years ago (95%) (Lo and Friedman 2002).

Of obvious concern here is that some of the medications currently prescribed to pregnant women may in fact be unsafe for the fetus. Consider ACE inhibitors—a medication widely prescribed for the treatment of hypertension. ACE inhibitors were of known contraindication in the second and third trimesters but had unknown risk status in the first trimester until a 2006 study published in the *New England Journal of Medicine* linked the antihypertensive drug to a small but statistically significant increased risk of fetal cardiovascular and neurological abnormalities (Cooper et al. 2006). The rub, in this case, is that if researchers had studied the drug in pregnancy earlier on, the congenital anomalies that resulted from the three decades of use since the approval of the drug could have been prevented.

For another example, consider the thalidomide disaster. Some of the resistance to the idea of clinical research with pregnant women almost certainly can be traced to the long shadow cast by this devastating episode. But the thalidomide example is in fact instructive. We must remember that the widespread birth defects experienced from its use were *not* the result of women's participation in research trials, but rather the result, at least in part, of inadequate research standards preceding distribution and marketing (Levine 1993). Careful and responsible research might well have attenuated the magnitude of the disaster. Yet the response of policymakers was instead to exclude nearly all women of reproductive potential from future research.

Reticence to Use: The Cost of Uncertainty

Worries about fetal safety obviously loom large not only for researchers, but for pregnant women and their health care providers. These concerns have led some clinicians or patients not to treat, or to undertreat, illnesses that continue or emerge during pregnancy. But the failure to treat illness *also* can lead to significant harm to women and their fetuses—indeed, harm that easily can outweigh the possible risks that might accompany use of medication during pregnancy. These issues point to the third reason that responsible research in pregnancy is required: lack of information can lead to worrisome reticence to treat dangerous medical conditions.

Consider depression, for example. Treatment for depression during pregnancy has been characterized by considerable reticence, despite significant harm that untreated mental illness can entail. The Web site for the National Alliance on Mental Illness (NAMI) admonishes women to "if possible, stop using the drugs before trying to conceive [and] do everything possible to avoid medication in the first trimester of pregnancy" (National Alliance on Mental Health 2008).[3] Yet women who discontinue medication have significantly higher rates of relapse of major depression than those who continued medication (68% compared to 25%) (Cohen et al. 2006). Untreated depression is problematic for pregnant women and the fetuses they carry: it is associated with premature birth, low birth weight, fetal growth restriction, and postnatal complications. It also is associated with decreased social support, poor weight gain, and alcohol and drug use, all of which adversely affect outcomes for women and infants alike (Orr et al. 2007; American College of Obstetricians and Gynecologists 2007).

Women with asthma, too, sometimes are treated suboptimally for fear of fetal exposure to medications (Dewyea and Nelson 2005). Halting medication brings many dangers to maternal health: poorly controlled asthma places a pregnant woman at higher risk of hypertension, preeclampsia, and uterine hemorrhage (Dombrowski 2006; American College of Obstetricians and Gynecologists 2008). Moreover, halting medication for the mother is risky for the fetus. Poorly controlled asthma is associated with fetal growth restriction, premature birth, and low birth weight; in contrast, women with asthma that is well controlled by medication have perinatal outcomes as good as comparable groups without asthma (Tan and Thomson 2000). And sometimes, the results of undertreatment are tragic: women—and the fetuses they carry—have died in emergency situations because physicians are insufficiently aggressive with medications out of concerns for fetal harm.[4]

Here we see the tendency in pregnancy (more accurately, the tendency until we get to labor and delivery) to notice the risks of intervening to the exclusion of noticing the risks to woman and the fetus of *not* intervening (Lyerly et al. 2007). A classic example is the trainee who hesitates, in the midst of resuscitating a pregnant woman who has had a heart attack—a woman whose small chance for life depends on decisive and optimal care—over concerns about whether a cardiac drug is teratogenic.[5] Another example is that of the radiologist who hesitates or refuses to perform standard imaging on a pregnant woman with suspected appendicitis, despite the fact that delayed diagnosis and appendicle rupture carries a ten-fold risk of miscarriage (Mazze and Kallen 1991). When a medical problem emerges or persists in pregnancy, many—sometimes patients, sometimes providers—feel concern about taking a medication, without appropriately weighing the risks of *not* taking it.

Pregnancy is in this respect no different than other arenas of life. The need to make calculated risks and trade-offs in the context of pregnancy is inevitable. Indeed, even for medications with known teratogenicity, calculated trade-offs may still be a fact of life. For instance, a pregnant woman with a mechanical heart valve who is insufficiently treated with heparin, may be strongly recommended to take warfarin (a blood thinner with a 30% risk of fetal anomaly), given the high risk of maternal (and needless to say, fetal) death entailed by inadequate anticoagulation (James, Abel, and Brancazio 2006).

The third reason to move toward responsible inclusion of pregnant women in clinical trials, then, is to counter unreasoned opposition to treating important medical conditions. If research is important to tell us when medications are unsafe, it is also important to reassure us when drugs *are* safe. The point is worth underscoring. For every drug that is found worrisome, it is likely that many more will bring news of welcome reassurance. Of the 468 drugs approved by the U.S. Food and Drug Administration in the last twenty years, only three drugs approved were judged to pose a "high" teratogenic risk; only eleven are believed to pose any teratogenic risk (Lo and Friedman 2002). Further, for the 6.4 percent of medications categorized as safe, it took an average of more than nine (ranging from two to nineteen) years from the time of FDA approval to ascribe a designation of low or minimal risk (Lo and Friedman 2002). And of course, research also can help us to quantify the risks of medications like warfarin or ACE inhibitors, so that we can proceed with more confidence when faced with the need to make difficult trade-offs in risk.

Access to the Prospect of Direct Benefit

The fourth reason to enhance clinical research of medical treatment during pregnancy has to do with an important subset of trials: those that carry the prospect of direct benefit to participants. Some trials, especially Phase I trials, are designed primarily to gather preliminary information, such as data about the safety, pharmacokinetics, and pharmacodynamics of a drug. These trials, although important for the advance of scientific knowledge, present no prospect of direct medical benefit to participants. But other trials do. Many Phase II and III trials are meant to see whether a given drug is, as hoped, therapeutic for a given medical condition. Those who participate in the active arm of these trials could end up with a significant medical benefit. This means that restriction of trials to non-pregnant individuals excludes a class of potential beneficiaries and places them at an unfair disadvantage when it comes to health and well-being.

Consider an example from current international HIV/AIDS research. Vaginal microbicides were identified as a promising means for women in developing countries to protect themselves from sexual transmission of HIV (Doncel and Mauck 2004). Because pregnancy is a marker of unprotected sexual activity, understanding the effects of a medication aimed at mitigating the risks of such exposure is particularly important for this group. Indeed, any possible teratogenic risk from the gel must be considered in the context of a very clear, real, and life-threatening risk that microbicides aim to prevent—namely, maternal and fetal exposure to HIV infection. Yet pregnant women have been summarily excluded from microbicide trials. In fact, high pregnancy rates in study populations were accompanied by *increased* efforts to exclude pregnant women and to terminate enrollment for participants who do become pregnant (Raymond 2006)—this despite the fact that animal studies have not shown adverse effects of microbicides

on fetal development, and the vaginal products do not seem to be systemically absorbed (Lard-Whiteford et al. 2004). And finally, given that pregnant women will certainly be among the consumers of microbicides if they prove effective, reassurance of the product's efficacy, as well as safety, would be useful.

In this example, the prospect of medical benefit extends to woman and fetus alike. If the microbicide turns out to decrease the transmission of HIV, both women and fetuses in the active arm will benefit. Other trials present more difficult issues, offering the prospect of direct medical benefit only to the fetus or only to the woman. Clearly, there must be strong limits on the risk that research may impose on the fetus, who cannot consent, for the potential medical benefit of the woman. But the current practice—the de facto exclusion of women from participation, even when participation holds a genuine prospect of direct benefit—goes beyond what would be considered reasoned limits and suggests alarm at the prospect of *any* fetal risk whatsoever.

Indeed, some theorists have noted a "cultural anxiety" about the very idea of placing risk on the fetus for the sake of the pregnant woman (Merton 1996). Often, of course, the idea of a conflict is overstated to begin with. Physically, the woman and fetus are interconnected, the health or illness of one influencing the same in the other. More than that, the future well-being of each is, in the usual case, deeply connected. Children are affected by their parents' health and happiness; parents are affected by their children's well-being—and not just contingently, but constitutively. The fact that stopping anti-depressant use during pregnancy increases the woman's chance of severe post-partum depression is not just a "maternal" risk; the fact that lead exposure during pregnancy increases a child's risk of learning disabilities is not just a "fetal" risk.

Nonetheless, just as the bodies are not identical, neither are the goods, projects, and interests. Trade-offs between risks to the woman and the fetus can be real, and decisions about responsible and reasonable trade-offs are critical. Yet the need for thoughtful criteria has been eclipsed by a social tendency to regard the very idea of trading off risks between the woman and her fetus— however well demonstrated and large the former, however theoretical or small the latter— as anathema. Exposing a fetus to a small, even miniscule, risk in the context of research that may entail even a large direct benefit to a woman (and probably to both woman and fetus) has seemed an unreasonable risk to some researchers and policy-makers contemplating categories for inclusion.

This form of reasoning carries a worrisome double standard. It holds pregnant women to a standard we do not hold fathers to; more than that, it holds pregnant women to a standard we do not hold mothers to. We accept small risks to our children for our own sakes every day. We believe it reasonable to impose the small risk of fatality introduced every time we put our children in the car (safely restrained in a car seat), even if our errand is mundane. To be sure, balancing such risks can be among the most challenging tasks of parenthood. But as parents and members of families, we recognize that rea-soning about risk is inevitable, that thoughtful, responsible trade-offs are a fact of life, and that there are times when benefit to one member of a family comes at the price of a risk to another.

The fourth reason to address the challenges of responsible inclusion of pregnant women in clinical trials, then, is an issue of justice. As scholars have noted in discussions of other underrepresented populations, *access* to research, not just protection from its risks, is a constitutive part of the ethical mandates governing clinical research (Mastroianni, Faden, and Federman 1994). Whereas no one would suggest that justice requires admitting pregnant women to all trials regardless of their risks and benefits, justice does call into question the de facto summary exclusion of pregnant women in research without justifica-tion in terms of those risks and benefits.

RISK AND RESPONSIBILITY

We suggested that there are profoundly impor-tant reasons to enhance clinical research of medical treatment in pregnancy. We also noted

that such research raises significant cultural unease: the intersection of risk and the fetus is an uncomfortable one.

Of course, part of the concern has to do with the fetus's inability to consent. But pregnancy is not the only context that raises this ethical issue. Pediatrics has a long history of confronting the need to study a population that cannot consent meaningfully. The fact introduces complexity, and the need for special safeguards, to be sure; what it does not mean is a firewall against research on the population. As a recent report of the Institute of Medicine on research with children pointed out, studies involving that vul-nerable population are "essential to the health of future children—and future adults"(Field and Berman 2004). After all, young children also do not consent to being treated with medication that has not been adequately tested on physiolo-gies resembling their own and thus, whose effi-cacy and risks, for them, are largely unknown. Whereas the details are complex, the bottom line is simple: if a population is going to use a drug, then we need to study that drug *in* that population (Brent 2004; Field and Berman 2004; Zajicek and Giacoia 2007).

But when it comes to reasoning about risk and the pregnant body, the cultural tendency is to retreat from the idea of risk rather than con-front the need to make reasoned and responsible decisions about it. The specter of risk can cast an eclipsing shadow over rational decision making. For example, in discussions about pregnancy, evidence that one thing or behavior carries quan-tifiable risk—say, exposure to oil-based paint or moderate caffeine consumption—can quickly taint another where there is no such evidence— for example, exposure to latex-based paint, or again, modest caffeine consumption. Indeed, the effect can persist even in the face of reassuring findings. For a recent example, we can look to the well-publicized findings of a study designed to explore the possible link of caffeine consump-tion and early pregnancy loss (Weng, Odouli, and Li 2008). Evidence of a modest increase in miscarriage risk with moderate caffeine con-sumption in the first trimester was touted as reason to "stop or reduce caffeine intake during pregnancy," even when the self-same study found that caffeine consumption under two cups was found to carry no increase in the miscarriage rate. Rather than reporting reassurance that low caffeine use was demonstrated to be safe, researchers took the finding of risk associated with moderate consumption and extended it against findings of safety.

Cultural reasoning about risk in pregnancy, in short, tends to invoke the precautionary principle in a particularly unfettered way. "Better safe than sorry" is a fine aphorism in general, and a particularly good one to take during pregnancy, where untoward effects on the fetus can be permanent. But when applied without sensitivity to evidence or appreciation of the *cost* of caution—when applied myopically, without due recognition of the long-term price of one's policy—it could turn out that a policy of "better safe than sorry" is the opposite of safe. It can, in fact, lead to significant harm to women and fetuses alike. Applied here, it collides with the animating purpose of the enterprise of clinical research, which is to take responsible, limited, and calculated risks in order to *garner* evidence, lest we visit more risk on more people in the future.

GOING FORWARD

Confronting the challenges of research with pregnant women is a critical if complex project. Going forward will require a number of steps. Some are obvious and morally straightforward. These include increasing funding for the OPRU and other groups to perform opportunistic studies involving women already taking medication during pregnancy. Because women in opportunistic studies already have made a decision to take medication outside of the research context, simple blood draws to measure pharmacokinetic and pharmacodynamic parameters introduce minimal risk and none of the onerous trade-offs that demand a novel ethical framework for inclusion. Also required is funding for research to determine the public health impact of the current lack of knowledge around medications in

pregnancy. Such funding could help to answer questions critical to decision making about research priorities: what is the current burden of disease for both pregnant women and their babies that results from the need to make treatment decisions in the absence of any relevant data? What are the emotional and psychological burdens of the anxiety and stress that treatment decisions in pregnancy engender? As newer approaches to treatment in the non-pregnant population are developed, what is the comparative cost of restricting pregnant women to the older medications that obstetrical providers are accustomed to using? For example, is there a health-related cost to the usual practice of replacing new antihypertensive medications with older medications such as methyldopa, which has been prescribed during pregnancy for decades? In both of these efforts, moving forward will involve developing legislative strategies modeled on those that have created incentives to include women and children in research.

Other steps will be considerably more complex and controversial. For instance, addressing the liability concerns that animate so much of the behaviour around research and drug development during pregnancy will require substantial efforts at both state and federal levels. Just as importantly, considerable efforts will be required to develop guidance for IRBs. Although IRBs are often and understandably focused on safety and protection from the harm of participation, in many ways they are the gatekeepers of access to research. As others have noted, IRB members may lack training or guidance regarding how to recognize or respond to the potential harm of exclusion (Chronic Disease Prevention and Control Research Center at Baylor College of Medicine and Intercultural Cancer Council 2008).

To make progress, we need an adequate ethical framework for determining what are and are not suitable justifications for exclusion of pregnant women from research. Some criteria can be borrowed from approaches to disparities in other underrepresented research populations. For instance, as with women generally, considerations of cost are not adequate justification for exclusion of underrepresented populations. When population-specific evidence is required to treat a particular group, the cost of research is one that must be borne in order to provide responsible, safe, and effective medical care to those who need it. For instance, the fact that sample size must be increased to adequately power a study that includes pregnant participants should not be accepted as valid criteria for their exclusion.

Other issues, though, will require a framework specific to pregnancy. Given the intermingled physiologies distinctly present in pregnancy, and the implications for what are potentially two rather than one person, thoughtful analysis is required to sort through the complex questions of the levels of risk the fetus—or for that matter, the woman—can be subjected for purposes of research that may benefit the other. A number of factors will be relevant, including the applicability of data from animal studies on fetal safety, data about the degree to which "borrowed knowledge" is possible, the balance of direct benefits of participation to the woman and the fetus with any potential harm, and the prevalence and seriousness of the condition in the pregnant population.

Details notwithstanding, we believe the core lesson is a simple one. As with other traditionally excluded populations, progress will not happen until we shift the burden of justification from inclusion to exclusion. There are many trials in which that burden may be met. To give an obvious example, pregnant women are not needed in trials of hormone therapies for prostate cancer. More broadly, and as with pediatric research, we do not include a population that introduces special ethical complexities into trials for medications of marginal medical importance (pharmacologic treatments for fungal infections of the nail bed). Special attention always must be given to the relevance of the goal in the population under consideration—for instance, new lipid-lowering drugs, of potential benefit to the broad population, are inappropriate for testing during early pregnancy, when the body significantly and importantly increases the production of cholesterol and triglycerides, high levels of which are considered adaptive to maternal and fetal nutritional needs and placental functioning. The claim then, is not that pregnant women belong in all trials. Rather, the claim is that decisions about whether pregnant women belong in a given trial, or type of trial, should be just that—*decisions*—made on the basis of reasoned criteria, reflecting balanced consideration of not only the risks of teratogenicity, but the potential importance of the medication for the health of women and the fetuses they carry. As with other underrepresented populations, it is exclusion, not inclusion, that requires justification.

But such justification is not currently required. Presently, Department of Health and Human Services regulations outline ten criteria that must be met if pregnant women are to be included in research protocols (U.S. Department of Health and Human Services 2005). Without any legislative or regulatory pressure to include pregnant women, all the incentives line up in favor of excluding pregnant women from clinical research. It is easier for researchers to simply side-step the questions and regulatory burden they represent by not including pregnant women. Until *that* decision *also* requires justification, we will continue to lack data on how to effectively and safely treat pregnant women.

In the absence of information about the safety and efficacy of medications, pregnant women and their providers are left with two unsavory options—take a drug, with unknown safety and efficacy; or fail to treat the conditions, thus leaving the woman and fetus vulnerable to the consequences of the underlying medical problems. They deserve better. Clinical research with pregnant women is morally challenging, but it is a challenge we must confront. For the alternative to responsible research in pregnancy is relegating pregnant women to second-class medical citizens—something, it turns out, that is not good for pregnant women nor the fetuses they carry.

Notes

1. Personal communication with M. Little during meeting of the Obstetric-Fetal Pharmacology Research Unit, Washington DC, November 2006.

2. The U.S. Food and Drug Administration classifies medications in one of the following five categories: (a) adequate and well-controlled studies have failed to demonstrate a risk to the fetus in the first trimester of pregnancy (and there is no evidence of risk in later trimesters); (b) animal reproduction studies have failed to demonstrate a risk to the fetus and there are no adequate and well-controlled studies in pregnant women; (c) animal reproduction studies have shown an adverse effect on the fetus and there are no adequate and well-controlled studies in humans, but potential benefits may warrant use of the drug in pregnant women despite potential risks; (d) there is positive evidence of human fetal risk based on adverse reaction data from investigational or marketing experience or studies in humans, but potential benefits may warrant use of the drug in pregnant women despite potential risks; (e) studies in animals or humans have demonstrated fetal abnormalities and/or there is positive evidence of human fetal risk based on adverse reaction data from investigational or marketing experience, and the risks involved in use of the drug in pregnant women clearly outweigh potential benefits. See Andrade et al. 2004; Cragan et al. 2006; U.S. Food and Drug Administration 2006.

3. We are grateful to Andrea Kalfoglou for bringing this to our attention.

4. Personal communication of Dr. David Grimes, Clinical Professor of Obstetrics and Gynecology, University of North Carolina Chapel Hill (Chapel Hill, NC) with A. Lyerly on August 31, 2005 via email.

5. Personal experience of A. Lyerly.

References

American College of Obstetricians and Gynecologists. 2002. ACOG Committee Opinion.

Number 268, February 2002. Management of asymptomatic pregnant or lactating women exposed to anthrax. *Obstetrics and Gynecology* 99 (2): 366–68.

———. 2007. ACOG Practice Bulletin No. 87: Use of psychiatric medications during pregnancy and lactation. *Obstetrics and Gynecology* 110 (5): 1179–98.

———. 2008. ACOG Practice Bulletin No. 90: Asthma in pregnancy. *Obstetrics and Gynecology* 111 (2): 457–64.

Andrade, Susan E., Jerry H. Gurwitz, Robert L. Davis, K. Arnold Chan, Jonathan A. Finkelstein, Kris Fortman, Heather McPhillips et al. 2004. Prescription drug use in pregnancy. *American Journal of Obstetrics and Gynecology* 191 (2): 398–407.

Andrew, M. A., T. R. Easterling, D. B. Carr, D. Shen, M. L. Buchanan, T. Rutherford, R. Bennett, P. Vicini, and M. F. Hebert. 2007. Amoxicillin pharmacokinetics in pregnant women: Modeling and simulations of dosage strategies. *Clinical Pharmacology and Therapeutics* 81 (4): 547–56.

Brent, Robert L. 2004. Utilization of animal studies to determine the effects and human risks of environmental toxicants (drugs, chemicals, and physical agents). *Pediatrics* 113 (4): 984–95.

Chronic Disease Prevention and Control Research Center at Baylor College of Medicine and Intercultural Cancer Council. 2008. Major deficiencies in the design and funding of clinical trials: A report to the nation improving on how human studies are conducted: Findings of the eliminating disparities in clinical trials project (EDICT). http://www.bcm.edu/cdrc/home.html (accessed 29 April 2008).

Cohen, Lee S., Lori L. Altshuler, Bernard L. Harlow, Ruta Nonacs, D. Jeffrey Newport, Adele C. Viguera, Rita Suri et al. 2006. Relapse of major depression during pregnancy in women who maintain or discontinue antidepressant treatment. *Journal of the American Medical Association* 295 (5): 499–507.

Cooper, William O., Sonia Hernandez-Diaz, Patrick G. Arbogast, Judith A. Dudley, Shannon Dyer, Patricia S. Gideon, Kathi Hall, and Wayne A. Ray. 2006. Major congenital malformations after first-trimester exposure to ACE inhibitors. *New England Journal of Medicine* 354 (23): 2443–51.

Cragan, Janet D., J. M. Friedman, Lewis B. Holmes, Kathleen Uhl, Nancy S. Green, and Laura Riley. 2006. Ensuring the safe and effective use of medications during pregnancy: Planning and prevention through preconception care. *Maternal and Child Health Journal* 10 (Suppl. 7): 129–35.

Dewyea, Victor A., and Michael R. Nelson. 2005. Asthma in pregnancy. *Allergy and Asthma Proceedings* 26 (4): 323–26.

Dombrowski, Mitchell P. 2006. Asthma and pregnancy. *Obstetrics and Gynecology* 108 (3): 667–81.

Doncel, G., and C. Mauck. 2004. Vaginal microbicides: A novel approach to preventing sexual transmission of HIV. *Curr HIV/AIDS Rep* 1 (1): 25–32.

Field, Marilyn J., and Richard E. Berman, eds. 2004. Ethical conduct of research involving children. Washington DC: National Academies Press.

Finer, Lawrence B., and Stanley K. Henshaw. 2006. Disparities in rates of unintended pregnancy in the United States, 1994 and 2001. *Perspectives on Sexual and Reproductive Health* 38 (2): 90–96.

General Accounting Office. 1992. Women's health: FDA needs to ensure more study of gender differences in prescription drug testing. Washington DC: GAO.

———. 2001. Women's health: Women sufficiently represented in new drug testing, but FDA oversight needs improvement.

Haire, Doris. 2001. FDA approved obstetrics drugs: Their impact on mother and baby. National Women's Health Alliance. http://nwhalliance.org/FDAAPPROVED.htm (accessed 17 June 2008).

James, Andra H., David E. Abel, and Leo R. Brancazio. 2006. Anticoagulants in pregnancy. *Obstetrical and Gynecological Survey* 61 (1): 59–69.

Jirtle, Randy. 2008. Randy L. Jirtle, Ph.D.: Epigenetics a window on gene dysregulation, disease. Interview by Bridget M. Kuehn. *Journal of the American Medical Association* 299 (11): 1249–50.

Lard-Whiteford, S. L., D. Matecka, J. J. O'Rear, I. S. Yuen, C. Litterst, and P. Reichelderfer.

2004. Recommendations for the nonclinical development of topical microbicides for prevention of HIV transmission: An update. *Journal of Acquired Immune Deficiency Syndromes* 36 (1): 541–52.

Lee, Euni, Mary Maneno, Leah Smith, Sheila Weiss, Ilene H. Zuckerman, Anthony Wutoh, and Zhenyi Xue. 2006. National patterns of medication use during pregnancy. *Pharmacoepidemiology and Drug Safety* 15 (8): 537–45.

Levine, Carol. 1993. Women as research subjects: New priorities, new questions. In *Emerging issues in biomedical policy: An annual review*. Vol. 2, ed. R. H. Blank and A. Bonnicksen. New York: Columbia University Press.

Little, Bertis B. 1999. Pharmacokinetics during pregnancy: Evidence-based maternal dose formulation. *Obstetrics and Gynecology* 93 (5): 858–68.

Lo, W. Y., and J. M. Friedman. 2002. Teratogenicity of recently introduced medications in human pregnancy. *Obstetrics and Gynecology* 100 (3): 465–73.

Lyerly, Anne D., Lisa M. Mitchell, Elizabeth M. Armstrong, Lisa H. Harris, Rebecca Kukla, Miriam Kuppermann, and Margaret O. Little. 2007. Risks, values, and decision making surrounding pregnancy. *Obstetrics and Gynecology* 109 (4): 979–84.

Martin, Joyce A., Brady E. Hamilton, Paul D. Sutton, Stephanie Ventura, Fay Menacker, Sharon Kirmeyer, and Martha L. Munson. 2007. National Vital Statistics Reports. Births: Final data for 2005. Atlanta: CDC.

Mastroianni, Anna C., Ruth R. Faden, and Daniel Federman, eds. 1994. *Women and health research: Ethical and legal issues of including women in clinical studies*. Washington DC: National Academy Press.

Mattison, D., and A. Zajicek. 2006. Gaps in knowledge in treating pregnant women. *Gender Medicine* 3:169–82.

Mazze, R. I., and B. Kallen. 1991. Appendectomy during pregnancy: A Swedish registry study of 778 cases. *Obstetrics and Gynecology* 77 (6): 835–40.

Merton, Vanessa. 1996. Ethical obstacles to the participation of women in biomedical research. In *Feminism and Bioethics: Beyond reproduction*, ed. S. Wolf. New York: Oxford University Press. National Alliance on Mental Health. 2008. *Pregnancy pointers for women with psychiatric history* 2008 [cited 15 February 2008]. http://www.nami.org/Content/ContentGroups/Helpline1/Pregnancy_Pointers_for_Women_with_Psychiatric_History.htm.

National Institute of Child Health and Human Development. 2003. *Request for applications for obstetric-fetal pharmacology research units* (HD-03-017) [cited 18 February 2008]. http://grants.nih.gov/grants/guide/rfa-files/RFA-HD-03-017.html.

National Institutes of Health (NIH) Revitalization Act of 1993, Pub L No. 103–43. Orr, Suezanne T., Dan G. Blazer, Sherman A. James, and Jerome P. Reiter. 2007. Depressive symptoms and indicators of maternal health status during pregnancy. *Journal of Women's Health* 16 (4): 535–42.

Raymond, E. 2006. Issues related to pregnancies in microbicide effectiveness trials. Paper presented at Microbicides Conference, in Cape Town, South Africa.

Tan, K. S., and N. C. Thomson. 2000. Asthma in pregnancy. *American Journal of Medicine* 109 (9): 727–33.

United States Department of Health and Human Services. Code of federal regulations at 45CFR46.204. http://www.hhs.gov/ohrp/humansubjects/guidance/45cfr46.htm#subpartb (accessed 17 June 2008).

United States Food and Drug Administration. 2006. Requirements on content and format of labeling for human prescription drug and biological products. *Federal Register* 71: 3921–3997.

Weng, Xiaoping, Roxana Odouli, and De-Kun Li. 2008. Maternal caffeine consumption during pregnancy and the risk of miscarriage: A prospective cohort study. *American Journal of Obstetrics and Gynecology* 198 (3): 279.e1–8.

Zajicek, A., and G. P. Giacoia. 2007. Obstetric clinical pharmacology: Coming of age. *Clinical Pharmacology and Therapeutics* 81 (4): 481–82.

Dancing with the Porcupine: Rules for Governing the University–Industry Relationship

Steven Lewis, Patricia Baird, Robert G. Evans, William A. Ghali, Charles J. Wright,
Elaine Gibson, and Françoise Baylis

Universities have long been involved in the creation and evaluation of pharmaceutical products. In its best form, academic participation in drug-related science both spurs innovation and, through the disinterest and skepticism that are hallmarks of the academic mission, provides a check on the premature enthusiasms of industry. In this commentary we examine the logic and behaviour of the pharmaceutical industry in pursuit of its interests and propose rules to govern university–industry partnerships that reflect the public interest.

The duty of universities is to seek truth. The duty of pharmaceutical companies is to make money for their shareholders. Drug companies that fail to do so go out of business. Universities that subordinate the disinterested search for truth to other ends lose credibility and their claim to a privileged status in society. If either abandons its fundamental mission, it ultimately fails. At times, institutional imperatives are bound to conflict.[1, 2]

Research can either serve or subvert the public interest. Its findings may advance knowledge and support useful innovation, or be filtered and twisted to support prejudices or gain commercial advantage. The capacities and integrity of researchers, and their universities, can be enhanced or corrupted in the process. Some partnerships are united by an open-minded quest for discovery; others are unholy alliances whereby researchers and universities become handmaidens of industry. Whatever ethical bed we make, we lie in.

There is abundant evidence that many such partnerships place industry imperatives above both the public interest and the fundamental ethos of the university. The evidence includes major variation in disclosure requirements,[3] insufficient protection of the right to publish in a timely fashion[4] and researchers having financial interests in companies potentially affected by the outcomes of their research.[5] The creation of the Canadian Institutes of Health Research (CIHR) and its renewed commitment to excellence and expanded capacity for innovation and discovery have created unprecedented health research opportunities in Canada. With what ethical compass will Canada chart its health research course?

The outcome will depend on 3 key players: the federal government and its agencies, the universities, and industry. The recent history of government policy is a 3-part drama. In the late 1980s the federal government concluded that increased drug research and development by the private sector in Canada would contribute to the economy. Second, multinational drug companies indicated that their expansion of research and development activities in their Canadian branches would be contingent on favourable patent protection legislation. Third, in return for extending patent protection, the government exacted a commitment from industry to invest 10% of sales in Canadian-based research.

The Medical Research Council of Canada[6] (MRC, the forerunner of the CIHR) and many faculty members and universities supported these treasures. The MRC budget declined for 3 consecutive years beginning in 1995/96 and was essentially frozen during most of the decade.[6] Elsewhere, spending on health research rose significantly, most notably

Lewis, S., Baird, P., Evans, R.G., Ghali, W.A., Wright, C.J., Gibson, E. & Baylis, F. (2001) "Dancing with the Porcupine: Rules for Governing the University-Industry Relationship." *Canadian Medical Association Journal* 165(6): pp. 783–785.

in the United States, where federal funding alone doubled in real terms during the 1990s.[7] Science became more complex, expensive and competitive. To offset the severe restraints imposed on public funding of universities as part of the war on government deficits in Canada during the 1990s, researchers and universities had to look elsewhere for funding. Enter industry.

In 2000, "business enterprise," which was almost exclusively the pharmaceutical industry (although Statistics Canada does not break down the figures), accounted for about 43% of gross domestic expenditures on research and development in the health field (the amount includes $350 million from foreign sources spent on business enterprises in Canada, which we assume to be industry dollars).[8] Universities and teaching hospitals received $161 million from industry, which was more than the amount from provincial governments combined and over half the amount received from federal sources (largely the MRC-CIHR). Aside from being a major player on campus, industry exerts considerable influence on public policy by virtue of the $900 million it spends in-house on research and development.

What does industry expect for its $161 million invested in universities and teaching hospitals? Drug companies have a fiduciary duty to exploit the intellectual talent and ethical credibility of universities to advance their interests. The proximate goal is the publication of positive results of trials of new drugs, or evaluations that show that certain drugs are better than their competitors' products. The ultimate goal is sales. Negative findings often, and predictably, create an unhappy industry partner. Common sense suggests that universities must be vigilant about protecting their own, fundamentally different culture and orientation.

To date, they have not been. The new money and activity exploded onto the scene with inadequate oversight and no standardization of rules or mechanisms to resolve disputes. The results: some highly publicized aggres-

sions,[9] tarnished institutional reputations, one-sided marriages of convenience, and who knows how much unhelpful drug therapy and increased cost.

Unsettling incidents of this nature have occurred throughout the world.[10] These are not impersonal and civil corporate disagreements; they often involve intimidating tactics by industry that profoundly affect researchers' lives and careers. Canadian cases, the details of which we do not recount for reasons of space, include the Bristol-Myers Squibb lawsuit against the Canadian Coordinating Office on Health Technology Assessment (CCOHTA) to suppress its statin report,[11] and the AstraZeneca legal threat against McMaster University researcher Anne Holbrook for her review of medications for stomach disorders (personal communication 2001). Regardless of the outcome of these cases, industry harassment consumes time and energy (and in the CCOHTA case, 13% of its budget, for legal fees) and creates unease; these are of course the intended effects.

In other cases, the financial clout of industry may influence academic behaviour more subtly, or at least appear to do so. Witness the withdrawal of an offer of employment to Dr. David Healy by the Centre for Addictions and Mental Health (CAMH) in Toronto shortly after he made a speech critical of Prozac, whose manufacturer, Eli Lilly, donated $1.55 million to the CAMH in 2000.[12–14] There is no evidence of direct involvement by Eli Lilly in this decision, but the company did withdraw corporate funding of The Hastings Centre after its journal published a series of articles critical of antidepressant prescribing practices.[15]

Such cases demonstrate yet again that, when public and private interests conflict, at least some companies will fiercely protect their shareholders' interests. If the drugs they hoped would be breakthroughs turn out to be "me-toos," they must market them at the highest possible price in order to recoup the development costs, which can exceed US$100 million. If one company's drug is the therapeutic equivalent of other companies' drugs, it is obliged to try to persuade doctors, pharmacists and the public that its drug is actually better. In this, they are identical to car manufacturers and brewers of beer.

These inevitabilities demand prudent engagement. The warrant for prudence is not that something *will* go wrong; it is simply that something *may* go wrong, and *has* gone wrong in several cases. The intimidation and lawsuits are only the tip of the iceberg. Far more prevalent and insidious is the correlation between industry funding and research that shows a positive therapeutic effect.[16] In a landmark article researchers found that industry-sponsored studies of calcium-channel antagonists are more likely to be supportive of that therapy than independently funded research.[17] Similar findings emerged from a review of economic analyses of new oncology drugs.[18] The positive skew is not dependent on such high-risk and brazen strategies as falsification of data; it is achievable by framing the questions and the design of studies to increase the probability of a positive result.

Industry funding creates an incentive to promote the positive and suppress the negative. When drug companies control publication of results or simply delay unwelcome findings, truth is partially disclosed and therefore compromised. And if researchers' laboratories and career prospects depend on renewed industry funding, their interests may begin to align with those of their paymasters. Unhappily, disinterested scholarly editorial practices often exacerbate rather than counteract this bias,[19–21] reaffirming Francis Bacon's observation that "the human intellect ... is more moved and excited by affirmatives than negatives."[19]

What is to be done? We propose the rules in Box 1 as a starting point for governing partnerships. The rules need an institutional home.

BOX 1

Proposed rules for governing university–industry relationships

- A standard, Canada-wide contract governing university–industry relationships, enshrining the right of the academic to disclose potentially harmful clinical effects immediately, and publish freely after a modest interval.
- Guidelines to determine whether a proposed industry–university project is of sufficient intellectual originality and interest to qualify as academic activity. If the project does not qualify, it should be defined as a service or consulting contract and should be priced and managed as such.
- Mandatory filing of all university–industry agreements and contracts with the overseeing body, and registration of all clinical trials.
- Mandatory written debriefing signed by all parties at the conclusion of every university–industry agreement, to be filed with the provost or equivalent of the university and the overseeing body, with a hearings process to resolve disputes.
- A certification and rating system for industry that assesses such areas as scientific integrity, observance of contracts, commitment to intellectual freedom, degree of interference in the conduct of research and appropriateness of financial arrangements.
- A surtax levied on all university–industry contracts, the proceeds from which would help both to fund a core office and its oversight activities and to cover the costs of defending researchers against industry harassment or formal litigation as vigorously as the Canadian Medical Protective Association protects doctors against medical malpractice claims.
- The appointment of an ombudsperson to whom researchers and industry can refer concerns about partnerships.
- Participation in and endorsement of the refined and expanded set of rules based on these general principles and structures by all agencies funding health research.

One option would vest responsibility with the Association of Universities and Colleges of Canada. Health research is but a subset of all research, and the university, not its parts or affiliates, should be the institution of record. Any tendency for the health sciences to develop ethical standards in isolation must be resisted. "Academic separatism" flies in the face of the multidisciplinary and interdisciplinary collaboration that is heavily promoted as essential to the advancement of knowledge. Even more centrally, the university must not duck its responsibility to govern activities in its well-funded peripheries, including teaching hospitals.

Is a coordinated, national approach necessary? On the basis of the evidence to date, universities and researchers cannot be expected to protect their (and by extension the public's) interests with uniform sophistication and vigour.[22] Some US commentators have proposed precisely our form of remedy.[23] In May of this year the US National Bioethics Advisory Commission called for federal legislation to create the National Office for Human Research Oversight to oversee all research involving human subjects, including the definition, disclosure, and management of conflict of interest.[24]

Not infrequently, universities encounter challenges, veiled in the language of increased accountability, to their freedom of inquiry and expression. The claim that proposed constraints would be fatal to the academic mission becomes hypocrisy if universities allow industry to define the nature of inquiry, dictate methods and shackle expression. An industry–university contract is a transaction, and our proposed rules are designed principally to protect the university's most precious commodity: intellectual integrity.

We are not asking academic researchers to forswear all interactions with industry. We are merely proposing rules for exercising due diligence to protect the essence of academic inquiry. A positive effect of the proposed rules would be voluntarily improved industry behaviour, with enlightened companies adopting honourable codes of conduct that in time may mitigate the wariness and cynicism that recent aggressions have doubtless engendered.

Some bargains are Faustian, and some horses are Trojan. Dance carefully with the porcupine, and know in advance the price of intimacy.

Acknowledgement

Dr. Ghali is supported by a Population Health Investigator Award from the Alberta Heritage Foundation for Medical Research and by a Government of Canada Research Chair in Health Services Research.

Notes

1. Press E, Washburn J. The kept university. *Atlantic Monthly* 2000; 285. Available: www.theantlantic.com/issues/2000/03/press.htm (accessed 2001 Aug 20).

2. Weatherall D. Academia and industry: increasingly uneasy bedfellows. *Lancet* 2000; 355:1574.

3. Van McCrary S, Anderson CB, Jakovljevic J, Khan T, McCullough LB, Wray NP, et al. A national survey of policies on disclosure of conflicts of interest in biomedical research. *N Engl J Med* 2000; 343:1621–6.

4. Cho MK, Shohara R, Schissel A, Rennie D. Policies on faculty conflicts of interest at US universities. *JAMA* 2000; 284:2237–8.

5. Lo B, Wolf LE, Berkeley A. Conflict-of-interest policies for investigators in clinical trials. *N Engl J Med* 2000; 343:1616–20.

6. Medical Research Council of Canada. *Report of the president 1999–2000*. Ottawa: Canadian Institutes of Health Research; 2000. Cat no MR1-2000. Available (in pdf format): www.cihr.ca/news/publications/publications/report9900_e.pdf (accessed 2001 Aug 20).

7. Meeks RL. *Federal R&D funding by budget function: fiscal years 1999–2001, special report*. Arlington (VA): National Science Foundation, Division of Science Resources Studies; 2001. Report no NSF 01-316.

8. Estimates of total expenditures on research and development in the health field in Canada, 1988 to 2000. Ottawa: Statistics Canada; 2001. Cat no. 88F0006XIE01006.

9. Hailey D. Scientific harassment by pharmaceutical companies: time to stop. CMAJ 2000; 162(2):212–3. Available: www.cma.ca/cmaj/vol-162/issue-2/0212.htm

10. Morgan S, Barer ML, Evans RG. Health economists meet the fourth tempter: drug dependency and scientific discourse. *Health Econ* 2000; 9:659–67.

11. Skolnick AA. Drug firm suit fails to halt publication of Canadian health technology report. *JAMA* 1998; 280:683–4.

12. Boseley S. Bitter pill. *Guardian Weekly* 2001; 164(22):23.

13. Hospital denies that withdrawal of MD's job offer was related to drug-company funding. *CMAJ* 2001; 164(13):1879. Available: www.cma.ca/cmaj/vol-164/issue-13/1879a.asp.

14. Lead donor Eli Lilly Canada launches education centre. In: *Foundation progress report winter 2000.* Toronto: Centre for Addiction and Mental Health; 2000. Available: www.camh.net/foundation/newsletters/foundation_news_winter2000.html (accessed 2001 Aug 20).

15. Kaebnick G. What about the report? *Hastings Cent Rep* 2001; 31(2):16–7.

16. Davidson RA. Source of funding and outcome of clinical trials. *J Gen Intern Med*, 1986; 1:155–8.

17. Stelfox HT, Chua G, O'Rourke K, Detsky AS. Conflict of interest in the debate over calcium-channel antagonists. *N Engl J Med* 1998; 332:101–6.

18. Friedberg M, Saffran B, Stinson TJ, Nelson W, Bennett CL. Evaluation of conflict of interest in economic analyses of new drugs used in oncology. *JAMA* 1999; 282:1453–7.

19. Dickersin K. The existence of publication bias and risk factors for its occurrence. *JAMA* 1990; 263:1385–9.

20. Easterbrook PJ, Berlin JA, Gopalan R, Matthews DR. Publication bias in clinical research. *Lancet* 1991; 337:867–72.

21. Naylor CD. Meta-analysis and the meta-epidemiology of clinical research. *BMJ* 1997; 315:617–9.

22. Boyd EA, Bero LA. Assessing faculty financial relationships with industry: a case study. *JAMA* 2000; 284:2209–14.

23. Hall ZA, Scott C. University-industry partnership. *Science* 2001; 591:553.

24. National Bioethics Advisory Commission. *Ethical and policy issues in research involving human participants.* Rockville (MD): The Commission; 2001 May 18. Recommendations available: http://bioethics.gov/press/finalrecomm5-18.html (accessed 2001 Aug 20).

CASES

Halushka v University of Saskatchewan, (1965), 53 DLR (2d) 436, [1965] 52 WWR 608 (Sask CA)

Summary prepared by Matthew Herder

Mr. Halushka learned about a study at the University of Saskatchewan from the University's employment office in late August 1961. During his initial visit with one of the researchers (Dr. Wyant), he was told that the research involved a new drug that was "perfectly safe" and that "it had been conducted many times before," that electrodes would be put into his limbs and head, that an incision would be made in his arm and a catheter inserted. For his research participation he would receive $50. Mr. Halushka agreed to take part in the research and signed a consent form that included a waiver of liability for the University and the researchers in the event of any "untoward effects or accidents."

Two days later, Mr. Halushka arrived at the hospital. Unbeknownst to him, the anesthetic drug to be used in the research ("fluoromar") had never been tested before. The researchers administered the fluoromar, and positioned the catheter inside Mr. Halushka's heart chambers. Shortly thereafter,

---

Reprinted by permission of the author.

the level of the anesthetic became too deep and Mr. Halushka suffered a cardiac arrest. To resuscitate him, the researchers had to manually massage his heart after making a large incision in his chest.

Mr. Halushka was unconscious for four days, and was discharged 10 days after waking up. At that point Dr. Wyant gave Mr. Halushka $50. When Mr. Halushka asked whether that was all he was going to get, given the adverse event he had suffered, Dr. Wyant offered to give him more in exchange for a complete release of legal liability from Mr. Halushka's mother or older sister. Mr. Halushka did not accept this offer and ultimately sued for trespass on the person and negligence.

Discussion Questions

1. What standard of disclosure is required for informed consent to participate in medical research? Should this differ from the standard of disclosure used in clinical practice?

2. What level of understanding is required for informed consent to participate in medical research? Should this differ from the level of understanding required in clinical practice?

3. What factors should be relevant when selecting subjects for participation in research? How can researchers avoid taking advantage of vulnerable persons in the selection of research participants?

Abdullahi v Pfizer Inc, 562 F 3d 163, 2009 WL 214649 (2nd Cir 2009)

Summary prepared by Cheluchi Onyemelukwe

In 1996, there was a meningitis epidemic in Kano, a state in the northern part of Nigeria. Pfizer, one of the largest American pharmaceutical companies, sent in staff to conduct a trial of an antibiotic, Trovafloxacin (commonly called Trovan). In conjunction with Nigerian officials, Pfizer recruited about 200 sick children to participate in the trials. The trials took place at the Kano Infectious Diseases Hospital. Pfizer's main reason for conducting the clinical trials in Kano was to obtain approval for the drug from the United States Food and Drug Agency (FDA). The trial investigated whether the oral form of Trovan was more effective and efficient in treating children infected with meningitis than other treatments available at the time. In 1998, the FDA approved Trovan for use on adult patients only. Its use in the United States was eventually limited to adult emergency care following reports of liver failure in patients associ-

ated with the use of Trovan. In 1999, the European Union banned the use of the drug. Eleven children died and many more suffered significant harm.

In a lawsuit against Pfizer, the parents and the representatives of the children alleged that informed consent was not obtained from the parents and guardians of the children. They alleged that Pfizer did not disclose the fact that the use of the drug was merely experimental and was not primarily meant to provide treatment for the children. They also claimed that Pfizer did not explain, read, or offer to read the informed consent documents in English or Hausa (the local language) as required by the protocol. Pfizer also allegedly failed to inform the potential participants about the side effects of the drug, or the fact that the non-governmental organization Médecins Sans Frontières (Doctors Without Borders) was providing effective treatment against bacterial meningitis for free at the same site. Further, although Pfizer had earlier claimed to have received ethics approval from an ethics review committee at the Infectious Diseases Hospital, the hospital had no ethics review committee at the time. In addition, the parents and representatives claimed that Pfizer deliberately gave the children, who were in the Ceftriaxone control group, a low dose in order to misrepresent the efficacy of Trovan in relation to Ceftrixaone. They also claimed that Pfizer failed to provide or administer follow-up care after the trial.

Discussion Questions

1. When is it ethically acceptable to conduct research in a developing country? For instance, is it acceptable to conduct clinical trials for a drug in a country that likely would never be able to afford the drug in a treatment context (once proven safe and effective)?

2. The UNESCO Universal Declaration on Bioethics and Human Rights stipulates that "Benefits resulting from any scientific research and its applications should be shared with society as a whole and within the international community, in particular with developing countries." What should this require in practical terms?

3. Should multi-national pharmaceutical companies and other research sponsors that conduct research in developing countries adhere to the ethical standards that apply in their country of origin, the ethical standards that apply in the country where the research will be conducted, or both?

Useful Resources

ONLINE

Belmont Report: Ethical Principles and Guidelines for the Protection of Human Subjects of Research

This influential report was prepared by the (U.S.) National Commission for the Protection of Human Subjects of Biomedical and Behavioral Research (1979).

Canadian Association of University Teachers (CAUT)

The case of University of Toronto clinician, Dr. Nancy Olivieri, gained attention when her research at the Hospital for Sick Children led her to believe that a new drug treatment posed dangers to some patients. The case was reviewed by CAUT's Committee on Academic Freedom and Tenure. The Committee concluded that the issues raised were serious and that many questions remained unanswered by reviews conducted by other bodies. The full report, and various summaries and news articles, are provided on the CAUT website.

Council for International Organizations of Medical Sciences (CIOMS)

In coordination with the United Nations, CIOMS facilitates and promotes international activities in the field of biomedical services and serves the scientific interest of the biomedical community through initiating and coordinating long-term projects in the following fields: bioethics, health policy, ethics and human values, drug development and use, and international nomenclature of diseases.

Declaration of Helsinki

The World Medical Association's statement intended to provide ethical guidance to physicians and other participants in medical research involving human subjects.

Health Canada: Ethics Resources

This website provides links to a number of research ethics resources.

Health Canada: Requirements for Informed Consent Documents

This website provides science researchers with background information that will assist them in preparing applications to be submitted to Health Canada and the Public Health Agency of Canada's Research Ethics Board. The section on consent details the basic elements of the consent process as well as what is required to construct a proper consent form.

Interagency Panel on Research Ethics (PRE)

In 2001, Canada's three federal research agencies, The Canadian Institutes of Health Research (CIHR), the Natural Sciences and Engineering Research Council (NSERC), and the Social Sciences and Humanities Research Council (SSHRC), jointly created the Interagency Advisory Panel on Research Ethics (PRE or the Panel) as part of a collaborative effort to promote the ethical conduct of research involving human participants. The Panel develops, interprets, and implements the Tri-Council Policy Statement: Ethical Conduct for Research Involving Humans (TCPS2).

International Ethical Guidelines for Biomedical Research Involving Human Subjects (CIOMS)

"The 2002 CIOMS Guidelines are designed to be of use to countries in defining national policies on the ethics of biomedical research involving human subjects, applying ethical standards in local circumstances, and establishing or improving ethical review mechanisms. A particular aim is to reflect the conditions and the needs of low-resource countries, and the implications for multinational or transnational research in which they may be partners."

Tri-Council Policy Statement: Ethical Conduct for Research Involving Humans (TCPS2)

These guidelines describe the standards and procedures for research involving humans adopted by the three Canadian federal research granting Agencies: The Canadian Institutes of Health Research (CIHR), the Natural Sciences and Engineering Research Council of Canada (NSERC), and the Social Sciences and Humanities Research Council of Canada (SSHRC).

Updated Guidelines for Human Pluripotent Stem Cell Research

This framework aims to ensure ethical and scientific oversight of publicly funded human pluripotent stem cell research—research conducted by individuals, or in institutions, that receive funding from one or more of the federal research funding Agencies.

U.S. Code of Federal Regulations Title 45, Part 46 Protection of Human Subjects

Title 45, CFR, Part 46 Common Rule is federal human research subject protection policy, as mandated by the Executive Branch of the United States (revised as of October 1, 1999).

READINGS

Brown, B. (1988) Proxy consent for research on the incompetent elderly. In Thornton, J., Winkler, E. (Eds.) *Ethics and aging* (pp. 318–324).

Emanuel, E., Grady C., Crouch, R.A., Lie, R., Miller, F. & Wendler, D. (Eds). (2008) *The Oxford textbook of clinical research ethics*. Oxford: Oxford University Press.

Emanuel, E., Wendler, D., & Grady, C. (2000) What makes clinical research ethical? *Journal of the American Medical Association* 283(20), 2701–11.

Hawkins, J.S. & Emanuel E. (Eds). (2008) *Exploitation and developing countries: The ethics of clinical research.* Princeton: Princeton University Press.

Kimmelman, J. (2009) *Gene transfer and the ethics of first-in-human research: Lost in translation.* New York: Cambridge University Press.

Shamoo, A. E., & Resnik, D. B. (2009). *Responsible conduct of research* (2nd ed.). New York, NY: Oxford University Press.

HEALTH LAW

Weiss c Solomon (1989), 48 CCLT 280 (QS Qc)

The family of Julius Weiss, a research participant who died while enrolled in a clinical trial, sued the researchers and hospital (including the Research Ethics Board) for failing to disclose a rare but potentially fatal risk of participation in the trial.

CanLII

CanLII is a non-profit organization managed by the Federation of Law Societies of Canada. CanLII's goal is to make Canadian law accessible for free on the Internet.

Chapter 8 REPRODUCTION

INTRODUCTION

When health care providers think about women's reproductive health, they often think about the myriad ways in which it is possible to routinely intervene in pregnancy. For example, technologies are now available to interrupt pregnancy (e.g., abortion), to circumvent infertility (e.g., assisted human reproduction using donated eggs), and to monitor the developing fetus (e.g., prenatal testing and screening). Articles in this chapter explore aspects of each of these interventions and identify some of the relevant ethical questions concerning their widespread use.

Abortion is a legal, safe, and effective procedure widely endorsed by a majority of Canadians. Nonetheless, abortion remains an ethically and socially contentious issue in Canada. There are at least two facets to this debate—one facet concerns the moral status of abortion, the other concerns the appropriate legal status of the practice. The first of these debates looks at whether abortion is (ever, sometimes, or always) morally permissible, and if so, under what circumstances. The second debate focuses squarely on the right of access to abortion and looks at whether the state should in any way restrict abortion access or simply treat this as an elective medical procedure.

In the first article, Wayne Sumner offers a critical review of the leading positions on the fetus's moral standing (the so-called "liberal" and "conservative" approaches) and presents his own proposal for a developmental view of the fetus, an approach that allows certain sorts of abortions (those in the early stages of pregnancy) and prohibits others (those in the later stages of pregnancy). In the second article, Alister Browne and Bill Sullivan provide a brief summary of recent Canadian legal history showcasing the fact that Canada is one of very few countries to have decriminalized abortion. They note, however, that decriminalization does not mean ready access, and they recognize that women who want to terminate a pregnancy often face a number of barriers.

While some women want to rid themselves of unwanted pregnancies, other women and couples want to overcome their infertility and start a family. It is currently estimated that between 8–12 percent of women in North America are unable to conceive spontaneously. Of these, about half will seek medical care for their infertility. Whereas with the abortion debate a key issue is the right to terminate an unwanted pregnancy, with assisted human reproduction a key issue is the right to reproduce, and more specifically, the right to access reproductive technologies. But what about reproductive options for women and couples who do not have eggs available for fertilization and thus have need of donor eggs in order to pursue a reproductive project? In the United States, female university students are routinely enticed to sell their eggs. In sharp contrast, in Canada, the buying and selling of human eggs is illegal. Reports suggest, however, that there is an underground market for human eggs in Canada and that Canadians travel to the United States (and other countries) to purchase human eggs for reproductive purposes.

In the third article, Alison Motluk effectively highlights some of the ethical problems with the current Canadian policy on human egg donation. She describes the experience of a 25-year-old woman from Toronto who donated her eggs through a Canadian fertility clinic. Because of various shortcomings in Canadian law, fertility clinics are able to circumvent rules about payment (often by labelling the money as "compensation"). More to the point, though, this sort of circumvention may seem appropriate because of the significant burdens and harms to the egg donor. Altruism may not be enough to motivate women to donate eggs. The young woman from Toronto ended up suffering a significant adverse event after donating her eggs; this also highlights some of the shortcomings related to informed consent in this context. One commentator in the article suggests that egg donation often has a manipulative element that trades on young women's socialized commitment to care for others. There are, it would seem, complex ethical issues raised by this practice that go beyond the usual concerns of commercialization.

The last two articles in this chapter are on prenatal screening and testing. The first selection by Abby Lippman begins with a critical commentary on that which is typically accepted uncritically, namely that knowledge in human genetics will fundamentally alter our understanding of the concepts of health and disease. This article is important not only for signaling genetic technology's role in the process of "geneticization," but also for calling into question the touted benefits of prenatal screening and testing. It is widely held that these technologies provide women with reassurance, choice, and control, but according to Lippman, this is only half the story. After all, we shouldn't just accept that reassurance is good until we've asked why it is that women need reassurance about their pregnancies. What social conditions have shaped the need for reassurance? Further, bioethicists writing about other new technologies have drawn attention to the ways in which increased choice doesn't necessarily translate into greater autonomy. And finally, it isn't clear who really gains control, and from whom control is taken, in the context of new reproductive technologies. Lippman suggests that we would do well to remember that prenatal testing and screening are public health measures intended to ensure quality control over the product: the "baby."

In the final article, Janet Malek defends the use of reproductive genetic technologies against the expressivist argument according to which the use of reproductive genetic technologies expresses a disvaluing of persons with disabilities. In her view, the expressivist argument is not a persuasive reason not to use reproductive genetic technologies. She offers a thought experiment involving a decision about whether to cross a street, given the information that you will be struck by a car and lose the use of your legs. She argues that a decision not to cross the street in this case, in order to avoid the predicted outcome, expresses no disvalue of individuals who have paraplegia. In conjunction with various modified scenarios, Malek aims to use this thought experiment to overcome the expressivist argument to reproductive genetic technologies.

A Third Way

L. Wayne Sumner

The practice of abortion confronts us with two different sets of moral questions belonging to two different decision contexts. The primary context is that in which a woman chooses whether to have an abortion and a physician chooses whether to perform it; here the focus is on the moral quality of abortion itself. Because this context is one of individual decision we will call the set of moral questions which it contains the *personal* problem of abortion. The secondary

Sumner, L.W.; *Abortion and Moral Theory.* © 1981 Princeton University Press. Reprinted by permission of Princeton University Press.

context is that in which a society chooses how, or whether, to regulate abortions; here the focus is on the merits of alternative abortion policies. Because this context is one of social decision we will call the set of moral questions which it contains the *political* problem of abortion.

Although the two kinds of problem raised by abortion are distinct, they are also connected. A complete view of the morality of abortion will therefore offer connected solutions to them. In most countries in the West, public discussion of abortion has been distorted by the dominance of two such views. The liberal view, espoused by "pro-choice" groups, holds that (voluntary) abortion is always morally innocuous and (therefore) that the only acceptable abortion policy is one which treats abortion as another variety of minor elective surgery. The conservative view, espoused by "pro-life" groups, holds that abortion is always morally serious and (therefore) that the only acceptable abortion policy is one which treats abortion as another variety of homicide.

Because they define the extremities of the continuum of possible positions, and because each is sufficiently simple and forceful to be advocated by a powerful movement, these established views constitute the familiar reference points in our abortion landscape. Yet neither has managed to command the allegiance of more than a small minority of the public. For the rest of us who are unwilling to embrace either of the extreme options the problem has been the lack of a well-defined middle ground between them. In contrast to the power of the established views more moderate alternatives may appear both indistinct and indecisive.

Public distrust of the established views is well grounded: neither stands up under critical scrutiny.[1] If their demise is not to leave us without any credible view of abortion three tasks must be successfully completed. The first is to define a third way with abortion and to distinguish it from both of the views which it will supersede. The second is to give it an intuitive defense by showing that it coheres better than either of its predecessors with our considered moral judgments both on abortion itself and on closely related issues. Then, finally,

the third way must be grounded in a moral theory. The first two of these tasks will be undertaken here; the more daunting theoretical challenge is confronted elsewhere.[2]

1. SPECIFICATIONS

Despite their opposition, the two established views suffer from similar defects. Collating their failures will provide us with some positive guidelines to follow in building a more satisfactory alternative. The central issue in the morality of abortion is the moral status of the fetus. Let us say that a creature has *moral standing* if, for the purpose of moral decisionmaking, it must be counted for something in its own right. To count for nothing is to have no moral standing; to count for as much as possible (as much, that is, as any creature does) is to have full moral standing. We may, for the purpose of the present discussion, make this rather vague notion more precise by adopting the rights vocabulary favored by both of the established views. We will suppose that having (some) moral standing is equivalent to having (some) right to life. The central issue in the morality of abortion is then whether fetuses have moral standing in this sense.[3]

The conservative view, and also the more naive versions of the liberal view, select a precise point (conception, birth, etc.) as the threshold of moral standing, implying that the transition from no standing to full standing occurs abruptly. In doing so they rest more weight on these sudden events than they are capable of bearing. A view that avoids this defect will allow full moral standing to be acquired gradually. It will therefore attempt to locate not a threshold point, but a threshold period or stage.

Both of the established views attribute a uniform moral status to all fetuses, regardless of their dissimilarities. Each, for example counts a newly conceived zygote for precisely as much (or as little) as a full-term fetus, despite the enormous differences between them. A view that avoids this defect will assign moral status differentially, so that the threshold stage occurs sometime during pregnancy.

A consequence of the uniform approach adopted by both of the established views is that neither can attach any significance to the development of the fetus during gestation. Yet this development is the most obvious feature of gestation. A view that avoids this defect will base the (differential) moral standing of the fetus at least in part on its level of development. It will thus assign undeveloped fetuses a moral status akin to that of ova and spermatozoa, whereas it will assign developed fetuses a moral status akin to that of infants.

So far, then, an adequate view of the fetus must be gradual, differential, and developmental. It must also be derived from a satisfactory criterion of moral standing. Such a criterion must be general (applicable to beings other than fetuses), it must connect moral standing with the empirical properties of such beings, and it must be morally relevant. Its moral relevance is partly testable by appeal to intuition, for arbitrary or shallow criteria will be vulnerable to counter-examples. But the final test of moral relevance is grounding in a moral theory.

An adequate view of the fetus promises a morally significant division between early abortions (before the threshold stage) and late abortions (after the threshold stage). It also promises borderline cases (during the threshold state). Wherever that stage is located, abortions that precede it will be private matters, since the fetus will at that stage lack moral standing. Thus the provisions of the liberal view will apply to early abortions: they will be morally innocent (as long as the usual conditions of maternal consent, etc., are satisfied) and ought to be legally unregulated (except for rules equally applicable to all other medical procedures). Early abortion will have the same moral status as contraception.

Abortions that follow the threshold stage will be interpersonal matters, since the fetus will at that stage possess moral standing. Thus the provisions of the conservative view will apply to late abortions: they must be assessed on a case-by-case basis and they ought to be legally permitted only on appropriate grounds. Late abortions will have the same moral status as infanticide, except for the difference made by the physical connection between fetus and mother.

A third way with abortion is thus a moderate and differential view, combining elements of the liberal view for early abortion with elements of (a weakened version of) the conservative view for late abortions. The policy that a moderate view will support is a moderate policy, permissive in the early stages of pregnancy and more restrictive (though not as restrictive as conservatives think appropriate) in the later stages. So far as the personal question of the moral evaluation of particular abortions is concerned, there is no pressing need to resolve the borderline cases around the threshold stage. But a workable abortion policy cannot tolerate this vagueness and will need to establish a definite time limit beyond which the stipulated grounds will come into play. Although the precise location of the time limit will unavoidably be somewhat arbitrary, it will be defensible as long as it falls somewhere within the threshold stage. Abortion on request up to the time limit and only for cause thereafter: these are the elements of a satisfactory abortion policy.

A number of moderate views may be possible, each of them satisfying all of the foregoing constraints. A particular view will be defined by selecting (a) a criterion of moral standing, (b) the natural characteristics whose gradual acquisition during normal fetal development carries with it the acquisition of moral standing, and (c) a threshold stage. Of these three steps, the first is the crucial one, since it determines both of the others.

2. A CRITERION OF MORAL STANDING

We are assuming that for a creature to have moral standing is for it to have a right to life. Any such right imposes duties on moral agents; these duties may be either negative (not to deprive the creature of life) or positive (to support the creature's life). Possession of a right to life implies at least some immunity against attack by others, and possibly also some entitlement to the aid of others. As the duties may vary in strength, so may the corresponding rights. To have some moral standing is to have some right to life, whether or not it may be overridden by the rights of others. To have full moral standing is to have the strongest right to life possessed by anyone, the right to life of the paradigm person. Depending on one's moral theory, this right may or may not be inviolable and indefeasible and thus may or may not impose absolute duties on others.

To which creatures should we distribute (some degree of) moral standing? On which criterion should we base this distribution? It may be easier to answer these questions if we begin with the clear case and work outward to the unclear ones. If we can determine why we ascribe full standing to the paradigm case, we may learn what to look for in other creatures when deciding whether or not to include them in the moral sphere.

The paradigm bearer of moral standing is an adult human being with normal capacities of intellect, emotion, perception, sensation, decision, action, and the like. If we think of such a person as a complex bundle of natural properties, then in principle we could employ as a criterion any of the properties common to all normal and mature members of our species. Selecting a particular property or set of properties will define a class of creatures with moral standing, namely, all (and only) those who share that property. The extension of that class will depend on how widely the property in question is distributed. Some putative criteria will be obviously frivolous and will immediately fail the tests of generality or moral relevance. But even after excluding the silly candidates, we are left with a number of serious ones. There are four that appear to be the most serious: we might attribute full moral standing to the paradigm person on the ground that he/she is (a) intrinsically valuable, (b) alive, (c) sentient, or (d) rational. An intuitive test of the adequacy of any of these candidates will involve first enumerating the class of beings to whom it will distribute moral standing and then determining whether that class either excludes creatures that upon careful reflection we believe ought to be included or includes creatures that we believe ought to be excluded. In the former case the criterion draws the boundary of the moral sphere too narrowly and fails as a necessary condition of moral standing. In the latter case the criterion draws the boundary too broadly and fails as a sufficient condition. (A given criterion may, of course, be defective in both respects.) ...

A criterion of life (or teleology) is too weak, admitting classes of beings (animate and inanimate) who are not suitable loci for moral rights; being alive is necessary for having standing, but it is not sufficient. A criterion of rationality (or moral agency) is too strong, excluding classes of beings (human and nonhuman) who are suitable loci for rights; being rational is sufficient for having standing, but it is not necessary. A criterion of sentience (or consciousness) is a promising middle path between these extremes. Sentience is the capacity for feeling or affect. In its most primitive form it is the ability to experience sensations of pleasure and pain, and thus the ability to enjoy and suffer. Its more developed forms include wants, aims, and desires (and thus the ability to be satisfied and frustrated); attitudes, tastes, and values; and moods, emotions, sentiments, and passions. Consciousness is a necessary condition of sentience, for feelings are states of mind of which their owner is aware. But it is not sufficient; it is at least possible in principle for beings to be conscious (percipient, for instance, or even rational) while utterly lacking feelings. If rationality embraces a set of cognitive capacities, then sentience is rooted in a being's affective and conative life. It is in virtue of being sentient that creatures have interests, which are compounded either out of their desires or out of the experiences they find agreeable (or both). If morality has to do with the protection and promotion of interests, it is a plausible conjecture that we owe moral duties to all those beings capable of having interests. But this will include all sentient creatures.

Like rationality, and unlike life, it makes sense to think of sentience as admitting of degrees. Within any given mode, such as the perception of pain, one creature may be more or less sensitive than another. But there is a further sense in which more developed (more rational) creatures possess a higher degree of sentience. The expansion of consciousness and of intelligence opens up new ways of experiencing the world, and therefore new ways of being affected by the world. More rational beings are capable of finding either fulfillment or frustration in activities and states of affairs to which less developed creatures are, both cognitively and affectively, blind. It is in this sense of a broader and deeper sensibility that a higher being is capable of a richer, fuller, and more varied existence. The fact that sentience admits of degrees (whether of sensitivity or sensibility) enables us to employ it both as an inclusion criterion and as a comparison criterion of moral standing. The animal kingdom presents us with a hierarchy of sentience. Nonsentient beings have no moral standing; among sentient beings the more developed have greater standing than the less developed, the upper limit being occupied by the paradigm of a normal adult human being. Although sentience is the criterion of moral standing, it is also possible to explain the relevance of rationality. The evolutionary order is one of ascending intelligence. Since rationality expands a creature's interests, it is a reliable indicator of the degree of moral standing which that creature possesses. Creatures less rational than human beings do not altogether lack standing, but they do lack full standing.

An analysis of degrees of standing would require a graded right to life, in which the strength of the right varied inversely with the range of considerations capable of overriding it. The details of any such analysis will be complex and need not be worked out here. However, it seems that we are committed to extending (some) moral standing at least to all vertebrate animals, and also to counting higher animals for more than lower.[4] Thus we should expect the higher vertebrates (mammals) to merit greater protection of life than the lower (fish, reptiles, amphibia, birds) and we should also expect the higher mammals (primates, cetaceans) to merit greater protection of life than the lower (canines,

felines, etc.). Crude as this division may be, it seems to accord reasonably well with most people's intuitions that in our moral reasoning paramecia and horseflies count for nothing, dogs and cats count for something, chimpanzees and dolphins count for more, and human beings count for most of all.

A criterion of sentience can thus allow for the gradual emergence of moral standing in the order of nature. It can explain why no moral issues arise (directly) in our dealings with inanimate objects, plants, and the simpler forms of animal life. It can also function as a moral guideline in our encounters with novel life forms on other planets. If the creatures we meet have interests and are capable of enjoyment and suffering, we must grant them some moral standing. We thereby constrain ourselves not to exploit them ruthlessly for our own advantage. The kind of standing that they deserve may be determined by the range and depth of their sensibility, and in ordinary circumstances this will vary with their intelligence. We should therefore recognize as equals beings who are as rational and sensitive as ourselves. The criterion also implies that if we encounter creatures who are rational but nonsentient—who utterly lack affect and desire—nothing we can do will adversely affect such creatures (in morally relevant ways). We would be entitled, for instance, to treat them as a species of organic computer. The same obviously holds for forms of artificial intelligence; in deciding whether to extend moral standing to sophisticated machines, the question (as Bentham put it) is not whether they can reason but whether they can suffer.

A criterion of sentience also requires gentle usage of the severely abnormal. Cognitive disabilities and disorders may impair a person's range of sensibility, but they do not generally reduce that person to the level of a nonsentient being. Even the grossly retarded or deranged will still be capable of some forms of enjoyment and suffering and thus will still possess (some) moral standing in their own right. This standing diminishes to the vanishing point only when sentience is entirely lost or never gained in the first place. If all affect and responsivity are absent, and if they cannot be engendered, then (but only then) are we no longer dealing with a sentient creature. This verdict accords well with the contemporary trend toward defining death in terms of the permanent loss of cerebral functioning. Although such patients are in one obvious sense still alive (their blood circulates and is oxygenated), in the morally relevant sense they are now beyond our reach, for we can cause them neither good nor ill. A criterion of life would require us to continue treating them as beings with (full?) moral standing, whereas a criterion of rationality would withdraw that standing when reason was lost even though sensibility should remain. Again a criterion of sentience enables us to find a middle way.

Fastening upon sentience as the criterion for possession of a right to life thus opens up the possibility of a reasonable and moderate treatment of moral problems other than abortion, problems pertaining to the treatment of nonhuman animals, extraterrestrial life, artificial intelligence, "defective" human beings, and persons at the end of life. We need now to trace out its implications for the fetus.

3. THE MORALITY OF ABORTION

The adoption of sentience as a criterion determines the location of a threshold of moral standing. Since sentience admits of degrees, we can in principle construct a continuum ranging from fully sentient creatures at one extreme to completely nonsentient creatures at the other. The threshold of moral standing is that area of the continuum through which sentience fades into nonsentience. In phylogenesis the continuum extends from homo sapiens to the simple animals and plants, and the threshold area is the boundary between vertebrates and invertebrates. In pathology the continuum extends from the fully normal to the totally incapacitated, and the threshold area is the transition from consciousness to unconsciousness. Human ontogenesis also presents us with a continuum from adult to zygote. The threshold area will be the stage at which sentience first emerges, but where is that to be located?

A mental life is built upon a physical base. The capacity for sentience is present only when the necessary physiological structures are present. Physiology, and in particular neurophysiology, is our principal guide in locating a threshold in the phylogenetic continuum. Like a stereo system, the brain of our paradigm sentient being is a set of connected components. These components may be roughly sorted into three groups: forebrain (cerebral hemispheres, thalamus, hypothalamus, amygdala), midbrain (cerebellum), and brainstem (upper part of the spinal cord, pineal and pituitary glands). The brainstem and midbrain play no direct role in the individual's conscious life; their various parts regulate homeostasis (temperature, respiration, heartbeat, etc.), secrete hormones, make reflex connections, route nerves, coordinate motor activities, and so on. All of these functions can be carried on in the total absence of consciousness. Cognitive, perceptual, and voluntary motor functions are all localized in the forebrain, more particularly in the cerebral cortex. Sensation (pleasure/pain), emotion, and basic drives (hunger, thirst, sex, etc.) are controlled by subcortical areas in the forebrain. Although the nerves that transmit pleasure/pain impulses are routed through the cortex, their ultimate destination is the limbic system (amygdala, hypothalamus). The most primitive forms of sentience are thus possible in the absence of cortical activity.

Possession of particular neural structures cannot serve as a criterion of moral standing, for we cannot rule out encounters with sentient beings whose structures are quite different from ours. But in all of the species with which we are familiar, the components of the forebrain (or some analogues) are the minimal conditions of sentience. Thus the evolution of the forebrain serves as an indicator of the kind and degree of sentience possessed by a particular animal species. When we turn to human ontogenesis we may rely on the same indicator.

The normal gestation period for our species is 280 days from the onset of the last menstrual period to birth. This duration is usually divided into three equal trimesters of approximately thirteen weeks each. A zygote has no central nervous system of any sort. The spinal cord makes its first appearance early in the embryonic period (third week), and the major divisions between forebrain, midbrain, and brainstem are evident by the end of the eighth week. At the conclusion of the first trimester virtually all of the major neural components can be clearly differentiated and EEG activity is detectable. The months to follow are marked chiefly by the growth and elaboration of the cerebral hemispheres, especially the cortex. The brain of a seven-month fetus is indistinguishable, at least in its gross anatomy, from that of a newborn infant. Furthermore, by the seventh month most of the neurons that the individual's brain will contain during its entire lifetime are already in existence. In the newborn the brain is closer than any other organ to its mature level of development.

There is no doubt that a newborn infant is sentient—that it feels hunger, thirst, physical pain, the pleasure of sucking, and other agreeable and disagreeable sensations. There is also no doubt that a zygote, and also an embryo, are presentient. It is difficult to locate with accuracy the stage during which feeling first emerges in fetal development. The structure of the fetal brain, including the cortex, is well laid down by the end of the second trimester. But there is reason to expect the more primitive and ancient parts of that brain to function before the rest. The needs of the fetus dictate the order of appearance of neural functions. Thus the brainstem is established and functioning first, since it is required for the regulation of heartbeat and other metabolic processes. Since the mammalian fetus develops in an enclosed and protected environment, cognition and perception are not essential for survival and their advent is delayed. It is therefore not surprising that the cortex, the most complex part of the brain and the least important to the fetus, is the last to develop to an operational level.

Simple pleasure/pain sensations would seem to occupy a medial position in this priority ranking. They are localized in a part of the brain that is more primitive than the cortex, but they could have little practical role for a being that is by and large unable either to seek pleasurable stimuli or to avoid painful ones. Behavioral evidence is by its very nature ambiguous. Before the end of the first trimester, the fetus will react to unpleasant stimuli by flinching and withdrawing. However, this reaction is probably a reflex that is entirely automatic. How are we to tell when mere reflex has crossed over into consciousness? The information we now possess does not enable us to date with accuracy the emergence of fetal sentience. Of some judgments, however, we can be reasonably confident. First-trimester fetuses are clearly not yet sentient. Third-trimester fetuses probably possess some degree of sentience, however minimal. The threshold of sentience thus appears to fall in the second trimester. More ancient and primitive than cognition, the ability to discriminate simple sensations of pleasure and pain is probably the first form of consciousness to appear in the ontogenetic order. Further, when sentience emerges it does not do so suddenly. The best we can hope for is to locate a threshold state or period in the second trimester. It is at present unclear just how far into that trimester this stage occurs.

The phylogenetic and pathological continua yield us clear cases at the extremes and unclear cases in the middle. The ontogenetic continuum does the same. Because there is no quantum leap into consciousness during fetal development, there is no clean and sharp boundary between sentient and nonsentient fetuses. There is therefore no precise point at which a fetus acquires moral standing. More and better information may enable us to locate the threshold stage ever more accurately, but it will never collapse that stage into a point. We are therefore inevitably confronted with a class of fetuses around the threshold stage whose sentience, and therefore whose moral status, is indeterminate....

The moral issues raised by early abortion are precisely those raised by contraception. It is for early abortions that the liberal view is appropriate. Since the fetus at this stage has no right to life, early abortion (like contraception) cannot violate its rights. But if it violates no one's rights, early abortion (like contraception) is a private act. There are of course significant differences between contraception and early abortion, since the former is generally less hazardous, less arduous, and less expensive. A woman has, therefore, good prudential reasons for relying on contraception as her primary means of birth control. But if she elects an early abortion, then, whatever the circumstances and whatever her reasons, she does nothing immoral.[5]

The moral issues raised by late abortion are similar to those raised by infanticide. It is for late abortions that (a weakened form of) the conservative view is appropriate. Since the fetus at this stage has a right to life, late abortion (like infanticide) may violate its rights. But if it may violate the fetus' rights, then late abortion (like infanticide) is a public act. There is, however, a morally significant difference between late abortion and infanticide. A fetus is parasitic upon a unique individual in a manner in which a newborn infant is not. That parasitic relation will justify late abortion more liberally than infanticide, for they do not occur under the same circumstances.

Since we have already explored the morality of abortion for those cases in which the fetus has moral standing, the general approach to late abortions is clear enough. Unlike the simple and uniform treatment of early abortion, only a case-by-case analysis will here suffice. We should expect a serious threat to the woman's life or health (physical or mental) to justify abortion, especially if that threat becomes apparent only late in pregnancy. We should also expect a risk of serious fetal deformity to justify abortion, again especially if that risk becomes apparent (as it usually does) only late in pregnancy. On the other hand, it should not be necessary to justify abortion on the ground that pregnancy was not consented to, since a woman will have ample opportunity to seek an abortion before the threshold stage. If a woman freely elects to continue a pregnancy past that stage, she will thereafter need a serious reason to end it.

A differential view of abortion is therefore liberal concerning early abortion and conservative (in an extended sense) concerning late abortion. The status of the borderline cases in the middle weeks of the second trimester is simply indeterminate. We cannot say of them with certainty either that the fetus has a right to life or that it does not. Therefore we also cannot say either that a liberal approach to these abortions is suitable or that a conservative treatment of them is required. What we can say is that, from the moral point of view, the earlier an abortion is performed the better. There are thus good moral reasons, as well as good prudential ones, for women not to delay their abortions....

Settling on sentience as a criterion of moral standing thus leads us to a view of the moral status of the fetus, and of the morality of abortion, which satisfies the constraints set out in Section 1. It is gradual, since it locates a threshold stage rather than a point and allows moral standing to be acquired incrementally. It is differential, since it locates the threshold state during gestation and thus distinguishes the moral status of newly conceived and full-term fetuses. It is developmental, since it grounds the acquisition of moral standing in one aspect of the normal development of the fetus. And it is moderate, since it distinguishes the moral status of early and late abortions and applies each of the established views to that range of cases for which it is appropriate.

4. AN ABORTION POLICY

A differential view of the morality of abortion leads to a differential abortion policy—one that draws a legal distinction between early and late abortions. If we work within the framework of a liberal social theory, then it is understood that the state has no right to interfere in the private transaction between a woman and her physician. No regulation of this transaction will be legitimate unless it is also legitimate for other contractual arrangements between patients and physicians. It might be quite in place for the state to require that abortions be performed by qualified (perhaps licensed) personnel in properly equipped (perhaps licensed) facilities:

whether or not this is so will depend on whether the state is in general competent to regulate trade in medical skills. Both the decision to abort and the decision to use contraceptives are private ones on which a woman ought to seek medical advice and medical assistance. There is no justification in either case for restricting access to that advice or that assistance.

An abortion policy must therefore be permissive for early abortions. There is at this stage no question of inquiring into a woman's reason for seeking an abortion. Her autonomy here is absolute; the simple desire not to have a child (or not to have one now) is sufficient. Grounds for abortion become pertinent only when we turn to late abortions. Since virtually all such abortions will result in the death of a being that has a right to life (though not all will violate that right), the state has a legitimate role to play in governing trade in abortion at this stage. Legal grounds for late abortion are a special case of conditions for justifiable homicide. As much as possible (allowing for the unique relation between mother and fetus) these grounds should authorize abortion when killing would also be justified in relevantly similar cases not involving fetuses. Two general conditions for justifiable homicide will be applicable to abortions: self-defense and euthanasia.

The usual legal grounds for abortion provided by moderate policies may be divided into four categories: (a) therapeutic (threat to maternal life or health); (b) eugenic (risk of fetal abnormality); (c) humanitarian (pregnancy due to the commission of a crime, such as rape or incest); (d) socioeconomic (poverty, family size, etc.). If a moderate treatment of late abortion is coupled (as it should be) with a permissive treatment of early ones, only the first two categories are necessary. Therapeutic grounds for abortion follow from a woman's right of self-defense. The threat, however, must be serious in two different respects: the injury in prospect must be more than trivial and the probability of its occurrence must be greater than normal. The risks generally associated with pregnancy will not here suffice. Further, there must be good medical reason not

to delay until the fetus has a better chance of survival, and every effort must be made to save the fetus' life if this is possible. Thus late abortion for therapeutic reasons ought to be reserved for genuine medical emergencies in which no other course of action would qualify as proper care of the mother. In many putatively moderate policies therapeutic grounds for abortion (especially mental health clauses) are interpreted so liberally as to cover large numbers of cases that are not by any stretch of the imagination medical emergencies. This is the standard device whereby a policy moderate in principle becomes permissive in practice. Since the policy here advanced is permissive in principle (for early abortions), a strict interpretation of the therapeutic grounds for late abortions will be mandatory.

The same strictures will apply to eugenic grounds. When there is a substantial risk of some severe anomaly (rubella, spina bifida, Tay-Sachs disease, etc.), abortion may be the best course of action for the fetus. This is not obviously the case for less severe defects (Down's syndrome, dwarfism, etc.). Again there will be no justification for an interpretation of eugenic grounds so elastic that it permits abortion whenever the child is unwanted (because, say, it is the "wrong" sex). A rough rule of thumb is that late abortion for reasons of fetal abnormality is permissible only in those cases in which euthanasia for defective newborns would also be permissible. Probability will play a different role in the two kinds of case, since prenatal diagnosis of these conditions is often less certain than postnatal. But against this reason for delay we must balance the anguish of a woman carrying a fetus who may turn out at birth to be grossly deformed. Since diagnostic techniques such as ultrasound and amniocentesis cannot be employed until the second trimester, a permissive treatment of early abortions will not eliminate the need for late abortions on eugenic grounds....

There is no need for any special notice of humanitarian grounds. It is doubtful indeed whether incest ought to be a crime, except in those cases in which someone is being exploited. In any case, any woman who has become pregnant due to incestuous intercourse will have ready access to an early abortion. If she declines this opportunity and if there is no evidence of genetic abnormality, she may not simply change her mind later. The same obviously applies to pregnancy due to rape, including statutory rape. The practical problems should be approached by providing suitable counseling.

A permissive policy for early abortions will also render socioeconomic grounds redundant. Since social constraints do not normally create an emergency for which abortion is the only solution, and since women will be able to terminate pregnancies at will in the early stages, there is no need for separate recognition of social or economic justifications for abortion.

An adequate abortion policy is thus a conjunction of a permissive policy for early abortions and a moderate policy for late abortions. The obvious remaining question is where to draw the boundary between the two classes of cases. When we are dealing with the morality of abortion, borderline fuzziness is both inevitable and tolerable. Many moral problems turn on factors that are matters of degree. Where such factors are present, we cannot avoid borderline cases whose status is unclear or indeterminate. It is a defect in a moral theory to draw sharp lines where there are none, or to treat hard cases as though they were easy. But what makes for good morals may also make for bad law. An abortion policy must be enforceable and so must divide cases as clearly as possible. A threshold stage separating early from late abortions must here give way to a cut-off point.

Since there is no threshold point in fetal development, any precise upper limit on the application of a permissive policy will be to some extent arbitrary. Clearly it must be located within the threshold period, thus sometime in the second trimester. Beyond this constraint the choice of a time limit may be made on pragmatic grounds. If a permissive policy for early abortions is to promote their autonomy, women must have time to discover that they are pregnant and to decide on a course of action. This factor will tend to push the cutoff point toward the end of the second trimester. On the other hand, earlier abortions are substantially safer and more economical of scarce medical resources than later ones. This factor will tend to pull the cutoff point toward the beginning of the second trimester. Balancing these considerations would incline one toward a time limit located sometime around the midpoint of pregnancy. But it should not be pretended that there is a unique solution to this policy problem. Differential policies may legitimately vary (within constraints) in their choice of a boundary between permissiveness and moderation....

Notes

1. I will not be defending this assessment in the present paper. For the arguments see *Abortion and Moral Theory*, chs. 2 and 3.
2. *Abortion and Moral Theory*, chs. 5 and 6.
3. The adoption of this working definition of moral standing should not be construed as a concession that rights are the appropriate category for dealing with the moral issues posed by abortion. But since both of the established views employ the rhetoric of rights, there is some point to showing how that rhetoric is equally available to a moderate view. For a generalized notion of moral standing freed from all connection with rights see *Abortion and Moral Theory*, Section 23.
4. It is unclear at present whether invertebrates are capable of feeling pain, though the discovery of endorphins (opiates manufactured by the body) even in very simple organisms suggests that they may be. If so, then we are committed to extending (some) moral standing to invertebrates as well.
5. Unless there are circumstances (such as extreme underpopulation) in which contraception would also be immoral.

Abortion in Canada

Alister Browne and Bill Sullivan

Canada is one of the few countries in the world—China is another—that has decriminalized abortion. In Canada, there are no legislative or judicial restrictions whatsoever on abortion: When, where, and under what circumstances abortions can be performed are all unregulated. In sharp contrast, abortion is generally illegal in South American and predominantly Catholic countries, as well as in African and Muslim countries. And the countries that do allow legal abortions, including most in Europe along with America, Australia, and Russia, typically permit it only up to a certain time or make it subject to circumstances such as risk to the woman.[1] In what follows we will first explain how Canada came to decriminalize abortion and then go on to assess that position from an ethical point of view.

CANADIAN LAW

Canada is a federation where the powers to make laws in various areas were divided under the British North America Act of 1867 between the provincial governments and the federal government. Under this division, the federal government has exclusive jurisdiction over criminal law in Canada, and provincial governments generally have the right to pass laws in regard to healthcare.

Until 1969, abortion was a criminal act in Canada. In that year an exception was provided by amending Section 251 of the Criminal Code to permit abortions if they were performed in an accredited or approved hospital and approved by a three-physician therapeutic abortion committee from that hospital as necessary to protect the woman's life or health. If an abortion was carried out without such approval, the woman was liable

for imprisonment for 2 years, and the person carrying it out for imprisonment for life.

A challenge to Section 251 was heard by the Supreme Court of Canada in 1988 in the case of *Regina v. Morgentaler*.[2] The majority of the judges found that section to be in violation of Section 7 of the Canadian Charter of Rights on the ground that it infringed a woman's right to "life, liberty and the security of a person." In particular, it interfered with the "security of a person" because, as the Chief Justice put it: "At the most basic physical and emotional level, every pregnant woman is told by the section that she cannot submit to a generally safe medical procedure that might be of clear benefit to her unless she meets criteria entirely unrelated to her own priorities and aspirations." To this, Madame Justice Wilson added that it interfered with a woman's right to liberty, given that it prevented her from making her own choices, as well as her right to freedom of conscience, given that the choice in question is a moral one.

The Court held that such an infringement would be acceptable if "the principles of fundamental justice" were followed. But here they were not, for those principles require that criminal defenses to crimes not be illusory or almost illusory, and in the case of abortion they were. Abortions could only be done in an "accredited or approved hospital." But many hospitals were neither, and many of those that were did not perform abortions. The Court cited the Badgely Report,[3] which found that out of 1,348 civilian hospitals in Canada in 1976, only 559 met the requirements of Section 251, and only 271 (20% of all the hospitals) had a therapeutic abortion committee.

The Court did, however, say that the state can take a legitimate interest in the fetus, and that

Browne, A. & Sullivan, B., "Abortion in Canada", *Cambridge Quarterly of Healthcare Ethics* 14 (3), pp. 287–291, © 2005 Cambridge University Press. Reproduced with permission.

protecting it would be "a perfectly valid legislative objective." But, it insisted, that is a matter for an elected Parliament, not the appointed courts, to decide. This invitation to rewrite Section 251 was accepted by the House of Commons in 1989, and after acrimonious debate, legislation was proposed that again made abortion permissible only for therapeutic reasons, but which widened the grounds to include the psychological health of the woman and only required the approval of one doctor. This passed the House of Commons by a vote of 140 to 131. Before it could become law, however, it had to pass the Senate, and the Senate—ironically, an appointed body—refused to pass it. The vote was an unprecedented tie—43 to 43—and under Senate rules, that meant defeat. The government of the day then announced that it would not introduce any further abortion legislation, a decision followed by subsequent governments.

The Supreme Court in *Morgentaler* did not rule on whether the fetus had rights. In the next decade it considered that question in regard to the Quebec Civil Code, the Quebec Charter of Human Rights and Freedoms (the Quebec Charter), the common law as it applied in the other provinces, and the criminal law of Canada.

On July 7, 1989, [Chantal] Daigle's exboyfriend, Guy Tremblay, obtained an injunction from the Quebec Supreme Court prohibiting Ms. Daigle from having an abortion on the basis that the fetus was entitled to protection under Quebec law. The decision was upheld by the Quebec Court of Appeal on July 20, and a further appeal was heard by all the members of the Supreme Court of Canada on August 8.[4] During that hearing, the Court was told that Ms. Daigle had already obtained an abortion, but given the importance of the issue, the Court nevertheless continued the hearing and at the end immediately invalidated the injunction. In addition to a unanimous finding that neither the Quebec Civil Code nor the Quebec Charter provided for fetal legal rights, the Court found that in the common law provinces there was no fetal right until birth. In referring to various Anglo-Canadian court decisions, the Court said: "These courts have consistently reached the conclusion that to enjoy rights, a fetus must be born alive." The Supreme Court of Canada further clarified what is meant by "born alive" in a subsequent case,[5] holding that to be a human being deserving of legal protection, the child had to be in a "living state" when it had "completely proceeded" out of "the body of its mother."

In all, the Supreme Court of Canada has consistently refused to ascribe rights to the fetus or to sanction interference with women in matters relating to the fetus. Parts of these judgments in the landmark abortion cases of *Morgentaler* and *Daigle* read in substance and tone like feminist tracts, as do passages of that Court's judgments on related matters. For example, the Supreme Court of Canada refused to permit forced obstetrical intervention to prevent a woman from endangering her fetus.[6] After considering the difficulties in legalizing the right to interfere with a woman's autonomy based on lifestyle choices, the Court went on to say: "The difficulties multiply when the lifestyle in question is that of a pregnant woman whose liberty is intractably and inescapably bound to her unborn child." Likewise, the Supreme Court of Canada held that children have no right to sue their mothers for injuries received during pregnancy, commenting: "The imposition by courts of tort liability on mothers for prenatal negligence would restrict a pregnant woman's activities, reduce her autonomy to make decisions concerning her health and have a negative impact upon her employment opportunities. It would have a profound effect upon every woman who is pregnant or merely contemplating pregnancy and upon Canadian society in general."[7]

ETHICAL REFLECTIONS

Canada's legal position on abortion thus originated not from any societal decision, but from the courts striking down attempts to interfere with the liberty of women. The longer Parliament does not step in and fill the legal vacuum, however, the more that position becomes societally chosen. The question is whether it is well chosen. We will now sketch why we think it is.

It is hard to deny that a woman has some kind of right to control her body. But it is not clear what kind of right that is. If it is absolute, the question of the morality of abortion is settled, and Canada has exactly the proper legal position. On the other hand, if a woman's right to control her body is only a prima facie right, the morality and consequent legality of abortion will be settled by whether there is any consideration sufficient to cancel or restrict that right.

The most natural and common place to look for such a consideration is in the rights-status of the fetus. If the fetus has a full right to life, abortion will be permissible only in those circumstances in which an innocent full-fledged human being can be killed, that is, very seldom, and a woman's right to control her body would not generally if ever prevail in such a conflict. If it has a partial right, abortions will be permissible or not, depending on the strength of that right and the reason a woman has for wanting an abortion. Can either of these views be defended?

There are only four possible positions one can hold on the rights-status of the fetus: (1) The fetus lacks a right to life up to some point in its development—what point is a matter of dispute among those who hold this view—but gains a full right at that point (the middle theory); (2) a right to life begins to phase in at some point of fetal development, starting as a weak right and growing in strength as the fetus develops (the gradualist theory); (3) the fetus has a full right to life from the point of conception onward (the conservative theory); (4) the fetus does not have any right to life at any time in its development (the liberal theory).[8]

All these theories are beset by well-known difficulties. The middle theory is faced with the problem that, because there is no sharp discontinuity anywhere in fetal development, any point at which the line is drawn will be arbitrary. The gradualist theory has the same problem of when to start ascribing a right, and also the problem of giving operational significance to the development of that right, that is, identifying at what stages what reasons are necessary and sufficient to justify abortion. Conservatives are charged with being committed to opposing contraception and celibacy, for the only thing that could make it wrong to kill the zygote is that we thereby prevent a full-fledged human being from coming into existence, and those practices do the same. And liberals are accused of having to endorse infanticide, for there is nothing that a late-term fetus lacks that a newborn infant has.[9]

These are not, of course, decisive objections to the theories against which they are directed. Indeed, they just start the complicated series of objections and replies that characterizes the debate on the status of the fetus. But that series does not end with any clear victor, and this puts those who want to decriminalize abortion in a strong position. For the absence of a satisfactory defense of fetal rights undercuts the most powerful reason one could have to cancel or restrict a woman's right to control her body, and thus those who want a restrictive abortion policy must look to second-best considerations. Two stand out. First, one can try to exploit the absence of a clear proof of the liberal theory, and argue that either the fetus has a full right to life or it does not; we just cannot say which at this time. But, given the importance of not killing innocent beings with a full right to life, we should give it the benefit of the doubt and legislate as if it had such a right, that is, as if the conservative position were true.[10] Second, one can contend that if late-term abortions are allowed, there is a danger that this will lead to an unhealthy lowering of psychological barriers against killing and respect for life generally. Thus, we should legislate as if one of the middle theories were true.[11]

But it is not obvious that the mere possibility that controversial meta-ethical and moral views about the status of the fetus are true is sufficient to justify visiting certain and substantial hardship on women. And there is no firm evidence for the alleged callous-making effects of abortions. We are thus still left without any clear reason to restrict a woman's right to control her body in the matter of abortion. Absent this, one can either draw the conclusion that there should be no legal restrictions on abortion or appeal to nonrational considerations such as a free vote in

Parliament or a public referendum to determine what restrictions should be put on it. Appeal to popular opinion, however, is very unattractive. It is repugnant, especially in a country that prides itself on freedom of religion and conscience, to let the religious or personal moral views of some, however numerous or vociferous, control the lives of others. Thus Canada's decriminalization of abortion seems exactly right.

Decriminalization, however, does not mean access, and although there is relatively good access to abortion in Canada, some nonlegal obstacles exist. Abortions in Canada are provided free of charge—like any other medically necessary service—in hospitals. But not all hospitals perform abortions, and there are often long waiting lists. Some provinces fund abortions in independent clinics. But not all do, and there are not enough clinics—especially in rural areas—to meet the demand.[12] Until these barriers to access are removed, there will remain a correctable inequality between men and women—indeed, between women—in matters of reproduction, and an iteration of the argument for decriminalizing abortion suggests they should be removed. Pro-choice groups urge they should be; pro-life groups say the opposite; and this battle is the current frontier of the abortion debate in Canada.

Notes

1. Department of Economic and Social Affairs Population Division. *Abortion Policies: A Global Review.* New York: United Nations; 2001.
2. *R. v. Morgentaler,* [1988] 1 S.C.R. 30.
3. Canada. Department of Justice. *Report of the Committee on the Operation of the Abortion Law.* Ottawa: Minister of Supply and Services Canada; 1977.
4. *Tremblay v. Daigle,* [1989] 2 S.C.R 530.
5. *R. v. Sullivan, Lemay,* [1991] 1 S.C.R 489.
6. *Winnipeg Child and Family Services (Northwest Area) v. G. (D.F.),* [1997] 3 S.C.R. 925.
7. *Dobson (Litigation Guardian of) v. Dobson,* [1999] 2 S.C.R. 753.
8. Classic papers on these positions are conveniently collected in Feinberg J, ed. *The Problem of Abortion.* Belmont, Calif.: Wadsworth; 1984.
9. A helpful review of criticisms is Glover J. *Causing Death and Saving Lives.* Harmondsworth Middlesex, England: Penguin Books, 1979;Ch. 9:119–28.
10. This view is advocated by Woods J. *Engineered Death: Abortion, Suicide, Euthanasia and Senecide.* Ottawa: University of Ottawa Press, 1978;Ch. 4, Sec. 5:57–60.
11. For a discussion, see Glover J. Matters of life and death. *New York Review of Books* 1985;32(9):19–23.
12. For other obstacles and details on these, see Arthur J. Abortion in Canada: History, law, and access. Available at: http://www.prochoiceactionnetwork-canada.org/Canada.html.

The Human Egg Trade: How Canada's Fertility Laws are Failing Donors, Doctors, and Parents

Alison Motluk

In the spring of 2006, Heather Cox got an unexpected phone call from a Toronto fertility clinic. Three years earlier, she had donated eggs anonymously to a gay couple through the clinic. Now the same couple wanted a full sibling for their child. Would she consider providing eggs again?

She hesitated. Her first experience had been extremely unpleasant. A few days after the eggs were retrieved, her abdomen had filled with fluid. "I looked nine months pregnant," she says. After fainting in the shower, she called the clinic, and they advised her to come back in to have the

From *The Walrus*, April 2010. Reprinted by permission of the author.

fluid drained. She did, but it took a full week before she felt better.

The clinic, CReATe Fertility Centre, called her during her recovery. They wanted to know if she had a telephone number for her cousin, who had also been a donor, and whom they wanted to ask to donate again. Cox couldn't help them. "Well, would *you* be interested in donating again?" she recalls them asking. She said no.

This latest request, however, felt different. There was a child out there who had resulted from her egg, and she alone could help that child have a full genetic brother or sister. "I sympathized," she says. "I only have one full-blooded sibling." She agreed to do it, but with conditions: the eggs were to be used only by this one couple, and the clinic was to take extra care so she didn't end up producing so many eggs that she got sick again. She also made it clear that this would be her last time donating.

At the time, Cox was twenty-five years old, a massage therapy student and competitive kick-boxer with strawberry blond curls and enormous green eyes. She wasn't in a relationship and hadn't had any children of her own. She had first learned about donation when her cousin had given eggs to a friend of her mother's in 2000. Her cousin had gone on to donate several more times over the years. Even her mom had donated eggs once, when a cycle of in vitro fertilization produced more than she could use.

For her first donation, Cox had requested $5,000, but this time she asked for $7,000. For one thing, she was now what's known as a "proven" donor, because a healthy child had resulted from her egg. She had also heard from her mother's friend, who had received her cousin's eggs, that $7,000 was a fair rate.

The following year, on a summer break between her course-work and her certification exam, she began injecting herself with fertility drugs in preparation for the second donation. Stimulating her ovaries to produce many more than the usual single egg per month would give the couple plenty of eggs, increasing the odds that a pregnancy would result. The first drug she took was to shut down her reproductive system; the second stimulated egg growth. She was given the final drug, the "trigger shot," about thirty-six hours before the retrieval, prompting the eggs to ripen fully.

On the morning of August 17, 2007, she went in to have the eggs retrieved. She was lightly sedated, and the physician used an ultrasound-guided aspiration needle to pierce through the vaginal wall and up into her ovary. The needle was inserted into the follicles and the contents—some fluid and, with luck, an egg—gently sucked out into a test tube. Her ovaries were extremely swollen, however, and one had come to rest below the other, blocking the needle's path, so only about half of the thirty-odd eggs that had ripened could be harvested. The procedure lasted less than half an hour. Shortly after, while she recuperated in a lounge chair in the recovery room, a staff member came by with the cheque.

The logistics of donating were much the same as they'd been years earlier. But since Cox's first retrieval, the legal landscape for egg donation in Canada had changed dramatically. A long-awaited law, the Assisted Human Reproduction Act, had come into force in April 2004, expressly outlawing the purchase of human eggs. Technically, anyone involved in such a transaction, including doctors and parents, could now be fined $500,000 and be jailed for up to ten years.

In reality, however, the law had done little to stop Canadians from buying human eggs. If anything, with women waiting longer than ever to start their families and gay men increasingly interested in having children, demand had gone up and the market had grown. The law, such as it was, simply forced the activity underground, with unintended and undesirable consequences. Fertility specialists, lacking official guidance from the government, began drawing their own boundaries. Patients had only doctors to rely on for advice. Worst of all, donors became part of a shadow economy, aware they were part of something vaguely illicit and therefore reluctant to come forward when something went wrong. The rare woman who did speak up risked being made the scapegoat of the whole under-the-table arrangement—as Heather Cox was to learn.

The Assisted Human Reproduction Act was supposed to make fertility medicine safer. In

1989, Canada convened the Royal Commission on New Reproductive Technologies, which spent four years and $28 million investigating how best to harness developments like in vitro fertilization, prenatal genetic diagnosis, and research on embryos. Its report, *Proceed with Care,* was released in November 1993. Regarding payment for eggs, the commission was unequivocal: it was "never acceptable."

The recommendation was in keeping with Canadian practices for other body products, such as blood and organs, and followed from an ethical position that offering money for a kidney or a lobe of a liver—or an egg—might persuade some people to offer them up without thinking through the consequences. The potential for exploitation, it was felt, was too great.

More than a decade went by between the royal commission report and the passing of the legislation, and the process was in some ways atypical. Usually, a law-in-progress is scrutinized by a Commons committee only after it has been fully drafted, but because reproductive technology was so controversial, then minister of health Allan Rock simply handed the Commons health committee some draft proposals and asked it to take the pulse of the nation.

Committee members heard reams of testimony and argued bitterly among themselves. Some MPs, such as committee chair Bonnie Brown, sought to protect women and couples from the industry itself. She voiced particular concern for egg donors, at one point asking a fertility doctor, "Is there any other medical procedure that you know where either males or females ingest drugs for the purpose of preparing them for an invasive procedure during which something is removed from their body for which they are paid money?" Others, such as Liberal MP Carolyn Bennett, saw parents' needs as the highest priority. Many witnesses argued that donors would not come forward unless they were compensated, and that a shortage would result. This was especially likely in egg donation, they said, which, unlike sperm donation, involved much more than a trip to a private room with a girlie magazine.

Ultimately, the law reflected the royal commission's concern, stating, "No person shall purchase, offer to purchase or advertise for the purchase of sperm or ova from a donor or a person acting on behalf of a donor."

In the years since the act was passed, however, Canada has found itself in the uncomfortable position of banning the purchase of gametes in principle but not in practice. Other countries, such as the United Kingdom, also ban their purchase but have strict enforcement provisions backing the ban. The Canadian law, by contrast, was never completed. The sections dealing with prohibited activities, like the sale of eggs, are done and in force, but certain parts, dealing with activities that are allowed but "controlled"—including the reimbursement of donor expenses—can't be proclaimed until regulations are produced setting out the details of how the system will work. Those regulations are still pending six years later.

The unproclaimed sections of the law suggest that reimbursement will only be permitted for very specific expenses and by people expressly licensed for the purpose. However, without the regulations, the various players have been left to interpret the law on their own. Some would-be parents travel to countries where eggs can be legally purchased. Of those who stay in Canada, some still employ egg donors but rely on the grey areas in the law. The $7,000 Heather Cox was paid for her second donation, for instance, was called a reimbursement for concrete expenses—even though, according to her, she negotiated the fee up front and was never asked to provide receipts.

Another option, which takes advantage of the open market for eggs in parts of the United States, has also gained favour. Instead of finding donors through Canadian clinics, many parents work with US-based agencies, which match them up with young women—mostly American but some Canadian—who fly in days before the retrieval, their ovaries already ripe with eggs. Because the money has gone through a legitimate agency ostensibly outside the jurisdiction of Canadian law, this tactic has become, for many, the preferred solution to the domestic ban.

Shortly after "Ania" and her husband got married in 1998, they discovered that he was azoospermic, producing no live sperm at all. Initially, they assumed Ania's eggs were fine, but after perhaps a dozen artificial inseminations, a miscarriage, and a failed attempt at in vitro fertilization, they realized she was infertile, too. The Toronto-area couple decided to adopt instead, and soon became parents for the first time.

Two years later, they were on track to adopt a second child when, just days before the baby was expected to be born, the arrangement fell through. They were devastated. "I thought, 'I can't go through something like that again,' " Ania says. So they began to focus on using donor eggs and sperm to conceive.

Ania started calling clinics in January 2008 and was struck by the inconsistencies she encountered. "No two were the same," she says. One clinic said it didn't have access to donor eggs. Another had clients willing to "share" their eggs in return for a reduced fee. Another told her they could connect her with a paid donor in Canada, explaining that they had been "grandfathered in" under the new law. And others advised her to arrange for donor eggs through agencies based in the United States.

She understood that these agencies were essentially a way to get around the law, but she didn't feel she was actually breaking it. "It's basically circumventing," she says. She would pay the agency, and the agency would pay the egg donor; all the money changed hands elsewhere. Egg donation itself was not illegal, only the purchase of eggs, so she understood that the donor could fly in and have the eggs extracted here without risking a violation of the ban.

Sherry Levitan, a Toronto lawyer who specializes in what's commonly referred to as third-party reproductive law, says the legality of using an out-of-country agency to help commit an act that is illegal in this country isn't quite so clear. It would ultimately come down to how a judge interpreted the transaction—whether there was a purchase and where it was deemed to have happened. But none of the clinics Ania spoke with raised this risk. "They didn't mention anything about the legality at all," she says. "They just said, 'We do it.' "

The Canadian Fertility and Andrology Society, which provides leadership in the field of reproductive medicine, insists that no Canadian clinic would knowingly work with paid donors, regardless of where they were paid. Roger Pierson, a professor at the University of Saskatchewan and spokesperson for the CFAS, says that when Canadian fertility doctors find out a donor is being paid for more than just expenses, they're obligated to cancel the cycle. "There's no clinic in the country that would do that procedure with a paid donor," he told me, adding that, unfortunately, sometimes donors and couples don't tell the truth.

That wasn't Ania's experience. She and her husband had no trouble finding clinics happy to work with paid donors. They first went through ReproMed, a Toronto clinic, which put them in touch with an agency called Our Fairy Godmother, run out of Naples, Florida, by a Canadian woman named Cathy Ruberto who had been ReproMed's clinical director for fifteen years. She had been a witness during the drafting of the AHR Act and had argued strongly that without payment there would be no donors. The year the law was passed, she left the country and set up her agency south of the border.

She found Ania and her husband a potential donor, whose eggs they were to share with another couple. According to the invoice, their portion of the cost for the donor cycle was to be $2,500 (US). "We were paying for the services," Ania explains, "not the ova themselves," pointing out that they would be charged regardless of whether any eggs resulted. Officially, the payment was called a reimbursement, but it was clearly not to cover, for example, legal fees, a psychological consultation, accidental health insurance, cycle monitoring, airfare, a hotel, a thank-you gift, meals, or even miscellaneous expenses, as each of these was itemized separately on the same bill. The invoice was for a total of $12,287.75 (US).

In the end, Ania decided not to proceed with Our Fairy Godmother, switching to another agency and another clinic. She ended up at CReATe, the same clinic where Cox had donated. The director there, Dr. Clifford Librach, had told her that CReATe would work with whomever she wanted, but that it had a long-standing working relationship with the International Assisted Reproduction Center, an agency in Maple Grove, Minnesota. He showed Ania a sample donor profile, which gave extensive details about current health, family health history, educational background, hobbies, and appearance, and even a personal message to the parents.

After a careful search, she and her husband selected a young woman who IARC said was very reliable and had flown up to Canada before. All went according to plan, and the couple welcomed a new child into their home in 2009. Both IARC and CReATe, she says, were extremely professional and compassionate. But she resents the quagmire she had to navigate, which she says only adds to the hardship already faced by infertile couples.

Edward Ryan, a fertility doctor at Toronto West Fertility Center, casts the current system as "really ridiculous," and says, "The government has forced patients to use agencies in the States so that legally we can do what we have to do." He adds that it's completely unrealistic to expect altruism alone to motivate women to inject themselves with drugs, have half a dozen vaginal ultrasounds, and undergo a medical procedure that will require time off work. Doctors have patients who want donor eggs, and they know there are women out there who are willing to donate them for compensation. But for the moment, he says, they feel they have no choice but to go ahead with the charade. "There's nothing to say that we can't use donated eggs as long as they're presumed altruistic," he says. "We presume to think that it's all being done for free, but obviously it's not. It makes it uncomfortable for us. Patients ask, 'What does it cost?' We don't know, because we don't want to know. Please—don't tell us."

Canada does have a federal agency to administer and enforce the law, funded to the tune of $10 million a year. Assisted Human Reproduction Canada (AHRC, pronounced "arc"), formally established in January 2006, is headquartered in Vancouver, with offices in Ottawa. In the absence of regulations, the organization has become a bit of a farce—an "agency set up to do nothing," in MP Carolyn Bennett's words.

The organization finds itself unable or unwilling to answer basic questions about the law. Sherry Levitan, the Toronto lawyer, recalls that at the 2008 annual meeting of the Canadian Fertility and Andrology Society, during what was supposed to be an educational session led by AHRC and Health Canada, both bodies declined to answer a direct question from Dr. Librach about whether or not receipts were necessary for reimbursement of egg donors. Representatives from the two agencies passed the question back and forth, and no one answered clearly. "They played pinball," Levitan says. She ultimately took it upon herself to offer a response, saying that at present there was no such requirement. Later in the meeting, Elinor Wilson, the president of AHRC, told Dr. Librach she'd answer "offline."

Dr. Tom Hannam, who heads the Hannam Fertility Centre in Toronto and was present at the session, laments the uncertain state of affairs. "I'm a law-abiding citizen in a respectable field," he says. "I'm many layers away from feeling that I should be threatened with going to jail." He adds that the system actually provides a disincentive for cautious doctors like himself to work with donors, potentially leaving it to others who are less wary. And the more time that goes by without regulation and enforcement, the more of a free-for-all the industry is becoming. "We are drawing lines arbitrarily, according to our own risk aversion," says Hannam. "And that line has been shifting, because people do things and nothing happens."

Wilson, for her part, denies knowledge of widespread paid egg donation in Canada. "I do not know that a lot of this is going on in the country," she told me in her Ottawa office last June. "It's anecdotal. You know, what you hear on the street." She said she simply didn't have "solid numbers about the extent" of paid egg donation or other activities; this suggests that until the exact numbers are pinned down there's nothing AHRC can do.

Solid numbers would indeed be hard to obtain. But it takes only a couple of hours and a few phone calls to establish that purchasing eggs is a common practice for Canadians undergoing fertility treatment. Ruberto, for instance, says that last year Our Fairy Godmother coordinated about 135 donations in Canada, most of them in Ontario, where there's a concentration of fertility clinics. About a third of those donors were Canadian women, she says. IARC told me that it has arranged roughly 225 Canadian-based donations over the past three years. In addition, online marketplaces such as Craigslist and Kijiji routinely feature Canadian couples looking for eggs and Canadian women proffering them. They don't mention money, but neither do they usually emphasize altruistic motives.

Then there are the donor blogs. In one, a young woman named Sonja, who lives in Washington State, chronicles in detail her six egg donations, all in Canada, between March 2007 and June 2009. The first, she told me, was at CReATe, while the rest were at the Markham Fertility Centre, north of Toronto. Interestingly, what worried her most before her first donation was not the procedure itself but the border. "Getting through immigration was a little stressful," she writes. "I was told that they would ask for my reason for coming to Canada and that I should say 'medical treatment.'" She had a letter from the clinic supporting that story, just in case, but in the end she didn't need it. Each time, she confirmed with me, she got to name her compensation, which started at $3,000 and rose to $6,000 by the end.

Canadian donors, too, are travelling around the country to provide eggs. One woman I spoke with has twice been asked to fly from Toronto to Victoria, though she turned down both offers because the compensation wasn't high enough. "I would like to say something romantic," she told me, "but it really is the money." Another woman has flown from the Maritimes to Ontario more than once to donate.

These cases may be anecdotal, as Wilson asserts, but, combined with the numbers from American agencies, they confirm that purchases are indeed taking place. And as the market has moved underground, the risks have arguably increased. In this situation, Hannam says, "donors are so vulnerable."

In the recovery room just minutes after her second donation, Heather Cox started to feel a growing ache in her abdomen. "I'm pretty tolerant of pain," she says. "In sports, you get hurt a lot." But this pain became worse than anything she'd ever experienced. When she started to squirm, one of the other two donors in the room—an American woman who'd earlier claimed she was being paid $15,000—alerted the nurse.

Medical personnel took Cox back to an ultrasound room, where she was examined by a nurse and an ultrasound technician, and later by the doctor. She was given painkillers, she recalls, and discharged. Her sister met her in a waiting room and helped her walk outside, where they waited for their grandfather, who'd been circling the block to avoid parking fees. The three drove the thirty minutes home to Oakville.

Cox managed to fall asleep that night, but the pain woke her several times, and by the next morning it was unbearable. She asked her sister to take her to the nearest hospital. There, the ER staff gave her morphine, contacted CReATe, and arranged for her to be transferred by ambulance late that night to Women's College Hospital in Toronto, just around the corner from the clinic.

Of particular concern was a complication known as ovarian hyperstimulation syndrome, a condition in which plasma seeps out of the blood vessels that have been supplying the engorged, hyperstimulated ovaries, and collects in the abdominal cavity. OHSS is essentially an inflammatory response gone awry; diagnosing it can be a challenge. Serious cases need to be monitored closely, because they can result in kidney failure, breathing difficulties, rupture of the ovary, a blood clot, even death. It's not known what percentage of donors experience the syndrome, because their young age and the high number of eggs typically retrieved puts them at increased risk, but doctors say about 1 percent of all women undergoing ovarian stimulation will suffer it.

Cox was aware of the risk: not only had she been informed of the possibility of OHSS before her donations, she had suffered from it following the first one. Though she'd made it a stipulation of her second donation that extra care be taken to prevent it from happening again, the fact that she'd experienced it once made a recurrence more likely.

The day after being admitted to Women's College, she was taken by wheelchair to CReATe, where excess fluid was once again drained from her abdomen. According to hospital records, she was retaining fluid and gaining weight—symptoms indicative of OHSS. She was discharged after four days, with a primary diagnosis of "post-retrieval pain" and mild OHSS, and although the discharge notes say that "her pain resolved over the course of her stay," the clinic sent her home with a supply of the narcotic oxycodone.

She ended up missing two weeks of work and the certification exam that would have allowed her to practise as a registered massage therapist. To top it all off, she heard from the surrogate that none of the embryos had developed properly, so no sibling was conceived. All her suffering, she felt, had been for nothing.

Her mother, Bette, had been following the whole ordeal from the United States, where she now lived with her current husband, himself a physician, and their young child. Concerned, she started making calls on Heather's behalf. She had nothing against egg donation, having done it herself, and she wasn't particularly opposed to payment. But in her view, her daughter had felt pressured to donate again after a terrible first experience. "She went through a very bad time," she says. "She really didn't want to do it again."

On January 23, 2008, Bette spoke to Beth Pieterson, then director of licensing and regulations at AHRC. Within a week, Pieterson was back in touch, joined in a conference call by Véronique Lalonde, a compliance specialist with the agency. According to an email from AHRC, which documented the conversation,

Bette informed the agency that her daughter had been paid, that the payment had been made directly through the clinic, and that Heather had provided no receipts for expenses.

AHRC passed the complaint over to the RCMP. According to records obtained through the Access to Information Act, the RCMP was already investigating the same clinic over similar allegations. Heather Cox was interviewed by an officer from the force in late April 2008. As well as answering questions in a videotaped interview, she provided them with a cheque for $7,000, made out to her by CReATe and dated the day of her retrieval. (The cheque was original but had been accidentally given to her without a signature; she had already deposited the signed replacement into her account.) The RCMP also interviewed her cousin.

But records show that in October 2008, the RCMP decided not to pursue the case at that time. In June, the Quebec Court of Appeal had ruled that parts of the AHR Act were unconstitutional because health is a provincial matter. The constitutional challenge did not affect the ban on purchasing eggs, but it did call into question the penalties. The Crown prosecutors involved in Cox's complaint felt that the case would not go forward until the Supreme Court had ruled in the matter.... [(the Supreme Court of Canada rendered its decision December 2010; a brief summary of the case is provided below; a longer summary is provided in Chapter 2.)] Legally, there was little more Bette could do.

During this process, the matter also came to the attention of the College of Physicians and Surgeons of Ontario, the body charged with disciplining Ontario doctors in cases of wrong-doing. The complaint, which is still in the initial stages of review by the CPSO, outlined what Bette felt was the poor quality of care Heather had received and the issue of payment for eggs.

Dr. Librach, head of CReATe, declined to be interviewed for this article, but he and the two doctors involved in the second donation noted in letters to the CPSO that Cox was a voluntary donor, was fully informed of the risks, and was cared for appropriately. Regarding the allegation that Cox (who now goes by Heather Parker-Doughty) had been paid, Dr. Librach wrote in a letter to the CPSO, "Let me make it clear that we did not pay Ms. Parker-Doughty to allow the Centre to stimulate her ovaries, as your letter suggests." He went on to say that they take a donor's word that her expenses are genuine, and that they are not required to, nor do they, ask for receipts. He pointed out that expenses can range from transportation, accommodation, and lost wages to nutrition and child care. "I have no knowledge or information relating to the specific expenses for which Ms. Parker-Doughty was reimbursed in 2007…Ms. Parker-Doughty signed her receipt, and I attach it to this letter."

In other words, sometimes donors don't tell the truth.

Diane Beeson, a medical sociologist at California State University, East Bay, who studies the fertility industry, points out that such complaints are rare, in part because of the chill cast by the haziness of the Canadian law. "If women have any knowledge at all that this is not above board, it makes it difficult for them to complain about medical problems," she says, citing the experiences of two Canadian women she has interviewed. And as Heather Cox's case shows, it may not be worth the effort.

Beeson is also concerned about how little follow-up is done on donors' health. "Doctors have an ongoing relationship with women who get pregnant," she says. "But these women who donate eggs, they may never see them again. Often they have no contact after they walk out the door." She notes that donors commonly report ovarian cysts, uncontrollable weight gain, and irregular periods—though she admits her sample may be biased because she is often contacted by women who have had negative experiences. The few studies that have been done, mostly on women who underwent egg retrieval for their own pregnancies, haven't turned up any clear findings, but little research has been done on young, healthy donors, some of whom go through repeated and aggressive ovarian stimulations. Two lingering concerns are premature menopause and cancer. Beeson thinks the health risks and uncertainties are not always adequately emphasized when donors sign on.

Egg donation has a coercive element, she adds, which relies on both money and social pressure. "There is a very overt manipulation of young women's emotions," she says. "Women are socialized to be caring, to take care of other people, to do good deeds. It's not unusual for former donors to get a letter from a parent saying how important it is for the baby to have a biological sibling."

Last year, Cox received yet another surprise phone call, this time from a Canadian "liaison service," which was contacting her on behalf of the couple she had donated to. Although the terms of both her donations had specified that she remain anonymous, she'd never been entirely comfortable with the arrangement. So after the second donation, she'd written a letter to the couple, included her name and contact details, and given it to the clinic to pass on. The couple had in turn forwarded the information to the liaison service, which was helping coordinate their next attempt at parenthood.

"[They] asked me if I would be willing to do it again," says Cox. "I said I didn't know, that I would have to think about it." Shortly after, a letter from the couple arrived. They told her how grateful they were for what she'd done, about how wonderful the child was, and how they just wanted one last try at a sibling. They enclosed a photo of the child, who looked just like her. The letter, and the profound gratitude it expressed, made her cry. "Up until I read it, I wasn't going to do it," she says. "The letter swayed me."

She and one of the fathers spoke on the phone. Then the liaison service got back in touch. "So, how much is this going to cost?" she recalls them asking. She found the question mildly insulting—she and the father had already decided she would only be compensated for actual expenses. But the service insisted she name a price, she says. So she asked for $10,000. Taken aback by the apparent shift, the couple began to reconsider.

When Bette found out Heather was thinking of donating again, she was upset. She called around to find her daughter a counsellor and emailed the couple, detailing all that her daughter had suffered. She urged them to meet Heather in person, which one of the men did. The two met up at a coffee shop, then drove down to Lake Ontario, where they had a heart-to-heart. They decided to cut the liaison out of the arrangement and go for a reimbursement of real expenses incurred—expected to be about $3,000, all told.

In June 2009, both Heather and Bette met the couple and their child. "It got validated, the whole experience, by meeting them and actually knowing what I helped create," Heather recalls. "I helped create a family. They're wonderful. [What] a very lucky child." Later that month, she started injecting herself with fertility drugs yet again.

The surrogate, who'd also carried the first pregnancy, had since switched clinics and was now working with ReproMed. The couple instructed the new physician, Dr. Alfonso Del Valle, to be extremely careful that Cox not be overstimulated, and made it clear that her health came first.

Just days before the retrieval was scheduled to take place, Dr. Del Valle counted the eggs in Cox's ovaries. There were too many, he told her, and they weren't maturing at the necessary rate. He decided to call off the procedure, saying the risk of another round of OHSS was too great. Cox says she would have gone ahead if it had been up to her. She's glad it wasn't.

Prenatal Genetic Testing and Screening: Constructing Needs and Reinforcing Inequities

Abby Lippman

PRENATAL DIAGNOSIS: A TECHNICAL AND A SOCIAL CONSTRUCTION

Of all applied genetic activities, prenatal diagnosis is probably most familiar to the general population and is also the most used. Prenatal diagnosis refers to all the technologies currently in use or under development to determine the physi(ologi) cal condition of a fetus before birth. Until recently, prenatal diagnosis usually meant amniocentesis,[1] a second trimester procedure routinely available for women over a certain age (usually thirty-five years in North America),[2] for Down syndrome detection. Amniocentesis is also used in selected circumstances where the identification of specific fetal genetic disorders is possible.[3] Now, in addition to amniocentesis, there are chorionic villus sampling (CVS)[4] tests that screen maternal blood samples to detect a fetus with a neural tube defect or Down syndrome, and ultrasound screening.[5] Despite pro-

fessional guidelines to the contrary,[6] ultrasound screening is performed routinely in North America on almost every pregnant woman appearing for prenatal care early enough in pregnancy. And although ultrasound is not usually labeled as "prenatal diagnosis," it not only belongs under this rubric but was, I suggest, the first form of prenatal diagnosis for which informed consent is not obtained.[7]

Expansion of prenatal diagnosis techniques, ever widening lists of identifiable conditions and susceptibilities, changes in the timing of testing and the populations in which testing is occurring, and expanding professional definitions of what should be diagnosed *in utero*, attest to this technology's role in the process of geneticization.[8] But these operational characteristics alone circumscribe only some aspects of prenatal diagnosis. Prenatal diagnosis as a social activity is becoming an element in our culture and this aspect, which has had minimal attention, will be examined in depth.

From *The American Journal of Law & Medicine*, 17. 1991. Lippman, A, "Prenatal Genetic Testing and Screen: Construction Needs and Reinforcing Inequities", pp. 15–50. Reprinted with permission.

A. Prenatal Diagnosis and the Discourse of Reassurance

Contemporary stories about prenatal diagnosis contain several themes, but these generally reflect either of two somewhat different models.[9] In the "public health" model, prenatal diagnosis is presented as a way to reduce the frequency of selected birth defects.[10] In the other, which I will call the "reproductive autonomy" model, prenatal diagnosis is presented as a means of giving women information to expand their reproductive choices.[11] Unfortunately, neither model fully captures the essence of prenatal diagnosis. In addition, neither acknowledges the internal tension, revealed in the coexistence of quite contradictory constructions of testing that may be equally valid: 1) as an assembly line approach to the products of conception, separating out those we wish to discontinue;[12] 2) as a way to give women control over their pregnancies, respecting (increasing) their autonomy to choose the kinds of children they will bear;[13] or 3) as a means of reassuring women that enhances their experience of pregnancy.[14]

The dominant theme throughout the biomedical literature, as well as some feminist commentary, emphasizes the last two of these constructions.[15] A major variation on this theme suggests, further, that through the use of prenatal diagnosis women can avoid the family distress and suffering associated with the unpredicted birth of babies with genetic disorders or congenital malformations, thus preventing disability while enhancing the experience of pregnancy.[16] Not unlike the approach used to justify caesarean sections,[17] prenatal diagnosis is constructed as a way of avoiding "disaster."

The language of control, choice, and reassurance certainly makes prenatal diagnosis appear attractive. But while this discourse may be successful as a marketing strategy,[18] it relates a limited and highly selected story about prenatal diagnosis. Notwithstanding that even the most critical would probably agree prenatal diagnosis *can be* selectively reassuring[19] (for the vast majority of women who will learn that the fetus does not have Down syndrome or some other serious diagnosable disorder), this story alone is too simplistic. It does not take account of why reassurance is sought, how risk groups are generated and how eligibility for obtaining this kind of reassurance is determined. Whatever else, prenatal diagnosis *is* a means of separating fetuses we wish to develop from those we wish to discontinue. Prenatal diagnosis does approach children as consumer objects subject to quality control.

This is implicit in the general assumption that induced abortion will follow the diagnosis of fetal abnormality.[20] This assumption is reinforced by the rapid acceptance of CVS, which allows prenatal diagnosis to be carried out earlier and earlier in pregnancy when termination of a fetus found to be "affected" is taken for granted as less problematic.[21] The generally unquestioned assumption that pre-implantation diagnosis is better than prenatal diagnosis also undermines a monotonic reassurance rhetoric.[22] With pre-implantation (embryo) diagnosis, the selection objective is clear: only those embryos thought to be "normal" will be transferred and allowed to continue to develop.[23] Thus, embryo destruction is equated with induced abortion.[24] …

B. Constructing the "Need" for Prenatal Diagnosis

While reassurance has been constructed to justify health professionals' offers of prenatal diagnosis, genetic testing and screening have also been presented in the same biomedical literature as responses to the "needs" of pregnant women. They are seen as something they "choose." What does it mean, however, to "need" prenatal diagnosis, to "choose" to be tested?[25] Once again, a closer look at what appear to be obvious terms may illuminate some otherwise hidden aspects of geneticization and the prenatal diagnosis stories told in its voice.

We must first identify the concept of need as itself a problem and acknowledge that needs do not have intrinsic reality. Rather, needs are socially constructed and culture bound, grounded in current history, dependent on context, and, therefore, not universal.

With respect to prenatal diagnosis, "need" seems to have been conceptualized predominantly in terms of changes in capabilities for fetal diagnoses: women only come to "need" prenatal diagnosis after the test for some disorder has been developed. Moreover, the disorders to be sought are chosen exclusively by geneticists.[26] In addition, posing a "need" for testing to reduce the probability a woman will give birth to a child with some detectable characteristic rests on assumptions about the value of information, about which characteristics are or are not of value, and about which risks should or should not be taken. These assumptions reflect almost exclusively a white, middle-class perspective.[27]

This conceptualization of need is propelled by several features of contemporary childbearing.[28] First, given North American culture, where major responsibility for family health care in general, for the fetus she carries and for the child she births, is still allocated to a woman,[29] it is generally assumed that she must do all that is recommended or available to foster her child's health. At its extreme, this represents the pregnant woman as obligated to produce a healthy child. Prenatal diagnosis, as it is usually presented, falls into this category of behaviors recommended to pregnant women who would exercise their responsibilities as caregivers.[30] Consequently, to the extent that she is expected generally to do everything possible for the fetus/child, a woman may come to "need" prenatal diagnosis, and take testing for granted. Moreover, since an expert usually offers testing, and careseekers are habituated to follow through with tests ordered by physicians,[31] it is hardly surprising that they will perceive a need to be tested.[32] With prenatal diagnosis presented as a "way to avoid birth defects," to refuse testing, or perceive no need for it, becomes more difficult than to proceed with it.[33] This technology perversely creates a burden of not doing enough, a burden incurred when the technology is *not* used.[34]

A second feature, related to the first, is that women generally, and pregnant women specifically, are bombarded with behavioral directives[35] that are at least as likely to foster a sense of incompetence as to nourish a feeling of control.[36] ...

Third, prenatal diagnosis will necessarily be perceived as a "need" in a context, such as ours, that automatically labels pregnant women thirty-five years and over a "high risk" group.[37] ...

Fourth, as prenatal diagnosis becomes more and more routine for women thirty-five years and older in North America, the risks it seems to avoid (the birth of a child with Down syndrome) appear to be more ominous,[38] although the frequency of Down syndrome has not changed....

Fifth, on the collective level, prenatal diagnosis is generally presented as a response to the public health "need" to reduce unacceptably high levels of perinatal mortality and morbidity associated with perceived increases in "genetic" disorders. This reduction is of a special kind, in that prenatal diagnosis does not *prevent* the disease, as is usually claimed.[39] ...

"Needs" for prenatal diagnosis are being created simultaneously with refinements and extensions of testing techniques themselves.[40] In popular discourse—and with geneticists generally silent witnesses—genetic variations are being increasingly defined not just as problems, but, I suggest, as problems for which there is, or will be, a medical/technical solution. With but slight slippage these "problems" come to be seen as *requiring* a medical solution. This again hides the extent to which even "genetic" disease is a social/psychological experience as much as it is a biomedical one.[41] This process is likely to accelerate as gene mapping enlarges the numbers of individuals declared eligible for genetic testing and screening. Given the extent of human variation, the possibilities for constructing "needs" are enormous.

C. Prenatal Diagnosis and the Social Control of Abortion and Pregnancy

The third element in the prenatal discourse that I will consider here stems from the often told story that testing is an option that increases women's reproductive choices and control. This claim has had much attention in the literature and I will examine it only with respect to how some features of prenatal diagnosis do increase control, but allocate it to someone other than a pregnant woman herself. This is most apparent in the context of abortion.[42]

Without doubt, prenatal diagnosis has (re)defined the grounds for abortion[43]—who is justified in having a pregnancy terminated and why—and is a clear expression of the social control[44] inherent in this most powerful example of geneticization. Geneticists and their obstetrician colleagues are deciding which fetuses are healthy, what healthy means, and who should be born, thus gaining power over decisions to continue or terminate pregnancies that pregnant women themselves may not always be permitted to make.

To the extent that specialists' knowledge determines who uses prenatal diagnosis and for what reasons, geneticists determine conditions that will be marginalized, objects of treatment, or grounds for abortion.[45] Prenatal diagnosis is thus revealed as a biopolitical as well as a biomedical activity.[46] For example, an abortion may only be "legal" in some countries if the fetus has some recognized disorder,[47] and the justifying disorder only becomes "recognizable" because geneticists first decide to screen for it. Fuhrmann suggests that in Europe, in fact, geneticists significantly influenced legislators establishing limits within which abortion would be at all permissible, by arguing that access to abortion be maintained through a gestational age that reflected when results from amniocentesis might be available.[48] One wonders where limits might have been placed had first trimester chorionic villus sampling been available *before* amniocentesis? Would they have been more restrictive?...

V. CONCLUSION

... Prenatal testing and screening ... are most often presented as ways to decrease disease, to spare families the pain of having a disabled child, and to enhance women's choice. The best-selling stories about them speak of reassurance, choice, and control. As has also been suggested,

this discourse presents a child born with some disorder requiring medical or surgical care as (exhibiting) a "failure."[49] This failed pregnancy theme is reinforced in counseling provided to these families when counselors emphasize how most fetuses with an abnormality abort spontaneously during pregnancy, are "naturally selected," as it were, and how prenatal testing is merely an improvement on nature.

Just as there are several ways to construe reassurance, choice, and control, the birth of a child with a structural malformation or other problem, "genetic" or otherwise, can be presented in other than biomedical terms. Is the story claiming that the pregnancy has malfunctioned (by not spontaneously aborting),[50] resulting in a baby with a malformation, any "truer" than the story suggesting that *society* has malfunctioned because it cannot accommodate the disabled in its midst?[51] Social conditions are as enabling or disabling as biological conditions. Why are biological variations that create differences between individuals seen as preventable or avoidable while social conditions that create similar distinctions are likely to be perceived as intractable givens?[52]

While "many people don't believe society has an obligation to adjust to the disabled individual,"[53] there is nothing inherent in malformation that makes this so. Consequently, arguing that social changes are "needed" to enable those with malformations to have rich lives is not an inherently less appropriate approach. Actually, it may be more appropriate, since malformation, a biomedical phenomenon, requires a social translation to become a "problem." Expanding prenatal diagnostic services may circumvent but will not solve the "problem" of birth defects; they focus on disability, not on society's discriminatory practices.[54] They can, at best, make only a limited contribution to help women have offspring free of disabilities, despite recent articles proposing prenatal diagnosis and abortion as ways to "improve" infant mortality and morbidity statistics.[55] Thus, as sociopolitical decisions about the place of genetic testing and screening in the health care system are made, it will be important to consider how problems are named and constructed so that we don't mistakenly assume the story told in the loudest voice is the only one—or that the "best seller" is best.

Unarguably, illness and disability *are* "hard" (difficult) issues,[56] and no one wants to add to the unnecessary suffering of any individual. But being "hard" neither makes illness or disability totally negative experiences,[57] nor does it mean they must all be eliminated or otherwise managed exclusively within the medical system. Women's desire for children without disability warrants complete public and private support. The question is how to provide this support in a way that does no harm....

When amniocentesis was introduced, abortion subsequent to a diagnosis of fetal abnormality was presented as a temporary necessity until treatment for the detected condition could be devised.[58] Advocates assumed that this would soon be forthcoming. With time, however, the gap between characterization and treatment of disease has widened.[59] New information from efforts at gene mapping will certainly increase the ability to detect, diagnose, and screen, but not to treat. A human gene map will identify variations in DNA patterns. Genes that "cause" specific disease, as well as those associated with increased susceptibility to specific disorders, will be found. Simultaneously, prenatal screening and testing are evolving in a context where a "genetic approach" to public health is gaining great favor.[60] All the variations that will be mapped can become targets of prenatal testing. Which targets will be selected in the quest for improved public health? And who will determine that they have been reached? Given the extraordinary degree of genetic variability within groups of people, what does "genetic health" actually mean—and does it matter?...

Notes

1. In amniocentesis, a hollow needle is inserted through a woman's abdomen and into the amniotic sac in order to remove a small sample of the fluid that surrounds the developing fetus. The procedure is usually preceded by an ultrasound examination to document the age of the fetus and its location so that an appropriate site for insertion of the amniocentesis needle can be chosen. The fluid that is removed—amniotic fluid—contains cells from the fetus that, if allowed to divide in the laboratory, can then be analyzed. In particular, one can count the number of chromosomes in the cells, determine fetal sex and carry out biochemical and specific genetic analyses on these cells. Amniocentesis is performed at about sixteen to twenty weeks' gestation, the second trimester of pregnancy: before this time not enough fluid or enough cells are available. Once a fluid sample has been obtained, there is a further three to four week wait for the analyses to be completed and results to be available, since it takes this long to grow a sufficient number of cells for study. Thus, if a fetus is found to be affected with the condition for which testing was done and the woman chooses to abort the pregnancy, the abortion is not induced until about the twentieth week, which is halfway through the pregnancy. *See* E. Nightingale & M. Goodman, Before Birth: Prenatal Testing for Genetic Disease 32–35 (1990) [hereinafter Before Birth]. R$_e$cent technical developments that allow diagnoses to be made following amplification of the genetic materials in a single cell can shorten considerably the time needed to obtain results. *See infra* note 4 and accompanying text.

2. *See infra* note 37 and accompanying text for a discussion of the social, rather than biological, bases for categorizing women over 35 as "at risk."

3. Over 150 "single gene" disorders can now be detected, and testing may be carried out for women who have a documented family history of one of these or who are otherwise known to be at increased risk. Testing is not carried out for these disorders without specific indications. *See generally* Antonarakis, *Diagnosis of Genetic Disorders at the DNA Level*, 320 New Eng. J. Med. 153 (1989) (reviewing recent progress in identifying single gene disorders).

4. In chorionic villus sampling (CVS), a small tube (catheter) is inserted through the vagina and cervix. It is then advanced, under ultrasound guidance, until it reaches the placenta, from which a small amount of tissue (chorionic villi) is removed. Some obstetricians now obtain a sample through a needle inserted into the abdomen instead. Any chromosomal or biochemical disorder can, in theory, be diagnosed with tissues obtained by CVS, because the cells of the fetus and placenta (which are formed from chorionic villi) are genetically the

same. *See* Vekemans & Perry, *Cytogenic Analysis of Chorionic Villi: A Technical Assessment*, 72 HUM. GENETICS 307 (1986). This procedure was first used successfully in China as early as 1975 to determine fetal sex. Tietung Hosp. Dep't of Obstetrics & Gynecology, *Fetal Sex Prediction by Sex Chromatin of Chorionic Villi Cells During Early Pregnancy*, 1 CHINESE MED. J. 117 (1975). CVS can be done as early as eight or nine weeks after a woman's last menstrual period and, while the results of tests carried out on the placental tissue can be available within hours, a two or three day waiting period is usually required. *See* BEFORE BIRTH, *supra* note 1, at 35–36. If a woman chooses to abort the pregnancy following CVS, the abortion can be carried out in the first trimester. Finally, CVS does not appear more likely to cause a spontaneous abortion than amniocentesis. Canadian Collaborative CVS – Amniocentesis Clinical Trial Group. *Multicentre Randomised Clinical Trial of Chorion Villus Sampling and Amniocentesis*, 1 LANCET 1, 4 (1989).

5. During an ultrasound examination, high frequency sound waves are projected into the uterus; the sound waves that are reflected back are resolved visually to allow one to "see" the fetus on a television-like display screen. A. Oakley, THE CAPTURED WOMB: A HISTORY OF THE MEDICAL CARE OF PREGNANT WOMEN 155–68 (1984).

6. See BEFORE BIRTH, *supra* note 1, at 31–32. A consensus development conference in the United States recently recommended reserving the use of ultrasound for pregnancies that may require it for specific medical reasons. PUB. HEALTH SERV., U.S. DEP'T OF HEALTH & HUM. SERVS., CONSENSUS DEVELOPMENT CONFERENCE: DIAGNOSTIC ULTRASOUND IMAGING IN PREGNANCY 11 (National Inst. Of Health Publications No. 667, 1984). This recommendation is clearly not being followed and, at present, in many major North American teaching hospitals, almost all pregnant women are referred for two "routine" ultrasound examinations—one before the twentieth week and one in the third trimester—for purposes of dating the pregnancy, even though the benefits of such a policy have not been established. Even more frequent scans are considered routine in France. As a specific tool for prenatal diagnosis, ultrasound can be used to identify certain malformations such as neural tube defects, cleft lip, or limb shortening in fetuses known to be at risk for one of the abnormalities. It can also be used to identify fetal sex. Most subtle malformations will not be identified when ultrasound is applied

routinely on a non-diagnostic basis, however; the detailed examination that would be necessary requires more than the time that is usually allowed (or the machinery that is employed) when the primary goal is pregnancy dating. Nevertheless, some fetal problems can be diagnosed and their recognition may influence subsequent decisions about how pregnancy is managed.

7. *See* Chervenak, McCullough & Chervenak, *Prenatal Informed Consent for Somogram.* 161 AM. J. OBSTETRICS & GYNECOLOGY 857, 860 (1989); Lippman, *Access to Prenatal Screening: Who Decides?* 1 CANADIAN J. WOMEN L. 434 (1986) [hereinafter *Who Decides?*]. Chervenak and colleagues have recently called attention to the issue of informed consent for ultrasound, but their conclusions are troublesome. They consider the pregnant woman "the patient's fiduciary," the "patient" to them being the fetus. Chervenak, McCullough & Chervenak, *supra*, at 858. This suggests that the consent process they propose will be coercive. It is also worth noting that ultrasound is no longer the only genetic technology applied without prior consent. Screening for carriers of hemoglobin disorders, for example, is also done unbeknownst to the individuals being tested in certain jurisdictions. *See* Rowley, Loader, Sutera & Walden, *Do Pregnant Women Benefit from Hemoglobinopathy Carrier Detection?* 565 ANNALS N.Y. ACADEMY SCIENCES 152, 153 (1989) [hereinafter Rowley]. These authors noted that consent for sickle cell and other hemoglobinopathies was not obtained because: "Consent for screening was not routinely sought; providers agreed that obtaining timely informed consent required counseling approaching that to be provided to identified carriers and many providers declined to participate if they had to obtain it." Rowley, *supra,* at 153.

8. *See generally Who Decides?*, *supra* note 7, at 434.

9. *Id.*

10. *See, e.g.,* Kolker, *Advances in Prenatal Diagnosis: Social-psychological and Policy Issues,* 5 INT'L J. TECH. ASSESSMENT HEALTH CARE 601 (1989); see also Dalgaard & Norby, *Autosomal Dominant Polycystic Kidney Disease in the 1980s,* 36 CLINICAL GENETICS 320, 324 (1989) (placing importance on "selective reproduction prevention").

11. *See* PRESIDENT'S COMM'N FOR THE STUDY OF ETHICAL PROBLEMS IN MEDICAL AND BIOMEDICAL AND BEHAVIORAL RESEARCH, SCREENING AND COUNSELING FOR GENETIC CONDITIONS: THE ETHICAL, SOCIAL, AND LEGAL IMPLICATIONS OF GENETIC SCREENING, COUNSELING, AND EDUCATION PROGRAMS 55 (1983)

[hereinafter PRESIDENT'S COMM'N]. ("In sum, the fundamental value of genetic screening and counseling is their ability to enhance the opportunities for the individual to obtain information about their personal health and childbearing risks and to make autonomous and noncoerced choices based on that information.")

12. *See* B. Rothman, RECREATING MOTHERHOOD: IDEOLOGY AND TECHNOLOGY IN A PATRIARCHAL SOCIETY 21 (1989) (describing the "commodification of life, towards treating people and parts of people … as commodities…. We work hard, some of us, at making the perfect product, what one of the doctors in the childbirth movement calls a 'blue ribbon baby.' "). *See also* Ewing, *Australian Perspectives on Embryo Experimentation: An Update,* 3 ISSUES REPRODUCTIVE & GENETIC ENGINEERING 119 (1990); Rothman, *The Decision to Have or Not to Have Amniocentesis for Prenatal Diagnosis,* in CHILDBIRTH IN AMERICA: ANTHROPOLOGICAL PERSPECTIVES 92, 92–98 (K. Michelson Ed. 1998) [hereinafter CHILDBIRTH IN AMERICA].

13. See Hill, *Your Morality or Mine? An Inquiry into the Ethics of Human Reproduction,* 154 AM. J. OBSTETRICS & GYNECOLOGY 1173, 1178–80 (1986).

14. *See generally* Royal College of Physicians of London, PRENATAL DIAGNOSIS AND GENETIC SCREENING: COMMUNITY AND SERVICE IMPLICATIONS (1989).

15. *See, e.g.,* WOMEN'S RIGHTS LITIGATION CLINIC, REPRODUCTIVE LAWS FOR THE 1990S: A BRIEFING HANDBOOK (1987); *Who Decides?, supra* note 7, at 438.

16. McDonough, *Congenital Disability and Medical Research: The Development of Amniocentesis,* 16 WOMEN & HEALTH 137, 143–44 (1990). McDonough notes that three rationales for amniocentesis emerged from her survey: "The procedure offered those at risk the possibility of 'health' … [it] provided parents with reassurance and avoided abortion… [and it] prevent[ed] disease and disability." *Id.*

17. *See e.g.,* McClain, *Perceived Risk and Choice of Childbirth Service,* 17 SOC. SCI. & MED. 1857, 1862 (1983).

18. There is no evidence that control, autonomy, and reassurance are actually enhanced and not merely assumed to occur. In fact, there have been very few in-depth studies in this area, and the conclusions of these investigations seem to vary with the orientation of the investigator. Studies reported in the social science and feminist literature suggest that prenatal diagnosis removes control; studies reported in the biomedical literature are interpreted to show how reassurance is provided. For an

overview of these studies, see Lippman, *Research Studies in Applied Human Genetics: A Quantitative Analysis and Critical Review (Biomedical) Literature,* to be published in AM. J. MED. GENETICS (1991). Much more ethnographic work in this area is required.

19. *See infra* text accompanying notes 48–51 [in original] for a reconstruction of the notion of reassurance.

20. *See supra* notes 12–13 and accompanying text.

21. This issue is discussed in A. Lippman, Led Astray by Genetic Maps (speech given, Ottawa, Canada, 1991). Treatment, often said to be a goal of early identification of affected fetuses, becomes even less likely with CVS. Pharmaceutical companies will not be motivated to invest in developing treatments for conditions that "need not occur." Rarely will they base business decisions on their social worth rather than on their financial value. This situation contains elements of an unusual conflict. Increasingly, geneticists are promising to have treatments available for a wide range of disorders and, for some conditions, therapeutic developments have occurred which make them far more benign than previously. The promises, and the available examples, are likely to be sufficiently persuasive that women "at-risk" may either make use of prenatal diagnosis less frequently or see less reason to abort an affected fetus than today. Yet, at the same time, the very availability of prenatal diagnosis and abortion may be seen as justifications for *not* investing in the further development of these therapies that parents will have been led to expect. *Cf.* Varekamp, Suurmeijer, Bröcker-Vriends, Van Dijck, Smit, Rosendaal & Briët, *Carrier Testing and Prenatal Diagnosis for Hemophilia: Experiences and Attitudes of 549 Potential and Obligate Carriers,* 37 AM. J. MED. GENETICS 147, 153 (1990) [hereinafter Varekamp] (noting decrease in hemophilia screening as treatment capabilities increased).

22. *See* Bell, *Prenatal Diagnosis: Current Status and Future Trends*, in HUMAN GENETIC INFORMATION: SCIENCE, LAW & ETHICS 1836 (Ciba Foundation Series 1990). *See also* Kolker, *supra* note 10, at 612 (prevention is "clearly cheaper than providing services for those with genetic disorders"); Modell, *Cystic Fibrosis Screening and Community Genetics,* 27 J. MED. GEN. 475, 476 (1990) ("undesirable [diseases] may be all but eradicated"); Dalgaard & Norby, *supra* note 10, at 323–24 ("access to selective reproductive prevention" is important).

23. S. Wymelenberg, Science and Babies: Private Decisions, Public Dilemmas 130 (1990).

24. In fact, some consider the combined procedures of *in vitro* fertilization and embryo diagnosis to be "ethically better" than prenatal diagnosis for detecting problems because it "avoids" abortion. *See* Michael & Buckle, *Screening for Genetic Disorders: Therapeutic Abortion and IVF*, 16 J. Med. Ethics 43 (1990). *But see* J. Testart, Le Monde Diplomatique 24 (1990) (suggesting that it is the very need to consider abortion ["de terribles responsabilités"] that is perhaps the best safeguard against ordinary eugenics ["l'eugenisme ordinaire"]).

25. While those in need are identified explicitly as (certain) pregnant women, it is worth noting that clinical geneticists, themselves, have a need for this technology, too. For instance, when a child is born with a malformation, geneticists likely feel most "helpful" when prenatal diagnosis, a technological palliative for the pains of etiologic ignorance, can be offered. Saying that the malformation is not likely to happen again, given the usually low empiric recurrence risks associated with most of these problems, is not nearly as comforting for genetic counselors as is offering *in utero* detection. Counselors "need" this technique for the satisfactory performance of their jobs no less than they believe a family "needs" prenatal diagnosis to prevent the birth of a second affected child.

26. *See* Lippman, *Prenatal Diagnosis: Reproductive Choice? Reproductive Control?* [hereinafter *Reproductive Choice?*], in The Future of Human Reproduction 182, 187 (C. Overall ed. 1989) [hereinafter The Future of Human Reproduction] (consideration of prenatal diagnosis as a professional resource).

27. *See* Nsiah-Jefferson, *Reproductive Laws, Women of Color and Low Income Women* in Reproductive Laws for the 1990s 17, 17–58 (S. Cohen & N. Taub eds. 1988) [hereinafter Reproductive Laws for the 1990s] (discussing potential areas of cultural conflict in genetic counseling).

28. There is an extensive literature on "medicalization" in general and on the medicalization of pregnancy and childbirth *per se* in which this discussion is rooted and from which it derives guidance. *See, e.g.,* A. Oakley, *supra* note 5, at 275. ("The medicalization of everyday life is a phenomenon described in many radical and liberal critiques of medicine."); *id* at 276 ("For both birth and death normal signs have become neon lights flagging risks which demand and validate medical intervention."); Raymond, *Feminist Ethics, Ecology, and Vision*, in Test-Tube Women 427, 427–37 (R. Arditti, R. Klein & S. Minden eds. 1984) [hereinafter Test-Tube Women]; I. Zola, *Healthism and Disabling Medicalization*, in I. Illich, I. Zola, J. McKnight, J. Caplan & H. Shaiken, Disabling Professions 41 (1977); Zola, *In the Name of Health and Illness: On Some Socio-Political Consequences of Medical Influence*, 9 Soc. Sci. & Med. 83, 85–87 (1975) (noting that control by medical value not achieved through political means but by "medicalization"); Zola, *Medicine as an Institution of Social Control*, 20 Sociology Rev. 487 (1972); *see also* Lewin, *By Design: Reproductive Strategies and the Meaning of Motherhood*, in Sexual Politics or Reproduction 123, 123–38 (H. Homans ed. 1985) [hereinafter The Sexual Politics of Reproduction] (women "must adapt" to "motherhood" but can also approach it as "active strategists").

29. See Oakley, *Smoking in Pregnancy: Smokescreen or Risk Factor? Towards a Materialist Analysis*, 11 Sociology Health & Illness 311 (1989).

30. See Farrant, *supra* note 50 [in original], at 96; Oakley *supra* note 29, at 311.

31. *See* R. Hatcher & H. Thompson, Satisfaction with Obstetrical Care Among Canadian Women (Health Servs. Res. Unit, Department of Community Health, Queen's Univ., Kingston, Ontario 1987) (results of a survey showing pregnant women's reluctance to question medical authority).

32. *See* Lippman, *supra* note 26, at 182. Physicians may pressure women into being tested, even using false information to do so. Marteau, Kidd, Cook, Michie, Johnston, Slack & Shaw, *Perceived Risk not Actual Risk Predicts Uptake of Amniocentesis*, 96 Brit. J. Obstetrics & Gynaecology 739 (1989).

33. See Hubbard & Henifin, *Genetic Screening of Prospective Parents and of Workers: Some Scientific and Social Issues*, 15 Int'l. J. Health Servs. 231 (1985); Rothman, *The Meaning of Choice in Reproductive Technology*, in Test-Tube Women, *supra* note 28, at 23. I have previously discussed the "burden" of decisionmaking in the context of genetic counseling and a similar "burden" would seem to exist here. See Lippman-Hand & Fraser, *Genetic Counseling I: Parents' Perceptions of Uncertainty*, 4 Am. J. Med. Genetics 51, 5863 (1979) [hereinafter *Genetic Counseling I*]; Lippman-Hand & Fraser, *Genetic Counseling II: Making Reproductive Choices*, 4 Am. J. Med. Genetics 73 (1978) [hereinafter *Genetic Counseling II*]. This theme is present in contemporary literature as demonstrated by Goldstein's reference to the "momentous decision"

that childbearing now involves. R. Goldstein, THE MIND-BODY PROBLEM 200 (1983). Hubbard and Henifin, in fact, identify a "new Catch-22" wherein participating in a genetic screening program may lead to a person's being identified as a "genetic deviant," but failure to participate (or to abort a fetus diagnosed with a disorder *in utero*) may lead to her being labeled as a "social deviant." Hubbard & Henifin, *supra.* At 231–48.

34. The degree of this burden is demonstrated by the frequency with which women queried about their reasons for having prenatal diagnosis say that they "had no choice." Sjögren & Uddenberg, *Decision Making During the Prenatal Procedure,* 8 PRENATAL DIAGNOSIS 263 (1988). *See* Kirejczyk, *A Question of Meaning? Controversies About the NRT's in the Netherlands,* 3 ISSUES REPRODUCTIVE & GENETIC ENGINEERING 23 (1990) (individuals often accept a medical technique because of fear that they might later regret not having done so); *see also* A. Finger, PAST DUE: A STORY OF DISABILITY, PREGNANCY AND BIRTH (1990); Beck-Gernsheim, *From the Pill to Test-Tube Babies: New Options, New Pressures in Reproductive Behavior,* in HEALING TECHNOLOGY: FEMINIST PERSPECTIVES 23 (1988) [hereinafter HEALING TECHNOLOGY]; Rapp, *Moral Pioneers: Women, Men and Fetuses in a Frontier of Reproductive Technology,* 13 WOMEN & HEALTH 101 (1987).

35. B. Rothman, *supra* note 12, at 92–97. Women are expected to behave in accordance with norms set up by those in power. *See* Rodgers, *Pregnancy as Justifications for Loss of Judicial Autonomy,* in THE FUTURE OF HUMAN REPRODUCTION, *supra* note 26, at 174.

36. *See e.g.,* Fleischer, *Ready for Any Sacrifice? Women in IVF Programmes,* 3 ISSUES REPRODUCTIVE & GENETIC ENGINEERING 1 (1990) (referring to a "code of good conduct" pregnant women ought to follow); *see also* M. De Koninck & F. Saillant, ESSAI SUR LA SANTÉ DES FEMMES (Conseil du Statut de la femme 1981); A. Quéniart, LE CORPS PARADOXAL: REGARDS DE FEMMES SUR LA MATERNITÉ (1988); Simkin, *Childbearing in Social Context,* 15 WOMEN & HEALTH 5 (1989) (all discussing the ideology of risk and behavioral expectations in pregnancy).

37. *See* Fuhrmann, *Impact, Logistics and Prospects of Traditional Prenatal Diagnosis,* 36 CLINICAL GENETICS 378, 380 (1988). This categorization is more a cultural than biological creation. *See* Bourret, *Le temps, l'espace en Génétique: Intervention Médicale et Géographique Sociale du gène,* 6 SCIENCES SOCIALES ET SANTÉ 171 (1988);

A. Lippman, The Geneticization of Health and Illness: Implications for Social Practice (manuscript in preparation based on presentation at National Ass'n for Science, Tech. & Soc'y, Washington, D.C., Feb. 2, 1991). It reflects prevailing ideas about the kinds of children women should have and when the probability for them is or is not diminished. *See* Finkelstein, *Biomedicine and Technocratic Power,* HASTINGS CENTER REP. 1990, at 13, 14–16; *see also infra* note 43 for a discussion of the role of genetics in creating these ideas. Age has thus become more than an event, a birthday; it has been redefined as a marker, a risk, although nothing inherent in it makes it so. *See* Fuhrmann, *supra.* at 380 (35 is the crucial age in North America); J. Moatti, J. Lanoë, C. LeGalés, H. Gardent, C. Julian & S. Aymé, Economic Assessment of Prenatal Diagnosis in France (unpublished manuscript presented at Joint Meeting of European Health Economic Societies, Barcelona, Spain. Sept. 21–23, 1989) (age 38 in France); Sjögren & Uddenberg, *supra* note 34, at 263 (age 37 in Sweden). This age marker may even serve to stigmatize the "older" woman. *See* Hubbard & Henifin, *supra* note 33, at 238 (1985). Further discussion of the arbitrariness of age 35 as a criterion for access to prenatal diagnosis can be found in *Who Decides?, supra* note 7, at 434; Vekemans & Lippman, *Letter to the Editor: Eligibility Criteria for Anmiocentesis,* 17 AM. J. MED. GENETICS 531 (1986).

38. This may be an example of what Tversky and Kahnemann have called the "availability" heuristic. Tversky & Kahneman, *Availability: A Heuristic for Judging Frequency and Probability,* 5 COGNITIVE PSYCHOLOGY 207 (1973). That is, having become familiar through constant reference to it and to prenatal diagnosis, Down syndrome may be perceived by the general population as "worse" and as more frequent than it is statistically.

39. *See, e.g.* Modell, *Cystic Fibrosis Screening and Community Genetics,* 27 J. MED. GENETICS 475 ("Cystic fibrosis … is fast becoming preventable … [because] [t]he gene in which mutation can lead to CF … has recently been identified.… [This creates] an imminent need to set up population screening for CF carriers.").

40. These techniques are likely to be driven by financial considerations of the pharmaceutical companies developing them. *See, e.g.,* D. Nelkin & L. Tancredi, DANGEROUS DIAGNOSTICS: THE SOCIAL POWER OF BIOLOGICAL INFORMATION 33–36 (1989); A. Lippman, *supra* note 21; *cf.* Note, *Patents for Critical Pharmaceuticals: The AZT Case,* 17 AM. J.L. & MED. 145 (1991) (analyzing the validity of

pharmaceutical companies' claims that without a federally granted monopoly, they would not have the incentive to research and develop orphan drugs).

41. *See* Shiloh, Waisbren & Levy, *A Psychosocial Model of a Medical Problem: Maternal PKU,* 10 J. Primary Prevention 51 (1989).

42. For thorough analyses of the question of women's control, see generally Rapp, *Chromosomes and Communication: The Discourse of Genetic Counseling.* 2 Med. Anthropology Q. 143 (1988).

43. In fact, the availability of amniocentesis "influenced legislation so that the upper limit of gestational age for legally tolerated termination of pregnancy was adjusted to the requirements of second trimester prenatal diagnosis in several countries." Fuhrmann, *supra* note 37, at 378. Evidently, geneticists can accomplish what women's groups cannot: a revisioning of abortion.

44. The term "social control" is used in accord with its original use to embrace "the widest range of influence and regulation imposed by society upon the individual." D. Gordon, *Clinical Science and Clinical Expertise: Changing Boundaries Between Art and Science in Medicine*, in Biomedicine Examined 257 (M. Lock & D. Gordon eds. 1988).

45. *Reproductive Choice? supra* note 26, at 187–192.

46. Finkelstein, *Biomedicine and Technocratic Power,* Hastings Center Rep. 1990, at 14–16.

47. Fetal abnormality as grounds for abortion is of fairly recent vintage, having first become "legal" in the United States in 1967 in response to a rubella epidemic. The Canadian Medical Association gave its approval the same year. Beck, *Eugenic Abortion: An Ethical Critique*, 143 Canadian Med. Ass'n J. 181, 181–84 (1990). Today, members of the general population as well as physicians regularly and strongly agree that fetal abnormality is a justification for abortion. *See* Annas, *The Supreme Court, Privacy and Abortion*, 321 New Eng. J. Med. 1200 (1989); Breslau, *Abortion of Defective Fetuses: Attitudes of Mothers of Congenitally Impaired Children,* 49 J. Marriage Family 839 (1987); Varekamp, *supra* note 21, at 147.

48. *See* Fuhrmann, *supra* note 37, at 383–84. A recent example of the use of genetics to set social policy in this area is the position taken by the American Society of Human Genetics with respect to possible restrictions on abortion under consideration in various parts of the United States. This professional group has proposed as model legislation that any pregnant female whose pregnancy has not reached the point of viability and who has been informed by a licensed or certified health care professional that her fetus (or fetuses) is/are likely to have a serious genetic or congenital disorder shall have the right, among other options, to choose to terminate her pregnancy. This right shall extend to situations where the female is at significantly increased risk for bearing a child with a serious disorder for which precise prenatal diagnosis is not available. Letter from Phillip J. Riley to the author. The merits for/against this position aside, it certainly demonstrates how geneticists seek to influence the resolution of fundamentally political, legal (and ethical) problems.

49. Dunstan, *Screening for Fetal and Genetic Abnormality: Social and Ethical Issues,* 25 J. Med. Genetics 290 (1988).

50. Dunstan thus sees genetic screening and "selective abortion" as a "rationalized adjunct to natural processes" in which "defective products" (babies) are "discard[ed] spontaneously." *Id.* at 292.

51. For a full development of these ideas, see Asch, *Reproductive Technology and Disability,* in Reproductive Laws for the 1990s, *supra* note 27, at 69; Asch & Fine, *Shared Dreams: A Left Perspective on Disability Rights and Reproductive Rights*, in Women with Disabilities 197 (M. Fine & A. Asch eds. 1988).

52. There would seem to be similar assumptions beneath the transformation of problems with dirty workplaces into problems with women workers who may become pregnant. *See, e.g.,* Bertin, *Women's Health and Women's Rights: Reproductive Health Hazards in the Workplace*, in Healing Technology, *supra* note 34, at 289, 297 (advocating legislation requiring safe workplaces and prohibiting sterility requirements); Woolhandler & Himmelstein, *Ideology in Medical Science: Class in the Cliinic,* 28 Soc. Sci. & Med. 1205 (1989).

53. Levin, *International Perspectives on Treatment Choice in Neonatal Intensive Care Units,* 30 Soc. Sci. & Med. 901, 903 (1990) (citation omitted).

54. For a further discussion on this, see McDonough, *supra* note 16, at 149.

55. Powell-Griner & Woolbright, *Trends in Infant Deaths from Congenital Anomalies: Results from England and Wales, Scotland, Sweden and the United States,* 19 Int'l. J. Epidemiology 391, 397 (1990) (probable that level of infant mortality will be influenced by prenatal screening and selective abortion); Saari-Kemppainen, Karjalainen, Ylostalo & Heinonen, *Ultrasound Screening and Prenatal Mortality: Controlled Trial of Systematic One-Stage Screening in Pregnancy,* 336 Lancet 387, 391 (1990) (Researchers of ultrasound screening in Helsinki, Finland concluded that "[t]he decrease in perinatal mortality of about half in this trial can

be explained mainly by the detection of major fetal anomalies by ultrasound screening and the subsequent termination of these pregnancies.").

56. Lippman, *Genetics and Public Health: Means, Goals and Justices,* to be published in AM. J. HUM. GENETICS (1991). *See* A. Finger, *supra* note 34; P. Kaufert, The Production of Medical Knowledge: Genes, Embryos and Public Policy (paper presented at *Gender, Science and Medicine II* conference, Toronto, Ontario, Nov. 2, 1990). Moreover, illness and disability are *hard* (i.e., difficult) issues partly because society defines them as such, in its decisions about how (not) to allocate resources to deal with them. Unfortunately, since resources are always "scarce," the programs or projects that do (not) get supported will merely be those which policymakers choose (not) to fund. No specific choice is inherent in the limited budgets available, although the requirement that choices be made is. In choosing how to deal with health problems, budget limitations may sometimes be secondary to limitations in our visions about what to do. And, in choosing how to approach (even) "hard" issues, genetic prevention is but one possibility.

57. Asch, *Reproductive Technology and Disability, supra* note 51, at 70.

58. See Friedmann, *Opinion: the Human Genome Project—Some Implications of Extensive "Reverse Genetic" Medicine,* 46 AM. J. HUM. GENETICS 407, 412 (1990).

59. *Id.* at 411.

60. Lippman, Messing & Mayer, *Is Genome mapping the Way to Improve Canadians' Health?* 81 CANADIAN J. PUB. HEALTH 397 (1990).

Deciding Against Disability: Does the Use of Reproductive Genetic Technologies Express Disvalue for People with Disabilities?

Janet Malek

INTRODUCTION

The increasing range of assisted reproductive and genetic technologies offers potential parents unprecedented control over the characteristics of their future children. A couple can use sperm-sorting technology to significantly increase the likelihood that they will conceive a girl in order to avoid having a child affected by haemophilia. A woman who carries the dominant gene for Huntington's disease can use in vitro fertilisation and preimplantation genetic diagnosis (PGD) to ensure that she will not pass the gene on to her offspring by transferring back only embryos that do not carry that gene. Potential parents can use chorionic villus sampling to determine whether their 11-week-old fetus has trisomy 18. At present, such reproductive genetic technologies (RGTs) are used primarily to select against certain traits; that is, they are used to prevent future children from having particular genetic conditions.

An array of ethical concerns has been raised about the use of these technologies. Some scholars have worried whether these technologies are safe for women and for the children they produce. Some have argued that such technologies are unnatural and that they may produce unintended consequences. Others have suggested that the routine use of RGTs could lead to diminished support for those with disability or that condoning such use will lead to a revival of Nazi-like eugenic programmes. This paper will focus on just one of the many objections to the use of RGTs: the argument known as the expressivist objection. According to this argument, selecting against embryos or fetuses with conditions that will lead to disability expresses disvalue for individuals who currently have those disabilities. Many have been persuaded by this impassioned perspective. In this paper I use a series of thought experiments to show that this argument is misguided and so does not constitute a sound objection to the use of RGTs to prevent disability in future children.

THE ARGUMENT

According to Parens and Asch, 'tests to select against disabling traits express a hurtful attitude about and send a hurtful message to people who have those same traits'.[1] In other words, the choice to use reproductive genetic technologies to prevent the birth of individuals with disabilities is an expression of disvalue for existing people with disability. The meaning of such a choice, proponents argue, is that people with disabilities are less valuable than people without disabilities. That choice therefore communicates a negative message to those existing people who have disabilities.

This conclusion seems to be built on the following reasoning: the choice to use RGTs to select against an embryo or fetus with a particular genetic trait implies that the value of that future child can be judged on a single characteristic. That choice therefore represents a problematic, reductionist understanding of the value of individuals in which their 'worth' is determined exclusively by the presence or absence of a disease trait. As Adrienne Asch, a consistent proponent of this position, has put it, such testing is 'a clear case of first impression ... that first impression includes a decision never to learn about the rest of who that embryo or fetus could become after its birth'.[2] Selecting against a future child on the basis of a disability signals that a disabling trait can be so significant and so undesirable that it eclipses all of the individual's other traits. According to proponents of the expressivist argument, this negative evaluation of the lives of people with disability applies equally to future and present persons. Therefore, the choice to use RGTs communicates to people with disabilities that their disability is so impor-

tant that it outweighs their other characteristics, a negative and hurtful message that reflects a lack of value for those individuals.

As Søren Holm has helpfully observed, proponents and critics have fleshed out the expressivist argument in a variety of ways.[3] Two points of clarification will help ensure that the argument is clearly and charitably understood for the purposes of the discussion below. First, there is some ambiguity about which types of practice generate the ethically worrisome messages in question. One version of the argument claims that individual choices to use RGTs send negative messages to those with disabilities.[1,4] An alternative version holds that it is only when medical professionals promote the use of RGTs or when such choices are promoted on a societal level that such messages are conveyed.[5] The distinction between these two versions is important, because they identify different practices as morally problematic. However, I believe the rebuttal laid out below applies equally to both versions of the argument. I will therefore discuss the two versions together in the arguments to follow.

Second, proponents and critics of this argument have both been less than clear about the nature of the message that is purportedly sent by the use of RGTs to prevent disability. It has sometimes been argued that the use of RGTs is discriminatory towards those with disability,[1,6] while in other cases authors have claimed that it simply reflects a negative attitude towards those individuals.[3,7,8] In the following pages, I will assume the weaker form of the argument that such choices reflect a negative attitude rather than a discriminatory one. Discriminatory actions or policies reflect negative attitudes towards those people who are being discriminated against. The negative-attitudes version of the argument therefore encompasses the discriminatory-attitudes version. This weaker version also sets a lower threshold at which the argument is successful. It is therefore the more plausible version of the argument.

In what follows, I will first identify a few responses that may be sound but not completely convincing to proponents of the expressivist position. I will then describe a thought experiment designed to demonstrate more clearly that choosing to use (or encouraging the use of) RGTs to prevent disability in future children does not convey a negative message about people who have disabilities. I will take the reader through a series of cases and show how each is morally equivalent to the previous one regarding the extent to which it expresses disvalue for such individuals. In doing so, I will also identify differences that one might be tempted to view as morally relevant to the question at hand and argue that each does not, in fact, affect the moral evaluation of the cases considered.

SOME POSSIBLE RESPONSES

Some authors have argued on semantic grounds that such a choice does not, in and of itself, communicate anything about people with disability and may not communicate anything at all. Buchanan[9] holds that, in order for an action to send a message, the action must logically dictate that the agent is motivated by the beliefs that correspond to the message supposedly sent. Further, the action must be rational *only* if the agent holds those beliefs. A choice to use RGTs to prevent disability in future children does not necessarily meet these two conditions. That is, an individual or couple could choose to use these technologies for any number of reasons that have nothing to do with the lives of those with disability, and in such cases the choice does not communicate anything about those individuals. A related argument has been made by Nelson, who claims that actions or practices are 'not semantically well-behaved enough to send any particular message'.[4] Following Wittgenstein, he suggests that in order for a choice to convey meaning, it must have an established and shared significance. The choice to use RGTs to prevent disability has no such publicly settled meaning and so may convey nothing at all. These rebuttals may be sound. But they may not be convincing to proponents of the expressivist argument, because they rest on semantic technicalities. They derive from real-world ambiguities and contingencies rather than

principled distinctions. A more robust response would therefore be helpful for an adequate rebuttal of the expressivist argument.

Another possible way of responding to this position would be to allow that the choice to use RGTs may convey a message but claim that the message need not be a negative one. Rather than viewing the use of these technologies as a choice *against* a disabled child, the decision could be understood as a choice *for* a healthy child. Viewed this way, the choice expresses value for normal traits but communicates nothing about disabling ones. This argument, however, seems too easy. Inherent in a choice to favour one option is at least *relative* disvalue for the choice not taken. Even if the choice is based on a positive evaluation rather than a negative one, that decision communicates that more value is placed on one option than the other, and so indicates that that second option is less valuable.

These arguments may be persuasive to some. However, for readers who are not yet convinced, let's assume that the decision to use RGTs to prevent disability *does* convey a message and that message is a negative one. Even given these assumptions, I will show in the following thought experiment that the expressivist objection can be refuted.

A THOUGHT EXPERIMENT

Scenario 1

Consider the following scenario: you are walking down the street one sunny morning to your local coffee shop. The walk signal flashes and you are about to enter the intersection when everything around you suddenly freezes. A disembodied voice claiming to be a guardian angel informs you that a driver approaching the intersection will momentarily be blinded by the early morning sun and run the red light; you will be hit by the driver in the crosswalk and paralysed from the waist down. Time then restarts and you are faced with the choice of when to cross the street. What would you do? Assuming that you can get on board with the idea that you have a guardian angel with the ability to freeze time, it seems safe to say that you would stay put on the sidewalk.

By choosing to wait to enter the intersection, you are choosing one possible future over another. More specifically, you are choosing a future self without disability (assuming all other things are equal) instead of a future self with a serious disability. Would this choice send a negative message about those people who are paraplegic? I don't believe that it would. The decision suggests that there is something negative associated with disability that you hope to avoid by not walking into the path of an oncoming car. It may therefore constitute an expression of disvalue for the inability to use one's legs. The expression of disvalue for a *disability,* however, is not the same as the expression of disvalue for a *person* who has a disability. The choice to stay on the sidewalk would not suggest that a person who cannot walk is any more or less valuable than a person who can. It would not mean that you would think any less of yourself as a person were you to fall down a manhole on the other side of the street and lose the use of your legs. Does this choice express disvalue for other individuals who have paraplegia? Just as trying to prevent the occurrence of disability in your own life does not imply that you would find your own life less valuable if you were to become disabled, seeking to prevent disability in your own life does not imply that the lives of others with disability are any less valuable. Given the opportunity, it seems highly likely that even those with (other) disabilities would make the same choice with a perfectly clear conscience. It would therefore be misguided to argue that the choice to wait to enter the intersection in the above scenario is ethically problematic because it expresses a negative attitude towards those with disabilities.

One might contend that the distinction between a disability and the person who has that disability is not as clear as this argument suggests. As Edwards has claimed, for some people with disability, 'disabling traits are, in fact, at least partly identity constituting'.[10] In other words, disabled individuals may consider their disability to be a central part of who they are. There are at least two reasons, however, to question whether this observation undermines the above distinction. First, Asch, the most consistent proponent of the expressivist argument, states that 'disability is not, and need not, be either a 'deep' or a valued part of identity for everyone who shares the disability critique'.[2] In fact, her primary objection to the use of RGTs to prevent disability in future children is that such use suggests a reduction of disabled people to their disabilities. She therefore clearly *rejects* the idea that disabled individuals should be defined by their disabilities. Second, even if a disabled person identifies strongly with his disability, such identification does not entail that the person and his disability are one and the same. The two can still be distinguished in a way that makes it possible to express a negative attitude towards one and not the other. Persons have inherent value that is independent of their characteristics or traits. Individuals are valued as persons to whatever extent they are persons, regardless of what else might be true of them. It is therefore perfectly consistent to express a negative attitude towards one of a person's traits without conveying a negative attitude towards the actual person. Because value as a person is independent of the person's characteristics or traits, the above distinction is defensible. It explains why choosing not to enter the intersection says nothing about people who have disabilities.

The above arguments have demonstrated that an individual would not convey a negative message about people who are paraplegic by choosing not to enter the intersection in the scenario above. But can this same conclusion be drawn about public policies or clinical guidelines intended to prevent similar disabilities? Yes, because analogous reasoning applies. A state law requiring drivers to wear seatbelts may reflect a negative attitude towards injuries caused by car accidents but does not send a message of disvalue to those people who have been injured in such accidents. When physicians encourage obese patients to lose weight they convey disvalue for the health complications caused by obesity, not for their overweight patients themselves. Such practices may express negative attitudes about certain traits but do not express negative attitudes about the persons who have those traits.

Scenario 2

You are walking down the street with your 9-year-old daughter to your local coffee shop. The walk signal flashes and the two of you are about to enter the intersection when everything around you suddenly freezes. A disembodied voice claiming to be a guardian angel informs you that a driver approaching the intersection will momentarily be blinded by the early morning sun and run the red light; your daughter will be hit by the driver in the crosswalk and paralysed from the waist down. Time then restarts and you are faced with the choice of when to cross the street.

The choice you must make in this case is different from the previous one because it involves making a decision on behalf of someone else rather than for yourself. Choosing to prevent a disability for another person suggests that the desire to avoid disability is not simply an idiosyncratic preference, but is based on a value that is presumed to be shared. The decision to prevent your daughter from entering the intersection in this scenario therefore suggests that having the ability to use one's legs is, all else being equal, a good thing. It could also be understood as presuming that an inability to use one's legs is, all else being equal, a bad thing. Even so, this variation does not introduce a negative attitude towards *persons* with paraplegia. The distinction made in the previous section applies to this case as well. Preventing your daughter from entering the intersection may signal that you associate something negative with paraplegia itself but does not send a negative message about persons who experience that condition.

As with the first case, the large-scale promotion of this type of choice through education campaigns, public policies or the development of professional practice guidelines is no more ethically problematic than individual decision-making with respect to the messages it may convey about the lives of people with disabilities. The 'Never Shake a Baby' campaign does not express disvalue for those babies who were shaken despite the fact that its goal is to prevent similar injuries to future children. When a physician encourages parents to vaccinate their children, that encouragement does not constitute an expression of a negative attitude towards children who have the diseases the vaccines are intended to prevent. Whether on the level of an individual or of a society, then, efforts to prevent disability on behalf of others do not express disvalue for those people who have disabilities.

Scenario 3

You are having a morning latte at your local coffee shop, thinking about when you and your partner should start trying to conceive a child. Everything around you suddenly freezes and a disembodied voice claiming to be a guardian angel informs you that if you conceive this month, your future child will have a congenital condition that will cause paraplegia. If you wait a month, however, your future child will not have this condition.

Would the decision to wait to conceive express a negative attitude towards persons with disability any more than a decision to prevent your daughter from entering the intersection would? In one case, you are acting to prevent future disability for your child when that child is 9 years old. In the other, you are acting to prevent future disability for your child before that child is conceived. The difference between the two choices is the point in the child's life at which the choice is made. Any negative attitude that may be expressed by the choice to prevent future disability is not dependent on temporal characteristics of that decision. In other words, the fact that these choices take place at different times in a child's life does not make a morally relevant difference to the issue of whether that choice expresses disvalue for those with disability. Therefore, if the choice to prevent your daughter from entering the intersection does not express such disvalue, the choice to wait to conceive doesn't either.

One might argue that this conclusion is unsound because there *is* a morally relevant difference between this scenario and the two above: in this third case, your choice changes the genetic identity of the individual who is brought into existence, whereas in the previous cases the same person (genetically defined) will continue to exist no matter which decision you make. It may be true that this is a difference between these two cases. However, this may not be a *morally relevant* difference, if the following reasoning is sound.

In ordinary decisions about conception, nothing specific is known about the characteristics of the possible future children. The decision to pick one possible future child over another is a choice between two unknowns. The choice is therefore a random one, just like the flip of a coin, with regard to the characteristics of those future children. (The decision would most likely be made on grounds unrelated to the characteristics of the future child, such as convenient timing for the parents.) The choice between two unknown possible future children does not express disvalue for people with disability.

In the scenario above, however, one piece of information about the characteristics of one of the possible future children is available. You know that if you choose to conceive this month, your future child will have a genetic condition that causes paraplegia. This is the only piece of information about that future child that you have. So a decision to wait to conceive could only be based on a negative attitude towards that disability and, as a result, reflects disvalue for the inability to use one's legs. However, the first two scenarios above established that the choice to select against a disabling trait, in and of itself, does not express disvalue for those with disability, but rather for the disability itself.

Putting these pieces together, it becomes apparent that the fact that the decision to conceive changes the genetic identity of the future child does not constitute a morally relevant difference for the purposes of this paper. That is,

it does not introduce an expression of disvalue for those with disability. The choice between one unknown possible future child and another does not reflect a negative attitude towards such individuals, nor does the choice to prevent the existence of a disabling condition. Essentially, because nothing is known about the other characteristics of the possible future children, it does not make sense to say that the presence of a disabling trait takes priority over or eclipses the future child's other traits; it is simply the sole piece of information available. The potential parents do not add up the future child's characteristics and decide to weigh that child's disability as more important than all the rest. Instead, they decide that, all else being equal (which it is, because of the lack of information about the possible future children), it is better for their future child to not have a disabling trait. The choice to wait to conceive, therefore, is similar to the cases above in the morally relevant ways, and so does not express disvalue for people who have disability.

But would the promotion of such choices on a societal level be different with respect to the messages they send people with disabilities? The March of Dimes, a non-profit organisation created to prevent birth defects, premature birth and infant mortality, works to educate women about the importance of taking folic acid before becoming pregnant in order to prevent neural tube defects. Obstetricians encourage potential mothers to quit smoking, get treatment for drug or alcohol abuse and taper off certain medications before becoming pregnant. Following any of these recommendations would be likely to cause a change in the genetic identity of the child conceived. But such recommendations are not discouraged on the grounds that they express negative attitudes about those who are disabled because their mothers made different choices.

Scenario 4

You have just come from your local coffee shop and have arrived at your appointment with a genetic counsellor. You and your partner are thinking about trying to conceive a child but are aware that you have a family history of a serious genetic condition that causes those who inherit a particular gene to become paraplegic. The counsellor informs you that it is possible to use PGD to ensure that your future child will not have this condition. If you choose to take this approach, several eggs will be fertilised in vitro and allowed to grow into embryos. Those embryos will be tested for the genetic condition in question, and only those embryos that do not carry that gene will be transferred and given the chance to develop. You and your partner decide to use PGD to ensure that your future child will not have the genetic condition.

The primary difference between the third and fourth scenarios is that in scenario three, a single future child is conceived, whereas in scenario four, numerous future children are conceived and those with the undesired trait are discarded or frozen indefinitely. Does this difference introduce negative attitudes towards those with disability? The difference between these scenarios is morally relevant only if the embryos in question have moral status. The moral status (or lack thereof) of embryos is a highly controversial issue that cannot be addressed in this paper. Fortunately, it is not necessary to resolve the issue to determine whether the choice in this scenario devalues people who are disabled. If embryos do have significant moral status, scenario four is importantly different from scenario three. However, if embryos have moral status, it is the destruction of those embryos that is morally problematic for the use of PGD in this case, not the decision to implant some embryos but not others. If, in contrast, embryos do not have moral status, the choice to use PGD in this fourth case is not morally different from the choice to wait to conceive in the third scenario above. The choice to discard or indefinitely freeze some embryos is analogous to waiting a month or two to conceive. If embryos do not have moral status, the two decisions are essentially the same: the choice to prevent one's future child from having a disabling trait. So, for the same reasons cited above, that choice

does not constitute an expression of disvalue for people with disability.

As argued above, the distinction between individuals choosing to use these technologies to prevent disability and the widespread promotion of such choices is a distinction without a moral difference. Analogous programmes and practices that are truly analogous to PGD are difficult to find, but if this distinction did not make a moral difference in the types of decisions discussed in scenarios 1, 2 and 3, it seems plausible to conclude that it also makes no moral difference in this fourth scenario.

Scenario 5

You have just come from your local coffee shop, and have arrived at your appointment with a genetic counsellor. You and your partner are 10 weeks pregnant and are aware that you have a family history of a serious genetic condition that causes those who inherit a particular gene to become paraplegic. The counsellor informs you that it is possible to use prenatal genetic testing to determine whether your future child will have this condition. You and your partner decide to undergo the testing, which shows that the fetus does have the unwanted gene. You decide to terminate the pregnancy and conceive again as soon as possible.

Once again, this scenario is morally equivalent to the preceding one with respect to the attitudes the potential parents' choice expresses about people with disabilities. In both cases, a few possible future children are conceived and testing is done to establish whether each future child will have a serious disabling condition. In scenario 4, the possible future children are conceived at the same time, whereas in scenario 5 they are conceived at different times. This temporal difference is a way of distinguishing the cases but is not a morally relevant difference for the purposes of this paper. There is nothing inherent in conceiving several possible future children over time that expresses disvalue for those people with disabilities if conceiving several possible children at one time does not. That is, the choice to spread out the conception of the possible future children does not introduce a negative attitude towards persons who are disabled.

The importance of the moral status question is even more obvious in this scenario than in the previous one. If the fetus has significant moral status, it is the destruction of that fetus (regardless of its genetic makeup) that is morally problematic. For those who take a gradualist position on moral status, holding that it increases gradually as the fetus develops, scenario 5 may be marginally more problematic than scenario 4 because the fetus is more developed. The objection, however, is generated by the inherent moral worth of the fetus at that stage of development and is unrelated to the fact that the fetus has a disabling condition. If, on the other hand, the fetus does not have moral status, there is a difference in kind between the fetus in this case and existing persons (whether disabled or not) who have full moral status. Because of this difference, the choice to terminate the pregnancy says nothing at all about those with disability.

CONCLUSION

In moving through the five scenarios above, I have argued that the choice to use reproductive genetic technologies to prevent disability in a future child is no different from the decision to protect oneself from becoming disabled with regard to the message that such a choice sends to those individuals who currently have disabilities. In each case, an individual is faced with making a choice between a life with a disability and one without. The choice to avoid creating a life with disability may reflect a negative view of the disability itself, but not of persons who have it.

It is worth emphasising that the expressivist argument is only one of several disability-based objections to the use of RGTs and that disability-based objections are only some of the many ethical considerations that must be taken into account in the ethical evaluation of these technologies. If the expressivist argument fails, there may be *other* good reasons to object to the use of RGTs to prevent disability. At the same time, if this rebuttal of the expressivist argument is not convincing, the soundness of that argument does not imply that the use of RGTs is, all things considered, a morally impermissible choice. Even if the use of these technologies does express a negative attitude towards people who have disabilities, that argument, in and of itself, may not be sufficient reason to avoid using RGTs. Other ethical considerations that support the use of these technologies may outweigh the force of the expressivist objection. As a result, the success or failure of the expressivist argument (and of its rebuttal) does not settle the question of whether the use of RGTs to prevent disability in future children is a morally acceptable practice.

I have argued that the choice to use RGTs to prevent disability in future children does not express disvalue for people who have disabilities. It would not be inconsistent with this argument to claim that people who have disabilities nonetheless feel disvalued by such choices. My conclusion must also be distinguished from the possibility that the routine use of such technologies will result in diminished support for people with disabilities. These are empirical issues that should be explored and taken into account in the overall ethical evaluation of the use of RGTs to prevent disability. However, the conclusion that such choices do not, in principle, communicate negative messages about people with disability shifts the burden of proof onto objectors. For their arguments to be persuasive, objectors will need to demonstrate that such negative effects will occur and that they cannot be ameliorated through any means other than refraining from the use of these technologies.

Acknowledgements

The author would like to thank the members of the Department of Medical Humanities at the Brody School of Medicine at East Carolina University for helpful comments on this paper.

Notes

1. Parens E, Asch A. The disability rights critique of prenatal genetic testing: reflections and recommendations. In: Parens E, Asch A, eds. *Prenatal testing and disability rights.* Washington, DC: Georgetown University Press, 2000:3–43.

2. Asch A. Why I haven't changed my mind about prenatal diagnosis: Reflections and refinements. In: Parens E, Asch A, eds. *Prenatal testing and disability rights.* Washington, DC: Georgetown University Press, 2000:234–58.

3. Holm S. The expressivist objection to prenatal diagnosis: Can it be laid to rest? *J Med Ethics* 2008;34:24–5.

4. Nelson JL. Prenatal diagnosis, personal identity, and disability. *Kennedy Inst of Ethics J* 2000;103:213–28.

5. Asch A. Disability equality and prenatal testing: Contradictory or compatible? *Fla State Univ Law Rev* 2003:318–42.

6. Shakespeare T. *Disability rights and wrongs.* New York, NY: Routledge, 2006.

7. Buchanan A, Brock DW, Daniels N, et al. *From chance to choice: Genetics and justice.* New York, NY: Cambridge University Press, 2000.

8. Nelson JL. The meaning of the act: Reflections on the expressivist force of reproductive decision making and policies. In: Parens E, Asch A, eds. *Prenatal testing and disability rights.* Washington, DC: Georgetown University Press, 2000:196–213.

9. Buchanan A. Choosing who will be disabled: Genetic intervention and the morality of inclusion. *Soc Philos Policy* 1996;13:18–46.

10. Edwards SD. Disability, identity and the "expressivist objection". *J Med Ethics* 2004;30:418–20.

CASES

R v Morgentaler, [1988] 1 SCR 30, 1988 CanLII 90 (SCC)

Summary prepared by Martina Munden

Under section 251 of the *Criminal Code of Canada,* a woman wishing to obtain an abortion had to receive a certificate from a therapeutic abortion committee at an accredited or approved hospital prior to a physician performing the abortion. These committees had the authority to issue a certificate stating that, in the opinion of a majority of the committee, the continuation of the pregnancy likely would endanger the pregnant woman's life or health. Once the certificate was given to a qualified medical practitioner, the practitioner was permitted to perform an abortion without either the physician or woman being subject to criminal liability. Failure of the woman to receive the medical approval for the abortion meant that the abortion was a criminal offence for both

the woman and the physician who provided the abortion. The therapeutic abortion committee would only provide a certificate when the s. 251 criterion was complied with, that being, a woman's life or health would or would likely be endangered by the pregnancy.

The physicians in this case (including Dr. Morgentaler) had set up a clinic to perform abortions for women who had not obtained a certificate from a therapeutic abortion committee of an accredited hospital as required by s. 251. The physicians had also made statements questioning the wisdom of the Canadian abortion law, asserting that a woman had an unfettered right to choose whether an abortion was appropriate in her individual circumstances. The physicians were charged with illegally performing an abortion. The physicians argued that s. 251 was contrary to the *Canadian Charter of Rights and Freedoms.*

Discussion Questions

1. Should abortion be treated differently from other medical treatments provided within the Canadian health care system?
2. What is the moral status of the fetus? Does the moral status of the fetus change as the fetus develops?

3. Even if the fetus was thought to have full moral status, it is sometimes argued that abortion is nonetheless morally permissible since the physical location of the fetus (within a particular woman's body) gives special moral weight to her views. How should the relationship between the pregnant woman and the fetus be understood? Is it necessarily adversarial in the case of unwanted pregnancies?

Raina v Shaw, 2006 BCSC 832, 150 ACWS (3d) 1137

Summary prepared by Tim Krahn

On April 3, 2006 Nidhi and Shankar Raina brought forward a negligence action against Dr. Lauren Shaw seeking compensation for the costs of raising their son who was born with Down syndrome. Ms. Raina alleged that Dr. Shaw failed to provide her with genetic counselling during her pregnancy, and argued that if she and her husband had been provided with information about prenatal testing and screening, they would have obtained relevant testing and made a decision to terminate the pregnancy.

The likelihood of a pregnancy being affected by Down syndrome increases as maternal age increases. Given that Ms. Raina was 37 during her pregnancy, she and her husband argued that the expected standard of care (in British Columbia) for an expectant mother of her age included genetic counselling. Dr. Shaw did not dispute this. What came under dispute was Dr. Shaw's claim to have provided counselling and materials on prenatal genetic testing at the first prenatal care appointment.

Importantly, Ms. Raina missed both her second and third prenatal care appointments. Ms. Raina claimed to have missed the first of these two appointments because she was preparing for a trip

to India, and the next because she was away on the trip. Ms. Raina testified that she had obtained Dr. Shaw's "permission" to make the trip; Dr. Shaw denied this and claimed that she would have "adamantly" advised against a trip to India. When Ms. Raina next visited Dr. Shaw, the window for prenatal testing had passed, and Dr. Shaw claimed that Ms. Raina confirmed at that time that she had chosen not to have prenatal testing.

Discussion Questions

1. Should all women and couples routinely be offered genetic counseling, or should this only be offered to women and couples who are at increased risk of having a child with a genetic anomaly?
2. Should physicians actively encourage women of advanced maternal age to pursue prenatal testing, or merely advise them of their options?
3. How much responsibility should patients have for the consequences of their decisions, whether a decision to refuse prenatal testing or a decision to miss a prenatal appointment?

Reprinted by permission of the author.

Useful Resources

ONLINE

American Society for Reproductive Medicine (ASRM)

"ASRM is a multidisciplinary organization dedicated to the advancement of the art, science, and practice of reproductive medicine." This professional organization regularly issues Ethics Committee Reports and Statements. These can be found in the section on News and Publications.

AnonymousUs.org

AnonymousUs.org is a website that invites anyone and everyone involved in reproductive technologies, but especially persons born via these practices, to write about their experiences and opinions anonymously. The aim is "to share the experiences of voluntary and involuntary participants in these technologies, while preserving the dignity and privacy for story-tellers and their loved ones."

Assisted Human Reproduction Canada (AHRC)

Federal responsibility for assisted human reproduction is shared by Health Canada and Assisted Human Reproduction Canada. Assisted Human Reproduction Canada (AHRC) is responsible for administering and enforcing the Act and its regulations.

Canadian College of Medical Geneticists (CCMG)

CCMG seeks to "maintain high quality professional and ethical standards of medical genetics services in Canada and to help ensure that the highest quality of service is delivered to the Canadian public." CCMG publishes position statements and reports on genetic testing, genetic screening, and genetic research that address a range of ethical issues.

Canadian Fertility and Andrology Society (CFAS)

CFAS regroups health professionals "in the field of assisted reproductive technologies and research in reproductive sciences." It "speaks on behalf of all interested parties in the field of assisted reproductive technologies and research in reproductive sciences."

Center for Genetics and Society (CGS)

The U.S. Center for Genetics and Society is a non-profit information and public affairs organization working to encourage responsible uses and effective societal governance of human genetic, reproductive, and biomedical technologies.

Joint Policy Statement: Ethical Issues in Assisted Reproduction (1999)

Joint Canadian Fertility and Andrology Society/Society of Obstetricians and Gynaecologists of Canada Report.

Health Canada, Assisted Human Reproduction

Federal responsibility for assisted human reproduction is shared by Health Canada and Assisted Human Reproduction Canada. Health Canada is responsible for developing policy and regulations under the *Assisted Human Reproduction Act.*

Human Fertilisation and Embryology Authority (HFEA)

"The HFEA is the U.K.'s independent regulator overseeing the use of gametes and embryos in fertility treatment and research. It licenses fertility clinics and centres carrying out in vitro fertilisation (IVF), other assisted conception procedures and human embryo research."

Society of Obstetricians and Gynaecologists of Canada (SOGC)

The SOGC's mission is "to promote excellence in the practice of obstetrics and gynaecology and to advance the health of women through leadership, advocacy, collaboration, outreach and education." The SOGC has an Ethics Committee that periodically issues ethics guidelines. As well, it is possible to find ethics articles published in the *Journal of Obstetrics and Gynaecology Canada* (JOGC) by performing a search using the keyword "ethics."

READINGS

Bankole, A., Singh, S., & Haas, T. (1998). Reasons why women have induced abortions: Evidence from 27 countries. *International Family Planning Perspectives,* 24(3), 117–152.

Ethics and Public Policy Committee, Canadian College of Medical Geneticists. (1991). Prenatal diagnosis: The medical genetics perspective. *Canadian Medical Association Journal,* 144(9), 1129–1132.

Glover, J. (2006). *Choosing children: The ethical dilemmas of genetic intervention.* New York, NY: Oxford University Press.

Harris, J., & Holm, S. (2000). *The future of human reproduction: Ethics, choice, and regulation.* New York, NY: Oxford University Press.

Levine, A. (2010). Self-regulation, compensation, and the ethical recruitment of oocyte donors. *Hastings Center Report,* 40(2), 25–36.

Marquis, D. (1989). Why abortion is immoral. *The Journal of Philosophy,* 86 (4), 183–202.

Overall, C. (1991). Access to *in vitro* fertilization: Costs, care and consent. *Dialogue,* 30(3), 383–397.

Parens, E., & Asch, A. (2000). *Prenatal testing and disability rights.* Washington, D.C.: Georgetown University Press.

Rodgers, S., & Downie, J. (2006). Abortion: Ensuring access [editorial]. *Canadian Medical Association Journal,* 175(1), 9.

Royal Commission on New Reproductive Technologies. (1993). *Proceed with care: Final report of the Royal Commission on New Reproductive Technologies* (Vols. 1 & 2). Ottawa: Minister of Supply and Services Canada.

Thomson, J. J. (1971). A defense of abortion. *Philosophy & Public Affairs*, 1(1), 47–66.

Tooley, M. (1972). Abortion and infanticide. *Philosophy & Public Affairs,* 2(1): 37–65.

Warren, M. A. (1973). On the moral and legal status of abortion. *Monist,* 57(1), 43–61.

Wilkinson, S. (2010). *Choosing tomorrow's children: The ethics of selective reproduction.* New York, NY: Oxford University Press.

HEALTH LAW

Winnipeg Child and Family Services (Northwest Area) v G(DF), [1997] 3 SCR 925, 1997 CanLII 336 (SCC)

Winnipeg Child and Family Services sought to detain a pregnant woman with an addiction to sniffing glue in order to treat her against her will for her addiction and thereby protect her fetus.

Arndt v. Smith, [1997] 2 S.C.R. 539

Ms. Arndt contracted chickenpox during the 12th week of her pregnancy, as a result of which her daughter was injured. Ms. Arndt sued her physician Dr. Smith for the costs associated with raising her daughter. She claimed that she would have aborted her fetus if she hadn't been reassured by her physician that the risks of fetal injury were very small.

Cameron v. Nova Scotia (Attorney General), 1999 CanLII 7243 (NS C.A.)

An infertile couple sought reimbursement of their costs for ICSI (intracytoplasmic sperm injection) under the provincial health insurance plan. They also sought a declaration to the effect that they were entitled to coverage for any further treatment, and an order directing the Nova Scotia Minister of Health to establish a mechanism for payment for IVF and ICSI procedures.

Reference re Assisted Human Reproduction Act, 2010 SCC 61

Shortly after the AHR Act was passed in 2004, the Québec government challenged the constitutionality of the legislation. The constitutional issue before the Court was whether the "pith and substance" (i.e., purpose and effects) of certain sections of the legislation were: (1) to protect morality, safety, and public health (which is a federal responsibility under the *Constitution Act, 1867*); or (2) to regulate and promote the benefits of medical practice and research related to assisted human reproduction (which is a provincial responsibility under the *Constitution Act, 1867*).

Pratten v British Columbia (Attorney General), 2011 BCSC 656

Ms. Pratten was conceived by donor insemination in 1981and as a young adult she wanted access to the records of the sperm donor. The physician who performed the insemination, Dr. Korn, was not legally required to keep a record of the donor's identity and claimed to have destroyed whatever records he had. Ms. Pratten charged the provincial government with failure to ensure that proper records of such procedures are maintained by physicians. Ms. Pratten argued that donor offspring should have the same ability as adopted children to access information about their origins.

CanLII
CanLII is a non-profit organization managed by the Federation of Law Societies of Canada. CanLII's goal is to make Canadian law accessible for free on the Internet.

Chapter 9 END-OF-LIFE ISSUES

INTRODUCTION

Providing care near the end of life and being involved in the ending of a life are two of the most troubling, agonizing challenges that individuals, families, and health care providers can confront. They implicate an array of moral, medical, and legal matters, but, more profoundly, they are about love and loss, intimacy, and spirituality. They engage our feelings and emotions as much as our reason and can exact a toll that only compassion, empathy, and understanding can lighten. Morality ultimately is about persons, and nowhere else is that reminder more needed than with matters concerning end-of-life.

End-of-life care also raises challenging public policy questions, most dramatically with respect to assisted suicide and euthanasia. Two landmark decisions from the Supreme Court of Canada, one on assisted suicide and one on euthanasia, are summarized in this chapter. In the former case, Sue Rodriquez, who had amyotrophic lateral sclerosis (also known as Lou Gehrig's disease), campaigned prominently and indefatigably for the legalization of assisted suicide. She lost by a 5-to-4 decision in the Supreme Court. In the latter case, the Supreme Court upheld the conviction of Robert Latimer, who ended the life of his severely disabled daughter, Tracy, to stop an unceasing sequence of surgeries on her and to relieve her unremitting pain.

Not surprisingly, the issue of who should decide, addressed in Chapters 5 and 6, also arises with respect to end-of-life matters, obliquely in debates about the notion of futility and directly in a recent case in Winnipeg. Doctors can refuse to provide or continue life-prolonging care when they regard it as "futile." But what does "futile" mean, and what kind of judgment are doctors making when they declare a treatment futile? Is this declaration a medical judgment that doctors are entitled to make unilaterally, or is it a moral judgment appropriately made by the patient and the patient's family? In the first article, Robert Truog, Allan Brett, and Joel Frader point out that claims of futility always are relative to a specific goal. So how, and by whom, the goal of care should be determined is critically important. Only thereafter can the likelihood of attaining that goal be assessed and possibly deemed futile. This and other problems lead the authors to call for a rejection of the concept of futility.

In Winnipeg physicians wanted to remove Mr. Golubchuk, an Orthodox Jew, from life support over the adamant objections of his family. The article by Alan Jotkowitz, Shimon Glick, and Ari Zivotofsky questions the moral and clinical justifications for the physicians' decision as well as their authority to make it. The companion piece by Pat Murphy, George Webster, and Brian Chaze, two of whom work as clinical ethicists in Winnipeg, notes similar controversies in the province and criticizes the position of the College of Physicians and Surgeons of Manitoba for "dressing up" assessments of the "appropriate" goals of treatment as medical judgments rather than ethical judgments.

The next three articles have a more theoretical orientation. Jocelyn Downie criticizes influential distinctions that pervade discussions of ending life, including acting vs. omitting to act (e.g, administering a lethal injection vs. not starting a life-prolonging procedure), dying from a natural cause vs. dying from an unnatural cause (e.g, dying from a disease vs. dying from the removal of life support), and intending to alleviate suffering vs. intending to end life (e.g., increasing the dose of a drug with the intention to reduce pain but foreseeing that the patient might die more quickly vs. injecting a drug with the intention of ending the patient's pain by killing the patient). Downie argues that these distinctions cannot do either the moral or legal work that their proponents expect them to do. The following two articles by Dan Brock and Daniel Callahan present opposing views about the legalization of voluntary active euthanasia. Brock argues in favour of legalization, primarily on the basis of individual self-determination or autonomy and individual well-being. Brock also holds that the potentially good consequences of legalization outweigh the potentially bad consequences, and he outlines the proper role of physicians in active euthanasia. Callahan criticizes the three central elements of Brock's position. He questions the meaning and extension of self-determination in this context; he disagrees with Brock's calculation of the likely consequences of legalization; and he contends that physicians have no responsibility and no right to try to relieve the kind of suffering—not pain—that motivates the desire to end one's life.

The final article discusses an approach to managing intractable pain or suffering that is taken to be preferable to assisted suicide and euthanasia: sedating a patient to unconsciousness until the patient dies. Because unconscious patients cannot eat or drink, however, they require artificial nutrition and hydration. Without artificial nutrition and hydration, a terminally sedated patient likely will die from dehydration within two weeks. With artificial nutrition and hydration, a terminally sedated patient will live much longer. Joseph Boyle reviews the history of the doctrine of double effect in Catholic moral casuistry and defends the doctrine and its use in bioethics. The doctrine holds that when an act has one consequence that is desirable and another consequence that is objectionable, the act is morally permissible only if the desirable consequence is intended and the objectionable consequence is merely foreseen. Increasing the dose of a drug to manage pain is a standard example. Higher doses of the drug could control the pain but also could depress respiration and thereby shorten the patient's life. Administering higher doses is permissible only if the intention of doing so is to relieve pain and the expedited death of the patient is merely foreseen. In Boyle's view, terminal sedation, unlike euthanasia, is not intentional killing. Even if he is correct, however, is the combination of terminal sedation and withholding artificial nutrition and hydration not intentional killing? More generally, can the moral distinction between consequences that are intended and consequences that are merely foreseen be sustained? Many health care professionals think the distinction makes sense, at least practically. Many philosophers (and Downie) think the distinction is indefensible. Who is right?

The Problem with Futility

Robert D. Truog, Allan S. Brett, and Joel Frader

"Futility" is one of the newest additions to the lexicon of bioethics. Physicians, ethicists, and members of the media are increasingly concerned about patients and families who insist on receiving life-sustaining treatment that others judge to be futile. A clear understanding of futility has proved to be elusive, however. Many clinicians view futility the way one judge viewed pornography: they may not be able to define it, but they know it when they see it.[1]

Truog, R., Brett, A., Frader, J., "The Problem with Futility", *New England Journal of Medicine* 326(23), pp. 1560–1564, © 1992 New England Journal of Medicine. Reprinted with permission from the publisher.

The notion of futile medical treatment may go back to the time of Hippocrates, who allegedly advised physicians "to refuse to treat those who are overmastered by their diseases, realizing that in such cases medicine is powerless."[2] More recently, the concept has appeared frequently in court decisions and policy statements.[3-6] The so-called Baby Doe law exempts physicians from providing treatment that would be "virtually futile."[7] The Council on Ethical and Judicial Affairs of the American Medical Association (AMA) recently concluded that physicians have no obligation to obtain consent for a do-not-resuscitate (DNR) order when cardiopulmonary resuscitation (CPR) is deemed futile.[8] The fact that this concept has appeared in law and policy may seem to indicate that it is clearly understood and widely accepted. In reality, however, the notion of futility hides many deep and serious ambiguities that threaten its legitimacy as a rationale for limiting treatment.

PARADIGMS OF FUTILITY

Contemporary discussions of futility have centered primarily on cases involving patients in a persistent vegetative state and those involving the use of CPR. A third type of case, involving organ-replacement technology, has received little attention but is helpful to our understanding of futility.

Futility and the Persistent Vegetative State

The first type of scenario involving the question of futility is represented by the recent Minnesota case of Helga Wanglie.[9] Mrs. Wanglie was an 86-year-old woman who had been dependent on mechanical ventilation and in a persistent vegetative state for more than a year. Her husband insisted that she believed in maintaining life at all cost, and that "when she was ready to go ... the good Lord would call her."[10] Her physicians, on the other hand, believed that the continued use of mechanical ventilation and intensive care was futile. When attempts to transfer her elsewhere failed, they sought to have a court appoint

an independent conservator with responsibility for making medical decisions on her behalf. The judge denied this petition and reaffirmed the authority of her husband as legal surrogate. Three days later, Mrs. Wanglie died.

Cases like that of Mrs. Wanglie seldom reach the courts, but they are probably not rare. A similar case involving a child with severe brain damage was concluded with a settlement favorable to the family before a judicial decision.[11]

Futility in Cases Involving CPR

The second prototypical scenario involves the use of DNR orders. Although the techniques of CPR were originally intended only for use after acute, reversible cardiac arrests, the current practice is to use CPR in all situations unless there is a direct order to the contrary. Since cardiac arrest is the final event in all terminal illness, everyone is eventually a candidate for this medical procedure. DNR orders were developed to spare patients from aggressive attempts at revival when imminent death is anticipated and inevitable. Nevertheless, patients or families sometimes request CPR even when care givers believe such attempts would be futile. Some have argued that in these circumstances a physician should be able to enact a DNR order without the consent of the patient or family.[12-14]

Futility and Organ-Replacement Technology

Although the bioethical debate over the question of futility has been most concerned with cases involving CPR and the treatment of patients in a persistent vegetative state, a third type of futility-related judgment has gone essentially unchallenged. It involves the increasingly large number of interventions that could possibly prolong the life of virtually any dying patient. For example, extracorporeal membrane oxygenation can replace heart and lung function for up to several weeks. Physicians now use this intervention when they expect organ systems eventually to recover or while they await organs for transplantation. However, it could prolong the life of almost anyone with cardiorespiratory failure, reversible or not. Patients thus kept alive may remain conscious and capable of communicating. Care givers do not now offer this therapy to terminally ill patients, presumably because it would be futile. This judgment has gone largely unchallenged, yet it is not obvious why a clinician's unilateral decision not to use "futile" extracorporeal membrane oxygenation is inherently different from a decision not to use "futile" CPR or "futile" intensive care. If all three treatments can be characterized as objectively futile, then unilateral decisions not to offer them should be equally justified.

As it is used in these three cases, the concept of futility obscures many ambiguities and assumptions. These can be usefully grouped into two categories: problems of value and problems of probability.

FUTILITY AND VALUES

It is meaningless simply to say that an intervention is futile; one must always ask, "Futile in relation to what?" The medical literature provides many examples in which the importance of identifying the goals of treatment has not been fully appreciated. The effectiveness of CPR, for example, is often discussed in terms of whether patients who require the procedure can survive long enough to be discharged from the hospital.[15] This definition of success usually implies that short-term survival is a goal not worth pursuing. Patients or family members may value the additional hours of life differently, however. Indeed, physicians and other care givers have repeatedly been shown to be poor judges of patients' preferences with regard to intensive care.[16–18]

Schneiderman and colleagues have argued that treatments that merely preserve permanent unconsciousness or that cannot end dependence on intensive medical care should be considered futile.[19] Although society may eventually endorse decisions to override the previously expressed wishes of patients or the desires of surrogates who demand such treatments, it does not follow that the treatments are futile. Mr. Wanglie would have rejected this conclusion, and there is no reason to dismiss his view out of hand. The

decision that certain goals are not worth pursuing is best seen as involving a conflict of values rather than a question of futility.

Certainly in this context, the plurality of values in our society makes agreement on the concept of futility difficult if not impossible. Several groups have therefore attempted to arrive at a value-free understanding of the concept.[20, 21] The most promising candidate thus far is the notion of "physiologic futility." As the guidelines on the termination of life-sustaining treatment prepared by the Hastings Center state, if a treatment is "clearly futile in achieving its physiological objective and so offer[s] no physiological benefit to the patient, the professional has no obligation to provide it."[20] For example, the physiologic objective of mechanical ventilation is to maintain adequate ventilation and oxygenation in the presence of respiratory failure, and the physiologic objective of CPR is to maintain adequate cardiac output and respiration in the presence of cardiorespiratory failure. The New York State Task Force on Life and the Law mistakenly concludes that CPR is physiologically futile when it will "be unsuccessful in restoring cardiac and respiratory function or [when] the patient will experience repeated arrest in a short time period before death occurs."[21] CPR is physiologically futile only when it is impossible to perform effective cardiac massage and ventilation (such as in the presence of cardiac rupture or severe outflow obstruction). Saying that CPR is physiologically futile when it will be unsuccessful in restoring cardiac function is like saying that mechanical ventilation is physiologically futile if it cannot restore respiratory function. The immediate physiologic effect of the intervention differs from the broader and more uncertain question of prognosis.

Physiologic futility, understood in narrow terms, comes close to providing a value-free understanding of futility. Unfortunately, it applies to a very small number of real cases involving CPR. Similarly, since in the case of Mrs. Wanglie mechanical ventilation could maintain adequate oxygenation and ventilation, her treatment could not be considered futile in the physiologic sense. Even the use of extracorporeal membrane oxygenation in terminally ill patients cannot be considered physiologically futile, since it can maintain circulation and ventilation. The concept of physiologic futility therefore falls short of providing guidance in most cases resembling those described above.

FUTILITY AND STATISTICAL UNCERTAINTY

In most medical situations, there is no such thing as never. Futility is almost always a matter of probability. But what statistical cutoff point should be chosen as the threshold for determining futility? The statement from the Council on Ethical and Judicial Affairs of the AMA concludes that physicians have no obligation to provide futile CPR, but it fails to specify any level of statistical certainty at which the judgment is warranted.[8] The AMA statement fails to acknowledge that this is even an issue. Should each physician decide independently what probability of success should be considered to indicate futility?

Even if we could agree on a statistical cutoff point for determining futility, physicians are often highly unreliable in estimating the likelihood of success of a therapeutic intervention. Psychological research[22, 23] has shown that estimates of probability are susceptible to "severe and systematic errors."[22] Empirical studies have corroborated the limitations of clinical assessment in estimating both prognosis[24] and diagnosis.[25] Even in theory, statistical inferences about what might happen to groups of patients do not permit accurate predictions of what will happen to the next such patient. In addition, the tendency to remember cases that are unusual or bizarre predisposes physicians to make decisions on the basis of their experiences with "miraculous" cures or unexpected tragedies.

Schneiderman and colleagues recently argued that a treatment should be considered futile when 100 consecutive patients do not respond to it.[19] But how similar must the patients be? In assessing the efficacy of mechanical ventilation to treat pneumonia, for example, is it sufficient simply to recall the 100 most recent patients who received artificial ventilation for pneumonia? Or must this group be stratified according to age, etiologic organism, or coexisting illness? Clearly, many of these factors will make an important difference.

FUTILITY AND RESOURCE ALLOCATION

Although medical practice has increasingly emphasized patients' autonomy, there is growing pressure on physicians to slow the increase in health care costs by foreclosing some options. Thus, we have a tension between the value of autonomy, exercised in the form of consent to use or omit various interventions, and the desirability of a more Spartan approach to the consumption of medical resources. We promote patients' freedom to request whatever the medical menu has to offer, but we also require that interventions be guided by considerations of cost and the likelihood of benefit.[26] Unfortunately, there is no consensus about what constitutes a just method of balancing the preferences of individual patients against the diverse needs of society.

To some, the concept of futility provides at least a partial solution to this dilemma: it offers a reason to limit therapy without the need to define a fair procedure for allocating resources. This approach allows treatments to be denied on the grounds that they are simply not indicated, apart from the matter of cost. Despite its attractions, there are good reasons why we should not use this concept to solve problems of allocation.

First, arguments based on the futility concept conceal many statistical and value-laden assumptions, whereas strategies based on resource allocation force these assumptions to be stated explicitly. Societies may choose to limit the use of therapies that may be of value and have a reasonable likelihood of success in some cases. For example, the much discussed Oregon plan for allocating Medicaid funds[27] seeks to reflect community values in ranking various health care goals (placing preventive care ahead of cosmetic surgery, for example). Since rationing policies make explicit the values and probabilities that futility-based arguments leave implicit, it is clearly preferable to develop and adopt them rather than use futility arguments as a cover for limiting the availability of scarce and expensive resources.

Another problem with invoking the idea of futility in the debate over allocation is that we have no reason to believe that it is applicable in enough cases to make a difference in the scarcity of medical resources. Although it may be true that beds in the intensive care unit (especially those used for extracorporeal membrane oxygenation) are relatively scarce, it seems unlikely that patients similar to Helga Wanglie occupy an important fraction of those beds, let alone account for a major proportion of the cost of medical care in the United States. From a macroeconomic perspective at least, we must remain skeptical that an appeal to the idea of futility will get us very far.

MOVING BEYOND FUTILITY

Our rejection of futility as a useful concept does not imply that we endorse patients' unrestricted demands for interventions such as those described in our prototypical scenarios. On the contrary, when providers oppose such demands they are usually acting from a profound sense that further treatment would be fundamentally wrong. Our task is to take account of that sense of wrongness without resorting to unilateral, provider-initiated declarations of futility.

In many of the situations in which questions of futility arise, providers believe that the treatment in question would not be in the patient's interests, even from the patient's perspective, and that any insistence by the patient (or surrogate) on further interventions is based on faulty reasoning, unrealistic expectations, or psychological factors, such as denial or guilt. In these circumstances, providers are obligated to make every effort to clarify precisely what the patient intends to achieve with continued treatment. If the patient's goals appear to reflect unrealistic expectations about the probable course of the underlying illness or the probable effect of medical interventions, providers should attempt to correct those impressions. Because inadequate or insensitive communication by providers probably accounts for a substantial proportion of unrealistic requests, such discussions will successfully resolve many conflicts.[14, 28] Empirical studies of ethics consultations have demonstrated precisely this point.[29, 30]

Although this appeal to the patient's interests may seem to contain some of the same ambiguities as arguments using the concept of futility, there is a subtle but important distinction between the two. Judgments about what is in the patient's interest are properly grounded in the patient's perspective, whereas judgments cast in the language of futility falsely assume that there is an objective and dispassionate standard for determining benefits and burdens. Nevertheless, even after providers make sustained attempts to clarify patients' preferences, some patients or surrogates will continue to demand life-sustaining interventions when the care givers feel deeply troubled about providing them. In many such cases, unrestrained deference to the wishes of the patient or surrogate conflicts with two other values that do not require a unilateral judgment of the futility of treatment: professional ideals and social consensus.

The ideals of medical professionals include respect for patients' wishes, to be sure, but they also include other values, such as compassionate action and the minimization of suffering. Consider, for example, a bedridden victim of multiple strokes who has contractures and bedsores and who "communicates" only by moaning or grimacing when she is touched. Physicians asked to perform chest compressions, institute mechanical ventilation, or use other life-sustaining interventions in such a patient may regard these actions as cruel and inhumane.[31] Moreover, physicians and other care givers have a legitimate interest in seeing that their knowledge and skills are used wisely and effectively. For example, if surgeons were repeatedly pressured to perform operations that they believed to be inappropriate, they would certainly suffer a loss of dignity and sense of purpose. Although appealing to professional ideals can serve as a convenient means of protecting the interests of physicians at the expense of patients' values, these ideals are legitimate factors to weigh against other values. To dismiss this perspective as irrelevant in decision making is to deny an essential part of what it means to practice medicine.

Although we believe that health care professionals should not be required to take part in care that violates their own morals, the law in this area remains uncertain. On the one hand, courts have upheld a state interest in protecting the ethical integrity of the medical profession. This may provide some basis for protecting doctors who wish to refrain from cruel or inhumane treatment, despite the wishes of the patient or surrogate.[32] On the other hand, in the two cases that have led to court decisions (those of Helga Wanglie[3] and of Jane Doe in Atlanta[33]) the judges upheld the surrogates' decision-making authority. Clearly, this area of the law remains to be defined.

Finally, social consensus is yet another expression of the values at stake in some medical decisions. In a pluralistic society, differences in personal values and interests occasionally run so deep that they cannot be resolved by the introduction of additional facts or by further private debate. At certain critical junctures, the resolution of these conflicts may require an explicit public process of social decision making.[34] Social consensus has been sought, for example, to address the issue of fair allocation of resources.[27] The involvement of society is also essential when the most highly charged questions of morality are at stake, as in the increasingly heated debate over euthanasia.[35]

In the prototypical scenarios described at the outset of this article, an ongoing attempt to achieve social consensus is perhaps most conspicuous with regard to the prolongation of life for patients in a persistent vegetative state. From a legal perspective, the relevant decisions began with the case of Karen Quinlan[36] and have extended through that of Nancy Cruzan.[37] These cases have increased awareness of the ethical issues raised by the situation of patients in a persistent vegetative state and have helped to consolidate the view that it is acceptable to withdraw life-sustaining treatment from patients in such a state. Controversy does remain about who has the ultimate authority to make these decisions. Some hold that the choice must remain with the patient or surrogate, whereas others believe that under some circumstances this prerogative may be overridden. For example, the Hastings Center[38] and the Society of Critical Care Medicine[39] have concluded that providing intensive care to patients in a persistent vegetative state is generally a misuse of resources, and the President's Commission stated that such patients should be removed from life support if such action is necessary to benefit another patient who is not in a persistent vegetative state.[40] It is unclear how this debate will conclude, but the confluence of medical, legal, and ethical thinking about the persistent vegetative state is an example of how social consensus may evolve.

In summary, the Wanglie case demonstrates how the resolution of these conflicts must proceed on many levels. Most such cases will benefit from sustained attempts to clarify the patient's values and the likelihood of the various relevant outcomes, and to improve communication with patients or their surrogates. When this approach fails, physicians and other care givers should ask themselves whether the care requested is consistent with their professional ethics and ideals. When these ideals appear to be violated, either alternative venues for such care should be found or the broader review could be provided through institutional mechanisms, such as the hospital's ethics committee, or by the courts. The public scrutiny that attends such cases will further the debate over the appropriate use of medical resources and foster the development of consensus through legislation and public policy.

CONCLUSION

In outlining the perspectives of the principal stakeholders—patients and their surrogates, physicians, and society—we have avoided the construction of a rigid formula for resolving conflicts over interventions frequently regarded as futile. Because of clinical heterogeneity, pluralistic values, and the evolutionary nature of social consensus, most clinical decision making on behalf of critically ill patients defies reduction to universally applicable principles.

The notion of futility generally fails to provide an ethically coherent ground for limiting life-sustaining treatment, except in circumstances in which narrowly defined physiologic futility can be plausibly invoked. Futility has been conceptualized as an objective entity independent of the patient's or surrogate's perspective, but differences in values and the variable probabilities of clinical outcomes undermine its basis. Furthermore, assertions of futility may camouflage judgments of comparative worth that are implicit in debates about the allocation of resources. In short, the problem with futility is that its promise of objectivity can rarely be fulfilled. The rapid advance of the language of futility into the jargon of bioethics should be followed by an equally rapid retreat.

Notes

1. *Jacobellis v. State of Ohio*, 84 S Ct 1676 (1964).
2. Hippocrates. The art. In: Reiser SJ, Dyck AJ, Curran WJ. eds. *Ethics in medicine: historical perspectives and contemporary concerns*. Cambridge. Mass.: MIT Press, 1977; 6–7.
3. Capron AM. In re Helga Wanglie. *Hastings Cent Rep* 1991; 21(5):26–8.
4. Lantos JD, Singer PA, Walker RM, et al. The illusion of futility in clinical practice. *Am J Med* 1989; 87:81–4.
5. Standards for cardiopulmonary resuscitation (CPR) and emergency cardiac care (ECC). V. Medicolegal considerations and recommendations. *JAMA* 1974; 227:Suppl:864–6.
6. Appendix A: the proposed legislation. In: *Do not resuscitate orders: the proposed legislation and report of the New York State Task Force on Life and the Law*. 2nd ed. New York: The Task Force, 1986; 83.
7. 1984 Amendments to the Child Abuse Prevention and Treatment Act. Pub Law 98-457. 1984.
8. Council on Ethical and Judicial Affairs. American Medical Association. Guidelines for the appropriate use of do-not-resuscitate orders. *JAMA* 1991; 265:1868–71.
9. Miles SH. Informed demand for "non-beneficial" medical treatment. *N Engl J Med* 1991; 325:512–5.
10. Brain-damaged woman at center of lawsuit over life-support dies. *New York Times*. July 5, 1991:A8.
11. Paris JJ, Crone RK, Reardon F. Physicians' refusal of requested treatment: the case of Baby L. *N Engl J Med* 1990; 322:1012–5.
12. Blackhall LJ. Must we always use CPR? *N Engl J Med* 1987; 317:1281–5.
13. Hackler JC, Hiller PC. Family consent to orders not to resuscitate: reconsidering hospital policy. *JAMA* 1990; 264:1281–3.
14. Murphy DJ. Do-not-resuscitate orders: time for reappraisal in long-term–care institutions. *JAMA* 1988; 260:2098–101.
15. Bedell SE, Delbanco TL, Cook EF, Epstein FH. Survival after cardiopulmonary resuscitation in the hospital. *N Engl J Med* 1983; 309:569–76.
16. Danis M, Gerrity MS, Southerland LI, Patrick DL. A comparison of patient, family, and physician assessments of the value of medical intensive care. *Crit Care Med* 1988; 16:594–600.
17. Danis M, Jarr SL, Southerland LI, Nocella RS, Patrick DL. A comparison of patient, family, and nurse evaluations of the usefulness of intensive care. *Crit Care Med* 1987; 15:138–43.
18. Danis M, Patrick DL, Southerland LI, Green ML. Patients' and families' preferences for medical intensive care. *JAMA* 1988; 260:797–802.
19. Schneiderman LJ, Jecker NS, Jonsen AR. Medical futility: its meaning and ethical implications. *Ann Intern Med* 1990; 112:949–54.
20. The Hastings Center. *Guidelines on the termination of life-sustaining treatment and the care of the dying*. Bloomington: Indiana University Press 1987:32.
21. Appendix C: New York Public Health Law Article 29-B — orders not to resuscitate. In: *Do not resuscitate orders: the proposed legislation and report of the New York State Task Force on Life and the Law*. 2nd ed. New York: The Task Force, 1986:96.
22. Tversky A, Kahneman D. Judgment under uncertainty: heuristics and biases. *Science* 1974; 185:1124–31.
23. Elstein AS. Clinical judgment: psychological research and medical practice. *Science* 1976; 194:696–700.
24. Poses RM, Bekes C, Copare FJ, Scott WE. The answer to "What are my chances, doctor?" depends on whom is asked: prognostic disagreement and inaccuracy for critically ill patients. *Crit Care Med* 1989; 17:827–33.

25. Poses RM, Cebul RD, Collins M, Fager SS. The accuracy of experienced physicians' probability estimates for patients with sore throats: implications for decision making. *JAMA* 1985; 254:925–9.

26. Aaron H, Schwartz WB. Rationing health care: The choice before us. *Science* 1990; 247:418–22.

27. Eddy DM. What's going on in Oregon. *JAMA* 1991; 266:417–20.

28. Youngner SJ. Who defines futility? *JAMA* 1988; 260:2094–5.

29. Brennan TA. Ethics committees and decisions to limit care: the experience at the Massachusetts General Hospital. *JAMA* 1988; 260:803–7.

30. La Puma J. Consultations in clinical ethics — issues and questions in 27 cases. *West J Med* 1987; 146:633–7.

31. Braithwaite S, Thomasma DC. New guidelines on foregoing life-sustaining treatment in incompetent patients: an anti-cruelty policy. *Ann Intern Med* 1986; 104:711–5.

32. Meisel A. *The right to die.* New York: John Wiley & Sons, 1989:104.

33. In re: Doe, Civil Action No. D93064 (Fulton County, GA, October 17, 1991).

34. Callahan D. Medical futility, medical necessity: the-problem-without-a-name. *Hastings Cent Rep* 1991; 21(4):30–5.

35. Misbin RI. Physicians' aid in dying. *N Engl J Med* 1991; 325:1307–11.

36. In the Matter of Karen Ann Quinlan, an alleged incompetent. 355 A.2d 647; or 70 NJ 10. March 31, 1976.

37. Annas GJ. Nancy Cruzan and the right to die. *N Engl J Med* 1990; 323:670–3.

38. The Hastings Center. *Guidelines on the termination of life-sustaining treatment and the care of the dying.* Bloomington: Indiana University Press, 1987:112.

39. Task Force on Ethics of the Society of Critical Care Medicine. Consensus report on the ethics of foregoing life-sustaining treatments in the critically ill. *Crit Care Med* 1990; 18:1435–9.

40. President's Commission for the Study of Ethical Problems in Medicine and Biomedical and Behavioral Research. *Deciding to forego life-sustaining treatment: ethical, medical, and legal issues in treatment decisions.* Washington, D.C.: Government Printing Office, 1983:188–9.

The Case of Samuel Golubchuk and the Right to Live

Alan Jotkowitz, Shimon Glick, and Ari Z. Zivotofsky

Samuel Golubchuk, an Orthodox Jew from Manitoba, Canada, who died on June 24, 2008, was unwittingly at the center of a medical controversy with important ethical ramifications. Mr. Golubchuk, an 84-year-old patient whose precise neurological level of function was subject to debate, was artificially ventilated and fed by a gastrostomy tube during the final months of his life. However, according to all reports he was neither brain dead nor in a vegetative state. The judge who ruled on the case twice indicated that these points are in agreement between the family and the hospital (Schulman 2008). Nevertheless, the physicians directly responsible for his care, with the backing of the hospital, requested that they be allowed to remove the patient from life support, actions that the patient's daughter and son vehemently opposed. The family also maintained that the patient himself would have opposed the removal of the life support, as this action would be contrary to Orthodox Jewish law, which does not allow the withdrawal of mechanical ventilation and tube feeding with the intent of hastening death. The family twice

"The Case of Samuel Golubchuk and the Right to Live", Jotkowitz, A., Glick, S., & Zivotofsky, A.Z., *The American Journal of Bioethics* 10(3) 2010, reprinted by permission of the publisher (Taylor & Francis Group, http://www.informaworld.com

obtained a legal injunction against the discontinuation of life support.

Concurrently the College of Physicians and Surgeons of Manitoba (2008) released a new guideline, which states that the final decision to withdraw life support lies with the physician regardless of the wishes of the family or the patient. According to this 2008 guideline, the criterion for maintaining life support is the ability of the patients to recover to a level at which they are aware of themselves, their environment, and their existence. If the family disagrees with this decision to terminate life support, the physician must consult with another physician. If the consulted physician agrees, therapy may be withdrawn over the objections of the patient/proxy/representative. Even if the minimum therapeutic goal is achievable, but the physician concludes nevertheless that life-sustaining therapy should be withdrawn, and he or she obtains a consultant's agreement, the physician may withdraw life support over the express opposition of the patient/proxy/representative, if the family is given 96 hours of notice before withdrawal of life support.

In our opinion, the actions of the physicians in the case of Samuel Golubchuk and the new guidelines are highly problematic ethically for a number of reasons.

1. They are in direct contradiction to the guiding principles of Western medical ethics that have developed and have been almost universally adopted during the last century. Modern bioethics strongly endorses the concepts of informed consent and autonomy. The principle of autonomy as the focal point of modern bioethics began in part as a response to the notorious experiments performed by Nazi doctors on concentration camp inmates. The organized medical community was profoundly shocked by the involvement of physicians in these crimes. The resultant international response led to the development of the Nuremberg Code, whose first principle states that "the voluntary consent of the human subject is absolutely essential" for any research

involving human subjects. This was followed by the World Medical Association's Declaration of Helsinki in 1964, which provided recommendations to physicians on research involving human subjects. It asserts that the subject "should be informed that he or she is at liberty to abstain from participating in the study and that he or she is free to withdraw his or her consent to participation at any time." These documents focus on research ethics and place major emphasis on the principle of autonomy and informed consent. The potential research subject has to be fully informed of the potential risks and benefits of the proposed research and must give his or her consent without undue coercion or pressure. In addition, there must exist no negative consequences of nonparticipation.

Bioethicists then brought the concepts of informed consent and patient autonomy to the bedside and to the doctor–patient relationship. In the not so distant past, patients had precious little say in medical decision making relating to their health and quality of life. This way of practicing medicine was viewed as an assault on human dignity and an affront to autonomy.

Clearly there is a difference between the relationship of the researcher to his or her subject and the relationship of the physician to his or her patient. The primary goal of the investigator is to advance science, while that of the doctor is to heal the patient. But for the application of the principle of patient autonomy this distinction makes little difference. In both instances the research subjects and the patients must give full consent for their treatment and anything less is unethical, even if the physician believes that he or she is acting in the best interest of the patient. According to this paradigm, not only do patients have to consent regarding their treatment but they should also play the role of primary decision maker regarding their care.

Based on this principle, in addition to deciding how he or she should be treated, the patient also has a number of fundamental human rights, including the right to die. Heretofore it had always been taken for granted that a patient has a right to live as well as a right to determine how he or she may die. Studies show that patients still prefer that the choice be theirs even though it may conflict with what the physician anticipates (Kobza and Erne 2007). The new guidelines represent a retreat from autonomy toward old-fashioned paternalism.

Because of the dominance of the autonomy principle there is virtually universal agreement that physicians may not impose even beneficial unwanted therapy on a patient. Autonomy trumps beneficence. But now in the converse situation in which the patient rather than the physician insists on treatment, autonomy suddenly loses its dominance. This turn of events represents a dramatic reversal of the tradition of medicine in which life has always been the default position.

The conflict between the Golubchuk family and their physicians mirrors the situation with the late Helga Wanglie, an 86-year-old Minneapolis woman who had been in a persistent vegetative state for over a year and whose physicians wanted her to be removed from a respirator against her husband's wishes. Mr. Golubchuk's condition is significantly better that was that of Helga Wanglie. In the Wanglie case the judge decided clearly in favor of Mr. Wanglie's position (*In re Helga Wanglie* 1991), and indeed his view coincided with that of many authorities in bioethics.

Marcia Angell (1991) in her editorial on the case stated, "Any other decision by the court would have been inimical to patient autonomy and would have undermined the consensus on the right to die that has been carefully crafted since the Quinlan case."

Alexander Capron stated (1991) that "the real peril is that physicians will unilaterally decide to limit or cease treatment (for example, to write a do-not-resuscitate [DNR] order) based on their own assessments of what outcomes are worth pursuing, without ever affording their patients or patients' surrogates the opportunity to join them in the process of making such decisions."

In the famous Terri Schiavo case that was the source of so much national debate and 12 years of court battles, the issue centered about the wishes of the patient in the vegetative state. But no one involved in the case even dared suggest that withdrawal of care could be considered if the patient had not so desired. It is hard not to be convinced about the realities of the so-called slippery slope, if one considers the slope between Kathryn Quinlan and Samuel Golubchuk.

As Daar (1995) pointed out in a U.S. legal review several years ago, "To date, in nearly every known case in which the patient has sought treatment and the doctor has objected on the grounds that the treatment offers no medical benefit, courts have found in favor of the patient,"

2. There has been much talk recently in medical education and medical ethics circles about the importance of teaching medicine and ethics from a culturally sensitive perspective (Klessig 1992). In addition, the impact of globalization on modern medicine mandates a broad cultural perspective. The AAMC and the ACGME now both require training with respect to the impact of culture on medical care. The position of Samuel Golubchuk's physicians and the new guidelines seem to act with a lack of appropriate sensitivity to their patient's particular culture:

a. Samuel Golubchuk comes from a culture that values life highly. Jewish tradition gives great weight to the concept of the sanctity of life, albeit not at all costs (Gesundheit et al. 2009). The leading American Jewish Orthodox ethical authority of the past century, the late Rabbi Moshe Feinstein (d. 1986), maintained that one is not required to initiate life support to a suffering terminally ill patient, but withdrawal of such is not sanctioned. This differentiation between withholding and withdrawing has been referred to as a myth (Meisel, Snyder, and Quill 2000) and is dismissed by leading ethicists. Nevertheless, in the same issue of the journal in which the differentiation is referred to as a myth, a poll of neonatologists in 10 European countries revealed that about two-thirds of them felt that there was a difference from an ethical point of view (Rebagliato et al. 2000). This distinction was recently observed among German intensive care unit (ICU) physicians as well (Beck S van de Loo and Reiter-Theil 2008). Many other religions and traditions would also have similar attitudes toward end-of-life care. To override these attitudes by the medical establishment might well be characterized as cultural imperialism. Judaism, and until recently Western ethics as well, considers the decision to terminate life as an ethical, rather than purely a medical decision. The present Manitoba ruling represents a dramatic change, by granting physicians the unilateral authority to make the ultimate ethical decision.

b. Besides the religious aspects of the case, there are also other cultural factors that need to be considered. Mr. Golubchuk is a member of a society that was almost destroyed 60 years ago in the Holocaust. During that period physicians took upon themselves criminal liberties in depriving innocent humans of their lives. It is possible that these events that occurred during Mr. Golubchuk's lifetime may have contributed to the family's position. We offer this explanation not because we believe there is any moral or ethical connection between the events but simply as a possible cultural explanation of why many Jews attach so much importance to the sanctity of life.

If one accepts these new guidelines that take away decision-making power from the families and hand it over to physicians, it is incumbent upon us to recognize the potential negative impact this policy may have on the trust that deprived and underprivileged socioeconomic groups have for the medical establishment. It is well documented that certain lower socioeconomic groups have not been treated fairly by the medical community and are already suspicious of the health care system (Dula 1994).

What assurance do we have that these same groups will not be the first to be denied care under the new guidelines or that other groups will not develop similar distrust of the medical system?

3. Aside from purely ethical, philosophic, and societal considerations, there are also medical and physiological problems with the physicians' decisions. The ability of physicians to predict life expectancy in terminally ill patients has been shown repeatedly to be quite limited (Christakis 2000), and there have been many anecdotal reports of surprising degrees of patient recovery in spite of dire predictions by the best of physicians (Login 2001). In addition, even in the cases of patients in a persistent vegetative state, which does not describe Mr. Golubchuk, newer data have shown surprising degrees of awareness and even recovery (Owen et al. 2006) in such patients. Last year another Canadian, Zongwu Jin, 66, fell into a coma after falling and hitting his head. Doctors "determined" that his brain injury was so traumatic that they issued a DNR order with the agreement of the patient's family. He is now speaking and writing (Beauchamp 2007).

We can accept the prioritization of care based on chances for recovery, and certainly these decisions have to be made and are made daily in every intensive care unit in the world. The principle of justice mandates such an approach. Thus, it would be legitimate in our opinion to give Mr. Golubchuk's intensive care unit bed to another patient with higher priority. But we cannot accept positive interventions whose express intention is to put an end to Mr. Golubchuk's life.

It may also be incumbent upon societies with limited resources—and all societies are to some extent limited in what they can offer—to set societal priorities on what medical resources are to be provided at societal expense. But these are societal and not medical responsibilities. The physicians have the expertise and knowledge, which they provide to society's decision makers, but it is not they who may arbitrarily impose their values on their patients. This issue is of course more pressing in countries with some form of socialized medicine, such as Canada, but these decisions should not be solely in the hands of physicians. In response to these real financial pressures, countries such as Britain and Israel have begun to develop mechanisms to limit health care expenditures on the basis of a national discussion of health care priorities. Until a society undergoes this process, it is not the role of a physician to play God, legislator, or judge. Samuel Golubchuk should have been allowed to live according to his personal values and health care beliefs.

References

Angell, M. 1991. The case of Helga Wanglie—A new kind of "right to die" case. *New England Journal of Medicine* 325: 511–512.

Beauchamp, P. 2007. Court fight saved man's life, family says: Do-not-resuscitate order fought. *Calgary Herald* November 24.

Beck S van de Loo, A., and S. Reiter-Theil. 2008. A "little bit illegal"? Withholding and withdrawing of mechanical ventilation in the eyes of German intensive care physicians. *Medicine, Health Care and Philosophy* 11: 7–16.

Capron, A. M. 1991. In re Helga Wanglie. *Hastings Center Report* September–October: 26–28.

Christakis, N. A. 2000. Extent and determinants of error in doctors' prognoses in terminally ill patients: A cohort study. *British Medical Journal* 320: 469–473.

College of Physicians and Surgeons of Manitoba. 2007. Withholding and withdrawing life-sustaining treatment. Statement no. 1602. Available at www.cpsm.mb.ca/statements/st1602 (accessed January 20, 2010). 52

Daar, J. F. 1995. Medical futility and implications for physician autonomy. *American Journal of Law and Medicine* 21: 221–240.

Dula, A. 1994. African American suspicion of the healthcare system is justified: what do we do about it? *Cambridge Quarterly of Healthcare Ethics* 3: 347–357.

Gesundheit, B., A. Steinberg, S. Blazer, and A. Jotkowitz. 2009. The Groningen Protocol—The Jewish perspective. *Neonatology* 96(1); 6–10.

In re Helga Wanglie. 1991. Fourth Judicial District (Dist. Ct. Probate Ct. Div) PX-91-283. Minnesota, Hennepin County.

Klessig, J. 1992 Cross-cultural medicine—A decade later. *Western Journal of Medicine* 157: 316–322.

Kobza, R., and P. Erne. 2007. End-of-life decisions in ICD patients with malignant tumors. *Pacing and Clinical Electrophysiology* 30: 845–849.

Login, I. S. 2001. Memoir: A miracle of Chanukah. *Neurology* 57: 2146–2147.

Meisel, A., L. Snyder, and T. Quill. 2000. Seven legal barriers to end-of-life care: Myths, realities and grains of truth. *Journal of the American Medical Association* 284: 2495–2501.

Owen, A. M., M. R. Coleman, M. Boly, M. H. Davis, S. Laureys, and J. D. Pickard. 2006. Detecting awareness in the vegetative state. *Science* 313: 1402.

Rebagliato, M., M. Cuttini, L. Broggin, et al. 2000. Neonatal end-of-life decision making: Physicians' attitudes and relationship with self-reported practices in 10 European countries. *JAMA* 284: 2451–2459.

Schulman, J. 2008. *Golubchuk v. Salvation Army Grace General Hospital*, Court of Queens's Bench of Manitoba, 2008 MBQB 49.

The Problem With Home Remedies:
Manitoba, Doctors and Unilateral Decisions
in End-of-Life Care

Pat Murphy, George C. Webster, and Brian Chaze

In, "The Case of Samuel Golubchuk and the Right to Live," Jotkowitz, Glick, and Zivotofsky (2010) add a new name to the litany of well-known cases of contested end-of-life care. While his is a local story, it follows a familiar storyline: a critically ill person represented by his family, whose opposition to recommendations that life-sustaining interventions be withdrawn leads to an impasse in need of adjudication. Furthermore, the authors note a twist in this story, namely, the concurrent public release by the College of Physicians and Surgeons of Manitoba (CPSM) of its "Statement on Withholding and Withdrawing Life-Sustaining Treatment" (2008a; 2008b).

The authors judge both "the actions of the physicians in the case of Mr. Samuel Golubchuk and the new guidelines" to be "highly problematic ethically" (Jotkowitz et al. 2010). As commentators, we elaborate by:

(a) Highlighting critical contextual features that gave rise to the CPSM Statement.
(b) Describing how the CPSM Statement inappropriately extends doctors' legitimate authority by disguising moral judgments as medical decisions.
(c) Identifying why the CPSM Statement's resort to unilateral decision making as the remedy to address impasse is ethically wanting.

The authors believe Mr. Golubchuk was "unwittingly at the center of a medical controversy with important ethical ramifications" (Jotkowitz et al. 2010). We believe Mr. Golubchuk

was unwittingly at the center of an ethical controversy with important medical ramifications. In Manitoba, this controversy predated, and survives, Mr. Golubchuk.

On January 30, 2008, when the CPSM announced the formal adoption of its statement, it asserted that the statement would "result in greater transparency, clarity and consistency in cases where the withholding or withdrawing of life-sustaining treatment is being considered" (CPSM 2008). This promise implied that such transparency, clarity and consistency was somehow lacking, and, that the CPSM Statement offered the corrective. Where did this come from? What was the "problem" in need of remedy?

On January 30, 2008, reports in the media portrayed the problem as "Who has the final word about stopping life-sustaining treatment?" Mr. Golubchuk's plight was the topic of heated exchanges. The parties involved were alternately praised for their courage and/or demonized for their unreasonableness. Understandably, the College's announcement appeared all too coincidental in its timing. Many did not know that the CPSM Statement was a long time in the making.

Winnipeg had already generated two notable court decisions addressing matters of conflicted end-of-life care, namely, *Child and Family Services of Central Manitoba v. Lavallee* (1997) and *Sawatzky v. Riverview Health Centre* (1998).

Lavallee (1997), addressed the matter of a do-not-resuscitate (DNR) order for an infant against the wishes of his parents (Sneiderman

---

1999). This decision set the stage for what would follow in the CPSM Statement 11 years later:

> Neither consent nor a court order in lieu is required for a medical doctor to issue a non-resuscitation direction where in his or her judgment the patient is in an irreversible vegetative state. Whether or not such a decision should be issued is a judgment call for the doctor to make having regard to the patient's history and condition and the doctor's evaluation of the hopelessness of the case. The wishes of the patient's family or guardian should be taken into account, but neither their consent nor the approval of a court is required.

Within a year, Winnipeg was again the focus of attention regarding Mr. Andrew Sawatzky, an elderly gentleman with Parkinson's disease, whose wife, Helene, sought an interim injunction when, having been effectively replaced as her husband's decision maker, she learned that a DNR order had been placed on her husband's health record without her knowledge. In granting the injunction, Justice Beard questioned whether the then current legal position, *Lavallee,* was definitive because it did not consider the application of existing human rights legislation, such as, the Canadian *Charter of Rights and Freedoms* or Manitoba's *Human Rights Code.*

In the years between *Sawatzky* and *Golubchuk,* the Manitoba Law Reform Commission invited comment on its "Discussion Paper on Withholding and Withdrawing Life-Sustaining Treatment" (MLRC 2003, 37), stating in the introduction:

> In order to satisfy the general public and the medical profession, the following broadly based issues need to be addressed:
>
> 1. In what circumstances is it appropriate to withhold or withdraw life-sustaining treatment?
> 2. Who should decide when it is appropriate?

The Manitoba Law Reform Commission's report made five recommendations but stopped short of recommending legislation. Notably, it recommended that the "sample policy" of the CPSM be amended to address suggestions in the report; that it be formulated as a statement of the College; and that it "be accepted by the health care system...as the definitive and authoritative template for end-of-life medical decision making" (MLRC 2003, 32). The "home remedy" was thus conceived, gestated some 48 months, and ultimately delivered at the height of the *Golubchuk* case.

The process outlined in the CPSM Statement contains all of the essential ingredients: clinical assessments; communication between physicians and patients or their representatives; development, implementation, and documentation of an agreed-upon care plan. However, in circumstances where there is an impasse, the remedy offered in the CPSM Statement fails, largely due to two ethically problematic ingredients: the "final say" problem and the "minimum goal of life-sustaining treatment" problem.

The "final say" problem emanates from the CPSM Statement's assertion that "physicians have the authority to make medical decisions to withhold or withdraw life-sustaining treatment from a patient without the consent of the patient or the patient's family" (CPSM 2008b, 15-S2). The CPSM Statement provides no substantive account of physicians' *moral* authority to act unilaterally. Their presumed *legal* authority is also in question. This point is underscored in Justice Schulman's ruling extending the injunction in *Golubchuk* (2008, 20):

> Contrary to the assertion of the defendants, it is not settled law that, in the event of a disagreement between a physician and his patient as to withdrawal of life supports, the physician has the final say.

The "announcement" of a conclusion about a difficult ethical question does not necessarily mean that it is the "right" answer. The conclusion announced to the public in the CPSM Statement is a matter far from resolved in law, bioethics, or social policy here in Manitoba or elsewhere.

One only needs to refer to the summary of the public forum held on June 9, 2008, in Winnipeg to see that disability scholars, ethicists, and legal scholars have serious concerns about the statement (VP-Net 2008).

The "minimum goal of life-sustaining treatment" (CPSM 2008b, 15-S3) problem is the most egregious ingredient in the College's "home remedy." The term, one that we were unable to reference in medical, legal, and/or bioethics literature, serves as the qualifying criterion for assessing whether or not life-sustaining treatment will be initiated, withheld, or withdrawn. It is defined as follows:

> Clinically, the minimum goal of *life-sustaining treatment* is to recover or maintain a level of function that enables the patient to achieve awareness of self and environment and to experience his/her own existence.

Assessments of "appropriate" goals of treatment are fundamentally ethical judgments, not clinical judgments. While physicians may properly assess the anticipated effectiveness of interventions, their medical expertise, per se, does not qualify them to assess the worthwhileness, or value, of interventions. By modifying the pivotal ingredient of its remedy as "clinically" defined, the CPSM Statement dresses up an ethical judgment as a medical decision. Such a ploy inevitably leaves patients subject to the personal or idiosyncratic views of physicians (Veatch 2009, 22).

Some will conclude that the "home remedy" in the CPSM Statement is the best that can be hoped for in an impasse. We hold that the harm to the integrity of all parties to such disputes requires a more thoughtful response. Given enduring ethical difference about "What kind of a life is a life worth living?," we would make the case for a more conciliatory approach than the one envisioned in the CPSM Statement. Instead of the "final" decision effectively defaulting to physicians, the community should require third-party mediation, dispute resolution, or court adjudication. The costs, in time and money, are a small price to pay to protect both the rightful place of patients and families in health care decision making and the integrity of the relationship between physicians and those entrusted to their care.

References

Child and Family Services of Central Manitoba v. R.L. and S.L.H. (1997), 154 D.L.R. (4th) 409; 123 Man. R. (2d) 135.

College of Physicians and Surgeons of Manitoba. 2008a. Withholding and withdrawing life-sustaining treatment. Statement no. 1602. Available at: www.cpsm.mb.ca/statements/st1602.pdf (accessed December 14, 2009).

College of Physicians and Surgeons of Manitoba. 2008b. *Process for withholding or withdrawing life-sustaining treatment released: Statement effective Feb. 1st, 2008—Binding on all Manitoba Physicians,* ed. General Public and Local Media. Press release. Winnipeg.

Golubchuk v. Salvation Army Grace General Hospital et al. (2008), 290 D.L.R. (4th) 46; 8W.W.R. 299; 227 Man. R. (2d) 209.

Jotkowitz, A., S. Glick, and A. Z. Zivotofsky. 2010. The case of Samuel Golubchuk and the right to live. *American Journal of Bioethics* 10(3): 50–53.

Manitoba Law Reform Commission. 2003. *Withholding or withdrawing life sustaining medical treatment (Report #109).* Winnipeg, Manitoba: MLRC.

Sawatzky v. Riverview Health Centre Incorporated (1998), 167 D.L.R. (4th) 359 (Man. Q.B.).

Sneiderman, B. 1999. A do not resuscitate order for an infant against parental wishes: A comment on the case of *Child and Family Services of Central Manitoba v. R.L. and S.L.H. Health Law Journal* 7: 205–231.

Veatch, R. 2009. *Patient, heal thyself: How the new medicine puts the patient in charge.* New York: Oxford University Press.

VP-Net. 2008. 2008 VP-Net end-of-life ethics and decision-making forum. University of Manitoba. Available at: www.umanitoba.ca/outreach/vpnet/about-events-ethicsevent.html (accessed December 14, 2009).

Unsustainable Distinctions

Jocelyn Downie

NATURE OF CONDUCT (ACT VS OMISSION)[1]

The acts/omissions distinction argument generally takes the following form: (1) to omit to save a life is acceptable whereas to act to end life is unacceptable; (2) the withholding and withdrawal of potentially life-sustaining treatment are omissions, but assisted suicide and euthanasia are acts; (3) therefore, the withholding and withdrawal of potentially life-sustaining treatment are acceptable but assisted suicide and voluntary euthanasia are not.[2]

There are at least two bases on which to lay a claim that the distinction between acts and omissions is not a sustainable distinction upon which to ground public policy with respect to assisted death. First, the withdrawal of potentially life-sustaining treatment is as much an act as assisted suicide and euthanasia are acts. Second, there is no moral significance to the distinction between acts and omissions.

First, consider my claim that the withdrawal of potentially life-sustaining treatment is an act. In the context of assisted death, something is an act when you *do* something knowing that, but for your action, the person would not die. Something is an omission when you *do not do* something knowing that, but for your omission, the person would not die.[3] When you withhold a necessary blood transfusion you are *not doing* something knowing that, but for your inaction, the person would not die. Therefore, withholding treatment is an omission. When you withdraw a respirator you are *doing* something knowing that, but for your act, the person would not die. Therefore, withdrawing treatment is an act. When you give a person a lethal injection you are *doing* something knowing that but for your act the person would not die. Therefore, euthanasia is an act. Therefore, it cannot be concluded that the withholding and withdrawal of potentially life-sustaining treatment are acceptable because they are omissions, and assisted suicide and euthanasia are unacceptable because they are acts. Withholding is an omission, while withdrawal, assisted suicide, and euthanasia are acts.

This is not to say that one cannot draw a distinction between the withholding and withdrawal of potentially life-sustaining treatment, on the one hand, and assisted suicide and euthanasia, on the other, and find significance in the distinction. It is simply to say that this distinction does not map onto the distinction between acts and omissions and that therefore one cannot hang the assessment of the withholding and withdrawal of potentially life-sustaining treatment versus assisted suicide and voluntary euthanasia on the distinction between acts and omissions.

Second, consider my claim that there is no significance to the distinction between acts and omissions.[4] James Rachels makes this argument through the following well-known, oft-repeated, and hotly contested illustration:

1. Smith stands to gain a large inheritance if anything should happen to his six-year-old cousin. One evening while the child is taking his bath, Smith sneaks into the bathroom and drowns the child, and then arranges things so that it will look like an accident.

2. Jones also stands to gain if anything should happen to his six-year-old cousin. Like Smith, Jones sneaks in planning to drown the child in his bath. However, just as he

Downie, J. (2004) "Chapter Eight: Unsustainable Distinctions." In Downie, J., *Dying Justice: A Case for Decriminalizing Euthanasia and Assisted Suicide in Canada* (pp. 89–107). Toronto: University of Toronto Press. Reprinted with permission of the publisher.

enters the bathroom Jones sees the child slip, hit his head, and fall face down in the water. Jones is delighted; he stands by, ready to push the child's head back under if it is necessary, but it is not necessary. With only a little thrashing about, the child drowns all by himself, 'accidentally,' as Jones watches and does nothing.[5]

To give a related example, suppose that we have the same Smith and Jones as above. The cousin is in hospital following a car accident. He is on a respirator but is expected to recover fully. In the first scenario, Smith enters the hospital room surreptitiously and disconnects the respirator. In the second scenario, Jones visits his cousin and watches as he has a violent seizure and accidentally disconnects the power supply to the respirator. In both scenarios, the young cousin dies. Although Smith acts and Jones omits to act, both the act and the omission are reprehensible but the distinction between acts and omissions plays no role in Smith's and Jones's culpability.

A number of arguments have been made in response to the conclusion that there is no morally significant distinction between acts and omissions.[6] These arguments all share a fatal flaw: they all end up relying upon a feature *in addition to* the acts and omissions feature. The feature itself may vary between the arguments (it might be intentionality, causation, or probability of death) but the addition of a feature is shared. The addition of a feature means that something other than the distinction between acts and omissions itself is critical. For example, it might be argued in response to these examples that both Smith and Jones are culpable but that while Jones is bad, Smith is worse. The distinction between acts and omissions therefore retains moral significance. However, this response only shows that, if anything, the distinction between acts and omissions is relevant to relative culpability. It does not establish that the distinction distinguishes morally acceptable from morally

unacceptable conduct. The distinction between acts and omissions alone does not do the work desired of it. An additional element is required. Potential additional elements will be considered, and rejected, in the subsequent sections of this chapter (e.g., cause of death, probability of death, and the intention to end life).

The distinction between acts and omissions has been widely relied upon to justify distinguishing between the withholding and withdrawal of potentially life-sustaining treatment and assisted suicide and voluntary euthanasia. However, for the reasons given above, it has been fairly described as 'backed by tradition but not by reason'[7] and as 'both morally and intellectually misshapen.'[8] I too conclude that the distinction between acts and omissions must not be permitted to shape the legal regime dealing with assisted death.

CAUSE OF DEATH (DISEASE/'NATURAL' VS ACTION/'UNNATURAL')

The argument frequently made with respect to cause of death is that when a health care provider withholds or withdraws treatment, the disease kills the patient, whereas when a health care provider performs euthanasia, a drug kills the patient. Framed another way, in the former, death results from 'natural causes,' whereas in the latter, it results from 'unnatural causes.'[9] So, for example, Yale Kamisar argues, 'in letting die, the cause of death is seen as the underlying disease process or trauma. In assisted suicide/euthanasia, the cause of death is seen as the inherently lethal action itself.'[10] However, this distinction does not map at all onto the line between the withholding and withdrawal of potentially life-sustaining treatment, on the one side, and assisted suicide and voluntary euthanasia, on the other.

As with assisted suicide and euthanasia, an 'unnatural cause' (the removal of a respirator) rather than a 'natural cause' (the underlying disease) can cause death in a case involving withdrawal of potentially life-sustaining treatment. An example should help to illustrate this point.

Consider someone who had polio as a child and requires a respirator for daily living. If a thief removed the respirator from that person, few would say that the polio killed the person or that the person died of 'natural causes.' Most, if not all, would say that the removal of the respirator killed the person and the person died of 'unnatural causes.' Consider also a person with a pacemaker. Someone intentionally releases a strong electromagnetic pulse when she enters a room, the pulse causes her pacemaker to stop working, and she dies. Did she die of natural causes? Was the agent of her death the underlying heart disease that required that she have a pacemaker or was it the electromagnetic pulse? Most, if not all, would say that the pulse killed the woman and that she died of 'unnatural causes,' and yet, this is ultimately an example of withdrawal of treatment.[11]

One could respond to these examples by denying the intuition that the person who took the respirator or released the electromagnetic pulse caused the death. One could claim that the person did not cause the death but was nonetheless culpable in the death. However, this manoeuvre will not rescue this distinction for the purposes of sustaining differential treatment of withholding and withdrawing life-sustaining treatment, on the one hand, and assisted suicide and euthanasia, on the other, because on this manoeuvre a person who withdraws treatment is culpable. Both culpable and nonculpable conduct will be found on both sides of the line drawn by causation.[12] Thus, even by denying the causal intuition, the distinction fails to do the work required of it. Again, something else is required to sustain the differential treatment.

PROBABILITY OF DEATH (CERTAINTY VS POSSIBILITY)

It might be argued that a distinction can be drawn between acts and omissions with a certainty of causing death and acts and omissions with just a possibility of causing death. This distinction might then be linked to the withholding and

withdrawal of potentially life-sustaining treatment, on the one hand, and assisted suicide and euthanasia, on the other. However, again, there can be as much certainty of death in a case involving the withdrawal of potentially life-sustaining treatment as there can be in a case of euthanasia. For example, when artificial hydration and nutrition are withdrawn from a patient in a persistent vegetative state, death is certain. Similarly, when a lethal dose of potassium chloride is given to a patient, death is certain. Again, this distinction fails to do the work expected or desired of it.

INTENTION (TO END LIFE VS TO ALLEVIATE SUFFERING)

Intention is frequently cited in an attempt to draw a distinction between the withholding and withdrawal of potentially life-sustaining treatment, on the one hand, and euthanasia, on the other. Some argue that the intention of withholding and withdrawal of potentially life-sustaining treatment is to alleviate suffering while the intention of assisted suicide and euthanasia is to end life. Hastening death with the intention of alleviating suffering is considered acceptable and hastening death with the intention of ending life is considered unacceptable. Therefore, they conclude, the withholding and withdrawal of potentially life-sustaining treatment are acceptable and assisted suicide and euthanasia are not.

One must, however, distinguish between two senses of intention: subjective foresight and motive or goal. Death is frequently a known consequence of the withholding and withdrawal of potentially life-sustaining treatment. Therefore, on this meaning of intention, the argument dissolves. Similarly, the motive or goal of all forms of assisted death is to alleviate suffering. Therefore, on this meaning of intention, the argument also dissolves. Consider each of these rejoinders in greater detail.

First, consider the issue of foresight. Just as when a health care provider injects a lethal dose of potassium chloride, when a health care provider withdraws artificial hydration and nutrition, he or she knows that a consequence of that action will be death. The subjective foresight test can be met by categories of assisted death on either side of the line between withholding and withdrawal of potentially life-sustaining treatment and assisted suicide and euthanasia.

Second, consider the issue of motive or goal. When a health care provider withdraws artificial hydration and nutrition, his or her motive is to alleviate suffering. When a health care provider injects a lethal dose of potassium chloride, his or her motive is to alleviate suffering. Again, the motive test can be met by categories of assisted death on either side of the line.

It is here that the principle of double effect must be considered. On this principle, 'it is sometimes permissible to bring about by oblique intention what one may not directly intend.'[13] However, this principle cannot ground a distinction between the categories of assisted death because it, too, captures some events on both sides of the line. Just as when a health care provider injects a lethal dose of potassium chloride, when he or she withdraws artificial hydration and nutrition at the request of a patient, no primary effect excuses the secondary effect. No effect of alleviating suffering exists apart from the effect of ending life. The intention to end life is direct rather than 'oblique,' and hence, on the principle of double effect, impermissible. And yet, as shown previously, the withdrawal of artificial hydration and nutrition from a patient is legally permissible. Therefore, the principle of double effect cannot be used to ground the distinction between the withholding and withdrawal of potentially life-sustaining treatment, on the one hand, and assisted suicide and voluntary euthanasia, on the other.

NATURE OF THE EFFECT OF THE PROHIBITION (VIOLATION OF BODILY INTEGRITY VS NO VIOLATION)

It might be argued that, in its effort to preserve individuals' lives, the state is willing to override autonomy unless that would require violating the patients' bodily integrity. On this view, treating competent individuals against their will violates bodily integrity and would therefore be unacceptable, but preventing third parties from assisting with a suicide or committing euthanasia does not violate the individual's bodily integrity and would therefore be acceptable. In the first type of case, by allowing third parties to treat patients against their wishes, the state would allow third parties to violate the patients' bodily integrity (evoking images of strapping an unwilling patient to an operating table). Whereas, in the second type of case, by not permitting third parties to provide patients with assisted suicide or euthanasia, the state is merely preventing third parties from doing something to the patients and is not allowing any violation of bodily integrity. Thus, it might be claimed, a bright line is drawn between the withholding and withdrawal of potentially life-sustaining treatment, on the one side, and euthanasia and assisted suicide, on the other.

This distinction does not, however, do the work required of it. Suicide and attempted suicide are legal and the state could prevent them without violating bodily integrity (e.g., by confining suicidal individuals). Potentially life-shortening palliative treatment is legal and the deaths caused by it could be prevented without violations of bodily integrity (by simply not allowing the provision of potentially life-shortening palliative treatment). These are two examples of situations in which the state could preserve individuals' lives without violating the individuals' bodily integrity—yet chooses not to.

Therefore, it can be concluded that the distinction based on violation of bodily integrity does not support permitting the provision of potentially life-shortening palliative treatment and the withholding and withdrawal of potentially life-sustaining treatment, on the one hand, and prohibiting assisted suicide and euthanasia, on the other.

OTHER AREAS OF LAW

It should be noted that these five distinctions are not uniformly applied in other areas of law to distinguish between culpable and non-culpable conduct. Acts that cause death are sometimes regarded as non-culpable conduct (e.g., shooting a person in self-defence or war) and omissions that cause death are sometimes regarded as culpable conduct (e.g., a lifeguard leaving a child to drown in a pool). Naturally caused death sometimes generates ascriptions of culpability (e.g., not taking a child with pneumonia to a physician for treatment) and unnaturally caused death sometimes fails to generate ascriptions of culpability (e.g., shooting a home invader who is trying to kill your child). Causing a certain death is sometimes regarded as non-culpable conduct (e.g., shooting a person who is threatening you with a gun). Causing an uncertain death is sometimes regarded as culpable conduct (shooting someone in the abdomen such that it is possible but not certain that he will die). Intending to end life (on both senses of intention) is not always culpable (e.g., shooting a person in self-defence). Ending life unintentionally is sometimes culpable (e.g., manslaughter). Violating bodily integrity is sometimes non-culpable (e.g., shooting in self-defence or war). Not violating bodily integrity is sometimes culpable (e.g., a lifeguard not saving a drowning swimmer or a parent not taking his child with pneumonia to a doctor). Clearly, these distinctions are not used on their own in the law to distinguish between culpable and non-culpable conduct. Something more is needed.

Notes

1. An excellent collection of articles on the distinction between killing and letting die is B. Steinbock and A. Norcross, eds., *Killing and Letting Die*, 2nd ed. (New York: Fordham University Press, 1994). This collection includes many of the classic articles in the field as well as nine original contributions.

2. The active/passive distinction has been the subject of much discussion in both the philosophical and legal literature. Leading proponents of the active/passive distinction include: Y. Kamisar, 'Against Assisted Suicide—Even a Very Limited Form' (1995) *U. Det. Mercy L. Rev.* 735, and 'Euthanasia Legislation: Some Nonreligious Objections' in T. Beauchamp and S. Perlin, eds. *Ethical Issues in Death and Dying* (New York: Oxford University

Press, 1978) 222; and D. Callahan, 'Self-Extinction: The Morality of the Helping Hand' in R. Weir, ed., *Physician-Assisted Suicide* (Bloomington: Indiana University Press, 1997) 69.

3. Dan Brock characterizes the distinction in a similar manner: 'One kills when one performs an action that causes the death of a person (e.g., we are in a boat, you cannot swim, I push you overboard, and you drown), and one allows to die when one has the ability and opportunity to prevent the death of another, knows this, and omits doing so, with the result that the person dies (e.g., we are in a boat, you cannot swim, you fall overboard, I don't throw you an available life ring, and you drown).' D. Brock, 'Physician-Assisted Suicide Is Sometimes Morally Justified' in Weir, ed., supra, n2 at 86.

4. The most influential proponent of this position is James Rachels. See, e.g., his 'Euthanasia, Killing, and Letting Die' in J. Ladd, ed., *Ethical Issues Relating to Life and Death* (New York: Oxford University Press, 1979) at 146, which is a longer version of the more frequently cited 'Active and Passive Euthanasia' (1975) 292 *N.E.J.M.* at 78–80; and J. Rachels, *The End of Life* (Oxford: Oxford University Press, 1986). One of the most active proponents of this position is D. Brock; see, e.g., 'Voluntary Active Euthanasia,' (1992) 22 *Hastings Center Report* 10–22, and 'Physician-Assisted Suicide Is Sometimes Morally Justified' in Weir, ed., supra, n2 at 86; 'Forgoing Food and Water: Is It Killing?' in J. Lynn, ed. *By No Extraordinary Means: The Choice to Forgo Life-Sustaining Food and Water* (Bloomington: Indiana University Press, 1986); 'Moral Rights and Permissible Killing' in J. Ladd, ed., *Ethical Issues Relating to Life and Death* (Oxford: Oxford University Press, 1979). Other leading proponents include: M. Tooley, 'An Irrelevant Consideration: Killing versus Letting Die' in Steinbock and Norcross, *Killing and Letting Die*, supra, n1 at 103–11; and J. Bennett, 'Acting and Refraining,' (1967) 28 *Analysis* 30-1, and 'Shooting, Killing, Dying,' (1973) 2 *Can. J. Philosophy* 315–23.

5. J. Rachels, 'Euthanasia, Killing, and Letting Die,' supra, n4 at 154.

6. See, e.g.: T.D. Sullivan, 'Active and Passive Euthanasia: An Impertinent Distinction?' in Steinbock and Norcross, supra, n1 at 131-8; P. Foot, 'Killing and Letting Die' in J.L. Garfield and P. Hennessey, eds., *Abortion and Legal Perspectives* (Amherst: University of Massachussetts Press, 1984), and 'Killing, Letting Die, and Euthanasia: A Reply to Holly Smith Goldman' (1981) 41 *Analysis* 159–60.

7. Rachels, 'Euthanasia, Killing, and Letting Die,' supra, n4 at 153.

8. *Airedale* N.H.S. *Trust* v. *Bland*, [1993] Appeal Cases 789 at 887 per Lord Mustill.

9. Again, Kamisar and Callahan are among the most influential proponents of this distinction, supra, n2. This distinction was also embraced by the President's Commission for the Study of Ethical Problems in Medicine and Biomedical and Behavioral Research, *Deciding to Forego Life-Sustaining Treatment: A Report of the Ethical, Medical, and Legal Issues in Treatment Decisions* (Washington, DC: Government Printing Office, 1983).

10. Kamisar, supra, n2.

11. The pacemaker example is taken from P. Hopkins, 'Why Does Removing Machines Count as "Passive" Euthanasia?' (1997) 27 *Hastings Center Report* 29.

12. Examples of non-culpable causation of death are accidental killing and killing in self-defence.

13. P. Foot, 'The Problem of Abortion and the Doctrine of Double Effect' in Steinbock and Norcross, supra, n1 at 266. Foot continues at 267: 'The doctrine of double effect is based on a distinction between what a man foresees as a result of his voluntary action and what, in the strict sense, he intends. He intends in the strictest sense both those things that he aims at as ends and those that he aims at as a means to his ends. The latter may be regretted in themselves but nevertheless desired for the sake of the end, as we may intend to keep dangerous lunatics confined for the sake of our safety. By contrast a man is said not strictly, or directly, to intend the foreseen consequences of his voluntary actions where these are neither the end at which he is aiming nor the means to this end. Whether the word "intention" should be applied in both cases is not of course what matters: Bentham spoke of "oblique intention," contrasting it with the "direct intention" of ends and means, and we may as well follow his terminology. Everyone must recognize that some such distinction can be made, though it may be made in a number of different ways, and it is the distinction that is crucial to the doctrine of double effect. The words "double effect" refer to the two effects that an action may produce: the one aimed at, and the one foreseen but in no way desired. By "the doctrine of double effect" I mean the thesis that it is sometimes permissible to bring about by oblique intention what one may not directly intend.'

Voluntary Active Euthanasia

Dan W. Brock

Since the case of Karen Quinlan first seized public attention fifteen years ago, no issue in biomedical ethics has been more prominent than the debate about forgoing life-sustaining treatment. Controversy continues regarding some aspects of that debate, such as forgoing life-sustaining nutrition and hydration, and relevant law varies some from state to state. Nevertheless, I believe it is possible to identify an emerging consensus that competent patients, or the surrogates of incompetent patients, should be permitted to weigh the benefits and burdens of alternative treatments, including the alternative of no treatment, according to the patient's values, and either to refuse any treatment or to select from among available alternative treatments. This consensus is reflected in bioethics scholarship, in reports of prestigious bodies such as the President's Commission for the Study of Ethical Problems in Medicine, The Hastings Center, and the American Medical Association, in a large body of judicial decisions in courts around the country, and finally in the beliefs and practices of health care professionals who care for dying patients.[1]

More recently, significant public and professional attention has shifted from life-sustaining treatment to euthanasia—more specifically, voluntary active euthanasia—and to

Brock, D.W. (1992) "Voluntary Active Euthanasia." *Hastings Center Report* 22(2): pp. 10–22.

physician-assisted suicide. Several factors have contributed to the increased interest in euthanasia. In the Netherlands, it has been openly practiced by physicians for several years with the acceptance of the country's highest court.[2] In 1988 there was an unsuccessful attempt to get the question of whether it should be made legally permissible on the ballot in California. In November 1991 voters in the state of Washington defeated a widely publicized referendum proposal to legalize both voluntary active euthanasia and physician-assisted suicide. Finally, some cases of this kind, such as "It's Over, Debbie," described in the *Journal of the American Medical Association,* the "suicide machine" of Dr. Jack Kevorkian, and the cancer patient "Diane" of Dr. Timothy Quill, have captured wide public and professional attention.[3] Unfortunately, the first two of these cases were sufficiently problematic that even most supporters of euthanasia or assisted suicide did not defend the physicians' actions in them. As a result, the subsequent debate they spawned has often shed more heat than light. My aim is to increase the light, and perhaps as well to reduce the heat, on this important subject by formulating and evaluating the central ethical arguments for and against voluntary active euthanasia and physician-assisted suicide. My evaluation of the arguments leads me, with reservations to be noted, to support permitting both practices. My primary aim, however, is not to argue for euthanasia, but to identify confusions in some common arguments, and problematic assumptions and claims that need more defense or data in others. The issues are considerably more complex than either supporters or opponents often make out; my hope is to advance the debate by focusing attention on what I believe the real issues under discussion should be.

In the recent bioethics literature some have endorsed physician-assisted suicide but not euthanasia.[4] Are they sufficiently different that the moral arguments for one often do not apply to the other? A paradigm case of physician-assisted suicide is a patient's ending his or her life with a lethal dose of a medication requested of and provided by a physician for that purpose. A paradigm case of voluntary active euthanasia is a physician's administering the lethal dose, often because the patient is unable to do so. The only difference that need exist between the two is the person who actually administers the lethal dose—the physician or the patient. In each, the physician plays an active and necessary causal role.

In physician-assisted suicide the patient acts last (for example, Janet Adkins herself pushed the button after Dr. Kevorkian hooked her up to his suicide machine), whereas in euthanasia the physician acts last by performing the physical equivalent of pushing the button. In both cases, however, the choice rests fully with the patient. In both the patient acts last in the sense of retaining the right to change his or her mind until the point at which the lethal process becomes irreversible. How could there be a substantial moral difference between the two based only on this small difference in the part played by the physician in the causal process resulting in death? Of course, it might be held that the moral difference is clear and important—in euthanasia the physician kills the patient whereas in physician-assisted suicide the patient kills him- or herself. But this is misleading at best. In assisted suicide the physician and patient together kill the patient. To see this, suppose a physician supplied a lethal dose to a patient with the knowledge and intent that the patient will wrongfully administer it to another. We would have no difficulty in morality or the law recognizing this as a case of joint action to kill for which both are responsible.

If there is no significant, intrinsic moral difference between the two, it is also difficult to see why public or legal policy should permit one but not the other; worries about abuse or about giving anyone dominion over the lives of others apply equally to either. As a result, I will take the arguments evaluated below to apply to both and will focus on euthanasia.

My concern here will be with *voluntary* euthanasia only—that is, with the case in which a clearly competent patient makes a fully voluntary and persistent request for aid in dying. Involuntary euthanasia, in which a competent patient explicitly refuses or opposes receiving euthanasia, and nonvoluntary euthanasia, in which a patient is incompetent and unable to express his or her wishes about euthanasia, will be considered here only as potential unwanted side-effects of permitting voluntary euthanasia. I emphasize as well that I am concerned with *active* euthanasia, notwithholding or withdrawing life-sustaining treatment, which some commentators characterize as "passive euthanasia." Finally, I will be concerned with euthanasia where the motive of those who perform it is to respect the wishes of the patient and to provide the patient with a "good death," though one important issue is whether a change in legal policy could restrict the performance of euthanasia to only those cases.

A last introductory point is that I will be examining only secular arguments about euthanasia, though of course many people's attitudes to it are inextricable from their religious views. The policy issue is only whether euthanasia should be permissible, and no one who has religious objections to it should be required to take any part in it, though of course this would not fully satisfy some opponents.

THE CENTRAL ETHICAL ARGUMENT FOR VOLUNTARY ACTIVE EUTHANASIA

The central ethical argument for euthanasia is familiar. It is that the very same two fundamental ethical values supporting the consensus on patient's rights to decide about life-sustaining treatment also support the ethical permissibility of euthanasia. These values are individual self-determination or autonomy and individual well-being. By self-determination as it bears on euthanasia, I mean people's interest in making important decisions about their lives for themselves according to their own values or conceptions of a good life, and in being left free to act on those decisions. Self-determination is valuable because it permits people to form and live in accordance with their own conception of a good life, at least within the bounds of justice and consistent with others doing so as well. In exercising self-determination people take responsibility for their lives and for the kinds of persons they become. A central aspect of human dignity lies in people's capacity to direct their lives in this way. The value of exercising self-determination presupposes some minimum of decisionmaking capacities or competence, which thus limits the scope of euthanasia supported by self-determination; it cannot justifiably be administered, for example, in cases of serious dementia or treatable clinical depression.

Does the value of individual self-determination extend to the time and manner of one's death? Most people are very concerned about the nature of the last stage of their lives. This reflects not just a fear of experiencing substantial suffering when dying, but also a desire to retain dignity and control during this last period of life. Death is today increasingly preceded by a long period of significant physical and mental decline, due in part to the technological interventions of modern medicine. Many people adjust to these disabilities and find meaning and value in new activities and ways. Others find the impairments and burdens in the last stage of their lives at some point sufficiently great to make life no longer worth living. For many patients near death, maintaining the quality of one's life, avoiding great suffering, maintaining one's dignity, and insuring that others remember us as we wish them to become of paramount importance and outweigh merely extending one's life. But there is no single, objectively correct answer for everyone as to when, if at all, one's life becomes all things considered a burden and unwanted. If self-determination is a fundamental value, then the great variability among people on this question makes it especially important that individuals control the manner, circumstances, and timing of their dying and death.

The other main value that supports euthanasia is individual well-being. It might seem that individual well-being conflicts with a person's self-determination when the person requests euthanasia. Life itself is commonly taken to be a central good for persons, often valued for its own sake, as well as necessary for pursuit of all other goods within a life. But when a competent patient decides to forgo all further life-sustaining treatment then the patient, either explicitly or implicitly, commonly decides that the best life possible for him or her with treatment is of sufficiently poor quality that it is worse than no further life at all. Life is no longer considered a benefit by the patient, but has now become a burden. The same judgment underlies a request for euthanasia: continued life is seen by the patient as no longer a benefit, but now a burden. Especially in the often severely compromised and debilitated states of many critically ill or dying patients, there is no objective standard, but only the competent patient's judgment of whether continued life is no longer a benefit.

Of course, sometimes there are conditions, such as clinical depression, that call into question whether the patient has made a competent choice, either to forgo life-sustaining treatment or to seek euthanasia, and then the patient's choice need not be evidence that continued life is no longer a benefit for him or her. Just as with decisions about treatment, a determination of incompetence can warrant not honoring the patient's choice; in the case of treatment, we then transfer decisional authority to a surrogate, though in the case of voluntary active euthanasia a determination that the patient is incompetent means that choice is not possible.

The value or right of self-determination does not entitle patients to compel physicians to act contrary to their own moral or professional values. Physicians are moral and professional agents whose own self-determination or integrity should be respected as well. If performing euthanasia became legally permissible, but conflicted with a particular physician's reasonable understanding of his or her moral or professional responsibilities, the care of a patient who requested euthanasia should be transferred to another.

Most opponents do not deny that there are some cases in which the values of patient self-determination and well-being support euthanasia.

Instead, they commonly offer two kinds of arguments against it that on their view outweigh or override this support. The first kind of argument is that in any individual case where considerations of the patient's self-determination and well-being do support euthanasia, it is nevertheless always ethically wrong or impermissible. The second kind of argument grants that in some individual cases euthanasia may *not* be ethically wrong, but maintains nonetheless that public and legal policy should never permit it. The first kind of argument focuses on features of any individual case of euthanasia, while the second kind focuses on social or legal policy. In the next section I consider the first kind of argument.

EUTHANASIA IS THE DELIBERATE KILLING OF AN INNOCENT PERSON

The claim that any individual instance of euthanasia is a case of deliberate killing of an innocent person is, with only minor qualifications, correct. Unlike forgoing life-sustaining treatment, commonly understood as allowing to die, euthanasia is clearly killing, defined as depriving of life or causing the death of a living being. While providing morphine for pain relief at doses where the risk of respiratory depression and an earlier death may be a foreseen but unintended side effect of treating the patient's pain, in a case of euthanasia the patient's death is deliberate or intended even if in both the physician's ultimate end may be respecting the patient's wishes. If the deliberate killing of an innocent person is wrong, euthanasia would be nearly always impermissible.

In the context of medicine, the ethical prohibition against deliberately killing the innocent derives some of its plausibility from the belief that nothing in the currently accepted practice of medicine is deliberate killing. Thus, in commenting on the "It's Over, Debbie" case, four prominent physicians and bioethicists could entitle their paper "Doctors Must Not Kill."[5] The belief that doctors do not in fact kill requires the corollary belief that forgoing life-sustaining treatment, whether by not starting or by stopping treatment, is allowing to die, not killing.

Common though this view is, I shall argue that it is confused and mistaken.

Why is the common view mistaken? Consider the case of a patient terminally ill with ALS disease. She is completely respirator dependent with no hope of ever being weaned. She is unquestionably competent but finds her condition intolerable and persistently requests to be removed from the respirator and allowed to die. Most people and physicians would agree that the patient's physician should respect the patient's wishes and remove her from the respirator, though this will certainly cause the patient's death. The common understanding is that the physician thereby allows the patient to die. But is that correct?

Suppose the patient has a greedy and hostile son who mistakenly believes that his mother will never decide to stop her life-sustaining treatment and that even if she did her physician would not remove her from the respirator. Afraid that his inheritance will be dissipated by a long and expensive hospitalization, he enters his mother's room while she is sedated, extubates her, and she dies. Shortly thereafter the medical staff discovers what he has done and confronts the son. He replies, "I didn't kill her, I merely allowed her to die. It was her ALS disease that caused her death." I think this would rightly be dismissed as transparent sophistry—the son went into his mother's room and deliberately killed her. But, of course, the son performed just the same physical actions, did just the same thing, that the physician would have done. If that is so, then doesn't the physician also kill the patient when he extubates her?

I underline immediately that there are important ethical differences between what the physician and the greedy son do. First, the physician acts with the patient's consent whereas the son does not. Second, the physician acts with a good motive—to respect the patient's wishes and self-determination—whereas the son acts with a bad motive—to protect his own inheritance. Third, the physician acts in a social role through which he is legally authorized to carry out the patient's wishes regarding treatment whereas the son has

no such authorization. These and perhaps other ethically important differences show that what the physician did was morally justified whereas what the son did was morally wrong. What they do *not* show, however, is that the son killed while the physician allowed to die. One can either kill or allow to die with or without consent, with a good or bad motive, within or outside of a social role that authorizes one to do so.

The difference between killing and allowing to die that I have been implicitly appealing to here is roughly that between acts and omissions resulting in death.[6] Both the physician and the greedy son act in a manner intended to cause death, do cause death, and so both kill. One reason this conclusion is resisted is that on a different understanding of the distinction between killing and allowing to die, what the physician does is allow to die. In this account, the mother's ALS is a lethal disease whose normal progression is being held back or blocked by the life-sustaining respirator treatment. Removing this artificial intervention is then viewed as standing aside and allowing the patient to die of her underlying disease. I have argued elsewhere that this alternative account is deeply problematic, in part because it commits us to accepting that what the greedy son does is to allow to die, not kill.[7] Here, I want to note two other reasons why the conclusion that stopping life support is killing is resisted.

The first reason is that killing is often understood, especially within medicine, as unjustified causing of death; in medicine it is thought to be done only accidentally or negligently. It is also increasingly widely accepted that a physician is ethically justified in stopping life support in a case like that of the ALS patient. But if these two beliefs are correct, then what the physician does cannot be killing, and so must be allowing to die. Killing patients is not, to put it flippantly, understood to be part of physicians' job description. What is mistaken in this line of reasoning is the assumption that all killings are *unjustified* causings of death. Instead, some killings are ethically justified, including many instances of stopping life support.

Another reason for resisting the conclusion that stopping life support is often killing is that it is psychologically uncomfortable. Suppose the physician had stopped the ALS patient's respirator and had made the son's claim, "I didn't kill her, I merely allowed her to die. It was her ALS disease that caused her death." The clue to the psychological role here is how naturally the "merely" modifies "allowed her to die." The characterization as allowing to die is meant to shift felt responsibility away from the agent—the physician—and to the lethal disease process. Other language common in death and dying contexts plays a similar role; "letting nature take its course" or "stopping prolonging the dying process" both seem to shift responsibility from the physician who stops life support to the fatal disease process. However psychologically helpful these conceptualizations may be in making the difficult responsibility of a physician's role in the patient's death bearable, they nevertheless are confusions. Both physicians and family members can instead be helped to understand that it is the patient's decision and consent to stopping treatment that limits their responsibility for the patient's death and that shifts that responsibility to the patient.

Many who accept the difference between killing and allowing to die as the distinction between acts and omissions resulting in death have gone on to argue that killing is not in itself morally different from allowing to die.[8] In this account, very roughly, one kills when one performs an action that causes the death of a person (we are in a boat, you cannot swim, I push you overboard, and you drown), and one allows to die when one has the ability and opportunity to prevent the death of another, knows this, and omits doing so, with the result that the person dies (we are in a boat, you cannot swim, you fall overboard, I don't throw you an available life ring, and you drown). Those who see no moral difference between killing and allowing to die typically employ the strategy of comparing cases that differ in these and no other potentially morally important respects. This will allow people to consider whether the mere difference that one is a case of killing and the other of allowing to die matters morally, or whether instead it is other features that make most cases of killing worse than most instances of allowing to die. Here is such a pair of cases:

> **Case 1.** A very gravely ill patient is brought to a hospital emergency room and sent up to the ICU. The patient begins to develop respiratory failure that is likely to require intubation very soon. At that point the patient's family members and long-standing physician arrive at the ICU and inform the ICU staff that there had been extensive discussion about future care with the patient when he was unquestionably competent. Given his grave and terminal illness, as well as his state of debilitation, the patient had firmly rejected being placed on a respirator under any circumstances, and the family and physician produce the patient's advance directive to that effect. The ICU staff do not intubate the patient, who dies of respiratory failure.

> **Case 2.** The same as Case 1 except that the family and physician are slightly delayed in traffic and arrive shortly after the patient has been intubated and placed on the respirator. The ICU staff extubate the patient, who dies of respiratory failure.

In Case 1 the patient is allowed to die, in Case 2 he is killed, but it is hard to see why what is done in Case 2 is significantly different morally than what is done in Case 1. It must be other factors that make most killings worse than most allowings to die, and if so, euthanasia cannot be wrong simply because it is killing instead of allowing to die.

Suppose both my arguments are mistaken. Suppose that killing is worse than allowing to die and that withdrawing life support is not killing, although euthanasia is. Euthanasia still need not for that reason be morally wrong. To see this, we need to determine the basic principle for the moral evaluation of killing persons. What is it that makes paradigm cases of wrongful killing wrongful? One very plausible answer is that killing denies the victim something that he or she values greatly—continued life or a future. Moreover, since continued life is necessary for pursuing any of a person's plans and purposes, killing brings the frustration of all of these plans and desires as well. In a nutshell, wrongful killing deprives a person of a valued future, and of all the person wanted and planned to do in that future.

A natural expression of this account of the wrongness of killing is that people have a moral right not to be killed.[9] But in this account of the wrongness of killing, the right not to be killed, like other rights, should be waivable when the person makes a competent decision that continued life is no longer wanted or a good, but is instead worse than no further life at all. In this view, euthanasia is properly understood as a case of a person having waived his or her right not to be killed.

This rights view of the wrongness of killing is not, of course, universally shared. Many people's moral views about killing have their origins in religious views that human life comes from God and cannot be justifiably destroyed or taken away, either by the person whose life it is or by another. But in a pluralistic society like our own with a strong commitment to freedom of religion, public policy should not be grounded in religious beliefs which many in that society reject. I turn now to the general evaluation of public policy on euthanasia.

WOULD THE BAD CONSEQUENCES OF EUTHANASIA OUTWEIGH THE GOOD?

The argument against euthanasia at the policy level is stronger than at the level of individual cases, though even here I believe the case is ultimately unpersuasive, or at best indecisive. The policy level is the place where the main issues lie, however, and where moral considerations that might override arguments in favor of euthanasia will be found, if they are found anywhere. It is important to note two kinds of disagreement about the consequences for public policy of permitting euthanasia. First, there is empirical

or factual disagreement about what the consequences would be. This disagreement is greatly exacerbated by the lack of firm data on the issue. Second, since on any reasonable assessment there would be both good and bad consequences, there are moral disagreements about the relative importance of different effects. In addition to these two sources of disagreement, there is also no single, well-specified policy proposal for legalizing euthanasia on which policy assessments can focus. But without such specification, and especially without explicit procedures for protecting against well-intentioned misuse and ill-intentioned abuse, the consequences for policy are largely speculative. Despite these difficulties, a preliminary account of the main likely good and bad consequences is possible. This should help clarify where better data or more moral analysis and argument are needed, as well as where policy safeguards must be developed.

Potential Good Consequences of Permitting Euthanasia. What are the likely good consequences? First, if euthanasia were permitted it would be possible to respect the self-determination of competent patients who want it, but now cannot get it because of its illegality. We simply do not know how many such patients and people there are. In the Netherlands, with a population of about 14.5 million (in 1987), estimates in a recent study were that about 1,900 cases of voluntary active euthanasia or physician-assisted suicide occur annually. No straightforward extrapolation to the United States is possible for many reasons, among them, that we do not know how many people here who want euthanasia now get it, despite its illegality. Even with better data on the number of persons who want euthanasia but cannot get it, significant moral disagreement would remain about how much weight should be given to any instance of failure to respect a person's self-determination in this way.

One important factor substantially affecting the number of persons who would seek euthanasia is the extent to which an alternative is available. The widespread acceptance in the law, social policy, and medical practice of the right of a competent patient to forgo life-sustaining treatment suggests that the number of competent persons in the United States who would want euthanasia if it were permitted is probably relatively small.

A second good consequence of making euthanasia legally permissible benefits a much larger group. Polls have shown that a majority of the American public believes that people should have a right to obtain euthanasia if they want it.[10] No doubt the vast majority of those who support this right to euthanasia will never in fact come to want euthanasia for themselves. Nevertheless, making it legally permissible would reassure many people that if they ever do want euthanasia they would be able to obtain it. This reassurance would supplement the broader control over the process of dying given by the right to decide about life-sustaining treatment. Having fire insurance on one's house benefits all who have it, not just those whose houses actually burn down, by reassuring them that in the unlikely event of their house burning down, they will receive the money needed to rebuild it. Likewise, the legalization of euthanasia can be thought of as a kind of insurance policy against being forced to endure a protracted dying process that one has come to find burdensome and unwanted, especially when there is no life-sustaining treatment to forgo. The strong concern about losing control of their care expressed by many people who face serious illness likely to end in death suggests that they give substantial importance to the legalization of euthanasia as a means of maintaining this control.

A third good consequence of the legalization of euthanasia concerns patients whose dying is filled with severe and unrelievable pain or suffering. When there is a life-sustaining treatment that, if forgone, will lead relatively quickly to death, then doing so can bring an end to these patients' suffering without recourse to euthanasia. For patients receiving no such treatment, however, euthanasia may be the only release from their otherwise prolonged suffering and agony. This argument from mercy has always been the strongest argument for euthanasia in those cases to which it applies.[11]

The importance of relieving pain and suffering is less controversial than is the frequency with which patients are forced to undergo untreatable agony that only euthanasia could relieve. If we focus first on suffering caused by physical pain, it is crucial to distinguish pain that *could* be adequately relieved with modern methods of pain control, though it in fact is not, from pain that is relievable only by death.[12] For a variety of reasons, including some physicians' fear of hastening the patient's death, as well as the lack of a publicly accessible means for assessing the amount of the patient's pain, many patients suffer pain that could be, but is not, relieved.

Specialists in pain control, as for example the pain of terminally ill cancer patients, argue that there are very few patients whose pain could not be adequately controlled, though sometimes at the cost of so sedating them that they are effectively unable to interact with other people or their environment. Thus, the argument from mercy in cases of physical pain can probably be met in a large majority of cases by providing adequate measures of pain relief. This should be a high priority, whatever our legal policy on euthanasia—the relief of pain and suffering has long been, quite properly, one of the central goals of medicine. Those cases in which pain could be effectively relieved, but in fact is not, should only count significantly in favor of legalizing euthanasia if all reasonable efforts to change pain management techniques have been tried and have failed.

Dying patients often undergo substantial psychological suffering that is not fully or even principally the result of physical pain.[13] The knowledge about how to relieve this suffering is much more limited than in the case of relieving pain, and efforts to do so are probably more often unsuccessful. If the argument from mercy is extended to patients experiencing great and unrelievable psychological suffering, the numbers of patients to which it applies are much greater.

One last good consequence of legalizing euthanasia is that once death has been accepted, it is often more humane to end life quickly and peacefully, when that is what the patient wants. Such a death will often be seen as better than a more prolonged one. People who suffer a sudden and unexpected death, for example by dying quickly or in their sleep from a heart attack or stroke, are often considered lucky to have died in this way. We care about how we die in part because we care about how others remember us, and we hope they will remember us as we were in "good times" with them and not as we might be when disease has robbed us of our dignity as human beings. As with much in the treatment and care of the dying, people's concerns differ in this respect, but for at least some people, euthanasia will be a more humane death than what they have often experienced with other loved ones and might otherwise expect for themselves.

Some opponents of euthanasia challenge how much importance should be given to any of these good consequences of permitting it, or even whether some would be good consequences at all. But more frequently, opponents cite a number of bad consequences that permitting euthanasia would or could produce, and it is to their assessment that I now turn.

Potential Bad Consequences of Permitting Euthanasia. Some of the arguments against permitting euthanasia are aimed specifically against physicians, while others are aimed against anyone being permitted to perform it. I shall first consider one argument of the former sort. Permitting physicians to perform euthanasia, it is said, would be incompatible with their fundamental moral and professional commitment as healers to care for patients and to protect life. Moreover, if euthanasia by physicians became common, patients would come to fear that a medication was intended not to treat or care, but instead to kill, and would thus lose trust in their physicians. This position was forcefully stated in a paper by Willard Gaylin and his colleagues:

> The very soul of medicine is on trial... This issue touches medicine at its moral center; if this moral center collapses, if physicians become killers or are even licensed to kill, the profession—and, therewith, each physician—will never again be worthy of trust and respect as healer and comforter and protector of life in all its frailty.

These authors go on to make clear that, while they oppose permitting anyone to perform euthanasia, their special concern is with physicians doing so:

> We call on fellow physicians to say that they will not deliberately kill. We must also say to each of our fellow physicians that we will not tolerate killing of patients and that we shall take disciplinary action against doctors who kill. And we must say to the broader community that if it insists on tolerating or legalizing active euthanasia, it will have to find nonphysicians to do its killing.[14]

If permitting physicians to kill would undermine the very "moral center" of medicine, then almost certainly physicians should not be permitted to perform euthanasia. But how persuasive is this claim? Patients should not fear, as a consequence of permitting *voluntary* active euthanasia, that their physicians will substitute a lethal injection for what patients want and believe is part of their care. If active euthanasia is restricted to cases in which it is truly voluntary, then no patient should fear getting it unless she or he has voluntarily requested it. (The fear that we might in time also come to accept nonvoluntary, or even involuntary, active euthanasia is a slippery slope worry I address below.) Patients' trust of their physicians could be increased, not eroded, by knowledge that physicians will provide aid in dying when patients seek it.

Might Gaylin and his colleagues nevertheless be correct in their claim that the moral center of medicine would collapse if physicians were to become killers? This question raises what at the deepest level should be the guiding aims of medicine, a question that obviously cannot be fully explored here. But I do want to say enough to indicate the direction that I believe an appropriate response to this challenge should take. In spelling out above what I called the positive argument for voluntary active euthanasia, I suggested that two principal values—respecting patients' self-determination and promoting their well-being—underlie the consensus that competent patients, or the surrogates of incompetent patients, are entitled to refuse any life-sustaining treatment and to choose from among available alternative treatments. It is the commitment to these two values in guiding physicians' actions as healers, comforters, and protectors of their patients' lives that should be at the "moral center" of medicine, and these two values support physicians' administering euthanasia when their patients make competent requests for it.

What should not be at that moral center is a commitment to preserving patients' lives as such, without regard to whether those patients want their lives preserved or judge their preservation a benefit to them. Vitalism has been rejected by most physicians, and despite some statements that suggest it, is almost certainly not what Gaylin and colleagues intended. One of them, Leon Kass, has elaborated elsewhere the view that medicine is a moral profession whose proper aim is "the naturally given end of health," understood as the wholeness and well-working of the human being; "for the physician, at least, human life in living bodies commands respect and reverence—*by its very nature*." Kass continues, "the deepest ethical principle restraining the physician's power is not the autonomy or freedom of the patient; neither is it his own compassion or good intention. Rather, it is the dignity and mysterious power of human life itself."[15] I believe Kass is in the end mistaken about the proper account of the aims of medicine and the limits on physicians' power, but this difficult issue will certainly be one of the central themes in the continuing debate about euthanasia.

A second bad consequence that some foresee is that permitting euthanasia would weaken society's commitment to provide optimal care for dying patients. We live at a time in which the control of health care costs has become, and

is likely to continue to be, the dominant focus of health care policy. If euthanasia is seen as a cheaper alternative to adequate care and treatment, then we might become less scrupulous about providing sometimes costly support and other services to dying patients. Particularly if our society comes to embrace deeper and more explicit rationing of health care, frail, elderly, and dying patients will need to be strong and effective advocates for their own health care and other needs, although they are hardly in a position to do this. We should do nothing to weaken their ability to obtain adequate care and services.

This second worry is difficult to assess because there is little firm evidence about the likelihood of the feared erosion in the care of dying patients. There are at least two reasons, however, for skepticism about this argument. The first is that the same worry could have been directed at recognizing patients' or surrogates' rights to forgo life-sustaining treatment, yet there is no persuasive evidence that recognizing the right to refuse treatment has caused a serious erosion in the quality of care of dying patients. The second reason for skepticism about this worry is that only a very small proportion of deaths would occur from euthanasia if it were permitted. In the Netherlands, where euthanasia under specified circumstances is permitted by the courts, though not authorized by statute, the best estimate of the proportion of overall deaths that result from it is about 2 percent.[16] Thus, the vast majority of critically ill and dying patients will not request it, and so will still have to be cared for by physicians, families, and others. Permitting euthanasia should not diminish people's commitment and concern to maintain and improve the care of these patients.

A third possible bad consequence of permitting euthanasia (or even a public discourse in which strong support for euthanasia is evident) is to threaten the progress made in securing the rights of patients or their surrogates to decide about and to refuse life-sustaining treatment.[17] This progress has been made against the backdrop of a clear and firm legal prohibition of euthanasia, which has provided a relatively bright line limiting the dominion of others over patients' lives. It has therefore been an important reassurance to concerns about how the authority to take steps ending life might be misused, abused, or wrongly extended.

Many supporters of the right of patients or their surrogates to refuse treatment strongly oppose euthanasia, and if forced to choose might well withdraw their support of the right to refuse treatment rather than accept euthanasia. Public policy in the last fifteen years has generally let life-sustaining treatment decisions be made in health care settings between physicians and patients or their surrogates, and without the involvement of the courts. However, if euthanasia is made legally permissible greater involvement of the courts is likely, which could in turn extend to a greater court involvement in life-sustaining treatment decisions. Most agree, however, that increased involvement of the courts in these decisions would be undesirable, as it would make sound decisionmaking more cumbersome and difficult without sufficient compensating benefits.

As with the second potential bad consequence of permitting euthanasia, this third consideration too is speculative and difficult to assess. The feared erosion of patients' or surrogates' rights to decide about life-sustaining treatment, together with greater court involvement in those decisions, are both possible. However, I believe there is reason to discount this general worry. The legal rights of competent patients and, to a lesser degree, surrogates of incompetent patients to decide about treatment are very firmly embedded in a long line of informed consent and life-sustaining treatment cases, and are not likely to be eroded by a debate over, or even acceptance of, euthanasia. It will not be accepted without safeguards that reassure the public about abuse, and if that debate shows the need for similar safeguards for some life-sustaining treatment decisions they should be adopted there as well. In neither case are the only possible safeguards greater court involvement, as the recent growth of institutional ethics committees shows.

The fourth potential bad consequence of permitting euthanasia has been developed by David Velleman and turns on the subtle point that making a new option or choice available to people can sometimes make them worse off, even if once they have the choice they go on to choose what is best for them.[18] Ordinarily, people's continued existence is viewed by them as given, a fixed condition with which they must cope. Making euthanasia available to people as an option denies them the alternative of staying alive by default. If people are offered the option of euthanasia, their continued existence is now a choice for which they can be held responsible and which they can be asked by others to justify. We care, and are right to care, about being able to justify ourselves to others. To the extent that our society is unsympathetic to justifying a severely dependent or impaired existence, a heavy psychological burden of proof may be placed on patients who think their terminal illness or chronic infirmity is not a sufficient reason for dying. Even if they otherwise view their life as worth living, the opinion of others around them that it is not can threaten their reason for living and make euthanasia a rational choice. Thus the existence of the option becomes a subtle pressure to request it.

This argument correctly identifies the reason why offering some patients the option of euthanasia would not benefit then. Velleman takes it not as a reason for opposing all euthanasia, but for restricting it to circumstances where there are "unmistakable and overpowering reasons for persons to want the option of euthanasia," and for denying the option in all other cases. But there are at least three reasons why such restriction may not be warranted. First, polls and other evidence support that most Americans believe euthanasia should be permitted (though the recent defeat of the referendum to permit it in the state of Washington raises some doubt about this support). Thus, many more people seem to want the choice than would be made worse off by getting it. Second, if giving people the option of ending their life really makes them worse off, then we should not only prohibit euthanasia, but also take back from people the right they now have to decide about life-sustaining treatment. The feared harmful effect should already have occurred from securing people's right to refuse life-sustaining treatment, yet there is no evidence of any such widespread harm or any broad public desire to rescind that right. Third, since there is a wide range of conditions in which reasonable people can and do disagree about whether they would want continued life, it is not possible to restrict the permissibility of euthanasia as narrowly as Velleman suggests without thereby denying it to most persons who would want it; to permit it only in cases in which virtually everyone would want it would be to deny it to most who would want it.

A fifth potential bad consequence of making euthanasia legally permissible is that it might weaken the general legal prohibition of homicide. This prohibition is so fundamental to civilized society, it is argued, that we should do nothing that erodes it. If most cases of stopping life support are killing, as I have already argued, then the court cases permitting such killing have already in effect weakened this prohibition. However, neither the courts nor most people have seen these cases as killing and so as challenging the prohibition of homicide. The courts have usually grounded patients' or their surrogates' rights to refuse life-sustaining treatment in rights to privacy, liberty, self-determination, or bodily integrity, not in exceptions to homicide laws.

Legal permission for physicians or others to perform euthanasia could not be grounded in patients' rights to decide about medical treatment. Permitting euthanasia would require qualifying, at least in effect, the legal prohibition against homicide, a prohibition that in general does not allow the consent of the victim to justify or excuse the act. Nevertheless, the very same fundamental basis of the right to decide about life-sustaining treatment—respecting a person's self-determination—does support euthanasia as well. Individual self-determination has long been a well-entrenched and fundamental value in the law, and so extending it to euthanasia would not require appeal to novel legal values or principles. That suicide or attempted suicide is no longer a criminal offense in virtually all states indicates an acceptance of individual self-determination in the

taking of one's own life analogous to that required for voluntary active euthanasia. The legal prohibition (in most states) of assisting in suicide and the refusal in the law to accept the consent of the victim as a possible justification of homicide are both arguably a result of difficulties in the legal process of establishing the consent of the victim after the fact. If procedures can be designed that clearly establish the voluntariness of the person's request for euthanasia, it would under those procedures represent a carefully circumscribed qualification on the legal prohibition of homicide. Nevertheless, some remaining worries about this weakening can be captured in the final potential bad consequence, to which I will now turn.

This final potential bad consequence is the central concern of many opponents of euthanasia and, I believe, is the most serious objection to a legal policy permitting it. According to this "slippery slope" worry, although active euthanasia may be morally permissible in cases in which it is unequivocally voluntary and the patient finds his or her condition unbearable, a legal policy permitting euthanasia would inevitably lead to active euthanasia being performed in many other cases in which it would be morally wrong. To prevent those other wrongful cases of euthanasia we should not permit even morally justified performance of it.

Slippery slope arguments of this form are problematic and difficult to evaluate.[19] From one perspective, they are the last refuge of conservative defenders of the status quo. When all the opponent's objections to the wrongness of euthanasia itself have been met, the opponent then shifts ground and acknowledges both that it is not in itself wrong and that a legal policy which resulted only in its being performed would not be bad. Nevertheless, the opponent maintains, it should still not be permitted because doing so would result in its being performed in other cases in which it is not voluntary and would be wrong. In this argument's most extreme form, permitting euthanasia is the first and fateful step down the slippery slope to Nazism. Once on the slope we will be unable to get off.

Now it cannot be denied that it is *possible* that permitting euthanasia could have these fateful consequences, but that cannot be enough to warrant prohibiting it if it is otherwise justified. A similar *possible* slippery slope worry could have been raised to securing competent patients' rights to decide about life support, but recent history shows such a worry would have been unfounded. It must be relevant how likely it is that we will end with horrendous consequences and an unjustified practice of euthanasia. How *likely* and *widespread* would the abuses and unwarranted extensions of permitting it be? By abuses, I mean the performance of euthanasia that fails to satisfy the conditions required for voluntary active euthanasia, for example, if the patient has been subtly pressured to accept it. By unwarranted extensions of policy, I mean later changes in legal policy to permit not just voluntary euthanasia, but also euthanasia in cases in which, for example, it need not be fully voluntary. Opponents of voluntary euthanasia on slippery slope grounds have not provided the data or evidence necessary to turn their speculative concerns into well-grounded likelihoods.

It is at least clear, however, that both the character and likelihood of abuses of a legal policy permitting euthanasia depend in significant part on the procedures put in place to protect against them. I will not try to detail fully what such procedures might be, but will just give some examples of what they might include:

1. The patient should be provided with all relevant information about his or her medical condition, current prognosis, available alternative treatments, and the prognosis of each.
2. Procedures should ensure that the patient's request for euthanasia is stable or enduring (a brief waiting period could be required) and fully voluntary (an advocate for the patient might be appointed to ensure this).
3. All reasonable alternatives must have been explored for improving the patient's quality of life and relieving any pain or suffering.
4. A psychiatric evaluation should ensure that the patient's request is not the result of a treatable psychological impairment such as depression.[20]

These examples of procedural safeguards are all designed to ensure that the patient's choice is fully informed, voluntary, and competent, and so a true exercise of self-determination. Other proposals for euthanasia would restrict its permissibility further—for example, to the terminally ill—a restriction that cannot be supported by self-determination. Such additional restrictions might, however, be justified by concern for limiting potential harms from abuse. At the same time, it is important not to impose procedural or substantive safeguards so restrictive as to make euthanasia impermissible or practically infeasible in a wide range of justified cases.

These examples of procedural safeguards make clear that it is possible to substantially reduce, though not to eliminate, the potential for abuse of a policy permitting voluntary active euthanasia. Any legalization of the practice should be accompanied by a well-considered set of procedural safeguards together with an ongoing evaluation of its use. Introducing euthanasia into only a few states could be a form of carefully limited and controlled social experiment that would give us evidence about the benefits and harms of the practice. Even then firm and uncontroversial data may remain elusive, as the continuing controversy over what has taken place in the Netherlands in recent years indicates.[21]

The Slip into Nonvoluntary Active Euthanasia. While I believe slippery slope worries can largely be limited by making necessary distinctions both in principle and in practice, one slippery slope concern is legitimate. There is reason to expect that legalization of voluntary active euthanasia might soon be followed by strong pressure to legalize some nonvoluntary euthanasia of incompetent patients unable to express their own wishes. Respecting a person's self-determination and recognizing that continued life is not always of value to a person can support not only voluntary active euthanasia, but some nonvoluntary euthanasia as well. These are the same values that ground competent patients' right to refuse life-sustaining treatment. Recent history here is instructive. In the medical ethics literature, in the courts since Quinlan, and in norms of medical practice, that right has been extended to incompetent patients and exercised by a surrogate who is to decide as the patient would have decided in the circumstances if competent.[22] It has been held unreasonable to continue life-sustaining treatment that the patient would not have wanted just because the patient now lacks the capacity to tell us that. Life-sustaining treatment for incompetent patients is today frequently forgone on the basis of a surrogate's decision, or less frequently on the basis of an advance directive executed by the patient while still competent. The very same logic that has extended the right to refuse life-sustaining treatment from a competent patient to the surrogate of an incompetent patient (acting with or without a formal advance directive from the patient) may well extend the scope of active euthanasia. The argument will be, Why continue to force unwanted life on patients just because they have now lost the capacity to request euthanasia from us?

A related phenomenon may reinforce this slippery slope concern. In the Netherlands, what the courts have sanctioned has been clearly restricted to voluntary euthanasia. In itself, this serves as some evidence that permitting it need *not* lead to permitting the nonvoluntary variety. There is some indication, however, that for many Dutch physicians euthanasia is no longer viewed as a special action, set apart from their usual practice and restricted only to competent persons.[23] Instead, it is seen as one end of a spectrum of caring for dying patients. When viewed in this way it will be difficult to deny euthanasia to a patient for whom it is seen as the best or most appropriate form of care simply because that patient is now incompetent and cannot request it.

Even if voluntary active euthanasia should slip into nonvoluntary active euthanasia, with surrogates acting for incompetent patients, the ethical evaluation is more complex than many opponents of euthanasia allow. Just as in the case of surrogates' decisions to forgo life-sustaining treatment for incompetent patients, so also surrogates' decisions to request euthanasia for

incompetent persons would often accurately reflect what the incompetent person would have wanted and would deny the person nothing that he or she would have considered worth having. Making nonvoluntary active euthanasia legally permissible, however, would greatly enlarge the number of patients on whom it might be performed and substantially enlarge the potential for misuse and abuse. As noted above, frail and debilitated elderly people, often demented or otherwise incompetent and thereby unable to defend and assert their own interests, may be especially vulnerable to unwanted euthanasia.

For some people, this risk is more than sufficient reason to oppose the legalization of voluntary euthanasia. But while we should in general be cautious about inferring much from the experience in the Netherlands to what our own experience in the United States might be, there may be one important lesson that we can learn from them. One commentator has noted that in the Netherlands families of incompetent patients have less authority than do families in the United States to act as surrogates for incompetent patients in making decisions to forgo life-sustaining treatment.[24] From the Dutch perspective, it may be we in the United States who are *already* on the slippery slope in having given surrogates broad authority to forgo life-sustaining treatment for incompetent persons. In this view, the more important moral divide, and the more important with regard to potential for abuse, is not between forgoing life-sustaining treatment and euthanasia, but instead between voluntary and nonvoluntary performance of either. If this is correct, then the more important issue is ensuring the appropriate principles and procedural safeguards for the exercise of decisionmaking authority by surrogates for incompetent persons in *all* decisions at the end of life. This may be the correct response to slippery slope worries about euthanasia.

I have cited both good and bad consequences that have been thought likely from a policy change permitting voluntary active euthanasia, and have tried to evaluate their likelihood and relative importance. Nevertheless, as I noted earlier, reasonable disagreement remains both about the consequences of permitting euthanasia and about which of these consequences are more important. The depth and strength of public and professional debate about whether, all things considered, permitting euthanasia would be desirable or undesirable reflects these disagreements. While my own view is that the balance of considerations supports permitting the practice, my principal purpose here has been to clarify the main issues.

THE ROLE OF PHYSICIANS

If euthanasia is made legally permissible, should physicians take part in it? Should only physicians be permitted to perform it, as is the case in the Netherlands? In discussing whether euthanasia is incompatible with medicine's commitment to curing, caring for, and comforting patients, I argued that it is not at odds with a proper understanding of the aims of medicine, and so need not undermine patients' trust in their physicians. If that argument is correct, then physicians probably should not be prohibited, either by law or by professional norms, from taking part in a legally permissible practice of euthanasia (nor, of course, should they be compelled to do so if their personal or professional scruples forbid it). Most physicians in the Netherlands appear not to understand euthanasia to be incompatible with their professional commitments.

Sometimes patients who would be able to end their lives on their own nevertheless seek the assistance of physicians. Physician involvement in such cases may have important benefits to patients and others beyond simply assuring the use of effective means. Historically, in the United States suicide has carried a strong negative stigma that many today believe unwarranted. Seeking a physician's assistance, or what can almost seem a physician's blessing, may be a way of trying to remove that stigma and show others that the decision for suicide was made with due seriousness and was justified under the circumstances. The physician's involvement provides a kind of social approval, or more accurately helps counter what would otherwise be unwarranted social disapproval.

There are also at least two reasons for restricting the practice of euthanasia to physicians only. First, physicians would inevitably be involved in some of the important procedural safeguards necessary to a defensible practice, such as seeing to it that the patient is well-informed about his or her condition, prognosis, and possible treatments, and ensuring that all reasonable means have been taken to improve the quality of the patient's life. Second, and probably more important, one necessary protection against abuse of the practice is to limit the persons given authority to perform it, so that they can be held accountable for their exercise of that authority. Physicians, whose training and professional norms give some assurance that they would perform euthanasia responsibly, are an appropriate group of persons to whom the practice may be restricted.

Acknowledgements

Earlier versions of this paper were presented at the American Philosophical Association Central Division meetings (at which David Velleman provided extremely helpful comments), Massachusetts General Hospital, Yale University School of Medicine, Princeton University, Brown University, and as the Brin Lecture at The Johns Hopkins School of Medicine. I am grateful to the audiences on each of these occasions, to several anonymous reviewers, and to Norman Daniels for helpful comments. The paper was completed while I was a Fellow in the Program in Ethics and the Professions at Harvard University.

Notes

1. President's Commission for the Study of Ethical Problems in Medicine and Biomedical and Behavioral Research, *Deciding to Forego Life-Sustaining Treatment* (Washington, D.C.: U.S. Government Printing Office, 1983); The Hastings Center, *Guidelines on the Termination of Life-Sustaining Treatment and Care of the Dying* (Bloomington: Indiana University Press, 1987); *Current Opinions of the Council on Ethical*

and Judicial Affairs of the American Medical Association—1989: Withholding or Withdrawing Life-Prolonging Treatment (Chicago: American Medical Association, 1989); George Annas and Leonard Glantz, "The Right of Elderly Patients to Refuse Life-Sustaining Treatment," *Millbank Memorial Quarterly* 64, suppl. 2 (1986): 95–162; Robert F. Weir, *Abating Treatment with Critically Ill Patients* (New York: Oxford University Press, 1989); Sidney J. Wanzer et al., "The Physician's Responsibility toward Hopelessly Ill Patients," *NEJM* 310 (1984): 955–59.

2. M.A.M. de Wachter, "Active Euthanasia in the Netherlands," *JAMA* 262, no. 23 (1989): 3315–19.

3. Anonymous, "It's Over, Debbie," *JAMA* 259 (1988): 272; Timothy E. Quill, "Death and Dignity," *NEJM* 322 (1990): 1881–83.

4. Wanzer et al., "The Physician's Responsibility toward Hopelessly Ill Patients: A Second Look," *NEJM* 320 (1989): 844–49.

5. Willard Gaylin, Leon R. Kass, Edmund D. Pellegrino, and Mark Siegler, "Doctors Must Not Kill," *JAMA* 259 (1988): 2139–40.

6. Bonnie Steinbock, ed., *Killing and Allowing to Die* (Englewood Cliffs, NJ.: Prentice Hall, 1980).

7. Dan W. Brock, "Forgoing Food and Water: Is It Killing?" in *By No Extraordinary Means: The Choice to Forgo Life-Sustaining Food and Water,* ed, Joanne Lynn (Bloomington: Indiana University Press, 1986), pp. 117–31.

8. James Rachels, "Active and Passive Euthanasia," *NEJM* 292 (1975): 78–80; Michael Tooley, *Abortion and Infanticide* (Oxford: Oxford University Press, 1983). In my paper, "Taking Human Life," *Ethics* 95 (1985): 851–65, I argue in more detail that killing in itself is not morally different from allowing to die and defend the strategy of argument employed in this and the succeeding two paragraphs in the text.

9. Dan W. Brock, "Moral Rights and Permissible Killing," in *Ethical Issues Relating to Life and Death*, ed. John Ladd (New York: Oxford University Press, 1979), pp. 94–117.

10. P. Painton and E. Taylor, "Love or Let Die," *Time,* 19 March 1990, pp. 62–71; *Boston Globe/*Harvard University Poll, *Boston Globe,* 3 November 1991.

11. James Rachels, *The End of Life* (Oxford: Oxford University Press, 1986).

12. Marcia Angell, "The Quality of Mercy," *NEJM* 306 (1982): 98–99; M. Donovan, P. Dillon, and L. Mcguire, "Incidence and Characteristics of Pain in a Sample of Medical-Surgical Inpatients," *Pain* 30 (1987): 69–78.

13. Eric Cassell, *The Nature of Suffering and the Goals of Medicine* (New York: Oxford University Press, 1991).

14. Gaylin et al., "Doctors Must Not Kill."

15. Leon R. Kass, "Neither for Love Nor Money: Why Doctors Must Not Kill," *The Public Interest* 94 (1989): 25–46; cf. also his *Toward a More Natural Science: Biology and Human Affairs* (New York: The Free Press, 1985), chs. 6–9.

16. Paul J. Van der Maas et al., "Euthanasia and Other Medical Decisions Concerning the End of Life," *Lancet* 338 (1991): 669–74.

17. Susan M. Wolf, "Holding the Line on Euthanasia," Special Supplement, *Hastings Center Report* 19, no. 1 (1989): 13–15.

18. My formulation of this argument derives from David Velleman's statement of it in his commentary on an earlier version of this paper delivered at the American Philosophical Association Central Division meetings; a similar point was made to me by Elisha Milgram in discussion on another occasion. For more general development of the point see Thomas Schelling, *The Strategy of Conflict* (Cambridge, Mass.: Harvard University Press, 1960); and Gerald Dworkin, "Is More Choice Better Than Less?" in *The Theory and Practice of Autonomy* (Cambridge: Cambridge University Press, 1988).

19. Frederick Schauer, "Slippery Slopes," *Harvard Law Review* 99 (1985): 361–83; Wibren van der Burg, "The Slippery Slope Argument," *Ethics* 102 (October 1991): 42–65.

20. There is evidence that physicians commonly fail to diagnose depression. See Robert I. Misbin, "Physicians Aid in Dying," *NEJM* 325 (1991): 1304–7.

21. Richard Fenigsen, "A Case against Dutch Euthanasia," Special Supplement, *Hastings Center Report* 19, no. 1 (1989): 22–30.

22. Allen E. Buchanan and Dan W. Brock, *Deciding for Others: The Ethics of Surrogate Decisionmaking* (Cambridge: Cambridge University Press, 1989).

23. Van der Maas et al., "Euthanasia and Other Medical Decisions."

24. Margaret P. Battin, "Seven Caveats Concerning the Discussion of Euthanasia in Holland," *American Philosophical Association Newsletter on Philosophy and Medicine* 89, no. 2 (1990).

When Self-Determination Runs Amok

Daniel Callahan

The euthanasia debate is not just another moral debate, one in a long list of arguments in our pluralistic society. It is profoundly emblematic of three important turning points in Western thought. The first is that of the legitimate conditions under which one person can kill another. The acceptance of voluntary active euthanasia would morally sanction what can only be called "consenting adult killing." By that term I mean the killing of one person by another in the name of their mutual right to be killer and killed if they freely agree to play those roles. This turn flies in the face of a longstanding effort to limit the circumstances under which one person can take the life of another, from efforts to control the free flow of guns and arms, to abolish capital punishment, and to more tightly control warfare. Euthanasia would add a whole new category of killing to a society that already has too many excuses to indulge itself in that way.

The second turning point lies in the meaning and limits of self-determination. The acceptance of euthanasia would sanction a view of autonomy holding that individuals may, in the name of their own private, idiosyncratic view of the good life, call upon others, including such institutions as medicine, to help them pursue that life, even at the risk of harm to the common good. This works against the idea that the meaning and scope of our own right to lead our own lives must be conditioned by, and be compatible with, the good of the community, which is more than an aggregate of self-directing individuals.

The third turning point is to be found in the claim being made upon medicine: it should be prepared to make its skills available to individuals to help them achieve their private vision of the good life. This puts medicine in the business of promoting the individualistic pursuit of general human happiness and well-being. It would overturn the traditional belief that medicine should limit its domain to promoting and preserving human health, redirecting it instead to the relief of that suffering which stems from life itself, not merely from a sick body.

I believe that, at each of these three turning points, proponents of euthanasia push us in the wrong direction. Arguments in favor of euthanasia fall into four general categories, which I will take up in turn: (1) the moral claim of individual self-determination and well-being; (2) the moral irrelevance of the difference between killing and allowing to die; (3) the supposed paucity of evidence to show likely harmful consequences of legalized euthanasia; and (4) the compatibility of euthanasia and medical practice.

SELF-DETERMINATION

Central to most arguments for euthanasia is the principle of self-determination. People are presumed to have an interest in deciding for themselves, according to their own beliefs about what makes life good, how they will conduct their lives. That is an important value, but the question in the euthanasia context is, What does it mean and how far should it extend? If it were a question of suicide, where a person takes her own life without assistance from another, that principle might be pertinent, at least for debate. But euthanasia is not that limited a matter. The self-determination in that case can only be effected by the moral and physical assistance of another. Euthanasia is thus no longer a matter only of self-determination, but of a mutual,

Callahan, D. (1992) "When Self-Determination Runs Amok." *Hastings Center Report* 22(2): pp. 52–55.

social decision between two people, the one to be killed and the other to do the killing.

How are we to make the moral move from my right of self-determination to some doctor's right to kill me—from my right to his right? Where does the doctor's moral warrant to kill come from? Ought doctors to be able to kill anyone they want as long as permission is given by competent persons? Is our right to life just like a piece of property, to be given away or alienated if the price (happiness, relief of suffering) is right? And then to be destroyed with our permission once alienated?

In answer to all those questions, I will say this: I have yet to hear a plausible argument why it should be permissible for us to put this kind of power in the hands of another, whether a doctor or anyone else. The idea that we can waive our right to life, and then give to another the power to take that life, requires a justification yet to be provided by anyone.

Slavery was long ago outlawed on the ground that one person should not have the right to own another, even with the other's permission. Why? Because it is a fundamental moral wrong for one person to give over his life and fate to another, whatever the good consequences, and no less a wrong for another person to have that kind of total, final power. Like slavery, dueling was long ago banned on similar grounds: even free, competent individuals should not have the power to kill each other, whatever their motives, whatever the circumstances. Consenting adult killing, like consenting adult slavery or degradation, is a strange route to human dignity.

There is another problem as well. If doctors, once sanctioned to carry out euthanasia, are to be themselves responsible moral agents—not simply hired hands with lethal injections at the ready—then they must have their own independent moral grounds to kill those who request such services. What do I mean? As those who favor euthanasia are quick to point out, some people want it because their life has become so burdensome it no longer seems worth living.

The doctor will have a difficulty at this point. The degree and intensity to which people suffer from their diseases and their dying, and whether they find life more of a burden than a benefit, has very little directly to do with the nature or extent of their actual physical condition. Three people can have the same condition, but only one will find the suffering unbearable. People suffer, but suffering is as much a function of the values of individuals as it is of the physical causes of that suffering. Inevitably in that circumstance, the doctor will in effect be treating the patient's values. To be responsible, the doctor would have to share those values. The doctor would have to decide, on her own, whether the patient's life was "no longer worth living."

But how could a doctor possibly know that or make such a judgment? Just because the patient said so? I raise this question because, while in Holland at the euthanasia conference reported by Maurice de Wachter elsewhere in this issue, the doctors present agreed that there is no objective way of measuring or judging the claims of patients that their suffering is unbearable. And if it is difficult to measure suffering, how much more difficult to determine the value of a patient's statement that her life is not worth living?

However one might want to answer such questions, the very need to ask them, to inquire into the physician's responsibility and grounds for medical and moral judgment, points out the social nature of the decision. Euthanasia is not a private matter of self-determination. It is an act that requires two people to make it possible, and a complicit society to make it acceptable.

KILLING AND ALLOWING TO DIE

Against common opinion, the argument is sometimes made that there is no moral difference between stopping life-sustaining treatment and more active forms of killing, such as lethal injection. Instead I would contend that the notion that there is no morally significant difference between omission and commission is just wrong. Consider in its broad implications what the eradication of the distinction implies: that death from disease has been banished, leaving only the actions of physicians in terminating treatment as the cause of death. Biology, which used to bring about death, has apparently been displaced by human agency. Doctors have finally, I suppose, thus genuinely become gods, now doing what nature and the deities once did.

What is the mistake here? It lies in confusing causality and culpability, and in failing to note the way in which human societies have overlaid natural causes with moral rules and interpretations. Causality (by which I mean the direct physical causes of death) and culpability (by which I mean our attribution of moral responsibility to human actions) are confused under three circumstances.

They are confused, first, when the action of a physician in stopping treatment of a patient with an underlying lethal disease is construed as *causing* death. On the contrary, the physician's omission can only bring about death on the condition that the patient's disease will kill him in the absence of treatment. We may hold the physician morally responsible for the death, if we have morally judged such actions wrongful omissions. But it confuses reality and moral judgment to see an omitted action as having the same causal status as one that directly kills. A lethal injection will kill both a healthy person and a sick person. A physician's omitted treatment will have no effect on a healthy person. Turn off the machine on me, a healthy person, and nothing will happen. It will only, in contrast, bring the life of a sick person to an end because of an underlying fatal disease.

Causality and culpability are confused, second, when we fail to note that judgments of moral responsibility and culpability are human constructs. By that I mean that we human beings, after moral reflection, have decided to call some actions right or wrong, and to devise moral rules to deal with them. When physicians could do nothing to stop death, they were not held responsible for it. When, with medical progress, they began to have some power over death—but only its timing and circumstances, not its ultimate inevitability—moral rules were devised to set forth their obligations. Natural causes of death

were not thereby banished. They were, instead, overlaid with a medical ethics designed to determine moral culpability in deploying medical power.

To confuse the judgments of this ethics with the physical causes of death—which is the connotation of the word kill—is to confuse nature and human action. People will, one way or another, die of some disease; death will have dominion over all of us. To say that a doctor "kills" a patient by allowing this to happen should only be understood as a moral judgment about the licitness of his omission, nothing more. We can, as a fashion of speech only, talk about a doctor killing a patient by omitting treatment he should have provided. It is a fashion of speech precisely because it is the underlying disease that brings death when treatment is omitted; that is its cause, not the physician's omission. It is a misuse of the word *killing* to use it when a doctor stops a treatment he believes will no longer benefit the patient—when, that is, he steps aside to allow an eventually inevitable death to occur now rather than later. The only deaths that human beings invented are those that come from direct killing—when, with a lethal injection, we both cause death and are morally responsible for it. In the case of omissions, we do not cause death even if we may be judged morally responsible for it.

This difference between causality and culpability also helps us see why a doctor who has omitted a treatment he should have provided has "killed" that patient while another doctor—performing precisely the same act of omission on another patient in different circumstances—does not kill her, but only allows her to die. The difference is that we have come, by moral convention and conviction, to classify unauthorized or illegitimate omissions as acts of "killing." We call them "killing" in the expanded sense of the term: a culpable action that permits the real cause of death, the underlying disease, to proceed to its lethal conclusion. By contrast, the doctor who, at the patient's request, omits or terminates unwanted treatment does not kill at all. Her underlying disease, not his action, is the physical cause of death; and we have agreed to consider actions of that kind to be morally licit. He thus can truly be said to have "allowed" her to die.

If we fail to maintain the distinction between killing and allowing to die, moreover, there are some disturbing possibilities. The first would be to confirm many physicians in their already too-powerful belief that, when patients die or when physicians stop treatment because of the futility of continuing it, they are somehow both morally and physically responsible for the deaths that follow. That notion needs to be abolished, not strengthened. It needlessly and wrongly burdens the physician, to whom should not be attributed the powers of the gods. The second possibility would be that, in every case where a doctor judges medical treatment no longer effective in prolonging life, a quick and direct killing of the patient would be seen as the next, most reasonable step, on grounds of both humaneness and economics. I do not see how that logic could easily be rejected.

CALCULATING THE CONSEQUENCES

When concerns about the adverse social consequences of permitting euthanasia are raised, its advocates tend to dismiss them as unfounded and overly speculative. On the contrary; recent data about the Dutch experience suggests that such concerns are right on target. From my own discussions in Holland, and from the articles on that subject in this issue and elsewhere, I believe we can now fully see most of the likely consequences of legal euthanasia.

Three consequences seem almost certain, in this or any other country: the inevitability of some abuse of the law; the difficulty of precisely writing, and then enforcing, the law; and the inherent slipperiness of the moral reasons for legalizing euthanasia in the first place.

Why is abuse inevitable? One reason is that almost all laws on delicate, controversial matters are to some extent abused. This happens because not everyone will agree with the law as written and will bend it, or ignore it, if they can get away with it. From explicit admissions to me by Dutch proponents of euthanasia, and

from the corroborating information provided by the Remmelink Report and the outside studies of Carlos Gomez and John Keown, I am convinced that in the Netherlands there are a substantial number of cases of nonvoluntary euthanasia, that is, euthanasia undertaken without the explicit permission of the person being killed. The other reason abuse is inevitable is that the law is likely to have a low enforcement priority in the criminal justice system. Like other laws of similar status, unless there is an unrelenting and harsh willingness to pursue abuse, violations will ordinarily be tolerated. The worst thing to me about my experience in Holland was the casual, seemingly indifferent attitude toward abuse. I think that would happen everywhere.

Why would it be hard to precisely write, and then enforce, the law? The Dutch speak about the requirement of "unbearable" suffering, but admit that such a term is just about indefinable, a highly subjective matter admitting of no objective standards. A requirement for outside opinion is nice, but it is easy to find complaisant colleagues. A requirement that a medical condition be "terminal" will run aground on the notorious difficulties of knowing when an illness is actually terminal.

Apart from those technical problems there is a more profound worry. I see no way, even in principle, to write or enforce a meaningful law that can guarantee effective procedural safeguards. The reason is obvious yet almost always overlooked. The euthanasia transaction will ordinarily take place within the boundaries of the private and confidential doctor-patient relationship. No one can possibly know what takes place in that context unless the doctor chooses to reveal it. In Holland, less than 10 percent of the physicians report their acts of euthanasia and do so with almost complete legal impunity. There is no reason why the situation should be any better elsewhere. Doctors will have their own reasons for keeping euthanasia secret, and some patients will have no less a motive for wanting it concealed.

I would mention, finally, that the moral logic of the motives for euthanasia contain within them the ingredients of abuse. The two standard motives for euthanasia and assisted suicide are said to be our right of self-determination, and our claim upon the mercy of others, especially doctors, to relieve our suffering. These two motives are typically spliced together and presented as a single justification. Yet if they are considered independently—and there is no inherent reason why they must be linked—they reveal serious problems. It is said that a competent, adult person should have a right to euthanasia for the relief of suffering. But why must the person be suffering? Does not that stipulation already compromise the principle of self-determination? How can self-determination have any limits? Whatever the person's motives may be, why are they not sufficient?

Consider next the person who is suffering but not competent, who is perhaps demented or mentally retarded. The standard argument would deny euthanasia to that person. But why? If a person is suffering but not competent, then it would seem grossly unfair to deny relief solely on the grounds of incompetence. Are the incompetent less entitled to relief from suffering than the competent? Will it only be affluent, middle-class people, mentally fit and savvy about working the medical system, who can qualify? Do the incompetent suffer less because of their incompetence?

Considered from these angles, there are no good moral reasons to limit euthanasia once the principle of taking life for that purpose has been legitimated. If we really believe in self-determination, then any competent person should have a right to be killed by a doctor for any reason that suits him. If we believe in the relief of suffering, then it seems cruel and capricious to deny it to the incompetent. There is, in short, no reasonable or logical stopping point once the turn has been made down the road to euthanasia, which could soon turn into a convenient and commodious expressway.

EUTHANASIA AND MEDICAL PRACTICE

A fourth kind of argument one often hears both in the Netherlands and in this country is that euthanasia and assisted suicide are perfectly compatible with the aims of medicine. I would note at the very outset that a physician who participates in another person's suicide already abuses medicine. Apart from depression (the main statistical cause of suicide), people commit suicide because they find life empty, oppressive, or meaningless. Their judgment is a judgment about the value of continued life, not only about health (even if they are sick). Are doctors now to be given the right to make judgments about the kinds of life worth living and to give their blessing to suicide for those they judge wanting? What conceivable competence, technical or moral, could doctors claim to play such a role? Are we to medicalize suicide, turning judgments about its worth and value into one more clinical issue? Yes, those are rhetorical questions.

Yet they bring us to the core of the problem of euthanasia and medicine. The great temptation of modern medicine, not always resisted, is to move beyond the promotion and preservation of health into the boundless realm of general human happiness and well-being. The root problem of illness and mortality is both medical and philosophical or religious. "Why must I die?" can be asked as a technical, biological question or as a question about the meaning of life. When medicine tries to respond to the latter, which it is always under pressure to do, it moves beyond its proper role.

It is not medicine's place to lift from us the burden of that suffering which turns on the meaning we assign to the decay of the body and its eventual death. It is not medicine's place to determine when lives are not worth living or when the burden of life is too great to be borne. Doctors have no conceivable way of evaluating such claims on the part of patients, and they should have no right to act in response to them. Medicine should try to relieve human suffering, but only that suffering which is brought on by illness and dying as biological phenomena, not that suffering which comes from anguish or despair at the human condition.

Doctors ought to relieve those forms of suffering that medically accompany serious illness and the threat of death. They should relieve pain, do what they can to allay anxiety and uncertainty, and be a comforting presence. As sensitive human beings, doctors should be prepared to respond to patients who ask why they must die, or die in pain. But here the doctor and the patient are at the same level. The doctor may have no better an answer to those old questions than anyone else; and certainly no special insight from his training as a physician. It would be terrible for physicians to forget this, and to think that in a swift, lethal injection, medicine has found its own answer to the riddle of life. It would be a false answer, given by the wrong people. It would be no less a false answer for patients. They should neither ask medicine to put its own vocation at risk to serve their private interests, nor think that the answer to suffering is to be killed by another. The problem is precisely that, too often in human history, killing has seemed the quick, efficient way to put aside that which burdens us. It rarely helps, and too often simply adds to one evil still another. That is what I believe euthanasia would accomplish. It is self-determination run amok.

Medical Ethics and Double Effect: The Case of Terminal Sedation

Joseph Boyle

The ethics of the medical profession incorporates some application of the moral doctrine of the double effect, particularly to govern medical decisions whose outcomes include shortening a patient's life. Very roughly: double effect provides that it can be morally good to shorten a patient's life as a foreseen and accepted but unintended side effect of an action undertaken for a good reason, even if it is agreed that intentionally killing the patient or shortening the patient's life is wrong. The medical profession's use of this moral doctrine has some support in legal decisions.[1]

The use of terminal sedation to control the intense discomfort of dying patients appears to be an established procedure within palliative care. But sometimes the amount of sedative needed to control suffering has the effect of shortening the patient's life. This creates worries that the requirements of appropriate palliative care mandate actions indistinguishable from euthanasia, which is illegal and morally objectionable to many health care professionals. Invoking double effect addresses these worries: the intent of the physician prescribing the life-shortening analgesics is to control the suffering, not to shorten life. Evidence of physician intent can be found in notations on the patient's chart and in the recorded dosages and titration of analgesics. Consequently, this action is not euthanasia but palliative care.[2]

A consensus was reached among a small but representative group of Canadian intensivists and a similar group of coroners that this application of double effect provided proper ethical guidance concerning terminal sedation. Possibly, therefore, there is consensus or the prospect of the emergence of a consensus on this application of double effect among intensivists and other physicians, including those with oversight responsibility for deaths related to medical decisions.[3]

Whether or not the consensus reported in this study can be further validated or extended,

---

With kind permission from Springer Science + Business Media: *Theoretical Medicine and Bioethics*, Boyle, J., "Medical Ethics and Double Effect: The Case of Terminal Sedation", 25(1), pp. 51–60, © 2004.

it pointedly raises the central ethical issues involved in the prospect that this application of double effect could be an established part of medical ethics—and, consequently, legally enforced. Addressing these issues is distinct from determining the consensus of practitioners. The central issue is perhaps this: double effect is a general moral doctrine, not an *ad hoc* device to deal with terminal sedation or other difficult life and death decisions. This doctrine emerged within the casuistry of Roman Catholicism. How much of this distinctive moral view does the medical profession and the law implicitly accept by accepting this application of double effect? To answer this question it is useful to consider further the idea of double effect and its rationale within Catholic moral theology.

The expression "double effect" was first used by St. Thomas Aquinas (1225–1274) to refer to the duality of the results of a single human action. A person performing an action that is foreseen to have a multiplicity of results can have very different interests in them—from serious commitment to bringing about a result to reluctant acceptance of a result that is unwanted but unavoidable. Since actions are purposeful, at least one of the results of an action must be intended, but others, although knowingly and voluntarily caused, can be outside the agent's intention; these latter results I will call "accepted side effects." Aquinas made this distinction in discussing killing in self-defense: one who uses lethal force for defense against attack need not intend the assailant's death; that can be outside the agent's intention.[4]

Following Aquinas, Roman Catholic moral theology has attributed a specific, and very important, moral significance to this distinction between what a person intends in acting and what a person accepts as a side effect of intentionally acting for another result. The significance is this: the factors sufficient to make simply wrong actions involving the intention of some result are not also sufficient to make simply wrong actions involving accepting, but not intending, a result of the same kind. In other words, the impermissibility of an action that is based upon the agent's intention of a certain result does not render impermissible actions having a result of that kind, if the result is not intended, but accepted as a side effect. In Aquinas's example of killing in self-defense, the moral issue was framed by the acceptance of the Augustinian prohibition of killing in self-defense on the part of private persons, those lacking public authority to kill. That prohibition, Aquinas maintained, applied only to intentional killing, not to killing brought about and accepted as a side effect. Consequently, the acceptance of the Augustinian limitation on those who are permitted to kill does not imply the impermissibility of lethal self-defense, where the death is not intentional.

The manuals of moral theology of the nineteenth century refined and formulated Aquinas's reasoning into a set of rules useful for giving moral advice and conducting casuistry. These rules became [known] as the doctrine of double effect, or the principle of double effect. They were generally formulated as three or four necessary conditions for the permissibility of actions similar in some of their results to actions that are impermissible because of the general categories into which they fall. Thus, the classic formulation of the Jesuit moralist J.-B. Gury, in the mid-nineteenth century:

> It is licit to posit a cause which is either good or indifferent from which there follows a twofold effect, one good the other evil, if a proportionately grave reason is present, and if the end of the agent is honorable—that is, if he does not intend the evil.[5]

Gury elaborated these three conditions into four, by construing the condition of honorable intention as two. The first addressed the distinction between a means and a side effect: if the bad effect—that is, the result which would render that action simply wrong were it intended—is the means to the good effect, then it cannot be a side effect and is intended. Thus, the key requirement that the good effect be brought about "immediately," that is, not by means of the bad effect. The second of these extrapolated conditions—that one intend only the good effect—excludes cases in which the bad effect is not brought about as a means to the good effect, but is nevertheless intended because it functions as an independent goal. An example would be "bonus" effects—results that emerge as side effects of bringing about a goal but then recognized as independently useful or beneficial and so (ordinarily) intended.

Gury's first two conditions—that the "cause" be morally good or indifferent and that there be a proportionately grave reason for doing what brings about evil side effects—refer to the further moral considerations that are needed for a complete assessment of an action meeting the conditions for upright intention. These conditions address the two areas where Gury thought an action that cleared the intentionally focused conditions might still fail morally. The first area of concern arises from the possibility that, prior to any consideration of further results that might be intended or accepted as side effects but not intended, some actions might be simply wrong. Perhaps his thought here is that since the movements a person chooses for the sake of self-defense have both defensive and destructive results, one can distinguish the chosen performance from the results and ask of it whether that performance is morally permissible. In some cases, telling a lie or committing adultery, for example, the action is impermissible on account of considerations logically prior to those concerning intended or accepted results. In the case at hand, a physician's prescribing analgesics, described in just that way, is morally indifferent; therefore, the results, intentions and other circumstances of this chosen behavior will determine its permissibility or impermissibility. In this respect the action is unlike acts of adultery or lying, which as so described are wrong.

This condition may be strictly redundant (and perhaps also confused) since an intended result is intrinsic to an action as a chosen performance, as the lying and adultery cases indicate. Nevertheless, this condition highlights an important aspect of the style of moral reasoning

involved in double effect: if this condition, or either of the intentionally focused conditions is not met, then the act is simply and indefeasibly impermissible. These are absolute judgments that cannot be overturned by further considerations of the action's particular circumstances: thus, in Aquinas's example of killing in self-defense, for any person who is not publicly authorized, intentionally killing the assailant is simply, that is, indefeasibly, wrong; nothing further one can discover about the action will reverse that moral judgment.[6] This is the absolutism of double effect.

The second area of concern is that even if the intentional conditions are met, and the action is not excluded as simply wrong for some prior reason, the full consideration of its circumstances might still turn up a morally excluding factor. The requirement of a proportionately grave reason explicitly addresses this second area; it presupposes that bringing about as a side effect what would be wrong to bring about intentionally is likely harmful or otherwise morally suspect, and so in need of wider justification. Thus, the requirement is that any other considerations relevant to the moral assessment of the action should be brought to bear. In Aquinas's example of self-defense, two concerns were addressed: whether one defending oneself has a duty to refrain from harming the assailant, and the extent of the violence of the defensive action. He argued that one's duty to refrain is generally less pressing than the duty to protect one's life, and only that level of violence needed for the defense is justified.[7]

The determination of what constitutes a proportionately grave matter is not essential for assessing what is distinctive in the doctrine of double effect. That determination is likely to be as complex and as variable in outcome as any other reasoning leading to an all-things-considered assessment of the morality of an action.[8] But the existence of this condition, both in the manualist formulations and in Aquinas's reasoning in his classic statement, underlines the fact that double effect does not imply that it is permissible to bring about bad results if and only if they are not intended.

In the case of terminal sedation, this condition of proportionality seems to be easily met, and the existing consensus assumes that. The need for palliation of some dying patients is substantial and is assumed generally to justify terminal sedation if moral and legal worries about euthanasia are satisfactorily addressed.[9]

This brief survey of the Catholic sources of double effect shows what it means, and at least roughly how it works. But the summary does not provide a justification of the special moral significance attributed to the distinction between what a person intends in acting and accepts as a side effect (hereafter the intended/accepted distinction). That is because there appears to be no developed justification in the tradition. It seems that Aquinas and the theological tradition regarded the ethical significance of the intended/accepted distinction of double effect as simply obvious. Aquinas's unargued assertion that what is intended is morally *per se* and what is outside or beyond the intention is *per accidens* suggests as much.[10]

Some applications of double effect are certainly intuitively compelling, for example, those distinguishing terror bombing in warfare from carefully targeted bombing of military targets where some civilians will likely be killed as side effects. But such intuitive convictions are not readily generalized to all cases of double effect, particularly to those where peoples' normative convictions about the cases distinguished is more variable and uncertain than in the bombing cases.[11] The distinction between terminal sedation and euthanasia may distinguish just such cases: some may accept terminal sedation but regard efforts to distinguish it from euthanasia to be sleight of hand; some may, for reasons independent of reasoning about terminal sedation, accept euthanasia as morally legitimate and so fail to see the point of introducing double effect's distinctions.

Moreover, people's convictions about especially clear cases are not sufficiently focused to justify the precise significance double effect requires the intended/accepted distinction to bear. Thus, some think that double effect implies that the distinction between bad outcomes that are intended and those that are accepted is that

bringing about the former is, other things being equal, morally worse than bringing about the latter.[12] This is not obviously true: the reckless or unjustified inflicting of harm as a side effect is not clearly worse than inflicting it intentionally. More importantly, the implication of double effect is different: namely, that the wrongness of the former does not guarantee that of the latter.

Perhaps the moral significance of this distinction appeared obvious to older Catholic moralists because of its analogy to the structure of divine creative activity: God creates only good, but allows the evils of his creation—evils he does not intentionally cause but only permits as privations that flaw his good creation.[13] This analogue suggests a justification. Just as God creates only what is good, humans should voluntarily pursue in their actions only what is humanly good. And just as God permits the evils flawing his creation, so humans must accept some evil consequences they should not intend.

The idea is that God, if he is to create some universe he has good reason to create, must permit the evils which inevitably arise as side effects of his creating that universe—for example, the misuse of free will by rational creatures' immoral choices. Applied to human action, the analogy suggests that in acting humans can and should aim exclusively at the good, but that there will inevitably be some bad side effects of doing that.

Independently of the suggestive theological analogy, there is a limitation on the human capacity to pursue the good, and that limitation is precisely an incapacity to avoid evil side effects, not an incapacity to choose and intend only the good.

The limitation is this: in all the situations calling for human choice, no matter what a person chooses to do, some instance of a human good will be harmed, destroyed or at least knowingly neglected (hereafter I will refer to all such harms as simply "harming a good"). Thus, it is beyond human power to act in such a way that one's action does nothing more than promote human good; in all human action some instances of human goods are promoted and served while others are, at the very least, not promoted (as when a person leaves some of her talents undeveloped to pursue a career), or, very often, more or less harmed (as one risks health for the sake of sports), or in some cases even destroyed (as when one kills, whether intentionally or as a side effect).

This limitation is essentially a limitation on the human capacity to avoid some bad side effects of good choices, and not a limitation on the human capacity to avoid choosing precisely for the sake of bad goals. In the choice to act for some goal, namely, in an intentional action, it always remains in the agent's power to choose not to do it. So, when something humanly evil—harming a good—is the intended result of one's action, one always has the choice of not doing that action. But one does not have a choice about whether or not there will be some bad side effects of whatever one chooses to do. Accepting bad side effects, therefore, is unavoidable, choosing to pursue results that involve harming a good is always avoidable—though often at a high price.

Since some bad side effects are inevitable, a morality based on concern for the human good does not justify an impossible prohibition of bringing them about. Rather, the relevant moral guidance concerning bringing about bad side effects addresses questions such as which bad side effects are to be accepted and on whom the harms will fall—matters considered under the proportionality condition of double effect. But if the underlying moral principle is taken to be allegiance to the human good, a person's intentional actions can always be aimed at the good, since one can always choose to avoid any that are not. Prohibition against intentionally harming a human good is not an impossible prohibition.

As already noted above, the prohibitions against intentionally harming human goods presupposed by double effect are taken to be indefeasible or absolute. That puts the morality in which double effect developed at odds with much of current moral opinion. What now counts as common sense morality largely rejects indefeasible prohibitions of actions of generally described kinds; and consequentialism rejects moral absolutes as inadequate devices for promoting the good. But if allegiance to the good is morally basic, and if instances of goods are not commensurable

in goodness, then rational concern for the good readily justifies absolute prohibitions of intentionally harming them. For if instances of human goods are incommensurable in their goodness, the respect for each instance of such goodness is required because there cannot be any good or sum of goods that would capture precisely the goodness of that instance. On these assumptions, therefore, absolute prohibitions of harms to the most basic goods alone do justice to the reality of the human good.[14] But although double effect presupposes the truth of some such indefeasible norms, its function in moral thought is not to justify them but rather to limit their application to intentionally harming the goods of human beings.

If the preceding account of the justification of double effect's use of the intended/accepted distinction is sound, then within the framework of traditional morality as understood by the older Catholic moralists double effect is a legitimate moral doctrine. Within that context, it plainly is a moral doctrine, not a specifically Catholic or religious doctrine, since it is the implication of the character of a limitation in human action and willing joined with the implications of a kind of goods based ethical theory. Can the justification be exported from its strictly moral framework to the regulatory framework of medical ethics?

In one respect, double effect cannot be exported as is. A person's intentions in doing an action may be inferred from the action and other aspects of its context, most importantly, how a person explains his or her actions. But a person's intentions themselves are at least in part inaccessible to others, and sometimes difficult even for the acting person to articulate accurately and reflectively. Opponents of double effect argue that these epistemological difficulties are insurmountable, indeed, that they suggest that the basic concepts of double effect cannot be rationally applied.[15] However, difficult applications of double effect can be debated with the possibility of confident agreement, and not all applications are controversial. Moreover, an individual's efforts to make upright choices will involve personal moral scrutiny and discussion with others that can lead to judgments that are sufficiently confident to guide choices for many cases.[16]

But in the context of the regulation of behavior by law or by professional ethics, the third person perspective of judges and juries becomes more central, and concerns about people's deepest moral orientations less important. Here the relevant volitions are not those inaccessible in a person's heart, but only those of which there is evidence accessible to others besides the agent. For example, the evidence of intent in terminal sedation cases is the sum of notations on charts, dosages and titration of analgesics, and so on. A physician who would prefer to perform euthanasia but who remains constrained in his or her actions by the requirements of intent as publicly accessible indicates that he or she does not intend to end life, even if he or she wishes to do that. And that implies that those who cooperate with such a physician's action, are cooperating only in a common act of palliative care, not of euthanasia.

These considerations show that the question about the exportability of double effect to medical ethics must be reformulated. The inherent limitations involved in using a moral doctrine for public regulatory purposes must be recognized. The question remains: supposing they are recognized, can the moral doctrine be exported?

If there are some kinds of behavior which society or a profession judges unacceptable, then altogether banning that behavior may be tempting. But a general ban on behavior having certain results likely prohibits too much, for reasons already noted: for example, causing death or bodily harm is not reasonably prohibited by medical ethics when unavoidable, and such results are unavoidable in some clinical conditions. However, banning intentional killing is not prohibiting too much in this way.

Furthermore, there appear to be good reasons why the medical profession would want to uphold such a ban,[17] and, therefore, if practitioners are confident of their ability publicly to determine intent in the relevant cases, then such a prohibition would be as justified as the prohibitions in the strictly moral cases. The fact that the ban would not be justified if applied to the acceptance of side effects has, of itself, no tendency to call into question the narrower exclusion of intentional killing.

The logic of double effect, therefore, has application in medical ethics and the law, quite independently of the particular moral framework in which it was developed and has a natural function in moral reasoning. Double effect does not provide the justification of norms excluding intentionally harming a person's good, but reminds us that when such norms are taken as true or appropriate, whether as moral norms or social regulations, they cannot reasonably prohibit harming as a side effect. And so, the inference common in debates about euthanasia is not sound: it is not the case that the fact that we accept bringing about death or an earlier death as a side effect of choosing something else gives rational grounds for judging intentional killing to be justified.[18]

Notes

1. *Vacco v. Quill*, 117 Supreme Court Reporter 2293 (1997); J. Finnis, G. Grisez, and J. Boyle, "'Direct' and 'Indirect': A Reply to Critics of Our Action Theory," *The Thomist* 65 (2001): 1–44.
2. L. Hawryluck and W. Harvey, "Analgesia, Virtue, and the Principle of Double Effect," *Journal of Palliative Care* 16 supplement, October (2000): S24–S30.
3. L. Hawryluck, W. Harvey, L. Lemieux-Charles, and P. Singer, "Consensus Guidelines on [Analgesia] and Sedation in Dying Intensive Care Patients," *BMC Medical Ethics* (2002), http://www.biomedcentral.com/1472-6939/3/3.
4. St. Thomas Aquinas, *Summa Theologiae*, II-II, q. 64, a. 7.
5. J. Boyle, "Towards Understanding the Principle of Double Effect," *Ethics* 90 (1980): 527–538.
6. Cf. n. 4, above.
7. Cf. n. 4, above.
8. G. Grisez, *The Way of the Lord Jesus: Volume 3: Difficult Moral Questions*, Appendix 1: "Human Acts and Moral Judgments," (Quincy, IL: Franciscan Press, 1997), pp. 849–870.
9. Cf. n. 2 and n. 3, above.
10. Cf. n. 4, above.
11. J. Boyle, "Who is Entitled to Double Effect?" *The Journal of Medicine and Philosophy* 16 (1991): 475–494.
12. Cf. n. 11, above.

13. J. Boyle, "Intentions, Christian Morality and Bioethics: Puzzles of Double Effect," *Christian Bioethics* 3 (1997): 87–88.

14. J. Finnis, J. Boyle, and G. Grisez, "A Sounder Theory of Morality," in *Nuclear Deterrence, Morality and Realism.* (Oxford: Oxford University Press, 1987), pp. 275–296; See also n. 11 and n. 13, above.

15. T. Quill, R. Dresser, and D. Brock, "The Rule of Double Effect: A Critique of Its Role in End-of-Life Decision Making," *The New England Journal of Medicine* 337 (1997): 1768–1771.

16. J. Finnis, G. Grisez, and J. Boyle, "'Direct' and 'Indirect': A Reply to Critics of Our Action Theory," *The Thomist* 65 (2001): 1–44; See also n. 5, above.

17. D. Sulmasy and E. Pellegrino, "The Rule of Double Effect: Clearing Up the Double Talk," *Archives of Internal Medicine* 159 (1999): 545–550; See also *Vacco v. Quill*, n. 1, above.

18. Cf. D. Sulmasy and E. Pellegrino, "The Rule of Double Effect: Clearing Up the Double Talk," n. [17], above. See also n. [15], above.

CASES

Rodriguez v British Columbia (Attorney General), [1993] 3 SCR 519, 1993 CanLII 519 (SCC)

Summary prepared by Josephine Johnston

At the time of her appeal to the Supreme Court of Canada, Sue Rodriguez was a 42-year-old woman living in British Columbia. She had been diagnosed with amyotrophic lateral sclerosis, also known as Lou Gehrig's disease. As a result of this disease, Ms. Rodriguez's health was rapidly deteriorating such that she would soon be unable to swallow, speak, walk, or move without assistance. She would eventually lose the ability to breathe without a respirator or eat without a surgically placed feeding tube. She knew that she would soon die (at the time of her appeal, her life expectancy was estimated at between 2 and 14 months). Ms. Rodriguez did not wish to die while she could still enjoy her life. However, she wanted the option of ending her life at a time of her choosing and with the aid of a physician. To this end, she went to court to challenge the *Criminal Code* prohibition on assisted suicide.

Section 241(b) of the *Criminal Code of Canada* states that every person who "aids or abets a person to commit suicide" is guilty of an offence and liable for 14 years imprisonment. Under the section, any physician who set up technological means by which Ms. Rodriguez could end her life, if and when she chose to, would be guilty of aiding her to commit suicide. In light of this potential criminal liability, Ms. Rodriguez sought an order declaring section 241(b) of the *Criminal Code* invalid on the ground that it breached the *Canadian Charter of Rights and Freedoms*.

Discussion Questions

1. What, if anything, is the difference between pain and suffering?

2. Is there a morally relevant difference between allowing to die and helping to die? Between helping to die and killing?

3. If assisting suicide was morally permissible for Sue Rodriguez, should the criminal law be changed to make assisting suicide legally permissible for all individuals? Should what is morally right in one specific case determine what is legally right?

Reprinted by permission of the author.

R v Latimer, 2001 SCC 1, [2001] 1 SCR 3

Summary prepared by Maegen Giltrow

On Sunday, October 24, 1993, while Tracy Latimer's mother and siblings were at church, her father, Robert Latimer, sat Tracy in the cab of his pickup truck and siphoned exhaust into the cab. Tracy died of carbon monoxide poisoning.

Tracy had suffered a severe form of cerebral palsy; she was quadriplegic and immobile. She was said to have the mental capacity of a four-month-old baby, with the concomitant ability to communicate through facial expressions, laughter, and crying. She suffered five to six seizures daily, and it was thought that she experienced a great deal of pain. The pain could not be reduced through medication, as pain medication conflicted with her anti-epileptic medication, and because she had difficulty swallowing. The Latimers had rejected a feeding-tube option as being both intrusive, and as a first step toward preserving Tracy's life artificially.

Mr. Latimer made the decision to end Tracy's life when another in a long line of surgeries for Tracy had been scheduled. This one was to address her dislocated hip, and, it was hoped, to lessen her constant pain. The Latimers were told that the surgery, wherein Tracy's upper thighbone would be removed and her leg left connected only by soft tissue, would cause Tracy pain. They were also told that future surgery would be required to relieve the pain Tracy felt in various joints of her body. Mr. Latimer concluded that Tracy's death was an alternative favourable to constant surgery and constant pain.

Discussion Questions

1. What makes a life worth living?
2. Does allowing a severely disabled person to die, or killing a severely disabled person as Mr. Latimer did, demonstrate a lack of respect for the humanity and dignity of vulnerable disabled persons? Or, does it promote the equality of severely disabled persons by according them, on their own or through a surrogate decision maker, the same options non-disabled persons have to discontinue or refuse life-sustaining care or to commit suicide when the likely burdens of life outweigh the likely benefits?
3. How should decisions be made about care for severely disabled persons who are not capable of making decisions for themselves? How extensive should the authority of family members be, and what role should health care professionals play in this decision making?

Useful Resources

ONLINE

Canadian Association of Critical Care Nurses (CACCN), Providing End of Life Care in the ICU

The CACCN position statement on providing end of life care in the ICU.

Canadian Medical Association

Euthanasia and Assisted Suicide (update 1998). The CMA does not support euthanasia and assisted suicide. It urges its members to uphold the principles of palliative care.

Canadian Nurses Association

CNA Position Statement. 2008. Providing nursing care at the end of life.

Canadian Pain Society

Position Statement on Pain Treatment as a Human Right.

Euthanasia and Assisted Suicide in Canada

A review of legal issues related to euthanasia, aiding suicide, the right to refuse medical treatment, and advance directives written for the Parliamentary Information and Research Service of the Library of Parliament and revised on July 17, 2008.

Joint Statement on Resuscitative Interventions (Update 1995)

This joint statement includes: guiding principles for health care facilities when developing cardiopulmonary-resuscitation (CPR) policy; CPR as a treatment option; competence; the treatment decision, its communication, implementation and review; and palliative care and other treatment. This joint statement was approved by the Canadian Healthcare Association, the Canadian Medical Association, the Canadian Nurses Association and the Catholic Health Association of Canada and was developed in cooperation with the Canadian Bar Association.

Of Life and Death

A "Report of the Special Senate Committee on Euthanasia and Assisted Suicide" published in June 1995 that addresses issues of palliative care, pain control and sedation, advance directives, withholding and withdrawing life-sustaining treatment, assisted suicide, and euthanasia.

Palliative.info

"Palliative.info offers an organized, up-to-date collection of links to palliative care resources on the internet, as well as locally developed palliative care material." This website includes a link to Ethics, Position Statements
http://palliative.info/pages/Position.htm

READINGS

Battin, M. P., Rhodes, R., & Silvers, A. (1998). *Physician-assisted suicide: Expanding the debate*. New York, NY: Routledge.

Canadian Neurological Care Group. (1999). Guidelines for the diagnosis of brain death. *Canadian Journal of Neurological Sciences, 26*, 64–6.

Downie, J. (2004). *Dying justice: A case for decriminalizing euthanasia and assisted suicide in Canada*. Toronto: University of Toronto Press.

Gedge, E., Giacomini, M., & Cook, D. (2007). Withholding and withdrawing life support in critical care settings: Ethical issues concerning consent. *Journal of Medical Ethics, 33*(4), 215–218.

Hardwig, J. (1997). Is there a duty to die? *Hastings Center Report, 27*(2), 34–42.

Marquis, D. (2010). Are DCD donors dead? *Hastings Center Report, 40*(3), 24–31.

Rachels, J. (1975). Active and passive euthanasia. *New England Journal of Medicine, 292*(2), 78–80.

Shemie, S. D., Baker, A. J., Knoll, G. et al. (2006). National recommendations for donation after cardiocirculatory death in Canada. *Canadian Medical Association Journal,* 175 (Suppl), S1–S24.

HEALTH LAW

NB v Hôtel-Dieu de Québec (QCA) (1992), 86 DLR (4th) 385, 69 CCC (3d) 450 (Qc Sup Ct)

Nancy B. was diagnosed with Guillian-Barré syndrome, an irreversible disease that caused ascending paralysis but left her intellectual faculties intact. Because her respiratory muscles had atrophied, she needed mechanical assistance to breathe. Knowing that she would soon die, she requested that the respirator be removed. She applied to the court for an order to compel her physicians to stop providing treatment.

Child and Family Services of Central Manitoba v Lavallee et al (1997), 154 DLR (4th) 409, 1997 CanLII 3742 (Man CA)

The parents of an infant in a persistent vegetative state refused to consent to a Do Not Resuscitate (DNR) order. Child and Family Services in the province of Manitoba applied to the court for authorization of the placement of a DNR order on the infant's chart.

Golubchuk v Salvation Army Grace General Hospital et al, 2008 MBQB 49, 290 DLR (4th) 46

Physicians for Mr. Golubchuk wanted to remove him from life support care, ventilation, tube feeding, and medication. His family members disagreed with the decision to stop treatment and sought an injunction to compel the physicians to continue treatment.

CanLII

CanLII is a non-profit organization managed by the Federation of Law Societies of Canada. CanLII's goal is to make Canadian law accessible for free on the Internet.

Chapter 10 CONTESTED THERAPIES AND TECHNOLOGIES

INTRODUCTION

While many people enthusiastically embrace and celebrate technological opportunities to enhance the human body as well as the human condition, many others worry about the ways in which widespread use of technological interventions could potentially distort our understandings of not just human health and well-being but of what it means to be human. That disagreement reflects two different ways of thinking and arguing about technological enhancement. Supporters regard the use of these technologies as simply an extension of what long has been done in many ways. Surgery can repair a cleft palate, but surgery also can straighten a crooked nose and remove wrinkles that are distressing signs of aging, for example. Moreover, parents always have tried to provide abundant opportunities for their children by, for example, sending them to expensive private schools, arranging music lessons for them, and enrolling them in sports. Enhancement technologies that have emerged and will continue to emerge are, in this context, just a new means of pursuing the laudable goal of improving people's lives.

Opponents, however, raise some difficult philosophical and moral questions about the assumptions and implications of enhancement technologies. How is the intimate relationship between our self and our body to be understood? How might a change to a person's body alter that person's identity, and how could it affect his or her relationships with other people? Who should have access to these technologies? How should medically indicated uses of technologies be distinguished from their elective uses? If some enhancements are available to only those who can afford them, would there be even less equality of opportunity than there is now?

In the first article, Arthur Frank uses what he calls "Socratic bioethics" to broaden the scope of the disconcerting questions that can be asked about enhancement technologies, in particular, to raise questions about the nature of the good life and what kind of health is part of the good life. He starts with a personal observation about his "unworthy" reaction to seeing a person who had a physical feature that was normal but nevertheless prompted him to muse, "I'm glad my body's not like that.... [b]ut if it were, I could get that sort of thing fixed." Frank recognizes that the possibility of fixing forces the question of whether to fix, which in turn forces questioning about what we are "called upon to live not only *with* but *as*." He then explores the limits on surgical self-fixing with respect to three contested surgical interventions—limb lengthening for achondroplasia (genetic dwarfism), intersex surgery for anomalous genitalia, and craniofacial surgery for craniofacial deformities. In so doing, he enjoins us to think about more than the time, cost, effort, and possible pain involved with surgical modification. Also relevant, according to Frank, is the impact of surgical modification on one's individuality, identity, and community. As he notes, "none of us chooses anything consequential for 'herself'...as we choose for ourselves, we also confront others with choice." "Choosing" and the "context" in which choices are made are central themes in this chapter.

The second article, by Alice Dreger, examines some of the ethical issues associated with the surgical treatment of intersexuality, one of the three surgeries highlighted by Frank. Dreger begins with a provocative question: "What makes us 'female' or 'male,' 'girls' or 'boys,' 'women' or 'men'—our chromosomes, our genitalia, how we (and others) are brought up to think about ourselves, or all of the above?" In addressing this question, Dreger challenges the dominant conception of "normal" sexual anatomy and "normal" sexual behaviour used to justify reconstructive genital surgery aimed at "normalizing" an "abnormal" child. Ambiguous genitalia, Dreger argues, do not constitute a disease in need of fixing.

The next article, by Françoise Baylis, continues to widen the scope of questions about enhancement by suggesting that human cloning is not only about baby-making or family-making, but also about species-making. Cloning for reproductive purposes should thus be seen as both a reproductive and an enhancement technology—"only in recognizing the enhancement dimensions of cloning technology can we begin to…grapple with the threat/opportunity that cloning humans represents." The theme of species control is explored further (albeit from a somewhat different perspective) in the following article by Françoise Baylis and Jason Scott Robert who predict that the use of genetic technologies to enhance human capacities and traits is inevitable. They argue that despite the many sound reasons why humans ought not to pursue genetic enhancement, use of these technologies will become widespread. Couched in Frank's terms, the controversy about enhancement technologies will be narrowed to an individualistic analysis that focuses on cost and risk–benefit assessments, with the result that identifiable benefits to specific individuals will prevail over amorphous, speculative concerns about deleterious impacts on society and humanity. If Baylis and Robert are right, the challenge then becomes how best to direct relevant technological developments in pursuit of worthy goals.

The final two articles present technologies that need precisely that direction. One of these technologies, examined by Vince Cakic, is cognitive enhancement through the use of pharmaceuticals—so-called cosmetic neurology. Cakic assumes that "smart drugs" will be widely used by healthy individuals who hope to gain a competitive advantage. So how can a sound ethical framework for the use of cognitive enhancers (that is both "reasonable and realistic") be developed? Cakic suggests that much can be learned from efforts to control enhancement in sport.

Another technology that needs to be carefully directed is cell-based regenerative medicine. The article on stem cell transplantation by Olle Lindvall and Insoo Hyun complements the article in Chapter 3 by Gillian Crozier and Françoise Baylis on international medical travel. As reported there, one of the reasons patients travel to foreign destinations for treatment is to access unproven interventions that are not available in their home country, such as stem cell transplantation. Lindvall and Hyun appreciate that stem cell clinics around the world exploit desperate, seriously ill patients. They urge caution in responding to this problem, however, because it is not easy to distinguish between objectionable stem cell tourism and acceptable medical travel for legitimate, medically innovative stem cell therapies. They endorse stem cell-based innovative care as long as the care is responsible, which for them means that it must be combined with clinical trials because research provides the rigorous oversight and scientific integrity necessary in developing safe and effective therapies.

Emily's Scars: Surgical Shapings, Technoluxe, and Bioethics

Arthur W. Frank

...[O]ne day as I went for a walk, I passed a person with a physical characteristic that was normal enough but still precipitated my thinking, "I'm glad my body's not like that." And then without discernable pause: "But if it were, I could get that sort of thing fixed." At that point, moral and sociological sense returned and I noted that my judgmental reaction to another's body was shaped by my coincidental assessment that surgeons work on conditions like that. Judgment conflates the body itself with the quality of work done on that body or the potential to have that work done. The possibility of fixing renders inescapable the question of whether or not to fix....

My unworthy but useful reaction to my fellow walker led me to realize how uneasy my sense of boundaries is between what I consider fixable about my body and what I believe I am called upon to live not only *with* but *as*. I wash, groom, exercise, and reflect on my diet; I convince myself—or am I convinced by an increasingly undifferentiated mixture of commercial advertisements and health promotion campaigns—that these actions have not only practical benefits but moral implications: caring for myself in these ways enhances the person I am. It is a short step along the continuum to seeking medical advice on matters not only potentially critical but also mundane: physiotherapy and wart removal. These consultations seem to raise no ethical issues. But my fix-it reaction to my fellow walker raises the question of where to draw limits of self-fixing. My initial modernist reaction is to phrase the issue in individualist terms: Is there some core of me that I should work with, not work on, or are some body parts no more than unwanted contingencies, like warts, that temporarily intrude on my life? If the latter, is the decision to fix determined only by a comparatively simple cost- and risk-benefit assessment? Need I ask only whether the promised improvement will be worth the time, trouble, and pain to me that the fixing involves?

The bioethics appropriate to such cost-benefit questions is a kind of consumer protectionism; it insists, for example, on full disclosure of risks, preferably based on follow-up studies of how such fixings have worked, or not, in past interventions. *Protectionist bioethics* takes for granted the presuppositions of consumerism; thus it wants people to know exactly what is being delivered at what cost and with what risk. The ethical standards are liberal, requiring medical professionals to be responsible salespeople and then leaving the choice to patient-consumers.... On a less functional level, this kind of bioethics has trouble taking seriously how one individual's choice—not only what is chosen, but also being in a position to choose—affects others.

Of course, there has always been another kind of bioethics, which can be called *Socratic.* Socratic bioethics questions what protectionist bioethics takes for granted; it asks disconcerting questions about the good life and what kind *of health* is part of this good life. These questions widen the scope of concerned parties whose needs ought to count in any individual's health-related decisions. No one lives a good life alone.

Parens, Erik, ed. *Surgically Shaping Children: Technology, Ethics, and the Pursuit of Normality.* pp. 68–89. © 2006 The Johns Hopkins University Press. Reprinted with permission of The Johns Hopkins University Press.

In this Socratic mode, whether my fix-it reaction is conducive to the kind of person I want to be depends on whether my reaction is conducive to my participation in the communities that support my good life. I then have to specify which parts I play in which communities, and how those parts need to be played for those communities to be good—as I understand "good." My understanding of *good* is not fixed but remains perpetually open to questioning from all sides, with specific decisions responding to that questioning.

This [article] follows the Socratic approach to bioethics, but unlike the Platonic Socrates, I am more concerned with practices and experiences than with the logic of arguments. I start with the social context in which surgical modification makes sense as a solution to bodily conditions that are perceived as troubles. I then consider what people say about decisions for surgical modification. My objective is not to offer guidelines for practice; it seems more useful to open up the discourses in which people—both professionals and potential patients—are able to think about how their actions affect themselves and their communities.

Socratic bioethics seeks to offer alternative courses of action as real possibilities for people who face decisions. If consumer-protection bioethics can be beneficial to people's physical, emotional, and economic welfare, Socratic bioethics can be liberating, in the sense of helping people to realize they have more options for how they live than they had imagined.

THE CONTEXT IN WHICH CHILDREN ARE SURGICALLY SHAPED

Only at a certain historical and cultural moment do the surgeries...limb lengthening, intersex surgery, and craniofacial surgery—make sense.[1] The technologies of medical intervention presuppose the willingness to use these technologies in certain ways. The problem of who is willing to do what in order

to achieve what end is endemic to the culture of high modernity. The sociologist Emile Durkheim, writing in 1896 about the relation of suicide to modernity, raised the question, "how [to] determine the quantity of well-being, comfort and luxury legitimately to be craved by a human being?"....[2] What Durkheim understood clearly, more than a century ago, is that the energy of modernity is always toward *more:* the cultural impetus is to expand what it is legitimate to crave. In reacting as I did to my fellow walker, I was being no less than modern.

Three aspects of the contemporary context of [limb-lengthening, intersex, and craniofacial surgeries] can be singled out to suggest why these surgeries make sense to people: neoliberal medicine, the idea of the body as project, and the moral language of personal authenticity.

Neoliberal medicine denotes the political-economic ideology that considers it proper for the for-profit, corporate sphere to set the agenda for professional medicine.[3] This corporate agenda makes it increasingly commonsensical to understand medical services as *products*. Health maintenance organizations refer to the "product lines" that they sell, and that language diffuses into the way people think of delivering and receiving services. Recently I heard a radio interview with a physician who used the words *patient* and *client* interchangeably, so far as I could tell, with no apparent awareness of a distinction between them. Patients become consumers of medical products—a status that empowers those with sufficient resources and disenfranchises others who lack these resources.[4]

Within neoliberal medicine, the boundaries of professional medicine increasingly blur. During the past century these boundaries were fairly clear, but in the nineteenth century they were less clear,[5] so there is no reason to suppose that professional boundaries will remain as they have been. In the century we have now entered, physicians, especially but not exclusively American physicians, become the delivery agents of corporate products, and corporate entities deliver these physicians' time as a product. Physicians remain *privileged* delivery agents—privileged in what they can do and in how much they are paid for doing it—but they take their place as one category of *providers,* with increasing overlaps between what different providers can offer patients, who are also known as clients and customers.[6] Neoliberal medicine can be recognized by this breakdown of traditional labels for who people are: physicians become providers; patients become consumers. As new interests assert themselves, different sorts of actors have to be identified in ways that suggest their new roles and entitlements.

Neoliberal medicine happens at the same time that an increasing number of people regard their bodies *as projects.*[7] The flesh as God-given reality—for better or worse, this is how I am—gives way to the flesh as stuff to be worked with by various sorts of body workers—among whom physicians are but one, albeit privileged, type. Cosmetic surgery websites feature the image of the surgeon as "flesh artist."[8] At the interventionist extreme of the continuum of body projects is the French performance artist Orlan, who incites reflection on body modification by orchestrating surgeries to reshape herself. Orlan's reshaping has proceeded through a series of cosmetic surgeries that she directs while under local anesthetic. Her art is both her face itself and the videos of her surgeries. She treats surgeons as instruments of her art and speaks of *using* them, as a traditional artist would use a brush to paint or a chisel to sculpt. Orlan is sculpting herself, using surgery as her artistic medium.[9]

Neither most middle-class consumers of traditional cosmetic surgeries nor younger body modifiers among whom tattooing and discrete piercing are popular have ever heard of Orlan, but she affects the milieu that eventually, through layers of diffusion, makes a navel ring seem like a moderate choice for a suburban housewife. Orlan pushes to new extremes both the material use of her body as a project and the self as inextricably tied to how that project is realized. What she does with her body becomes as real a moral responsibility for her, in the twenty-first century, as what people did with their souls was real in earlier centuries.

The body as project extends the trajectory that Charles Taylor argues emerged in the late eighteenth century, when for the first time in history each individual life became something new, a *self.* Life became a project of finding each self's unique point; as Taylor writes, it became possible to miss the point of your life.[10] In other words, one's life became something— raw material—that people expected themselves to *do something* with. The contemporary twist on the modern project of the self is that many of us moderns—most observers agree the number is increasing—include doing things with our bodies among the ways to seek the unique point of our lives. At the extreme, the point of one's life can be the modification of one's body.[11]

Here lies the crucial difference between contemporary body projects and various forms of body modification that have been practiced in traditional societies since the beginning of humanity. Traditional body modification, including initiation ceremonies, marks the body's membership in a group; particular markings indicate a prescribed status in that group. Undergoing these modifications is not something that individuals decide upon or negotiate. Markings express, but they are not *expressive,* which is a modern concept requiring a post-Romantic self. Markings are a non-negotiable expectation, expressing such matters as a member's gender, family status, and age group (such as having attained puberty).[12,13] Those who elect contemporary body projects speak of these projects in a language *of personal* decision making and *individual* choice. At least in the eyes of the modifier, although not necessarily as perceived by others, tattoos and piercings (not to mention more extreme modifications like branding and scarification) are marks of *unique* individuality. When body modifications do express membership—such as when members of sports teams get a common tattoo at the end of the season—those affiliations are individually chosen and often competed for.[14] The tattoo or more extreme modification is understood to say something about the individual, since the affiliations are expressive of who the individual is. Contemporary individualism includes memberships, but the marks of membership are elective, not prescribed expectations.

To illustrate how these contextual elements of neoliberal medicine, body projects, and moral claims conjoin, and to complicate the question of what ought to be fixed by surgery, I offer a single example: feet. Looking at what people are doing with their feet, or more specifically, the cultural threshold of what it now makes sense to do with one's feet, is a provocative way to suggest the uses of surgery that already make sense to people when they find themselves confronted with decisions about surgically shaping children.

SURGICALLY SHAPING FEET

In March 2003, *Vogue* ran a story in its "beauty, health & fitness" section—a concatenation of topics typical of neoliberal medicine—titled "the flawless foot."[15] The story interviewed several New York podiatrists whose surgical practice includes shaping women's feet so that they can fit into and can look good wearing designer shoes. These shoes "require designer feet."[16] As *Vogue* told the story, surgical practice is being pushed by patient-consumers, who in turn are being pushed by shoe designs. Thus *Vogue* quoted a "Manhattan-based podiatrist and podiatric surgeon" who said: "Until recently, my patients would have surgery only to relieve painful foot deformities like ingrown toenails and plantar warts. Now they come in for a consultation, pull a strappy stiletto out of their bag, and say, 'I want to wear this shoe.'"[17] This scene is certainly not typical of twenty-first century medicine, but the description instigates a cultural expectation among *Vogue*'s many readers. Whether or not these readers actually have their feet reshaped, *Vogue* presents a potent lesson in

what patients are entitled to expect from their physicians, as well as what people should expect of their bodies.

The cultural resonance of *Vogue*'s story is suggested by the appearance of a similar—the unkind adjective would be *clone*—story that appeared in June 2003 in the "style" section of Toronto's *Globe & Mail,* one of Canada's two national newspapers.[18] The *Globe*'s story focuses on Suzanne Levine, the same New York podiatrist who is quoted extensively in *Vogue*'s story. Her statement expresses the taken-for-granted values of neoliberal medicine: "The shoes out there right now are like looking at jewelry. I just saw these sandals, with stones and gems... they're gorgeous. You want to be able to wear them. If your foot is unsightly, it detracts from the shoe." This statement lends a new twist to Martin Heidegger's critique of modern technology. In two of Heidegger's examples, technology causes the river to be seen as a source of hydroelectric power and the forest to be seen as a source of lumber. The water becomes "standing-reserve" for the power plant and the trees standing reserve for the sawmill.[19] Levine presents the foot as standing-reserve for surgery, which is how Heidegger describes patients in clinics.[20] But she then broadens the frame as she presents the practice of surgery as standing reserve for fashion. What comes first is the shoe, which then dictates the shape of feet. If the shoe does not fit, then perform surgery on the foot.

The moral justification of this ordering of priorities lies in what *Vogue* called "a woman's confidence." "I got tired of burying my toes in the sand when I went to the beach. It was humiliating," says a woman who had surgery to shorten several toes. Cinderella stories are ancient and culturally diffuse; this woman's description of the effect of surgery sounds like Peter Kramer's biotech version of the Cinderella plot, told in his best-selling *Listening to Prozac.*[21] Kramer describes patients who experience Prozac as a transformation of self. "At first I thought I was just being nit-picky," the podiatric patient says. "But the transformation is amazing. And I was back in high-heels in less than two months."[22] "It changed my life," says another woman, speaking not about medical podiatry but about the effect of treatments from those medical adjuncts whom *Vogue* describes as "expert pedicurists at Buff Spa in Manhattan's Bergdorf Goodman."[23] I note these *expert* pedicurists as an example of the point made earlier, that physicians practice as delivery agents of services within an array of agents offering complementary services. But my main point is the Prozac-like language of transformation and life change as a justification for surgery. These patients and *Vogue's* writer may well have read Kramer, but whether they have or not the diffusion of Kramer's language sets their rhetorical expectations, and they perpetuate the diffusion of this language.

Vogue refers to this form of podiatric practice as "technoluxe," a useful description of what neoliberal medicine brings about.[24] Technoluxe comprises both product lines and conditions of delivery. Neither discretionary medical services nor high-end delivery is new; when I was a boy, one floor in the local hospital was referred to as the gold coast. But in those days, the gold coast could offer little more—though no less—than more comfortable surroundings in which to receive the same medicine. What is new is the profusion—the sheer quantity and accessibility at different income levels, in different sites—of medical product lines. Technoluxe depends, first, on the increasing public and professional acceptance of the body as something to shape and life as a project of shaping. It depends equally on the idea that projects are realized through acts of consumption. Those who are disturbed by technoluxe have to ask a question that specifies the problem of modernity that Durkheim and Heidegger brooded over: What exactly is wrong with the aspiration to have, and to use medicine to produce, designer feet?

One objection is functional. *Vogue* quotes one sole medical dissenter, a podiatrist from Moline, Illinois, and the rhetoric of locating dissent there is interesting, since the other prosurgical podiatrists quoted in the article are all New Yorkers. "When I operate, my goal is to alleviate pain," says the Midwestern medical traditionalist. "The risk with all podiatric surgery, no matter how minor, is that it fundamentally alters the structure of the foot and the way you walk, which may cause new calluses and pain you didn't have to begin with."[25] Especially in the world of technoluxe medicine, caveat emptor applies. As the patient becomes more of a consumer—a buyer—the need to beware intensifies. But I do not regard the functional objection, important as it is, to be the most provocative, since it relegates the moral question of *should we?* to the level of whether it works.

If the only objection were functional, then it could be argued that the rich do the rest of us a favor by acting as guinea pigs for new medical technologies.[26] The objection I consider more significant for more people, more of the time, is that technoluxe medicine distorts the allocation of medical services and distracts medicine from its original and still-predominant purpose.[27] This purpose is clearly stated by the dissident podiatrist: "to alleviate pain." But pain is not what it used to be, and here I return to the moral justification of the satisfied medical consumer who says going to the beach pretreatment was "humiliating." I react to this statement as an inflation of the language of pain: if having unfashionable toes counts as humiliation, in what words can we describe the lives of people living with massive facial deformities? But as troubling as I find the usage of *humiliating* in this instance, it is important to hear the very real problem that this woman is working to express.

This woman exists, like all of us, in what Pierre Bourdieu calls a field.[28] What counts most about fields for the present argument is that positions within them are hierarchical, and one's place depends on possessing capital. Bourdieu delineates different forms of capital, including physical capital, and calls attention to how different forms of capital count in some fields but not others, and how some forms of capital hold their value between fields.[29] This woman's capital, in at least one of the multiple fields of her life, includes being able to go barefoot or wear sandals and have her feet look a certain way. The field determines what this *certain way* is. Fields set the terms of *what counts* as capital, and fields are also sites of perpetual *contest* between rival forms of capital. This woman, in her field, is doing with her feet what all members of any society, including bioethicists, do with our bodies and with our talents: we shape and allocate them in order to make them count as capital. Feet can be a form of capital not only in dating and marriage markets, but in job markets as well.

What counts as capital goes well beyond the feet themselves. Reshaped feet *display the willingness to reshape one's body* to conform to the demands of the field. The woman's feet mark her *ability to read properly* what counts as capital and to endure what has to be endured to accrue that capital. This interpretive skill and the complementary endurance are the woman's real capital. Any self-reshaping, whether of body, language (as in Shaw's *Pygmalion,* a resonant plot later adapted to become *My Fair Lady*), or skills (in education, certification and recertification) is properly brought off when and because it demonstrates the person's *attunement* to the demands of a specific field. In modernity, attunement is no longer an automatic corollary of membership. Members of traditional societies accepted being told when and how to reshape their bodies. Their decision was binary: either participate or leave the group. In contemporary society, each individual is responsible for choosing and effecting her *own* reshaping, thus demonstrating her fitness for membership within a given field. Hierarchical position depends on displaying attunement to the field, and what counts as capital changes; people have to anticipate shifts. Bourdieu emphasizes throughout his writing that playing in any field requires the correct assessment of what counts as capital *there,* and *then,* including what kind of body counts as

right. The right body demonstrates having made the right assessment of capital, and thus becomes a potent display of rights to participation and position.

If Bourdieu's argument stopped here, it would be a neoliberal defense of anyone doing anything that enhances his market position. This defense would effectively end ethical discourse, since our capacity to claim that some actions are good and others are not so good would be determined only by what counts as capital in specific fields. Nothing could be further from Bourdieu's point, which is to oppose neoliberalism. I lack space to pursue this argument, however. I use Bourdieu's ideas not to make technoluxe surgery legitimate, but only to show that it is plausible.

Recognizing the demands of capital and fields allows us to take a generous view of the podiatry patient who seeks designer feet, and it complicates the question of what's wrong with these feet. Unless this woman leads a charmed life, she will have other experiences that will shift her scale of what counts as humiliation. But for now she is doing what we all do: she is *trying to hold her own.* And so is her podiatrist. The website of Suzanne Levine, the podiatrist who wants to shape feet to fit designer shoes, tells us that only 8 percent of podiatrists are women, and Levine's success is singular for a woman in this field.[30] Although she may not be a feminist hero, she too, in her field, is working to hold her own.

...

IN THE GRAVITATIONAL FIELD OF TECHNOLUXE

The [enhancement] surgeries are not shaping children so that they can wear designer shoes; but the same basic equation applies: if the body does not fit, reshape it. The problem of how to respond to these surgeries is tied to this equation. The [enhancement] surgeries—most evidently, limb-lengthening surgery—can be presented as the leading edge of a slippery slope that relegates all medicine to technoluxe market values: those who have the most resources to put into their bodies can produce bodies that accrue the most capital in the most rewarding fields. The body is called forth as a site of investment and accrual, and in neoliberal society, those who have the most to invest have the first call on services. Alternatively, these surgeries can be defended as medicine in the cause of democratic humanism: they offer the best chance for people who have been allocated low physical capital to get back onto as level a playing field as possible. And who can say they should not have that chance?[31] Both perspectives have some merit, which is what makes bioethical response so difficult. A beginning is to consider the moral justifications people offer for each type of surgery.

The language of moral justification for limb-lengthening surgery is individualistic.[32] The following statement is taken from a long article posted on the website of the Little People of America (LPA). The author is a Little Person named Gillian Mueller, whose experience of limb-lengthening was the subject of a 1992 article in *People* magazine. Her updated story is posted on the LPA website, dated September 2002.[33] Mueller describes her near-total satisfaction with how limb-lengthening has affected her life. She concludes:

> Undergoing limb-lengthening was clearly the right decision for me. That is not to say it is the answer for everyone, or even a majority. It is a personal decision that every individual whose lives [*sic*] can be functionally improved by the procedure should be allowed to make for him/herself, without being judged by anyone for that decision.

This dual emphasis—that only the individual can decide for herself, and that no one else can judge that decision—is repeated in Internet chat groups of people who are planning or considering limb-lengthening surgery.[34] Moreover, Mueller's statement is entirely consistent with the language of people who practice both conventional and extreme body modification.[35]

Mueller's rationale for undergoing surgery appeals to mundane matters of convenience— she writes of driving an unmodified car and reaching objects on supermarket shelves. She downplays issues of identity, writing that before her surgery, "I knew I really was no different from anyone else, and I knew if I set my mind to it I could do anything any average person could do, if not more … My mother made sure I came home to a place where I knew I was loved for who I was, even though I was small." But the "even though" qualification is inescapable, and the decision to have surgery reinforces how much "even though" counts. By asserting how much better her life is since she made herself less small, she makes "even though" count for others as well. She necessarily poses a choice whether or not to make it count less. When being small is presented as a choice, the "even though" becomes a heavier weight.

That her choice affects others does not impugn the validity of what she chooses. When, as a young teenager, she is sent to a medical presentation on limb-lengthening, she too *cannot avoid* choosing. Some people's discovery of choices that they find liberating will force others to confront choices they would rather not have recognized in the first place; this chaining of possibilities seems inevitable. But Mueller should be aware that her choices affect other Little Peoples' ability to choose, and she should take responsibility for how she frames the choices that do affect others. The recognition that none of us chooses anything consequential "for herself" seems fundamental to moral participation in society. That means only that we must choose carefully, because as we choose for ourselves, we also confront others with choice.

The choice of limb-lengthening surgery is a form of normalization—fitting the body to the demands of society rather than calling on society to create accommodations for different bodies—and normalization has a bad name in an age of disability rights.[36] Yet who among us of normal height wants to tell Gillian Mueller that she has no right to a technology allowing her the advantages she claims? What, then, needs to be offered to those who are affected by the expectations that her decision generates in their lives? These questions are typical of modernity, a defining characteristic of which is the dislocation of people's lives by technologies. These dislocations have always brought benefits and losses, often to the same people. At this stage in modernity, bioethics can offer those who must choose the reflective observation that practices reinforce each other's acceptability; bioethics can heighten people's awareness of how their practices affect their sense of connection with other people.

Simply the reporting of technoluxe podiatry in *Vogue,* followed by various clone stories, regardless of how many feet are actually reshaped—even in Manhattan—affects the acceptability of surgically reshaping limbs. In a technoluxe context, achondroplasia is readily understood as another individual problem that requires medical fixing. Surgical intervention is one of a series of available choices for fixing some part of one's life—choices from pharmacology to promises of gene therapy.

In this framework of choice, living with achondroplasia becomes understood as *a choice of body projects*. This understanding can be either liberating or constraining, or both. What constitutes liberation and what constitutes constraint depends on values and politics and will remain contested. Participation in disability rights— claiming one's disability as a cultural difference, even as a positive value—is one available body project. Another project is to minimize disability through surgery. Many people—probably an increasing number—will mix both projects, since the projects are mutually exclusive in theory more than in practice. Decisions of which project to pursue—when to pursue it, how far to go, and to what extent that pursuit excludes other projects—depend on expectations that are constantly being conditioned. The conditioning of expectations is not unidirectional from technoluxe to disability; it cuts the other way as well: once limb-lengthening becomes known as a standard of surgical body modification in the cause of convenience, cosmetic podiatric surgeries like bunionectomies will seem like pedicures.

The consequences of normalization darken when we move from the legs to the genitals. Limb-lengthening surgery is performed on teenagers who participate in the decision for surgery, as Mueller carefully specifies she did. Intersex surgery is usually decided between parents and surgeons, excluding the child from the decision. Children are often considered too young to be informed—infants clearly are too young, but age of consent becomes contested as children grow older....[37] The stories of those who have been subjected to this surgery are filled with expressions of shame and recriminations for familial secrecy. Both academic research and the website of the Intersex Society of North America (ISNA) present stories of people who feel mutilated by surgeries that sought to correct differences in genitalia.[38] What we have been lacking are the stories of the decision makers....

[Observations suggest]...that surgeons present a threefold justification for their intersex-related interventions. First, surgeons believe that they carry out the wishes of the parents, who are the child's surrogate decision makers. When pressed as to why they operate on infants so soon after their birth, surgeons appeal to the level of parental distress and their responsibility to relieve it, a responsibility that is equated with intervening as fast as possible. Second, they claim to achieve the surgical outcome of normal-appearing genitalia and support that claim by showing numerous before-and-after slides. Third, their descriptions of their patients' lives foreground the risk of social humiliations— in locker rooms and other change rooms and in public bathrooms—that could make embarrassment over one's toes seem trivial. If patient stories are about shame and loss as the effects of surgery, surgeons' stories are about how surgery can prevent teasing, and they claim the moral responsibility to do so.

In intersex surgery as in technoluxe podiatry, it is no surprise that the need to reinforce self-esteem or confidence—whatever words are used—is presented as a moral trump. Self-esteem is a crucial resource for the modern self precisely because this self's uniqueness entails being out there by itself, on its own, responsible for itself. Surgeons have good reason to believe that medicine must use its resources to protect this self-esteem.[39]

Again there is a functional objection, this time expressed in personal accounts of loss of genital sensation as a result of surgery, as well as the trauma of repeated operations for more complex conditions. Too often professional surgery chooses not to hear these stories.... What is at stake is crucial for medicine: Whose opinion trumps in the determination of surgical success? And based on that question, whose opinion ought to count in decisions about future interventions? But again, surgeons have considerable justification for believing that they are doing what those around the intersexed person—if not that person himself—wants to have done.

In contrast to Mueller's story of limb-lengthening, people who have had surgery for intersex conditions believe that their families and society at large find them acceptable *only if* their anomaly is fixed. Many believe that the attempted fixing created only a crude simulacrum of normality. They remain marginalized from the society of normal genitalia, and they are alienated from the bodies they had been born with.

We can only speculate about why parents elect surgical correction for their children's intersex conditions. Those stories would be difficult to elicit....[40] As important as standards of practice for patient information are, the use of any information confronts an inherent limitation. Information always requires interpretation in order to be acted on, and even the most accurate, appropriate information will be interpreted within dominant cultural paradigms. Thus, any advice concerning surgery risks being understood within the same equation that applies to feet: failing to fit the fashion is humiliating, and surgery provides a fix. Most of these parents undoubtedly would feel they had failed to be responsible if they did not offer their children the more approximately normal future that surgery promises.

This same hope for a normal future pervades decisions around craniofacial surgeries. It may be easy to regard intersex surgery as medicine acting to police physiologies that threaten the conventional binaries of gender normality—and more threatening still, physiologies that people claim to take pleasure in—but this critique of surgical normalization is difficult to apply to ... craniofacial surgeries [as seen] through the conventional medical rhetoric of before-and-after slides, and these slides, like the word *deformity,* depend on normative visual convention, and those conventions need to be contested. Yet it would challenge most observers to see these pictures and not feel the appropriateness of this language of deformity. Faced with such faces, it is difficult not to affirm the value of surgery as at least an improvement in what are readily (perhaps too readily) perceived as life-impairing conditions. Moreover, there is no craniofacial group equivalent to ISNA: no survivors of craniofacial surgery protest what has been inflicted on them and claim they would have better lives if they had been left alone. The problem craniofacial surgery presents is not understanding why surgery is first undertaken. The question is deciding when, after years of operations, surgery ought to end.

Jeffrey Marsh, a craniofacial surgeon ... crystallized the issue when he said that after what is often more than a decade of operations, the current surgery is being undertaken to ameliorate the effects of earlier surgery. Candidates for continuing surgery eventually have to ask when is *enough.* Is the next surgical revision going to affect any improvement in appearance, or will it only rearrange past damage? Perhaps more to the point, the potential patient, much of whose life has been invested in undergoing surgery, eventually has to ask whether she *needs* that promised improvement (even if surgery achieves it) to get on with the life she needs to get on with. This life may not be the one that the person would prefer, and the difficulty lies in reconciling the difference between what has been hoped for with what now seems to be the reality.

[Enhancement medicine] becomes the business of rewriting what counts as reality. In response to any patient's condition, some surgeon somewhere will probably offer the possibility—which from another perspective is a fantasy—that the face and the life that goes with it could be a great deal better if only that last surgical revision is agreed to. When we asked why both craniofacial and intersex surgical interventions continued past a point when it seemed…that little could be gained and harm was being risked, the best answer we found was that the momentum of previous decisions made stopping difficult to consider as an option. Momentum reinforces the quality that intersex and craniofacial surgeries share with technoluxe: the promise of a better life—more particularly a better self—if *one more* medical step is taken.

Craniofacial surgery, like limb-lengthening and intersex surgery, takes place in the gravitational orbit of technoluxe. Many of the surgeons operating on what might be agreed on as facial deformity are or have been engaged in cosmetic surgery as well, and assumptions, like language, diffuse between activities. Yet craniofacial surgery differs from limb-lengthening and intersex surgery because among human body parts faces have a unique place.[41] Potential patients of cosmetic podiatry can choose to wear other shoes, even on the beach…. Living with a face that will attract horrified stares from strangers is where the word *humiliation* seems to find its most uninflated and unavoidable usage.[42] The public visibility of the face and the symbolic importance that links faces to character—exemplified by the aphorism attributed to Lincoln that after a certain age a person is responsible for his or her own face—make facial deformity a problem of a different magnitude, and that difference commands our respect.

Here we reach the crux of what makes responding to these surgeries difficult. How far do we expand the sphere of persons to whom we offer that respect? I believe that trying to compare forms of suffering—comparing the woman humiliated by her toes with a young person deformed by a facial hemangioma—is not useful. The attraction of such a comparison is that it promises apparently clear-cut medical guidelines for practice. Unfortunately, practice will have to confront a reality that is not clearly divisible into categories. The issue may be better thought of not in terms *of what suffering* we allow as legitimately in need of fixing, but rather *what form of decision making* we respect.

WHAT IS A BIOETHICAL RESPONSE TO SURGICAL SHAPINGS?

I suggested earlier that there are two forms of bioethics. Bioethics as consumer protection responds by recommending procedures that seek to protect those subject to surgical shaping; those protections include but are hardly limited to more fully informed consent. The need for whatever protection bioethics can instigate is most pressing in intersex surgery. What I have called Socratic bioethics poses questions about what sort of people we become by choosing to act as we do. My sociological Socraticism broadens the scope of those who are involved when questioning who we are becoming. It calls attention to connections: connections between practices, so that people recognize how one practice reinforces another, and also connections between people, breaking down the idea that any decision can be strictly *individual,* insofar as that word suggests that one person's decision does not affect how another person chooses. In conclusion I want to suggest another dimension of Socratic bioethics: the significance of dialogue. In Socratic dialogues, people are having a good deal more than a pleasant chat.

Dialogue lakes on a distinctive significance as a response to two features of neoliberal society and the medical practices that seem natural within it. One defining characteristic of neoliberalism is the absence of any alternative political-economic discourse that challenges it; the old Marxist-socialist alternative is effectively dead as any kind of opposition. The resulting fatalism is relieved by the glitz of consumerism, including technoluxe, and diverse panics, including epidemiological panics. Second, the pervasive myth of the market privileges an assumption that personal choice trumps in all matters. I suggested this language of personal choice in the discussion of rationales for limb-lengthening surgery as the individual's private decision. The personal is equated with the private. In this neoliberal context, *dialogue* means opening an oppositional space that is too often closed, and it means recognizing that the personal is communal. A Socratic bioethics can instigate dialogue that informs people's sense of how their particular trouble relates to others' troubles, and how their proposed solutions might cause others more trouble.

The technoluxe podiatry patient who is humiliated by her toes is, as I wrote, trying to hold her own, and such efforts are worth a certain respect. The limit of this respect depends on whether this person thinks about how her strategies for holding her own affect others' capacity to hold their own. If I am reluctant to call the woman's sense of humiliation trivial, I am willing to say she is not looking around very far or talking to a sufficient range of people. She is responding to her field, but only to *her* field and *her* need to position herself in this field. To paraphrase Michel Foucault, she knows what she is doing, but she seems to have little awareness or interest in what her doing does.[43] In a world in which medicine has more work than it can do alleviating pain, how far anyone is entitled to plead ignorance of the needs of others is questionable. It is questionable whether surgeons who operate on anomalous genitalia can ignore the testimony of those who have had these surgeries; this testimony may not take the form of controlled trials, but as organized by ISNA, it is a compelling aggregation. Technoluxe patients and overly aggressive surgeons both lack sufficient participation in dialogue as a process of testing their needs and assumptions against others' realities.

Lisa Hedley ... provides a specific illustration of dialogue as a kind of talk.[44] She writes about what it meant when her daughter, LilyClaire, was born with achondroplasia, an unknown condition in their family. One day soon after LilyClaire was born, Hedley saw a Little Person, approached him and told him—as a stranger—that her daughter was also a Little Person. I imagine him looking at her as people do when they are not sure on what basis strangers have approached them. He replied, "Right, well, is she healthy?" That simple question shifted Hedley's sense of her daughter's having achondroplasia. The question *repositioned* Hedley: her daughter's condition was no longer a problem, though problems might certainly occur related to that condition. Socratic bioethics recognizes that bodies and diseases are not there to be solved, but how one lives with them depends on how one positions oneself with respect to them. Of course, Hedley was already open to dialogue. The bioethical problem is to lead those not yet open to dialogue toward that openness.

Hedley's story suggests that Socratic bioethics often proceeds best through questions that are not especially clever; in that sense, my allusion to the philosophical Socrates is misplaced.[45] But Socrates remains a founding figure for this form of bioethics for several other reasons: he worked in the public square, where he talked to people about their everyday problems; he forced people to account for why they held the opinions they believed to be true; despite his cleverness, he operated in ordinary, accessible language; he did not make it the measure of his success to disturb people, but his questions did disturb; and, most important, he kept people focused on ideals of truth and the good while keeping the content of these ideals unfixed.[46] Truth and the good seem to have more to do with sustaining the *process* of dialogue than with being *outcomes* of dialogue.

Yet medicine, especially surgery, is about acting and producing an outcome; dialogical surgery can seem a contradiction in terms.... Surgery must be dialogical in order to be ethical: focused, mutual inquiry about what surgery can do must be open to multiple voices, and decisions need to be held open longer; these are recommendations for practice, though they are hard to wrestle into formal guidelines. In stories about surgical outcomes that [most bioethicists] felt were bad ... the trouble began when not enough people were involved in the conversation over a long enough time. The fullest range of possible outcomes, and their fullest range of consequences, were not considered, nor was the fullest range of alternatives explored. These alternatives include that posed implicitly by the Little Person who responds to Lisa Hedley by asking, in effect, why she thinks she has a problem.

Another distinction now cuts across my initial one between consumer-protection bioethics and Socratic bioethics. There are problems that arise *in the course of* medical practice—such as consent issues—and there are problems that arise *as a result of* the possibility of medical practice. Consumer-protection bioethics is more useful responding to the former sort of problems, since these problems seem amenable to solution. Socratic bioethics presents very different kinds of responses to the latter problems because these problems are ones that we cannot solve but instead must learn to live with. Medical technologies and science, almost instantaneously transformed into marketed commodities, will continue to present problems that require individuals and communities to rethink who they want to be, just as my reaction to the person I passed while walking—the story that begins this [article]—required me to rethink who I was becoming and whether I wanted to be that person.[47]

Limb-lengthening, intersex, and craniofacial surgeries all pose problems about what constitutes a good life, and about when medicine should be used and when refused in pursuit of the good life. In a neoliberal age it is difficult to convince people that they cannot lead good lives by themselves. The neoliberal subjectivity does not readily accept that "personal" decisions implicate others, because any person's good life depends on others also leading good lives.[48] At this point neoliberal economic thinking converges with a postmodern philosophical recognition—which probably finds its earliest, most explicit statement in Nietzsche—that there is no gold standard of the good....

...

It seems both politically and culturally naïve to believe that bioethics can respond to the [enhancement] cases by drawing lines between types of surgeries and giving some but not others an ethical seal of approval. We cannot adjudicate either what forms of suffering are sufficiently authentic to warrant medical intervention or what medical interventions are sufficiently effective to be ethical responses to that suffering. What seems useful is to show how decision making can proceed in ways that command respect.

CODA

...Emily Sullivan Sanford, a young woman [whom I met at meetings of the Hastings Center project on Surgically Shaping Children] had [limb-lengthening] surgery several years earlier....[49] She wore a sleeveless top, and on her upper arms were prominent rectangular scars where, during surgery, the bone had been broken and pins inserted, so that the bone's length could be increased by continually pulling the two fragments apart, preventing healing and generating new bone growth over several months. The scars were not neat, surgical scars. The skin looked well healed, but the past trauma was visible.

Emily talked about her scars at some point in our discussion. She said she had been encouraged to have a skin graft to remove them, but she refused. They were an emblem of the ordeal she had gone through. She was clear about her choice of word, *ordeal.* Her scars reminded me of an interview in *Habits of the Heart*, a major study of American values by Robert Bellah and his colleagues. They quote a woman whom they call Ruth Levy, who tells this story:

> The woman who took care of my daughter when she was little was a Greek Jew. She was very young, nine, ten, eleven, when the war broke out, and was lying at the crematorium door when the American troops came through. So that she has a number tattooed on her arm. And it was always like being hit in the stomach with a brick when she would take my baby and sit and circle her with her arm, and there was the number.[50]

Scars do hit us like a brick, as they connect immediate persons to imagined forms of suffering and thus render that suffering tangible.

Bellah and his colleagues use Ruth Levy's story as an example of what they call communities of memory,[51] a term that does not quite fit Emily's situation. Memory is one issue for Emily, but her scars also look forward to the person she is becoming; they hold her surgery as partial foundation of that becoming. What kind of community Emily and her scars will figure in remains unknown. We do not yet know what to call a community of those who will define themselves as sharing some aspect of Emily's experience, or what aspects of her experiences will be shared within different communities.

Emily is normalized in height; when I first saw her across a room I did not identify her as a Little Person. But to suggest that Emily underwent surgery to trade a disability identity for a normal identity—that her limb-lengthening is a form of "passing"—would underestimate both Emily's moral awareness and the complexity of surgical shaping. Emily negotiates multiple resources, including medicine, to live in multiple fields. She is aware that she does not act for herself alone.... Her moral freedom is embodied in her scars and her self-conscious decision not to fix them. Her scars keep open both her identity and the dialogue about disability and difference. That openness is good, for us all.

Acknowledgements

My thanks to my colleagues on the Surgically Shaping Children (SCC) project, especially to Erik Parens and Jim Edwards for specific advice on this essay, to Alice Dreger for her research on intersex surgeries, and to Lisa Hedley, Paul Miller, and Tom Shakespeare for help on limb-lengthening. Research materials on feet were generously provided by Rachael Meziere. A much shorter version of this article was presented at the "Vital Politics" conference, London School of Economics, September 2003; particular thanks to Monica Greco. The SSC project is funded by the National Endowment for the Humanities. Additional research support for my work is from the Social Sciences and Humanities Research Council of Canada. Perhaps most of all, thanks to Emily Sullivan Sanford for the quality of embodied witness that she, along with Cheryl Chase and Cassandra Aspinall, brought to the SSC meetings.

Notes

1. This paper was written as a contribution to the Hastings Center working group on Surgically Shaping Children, which studied these three types of surgeries.

2. E. Durkheim, *Suicide*, tr. J A. Spaulding and G. Simpson (New York: The Free Press, 1951), 247.

3. For an overview of neo-liberalism, see B. Smart, *Economy, Culture and Society: A Sociological Critique of Neo-Liberalism* (Buckingham and Philadelphia: Open University Press, 2003).

4. Given their emphasis on the primacy of the market, neo-liberals restrict the role of governments to reacting to corporate agendas. Government's most consequential role is that of a safety net that catches the least profitable, most expensive patients who would derail profits, if the corporate sphere were held responsible for them. For discussion of medical services as commodities, see S. Henderson and A. Petersen, eds., *Consuming Health: The Commodification of Health Care* (London: Routledge, 2002), including A.W. Frank, "What's Wrong with Medical Consumerism?" 13–30.

5. P. Starr, *The Social Transformation of American Medicine* (New York: Basic Books, 1982).

6. Among numerous examples of this language, see the Special Issue on Consumers and Collaborative Care, *Families, Systems & Health*, 18, no. 2 (Summer 2000).

7. If not the original source of "body projects," certainly one of the first discussions is C. Shilling, *The Body and Social Theory* (London: Sage, 1993).

8. I draw the term "flesh artist" from M. Atkinson, *Tattooed: The Sociogenesis of a Body Art* (Toronto: University of Toronto Press, 2003).

9. For discussions of Orlan and other body performance artists, see V. Pitts, *In the Flesh: The Cultural Politics of Body Modification* (New York: Palgrave Macmillan, 2003) and K. Davis, "'My Body Is My Art': Cosmetic Surgery as Feminist Utopia?" in K. Davis, *Dubious Equalities & Embodied Differences* (Lanham, MD.: Rowman & Littlefield, 2003), 105–116.

10. C. Taylor, *The Malaise of Modernity* (Concord, Ontario: Anansi, 1991) (published in the United States as *The Ethics of Authenticity*). For a complementary perspective, see U. Beck and E. Beck-Gernsheim, *Individualization: Institutionalized Individualism and its Social and Political Consequences* (London: Sage, 2002).

11. A frequently discussed example is Sam Fussell's autobiography of bodybuilding, see S.W. Fussell, *Muscle: Confessions of an Unlikely BodyBuilder* (New York: Avon Books, 1991). For a recent commentary, see C. Elliott, *Better Than Well: American Medicine Meets the American Dream* (New York: Norton, 2003). For other examples of making what is done with one's body the point of one's life, see Pitts, *In the Flesh.*

12. For examples and a more nuanced discussion of the relational aspects of body projects, see A.W. Frank, "Surgical Body Modification and Altruistic Individualism: A Case for Cyborg Ethics and Methods," *Qualitative Health Research,* 13, no. 10 (2003): 1407–418.

13. Nelson Mandela's autobiography uses such a language of external determination: "When I was sixteen, the regent decided that it was time that I became a man," which required ritual circumcision. "An un-circumcised Xhosa man is a contradiction in terms," Mandela continues; "for he is not considered a man at all, but a boy. For the Xhosa people, circumcision represents the formal incorporation of males into society." N. Mandela, *Long Walk to Freedom* (London: Abacus, 1995), 30. Compare Mandela's account to the language of those interviewed in contemporary studies like Atkinson, *Tattooed,* and Pitts, *In the Flesh.*

14. Ibid., 442.

15. E. Lamont, "The Flawless Foot," *Vogue,* March 2003, 437, 442, 444.

16. Ibid.

17. Ibid.

18. T. Pearce, "The new T & A," *The Globe & Mail,* June 24, 2003.

19. M. Heidegger, "The Question Concerning Technology," 311–41 in *Basic Writings,* ed. D.F. Krell, revised and expanded edition (New York: HarperCollins, 1993), 320–22.

20. In Heidegger's terms, Dr. Levine presents medicine as a technology with which fashion *sets upon* the body; medicine legitimates the capacity of fashion to *challenge* the body. The contested issue is whether and how this subordination of medicine to fashion affects the moral standing of medicine as a social enterprise. Part of what is contested is

how much moral standing medicine has anyway, and what sort of moral standing it ought to have.

21. P.D. Kramer, *Listening to Prozac* (New York: Viking, 1993). For discussion, see T. Chambers and C. Elliott, eds., *Prozac as a Way of Life* (Chapel Hill, N.C.: University of North Carolina Press, 2004).

22. E. Lamont, "The Flawless Foot," *Vogue,* March 2003, 437, 442, 444.

23. Ibid., 446.

24. The complementary term is *boutique medicine.* See, for example, D.C. Cascardo, "Boutique Medicine: A New Concept Based on Traditional Ideals," *Medscape Money & Medicine* 4, no. 2 (2003), www.medscape.com, accessed September 17, 2003.

25. Ibid., 446.

26. This argument is proposed by P. Baldi, *The Shattered Self. The End of Natural Evolution* (Cambridge, Mass.: MIT Press, 2001), 217 n13.

27. In Heideggerian language (see note 19, above), the conflict concerns what will enframe medicine: will medicine be called forth as relief of pain or as technoluxe?

28. See P. Bourdieu, *The Logic of Practice*, tr. Richard Nice (Stanford: Stanford University Press, 1990), and *Practical Reason: On the Theory of Action* (Stanford: Stanford University Press, 1998).

29. Bourdieu's ideas on physical capital are discussed by N. Crossley, *The Social Body: Habit, Identity, and Desire* (London: Sage, 2001).

30. www.footfacial.com, accessed August 2003.

31. Kathy Davis makes this argument by reviewing the career of the pioneering French cosmetic surgeon, "Madame Noel," who wrote eloquently about her women patients' fear "of losing their jobs as their faces begin to show the first signs of aging" (p. 27). Madame Noel considered her surgical practice an expression of her feminism—a self-image for which Davis provides considerable justification. K. Davis, "Cosmetic Surgery in a Different Voice," in *Dubious Equalities and Embodied Differences* (Lanham, MD: Rowman & Littlefield, 2003): 19–39.

32. Disability rights activists certainly express objections to limb lengthening, but in my search of publicly available materials—quick web hits—those voices are comparatively hidden behind issues of function that ask whether it will work, at what cost, and with what risk.

33. G. Mueller, "Extended Limb-lengthening: Setting the Record Straight." Revised posting, 09–27/02. http://www.lpaonline.org/library_ell-muelier.html, accessed August 31, 2003.

34. See Frank, "Surgical Body Modification and Altruistic Individualism."

35. See Atkinson, *Tattooed,* and Pitts, *In the Flesh.*

36. Among many critiques of normalization, see L. Davis, *Enforcing Normalcy: Disability, Deafness, and the Body* (London: Verso, 1995).

37. See P. Alderson, *Children's Consent to Surgery* (Buckingham and Philadelphia: Open University Press, 1993).

38. See A.D. Dreger, ed., *Intersex in the Age of Ethics* (Hagerstown, MD.: University Publishing Group, 1999).

39. Taylor, C. 1991. *The Malaise of Modernity.* Concord, ON: Anansi (published in the United States as *The Ethics of Authenticity*).

40. Another surgical rationale for quick, early intervention is that infants will be too young to remember the experience. Family secrecy begins in the parental hope that the intervention can effectively disappear, the child growing up as if she or he had been born with the genitals that surgery has recreated. Groups like ISNA never hear from those people for whom this strategy is effective.

41. These surgeons are acting in accordance with moral norms deeply ingrained in modernity that privilege the face. With reference to diffuse social usage, Goffman made the face his trope for that which members of a social group have a responsibility to protect; both their own face and the faces of other people. See E. Goffman, "On Face Work" (pp. 5–45) and "Embarrassment and Social Organization" (pp. 97–112) in *Interaction Ritual: Essays in Face-to-Face Behavior* (Garden City, N.J.: Anchor Books, 1967).

42. Erving Goffman defines stigma as that which spoils identity. Stigmas allow various kinds of management of the effects of this spoiling; at the extreme, "passing" as normal allows the condition to remain unnoticed. Goffman presents facial deformity as the exemplar of stigmatizing conditions that do not allow passing. See *Stigma: Notes on the Management of Spoiled Identity* (Englewood Cliffs, N.J.: Prentice Hall, 1963).

43. Quoted in H.L Dreyfus and P. Rabinow, *Michel Foucault: Beyond Structuralism and Hermeneutics*, second edition (Chicago, Ill.: University of Chicago Press, 1983), 187.

44. LA. Hedley, "A Child of Difference," *New York Times Magazine*, October 12, 1997; available at http://home.earth-link.net/-dkennedy56/dwarfism_nytmag.html, accessed September 21, 2003.

45. Perhaps I should call it Parzival bioethics, in honor of the wise simpleton who, alone among the Arthurian knights, has the moral sense to ask the wounded Fisher King the obvious but previously unasked question of what's wrong with him. This simple but profound question breaks the spell and relieves the King's suffering. Wolfram von Eschenbach, *Parzival*, tr. AT. Hatto (London: Penguin, 1980).

46. Socrates also sought the sort of universal attributes that my line of argument rejects. For an especially useful discussion, see B. Flyvbjerg, *Making Social Science Matter: Why Social Inquiry Fails and How It Can Succeed Again*, tr. S. Sampson (Cambridge: Cambridge University Press, 2001), especially 67–71. Flyvbjerg argues for an Aristotelian *phronesis* as the basis of social science. Bioethics can choose what it needs from both philosophers.

47. A.W. Frank, "The Bioethics of Biotechnologies: Alternative Claims of Posthuman Futures," in S.J. Williams, L. Birke, and G. Bendelow, eds., *Debasing Biology: Sociological Reflections on Health, Medicine, and Society* (London: Routledge, 2003), 261–70.

48. Thus Lisa Hedley writes: "Early on I learned that the way other people respond to a child of difference becomes integral to your experience of the world." Hedley, "A Child of Difference." If this statement falls at the personal end of a continuum, at the global end is the theological ideal, emphasized in but not exclusive to Buddhism, that no person's suffering can be fully relieved until everyone's suffering is relieved. You can read more from Lisa Hedley in her article *The Seduction of the Surgical Fix*, which can be found within Erik Parens edition of *Surgically Shaping Children: Technology, Ethics, and the Pursuit of Normality*, pp. 43–48. Baltimore: Maryland: Johns Hopkins University Press.

49. Emily's surgery is depicted in Lisa Abelow Hedley's film, "Dwarfs: Not a Fairy Tale." A project of the Children of Difference Foundation. Emily's name is used in this article with her permission. You can read more about Emily Sanford's experiences in her essay *My Shoe Size Stayed the Same: Maintaining a Positive Sense of Identity with Achondroplasia and Limb-Lengthening Surgeries* (2006), pp. 29–42, in Erik Parens edition of *Surgically Shaping Children: Technology, Ethics, and the Pursuit of Normality*, pp. 43–48. Baltimore: Maryland: Johns Hopkins University Press.

50. R.N. Bellah et al., Habits of the Heart: Individualism and Commitment in American Life, updated edition (Berkeley: University of California Press, 1996), 138.

51. Ibid., 152 ff.

"Ambiguous Sex"—or Ambivalent Medicine? Ethical Issues in the Treatment of Intersexuality

Alice Domurat Dreger

What makes us "female" or 'male," "girls" or "boys," "women" or "men"—our chromosomes, our genitalia, how we (and others) are brought up to think about ourselves, or all of the above? One of the first responses to the birth of a child of ambiguous sex by clinicians, and parents, is to seek to "disambiguate" the situation: to assign the newborns identity as either female or male, surgically modify the child's genitalia to conform believably to that sex identity, and provide other medical treatment (such as hormones) to reinforce the gender decided upon. The assumptions that underly efforts to "normalize" intersexual individuals and the ethics of "treatment" for intersexuality merit closer examination than they generally receive.

A number of events have lately aroused substantial public interest in intersexuality (congenital "ambiguous sex") and "reconstructive" genital surgery. Perhaps the most sensational of these is the recent publication of unexpected long-term outcomes in the classic and well-known "John/Joan" case.[1] "John" was born a typical XY male with a twin brother, but a doctor accidentally ablated John's penis during a circumcision at age eight months. Upon consultation with a team of physicians and sexologists at the Johns Hopkins Hospital (circa 1963) it was decided that given the unfortunate loss of a normal penis John should be medically reconstructed and raised as a girl—"Joan." Surgeons therefore removed John/Joan's testes and subsequently subjected Joan to further surgical and hormonal treatments in an attempt to make her body look more like a girl's. The team of medical professionals involved also employed substantial psychological counselling to help Joan and the family feel comfortable with Joan's female gender. They believed that Joan and the family would need help adjusting to her new gender, but that full (or near-full) adjustment could be achieved.

For decades, the alleged success of this particular sex reassignment had been widely reported by Hopkins sexologist John Money and others as proof that physicians could essentially create any gender out of any child, so long as the cosmetic alteration was performed early. Money and others repeatedly asserted that "Johns" could be made into "Joans" and "Joans" into "Johns" so long as the genitals looked "right" and everyone agreed to agree on the child's assigned gender. The postulates of this approach are summarized succinctly by Milton Diamond and Keith Sigmundson: "(1) individuals are psychosexually neutral at birth and (2) healthy psychosexual development is dependent on the appearance of the genitals"[2] While not a case of congenital intersexuality, the John/Joan case was nevertheless used by many clinicians who treat intersexuality as proof that in intersex cases the same postulates should hold. The keys seemed to be surgical creation of a believable sexual anatomy and assurances all around that the child was "really" the assigned gender.

But reports of the success of John/Joan were premature—indeed, they were wrong. Diamond and Sigmundson recently interviewed the person in question, now an adult, and report that Joan had in fact chosen to resume life as

---

Dreger, A., "Ambiguous Sex—or Ambivalent Medicine? Ethical Issues in the Treatment of Intersexuality", *Hastings Center Report* 28 (3), pp. 24–36. Published by the Hastings Center © 1998. Reprinted by permission.

John at age fourteen. John, now an adult, is married to a woman and, via adoption, is the father of her children. John and his mother report that in the Joan-years, John was never fully comfortable with a female gender identity. Indeed, Joan actively attempted to resist some of the treatment designed to ensure her female identity; for instance, when prescribed estrogens at age twelve, Joan secretly discarded the feminizing hormones. Depressed and unhappy at fourteen, Joan finally asked her father for the truth, and upon hearing it, "All of a sudden everything clicked. For the first time things made sense, and I understood who and what I was."[3] At his request, John received a mastectomy at age fourteen, and for the next two years underwent several plastic surgery operations aimed at making his genitals look more masculine.[4]

Diamond and Sigmundson are chiefly interested in using this new data to conclude that "the evidence seems overwhelming that normal humans are not psychosocially neutral at birth but are, in keeping with their mammalian heritage, predisposed and biased to interact with environmental, familial, and social forces in either a male or female mode."[5] In other words, sexual nature is not infinitely pliable; biology matters.

In their report, Diamond and Sigmundson also take the opportunity of publication to comment on the problem of the lack of long-term follow-up of cases like these. But what is also troubling is the lack of ethical analysis around cases like this—particularly around cases of the medical treatment of intersexuality, a phenomenon many orders of magnitude more common than traumatic loss of the penis. While there have been some brief discussions of the ethics of deceiving intersex patients (that discussion is reviewed below), the medical treatment of people born intersexed has remained largely ignored by ethicists. Indeed, I can find little discussion in the literature of any of the ethical issues involved in "normalizing" children with allegedly "cosmetically offensive" anatomies. The underlying assumption grounding this silence appears to be

that "normalizing" procedures are necessarily thoroughly beneficent and that they present no quandaries. This article seeks to challenge that assumption and to encourage interested parties to reconsider, from an ethical standpoint, the dominant treatment protocols for children and adults with unusual genital anatomy.

FREQUENCY OF INTERSEXUALITY

Aside from the apparent presumption that "normalizing" surgeries are necessarily good, I suspect that ethicists have ignored the question of intersex treatment because like most people they assume the phenomenon of intersexuality to be exceedingly rare. It is not. But how common is it? The answer depends, of course, on how one defines it. Broadly speaking, intersexuality constitutes a range of anatomical conditions in which an individual's anatomy mixes key masculine anatomy with key feminine anatomy. One quickly runs into a problem, however, when trying to define "key" or "essential" feminine and masculine anatomy. In fact, any close study of sexual anatomy results in a loss of faith that there is a simple, "natural" sex distinction that will not break down in the face of certain anatomical, behavioral, or philosophical challenges.[6]

Sometimes the phrase "ambiguous genitalia" is substituted for "intersexuality," but this does not solve the problem of frequency, because we still are left struggling with the question of what should count as "ambiguous." (How small must a baby's penis be before it counts as "ambiguous"?) For our purposes, it is simplest to put the question of frequency pragmatically: How often do physicians find themselves unsure which gender to assign at birth? One 1993 gynecology text estimates that "in approximately 1 in 500 births, the sex is doubtful because of the external genitalia."[7] I am persuaded by more recent, well-documented literature that estimates the number to be roughly 1 in 1,500 live births.[8]

The frequency estimate goes up dramatically, however, if we include all children born with what some physicians consider cosmetically "unacceptable" genitalia. Many technically non-intersexed girls are born with "big" clitorises, and many technically nonintersexed boys are born with hypospadic penises in which the urethral opening is found somewhere other than the very tip of the penis.

HISTORICAL BACKGROUND

I came to this topic as an historian and philosopher of science. My initial interest was actually in learning how British and French medical and scientific men of the late nineteenth century dealt with human hermaphroditism. The late nineteenth century was a time when the alleged naturalness of European social sex borders was under serious challenge by feminists and homosexuals and by anthropological reports of sex roles in other cultures. I wanted to know what biomedical professionals did, at such a politically charged time, with those who *inadvertently* challenged anatomical sex borders.

The answer is that biomedical men tried their best to shore up the borders between masculinity and femininity.[9] Specifically, the experts honed in on the ovarian and testicular tissues and decided that these were the key to any body's sexual identity. The "true sex" of most individuals thus by definition settled nicely into one of the two great and preferred camps, no matter how confusing the rest of their sexual anatomies. People with testicular tissue but with some otherwise "ambiguous" anatomy were now labeled "male pseudo-hermaphrodites"—that is, "true" males. People with ovarian tissue but with some otherwise ambiguous anatomy were labeled "female pseudo-hermaphrodites"—"true" females.

By equating sex identity simply with gonadal tissue, almost every body could be shown really to be a "true male" or a "true female" in spite of mounting numbers of doubtful cases. Additionally, given that biopsies of gonads were not done until the 1910s and that Victorian medical men insisted upon histological proof of ovarian and testicular tissue for claims of

"true hermaphroditism," the only "true hermaphrodites" tended to be dead and autopsied hermaphrodites.

Nevertheless, new technologies—specifically laparotomies and biopsies—in the 1910s made this approach untenable. It now became possible (and, by the standing rules, necessary) to label some living people as "true" hermaphrodites via biopsies, and disturbed physicians noted that no one knew what to do with such people. There was no place, socially or legally, for true hermaphrodites. Moreover, physicians found case after case of extremely feminine-looking and feminine-acting women who were shown upon careful analysis to have testes and no ovaries. The latter were cases of what today is called androgen-insensitivity syndrome (AIS), also known as testicular feminization syndrome. We now know that individuals with AIS (roughly 1/60,000[10]) have an XY ("male") chromosomal complement and testes, but their androgen receptors cannot "read" the masculinizing hormones their testes produce. Consequently, *in utero* and throughout their lives, their anatomy develops along apparently "feminine" pathways. AIS is often not discovered until puberty, when these girls do not menstruate and a gynecological examination reveals AIS. Women with AIS look and feel very much like "typical" women, and in a practical, social, legal, and everyday sense they are women, even though congenitally they have testes and XY chromosomes.

In the 1910s, physicians working with intersexuality realized that assigning these women to the male sex (because of their testes) or admitting living "true hermaphrodites" (because of their ovotestes) would only wreak social havoc. Consequently, in practice the medical profession moved away from a strict notion of gonadal "true sex" toward a pragmatic concept of "gender" and physicians began to focus their attentions on gender "reconstruction." Elaborate surgical and hormonal treatments have now been developed to make the sexual anatomy more believable, that is, more "typical" of the gender assigned by the physician.

DOMINANT TREATMENT PROTOCOLS

Thus the late twentieth century medical approach to intersexuality is based essentially on an anatomically strict psychosocial theory of gender identity. Contemporary theory, established and disseminated largely via the work of John Money[11] and endorsed by the American Academy of Pediatrics,[12] holds that gender identity arises primarily from psychosocial rearing (nurture), and not directly from biology (nature); that all children must have their gender identity fixed very early in life for a consistent, "successful" gender identity to form; that from very early in life the child's anatomy must match the "standard" anatomy for her or his gender; and that for gender identity to form psychosocially boys primarily require "adequate" penises with no vagina, and girls primarily require a vagina with no easily noticeable phallus.[13]

Note that this theory presumes that these rules *must* be followed if intersexual children are to achieve successful psychosocial adjustment appropriate to their assigned gender—that is, if they are to act like girls, boys, men, and women are "supposed" to act. The theory also by implication presumes that there are definite acceptable and unacceptable roles for boys, girls, men, and women, and that this approach *will* achieve successful psychosocial adjustment, at least far more often than any other approach.

Many parents, especially those unfamiliar with sex development, are bothered by their children's intersexed genitals and receptive to offers of "normalizing" medical treatments. Many also actively seek guidance about gender assignment and parenting practices. In the United States today, therefore, typically upon the identification of an "ambiguous" or intersexed baby teams of specialists (geneticists, pediatric endocrinologists, pediatric urologists, and so on) are immediately assembled, and these teams of doctors decide to which sex/gender a given child will be assigned. A plethora of technologies are then used to create and maintain that sex in as believable a form as possible, including, typically, surgery on the genitals, and sometimes later also

on other "anomalous" parts like breasts in an assigned male; hormone monitoring and treatments to get a "cocktail" that will help and not contradict the decided sex (and that will avoid metabolic dangers); and fostering the conviction among the child's family and community that the child is indeed the sex decided—"psychosocial" rearing of the child according to the norms of the chosen sex. Doctors typically take charge of the first two kinds of activities and hope that the child's family and community will successfully manage the all-critical third.

Clinicians treating intersexuality worry that any confusion about the sexual identity of the child on the part of relatives will be conveyed to the child and result in enormous psychological problems, including potential "dysphoric" states in adolescence and adulthood. In an effort to forestall or end any confusion about the child's sexual identity, clinicians try to see to it that an intersexual's sex/gender identity is permanently decided by specialist doctors within forty-eight hours of birth. With the same goals in mind, many clinicians insist that parents of intersexed newborns be told that their ambiguous child *does* really have a male or female sex, but that the sex of their child has just not yet "finished" developing, and that the doctors will quickly figure out the "correct" sex and then help "finish" the sexual development. As the sociologist Suzanne Kessler noted in her ground-breaking sociological analysis of the current treatment of intersexuality, "the message [conveyed to these parents] … is that the trouble lies in the doctor's ability to determine the gender, not in the baby's gender per se."[14] In intersex cases, Ellen Hyun-Ju Lee concludes, "physicians present a picture of the 'natural sex,' either male or female, despite their role in actually constructing sex."[15]

Because of widespread acceptance of the anatomically strict psychosocial theory of treatment, the practical rules now adopted by most specialists in intersexuality are these: genetic males (children with Y chromosomes) must have "adequate" penises if they are to be assigned the male gender. When a genetic male is judged to have an "adequate" phallus size, surgeons may operate, sometimes repeatedly, to try to make the penis look more "normal." If their penises are determined to be "inadequate" for successful adjustment as males, they are assigned the female gender and reconstructed to look female. (Hence John to Joan.) In cases of intersexed children assigned the female sex/gender, surgeons may "carve a large phallus down into a clitoris" (primarily attempting to make the phallus invisible when standing), "create a vagina using a piece of colon" or other body parts, "mold labia out of what was a penis," remove any testes, and so on.[16]

Meanwhile, genetic females (that is, babies lacking a Y chromosome) born with ambiguous genitalia are declared girls—no matter how masculine their genitalia look. This is done chiefly in the interest of preserving these children's potential feminine reproductive capabilities and in bringing their anatomical appearance and physiological capabilities into line with that reproductive role. Consequently, these children are reconstructed to look female using the same general techniques as those used on genetically male children assigned a female role. Surgeons reduce "enlarged" clitorises so that they will not look "masculine." Vaginas are built or lengthened it necessary, in order to make them big enough to accept average-sized penises. Joined labia are separated, and various other surgical and hormonal treatments are directed at producing a believable and, it is hoped, fertile girl.

What are the limits of acceptability in terms of phalluses? Clitorises—meaning simply phalluses in children labeled female—are frequently considered too big if they exceed one centimeter in length.[17] Pediatric surgeons specializing in treating intersexuality consider "enlarged" clitorises to be "cosmetically offensive" in girls and therefore they subject these clitorises to surgical reduction meant to leave the organs looking more "feminine" and "delicate."[18] Penises—meaning simply phalluses in children labeled male—are often considered too small if the stretched length is less than 2.5 centimeters (about an inch). Consequently, genetically male children born at term "with a stretched penile length less than 2.5 [centimeters] are usually given a female sex assignment?[19]

Roughly the same protocols are applied to cases of "true" hermaphroditism (in which babies are born with testicular and ovarian tissue). Whereas the anatomico-materialist metaphysics of sex in the late nineteenth century made true hermaphrodites an enormous problem for doctors and scientists of that time, clinicians today believe that "true hermaphrodites" (like "pseudo-hermaphrodites") can be fairly easily retrofitted with surgery and other treatment to either an acceptable male or acceptable female sex/gender.

One of the troubling aspects of these protocols are the asymmetric ways they treat femininity and masculinity. For example, physicians appear to do far more to preserve the reproductive potential of children born with ovaries than that of children born with testes. While genetically male intersexuals often have infertile testes, some men with micropenis may be able to father children if allowed to retain their testes.[20]

Similarly, surgeons seem to demand far more for a penis to count as "successful" than for a vagina to count as such. Indeed, the logic behind the tendency to assign the female gender in cases of intersexuality rests not only on the belief that boys need "adequate" penises, but also upon the opinion among surgeons that "a functional vagina can be constructed in virtually everyone [while] a functional penis is a much more difficult goal."[21] This is true because much is expected of penises, especially by pediatric urologists, and very little of vaginas. For a penis to count as acceptable—"functional"—it must be or have the potential to be big enough to be readily recognizable as a "real" penis. In addition, the "functional" penis is generally expected to have the capability to become erect and flaccid at appropriate times, and to act as the conduit through which urine and semen are expelled, also at appropriate times. The urethral opening is expected to appear at the very tip of the penis. Typically, surgeons also hope to see penises that are "believably" shaped and colored.

Meanwhile, very little is needed for a surgically constructed vagina to count among surgeons as "functional." For a constructed vagina to be considered acceptable by surgeons specializing in intersexuality, it basically just has to be a hole big enough to fit a typical-sized penis. It is not required to be self-lubricating or even to be at all sensitive, and certainly does not need to change shape the way vaginas often do when women are sexually stimulated. So, for example, in a panel discussion of surgeons who treat intersexuality, when one was asked, "How do you define successful intercourse? How many of these girls actually have an orgasm, for example?" a member of the panel responded, "Adequate intercourse was defined as successful vaginal penetration.[22] All that is required is a receptive hole.

Indeed, clinicians treating intersex children often talk about vaginas in these children as the absence of a thing, as a space, a "hole," a place to put something. That is precisely why opinion holds that "a functional vagina can be constructed in virtually everyone" because it is relatively easy to construct an insensitive hole surgically. (It is not always easy to keep them open and uninfected.) The decision to "make" a female is therefore considered relatively foolproof, while "the assignment of male sex of rearing is inevitably difficult and should only be undertaken by an experienced team" who can determine if a penis will be adequate for "successful" malehood.[23]

THE PROBLEM OF "NORMALITY"

The strict, conception of "normal" sexual anatomy and normal sex behavior that underlies prevailing treatment protocols is arguably sexist in its asymmetrical treatment of reproductive potential and definitions of anatomical "adequacy." Additionally, as Lee and other critics of intersex treatment have noted, "[d]ecisions of gender assignment and subsequent surgical reconstruction are inseparable from the heterosexual matrix, which does not allow for other sexual practices or sexualities. Even within

heterosexuality, a rich array of sexual practices is reduced to vaginal penetration."[24] Not surprisingly, feminists and intersexuals have invariably objected to these presumptions that there is a "right" way to be a male and a "right" way to be a female, and that children who challenge these categories should be reconstructed to fit into (and thereby reinforce) them.

Indeed, beside the important (and too often disregarded) philosophical-political issue of gender roles, there is a more practical one: how does one decide where to put the boundaries on acceptable levels of anatomical variation? Not surprisingly, the definition of genital "normality" in practice appears to vary among physicians. For example, at least one physician has set the minimum length of an "acceptable" penis at 1.5 centimeters.[25]

Indeed, at least two physicians are convinced (and have evidence) that any penis is a big enough penis for male adjustment, if the other cards are played right. Almost a decade ago Justine Schober (nee Reilly), a pediatric urologist now based at the Hamot Medical Center in Erie, Pennsylvania, and Christopher Woodhouse, a physician based at the Institute of Urology and St. George's Hospital in London, "interviewed and examined 20 patients with the primary diagnosis of micropenis in infancy" who were labeled and raised as boys. Of the post-pubertal (adult) subjects, "All patients were heterosexual and they had erections and orgasms. Eleven patients had ejaculations, 9 were sexually active and reported vaginal penetration, 7 were married or cohabitating and 1 had fathered a child."[26]

Schober and Woodhouse concluded that "a small penis does not preclude normal male role" and should not dictate female gender reassignment. They found that when parents "were well counseled about diagnosis they reflected an attitude of concern but not anxiety about the problem, and they did not convey anxiety to their children. They were honest and explained problems to the child and encouraged normality in behavior. We believe that this is the attitude that allows these children to approach their peers with confidence."[27]

Ultimately, Schober and Woodhouse agreed with the tenet of the psychosocial theory that assumes that "the strongest influence for all patients [is] the parental attitude." But rather than making these children into girls and trying to convince the parents and children about their "real" feminine identity, Schober and Woodhouse found that "the well informed and open parents…produced more confident and better adjusted boys." We should note that these boys were not considered "typical" in their sex lives: "The group was characterized by an experimental attitude to [sexual] positions and methods…. The group appears to form close and long-lasting relationships. They often attribute partner sexual satisfaction and the stability of their relationships [with women partners] to their need to make extra effort including nonpenetrating techniques."[28]

"Ambiguous" genitalia do not constitute a disease. They simply constitute a failure to fit a particular (and, at present, a particularly demanding) definition of normality. It is true that whenever a baby is born with "ambiguous" genitalia, doctors need to consider the situation a *potential* medical emergency because intersexuality may signal a potentially serious metabolic problem, namely congenital adrenal hyperplasia (CAH), which primarily involves an electrolyte imbalance and can result in "masculinization" of genetically female fetuses. Treatment of CAH may save a child's life and fertility. At the birth of an intersex child, therefore, adrenogenital syndrome must be quickly diagnosed and treated, or ruled out. Nonetheless, as medical texts advise, "of all the conditions responsible for ambiguous genitalia, congenital adrenal hyperplasia is the only one that is life-threatening in the newborn period," and even in cases of CAH the "ambiguous" genitalia themselves are not deadly.[29] As with CAH's clear medical issue, doctors now also know that the testes of AIS patients have a relatively high rate of becoming cancerous, and therefore AIS needs to be diagnosed as early as possible so that the testes can be carefully watched or removed. However, the genitalia of an androgen-insensitive person are not diseased. Again, while unusual genitalia may signal a present or potential threat to health, in themselves they just *look* different. As we have seen, because of the perception of a "social emergency" around an intersex birth, clinicians take license to treat nonstandard genitalia as a medical problem requiring prompt correction. But as Suzanne Kessler sums up the situation, intersexuality does not threaten the patient's life; it threatens the patient's culture.

PSYCHOLOGICAL HEALTH AND THE PROBLEM OF DECEPTION

Clearly, in our often unforgiving culture intersexuality can also threaten the patient's psyche; that recognition is behind the whole treatment approach. Nevertheless, there are two major problems here. First, clinicians treating intersex individuals may be far more concerned with strict definitions of genital normality than intersexuals, their parents, and their acquaintances (including lovers). This is evidenced time and again, for example, in the John/Joan case:

> John recalls thinking, from preschool through elementary school, that physicians were more concerned with the appearance of Joan's genitals than was Joan. Her genitals were inspected at each visit to The Johns Hopkins Hospital. She thought they were making a big issue out of nothing, and they gave her no reason to think otherwise. John recalls thinking: "Leave me be and then I'll be fine…. It's bizarre. My genitals are not bothering me; I don't know why it is bothering you guys so much."[30]

Second, and more basically, it is not self-evident that a psychosocial problem should be handled medically or surgically. We do not attempt to solve the problems many dark-skinned children will face in our nation by lightening their skins. Similarly, Cheryl Chase has posed this interesting question: when a baby is born with a severely disfigured but largely functional arm, ought we quickly remove the arm and replace it with a possibly functional prosthetic, so that the parents and child experience less psychological trauma?[31] While it is true that genitals are more psychically charged than arms, genitals are also more easily and more often kept private, whatever their state. Quoting the ideas of Suzanne Kessler, the pediatric urologist Schober argues in a forthcoming work that "Surgery makes parents and doctors more comfortable, but counseling makes people comfortable too, and [it] is not irreversible." She continues: "Simply understanding and performing good surgeries is not sufficient. We must also know when to appropriately perform or withhold surgery. Our ethical duty as surgeons is to do no harm and to serve the best interests of our patient. Sometimes, this means admitting that a 'perfect' solution may not be attainable."[32]

Ironically, rather than alleviating feelings of freakishness, in practice the way intersexuality is typically handled may actually produce or contribute to many intersexuals' feelings of freakishness. Many intersexuals look at these two facts: (1) they are subject, out of "compassion," to "normalizing" surgeries on an emergency basis without their personal consent, and (2) they are often not told the whole truth about their anatomical conditions and anatomical histories. Understandably, they conclude that their doctors see them as profound freaks and that they must really be freaks. H. Martin Malin, a professor in clinical sexology and a therapist at the Child and Family Institute in Sacramento, California, has found this to be a persistent theme running through intersexuals' medical experience:

> As I listened to [intersexuals'] stories, certain leit motifs began to emerge from the bits of their histories. They or their parents had little, if any, counseling. They thought they were the only ones who felt as they did. Many had asked to meet other patients whose medical histories were similar to their own, but they were stonewalled. They recognized themselves in published case histories, but when they sought medical records, were told they could not be located....

The patients I was encountering were not those whose surgeries resulted from life-threatening or seriously debilitating medical conditions. Rather, they had such diagnoses as "micropenis" or "clitoral hypertrophy." These were patients who were told—when they were told anything—that they had vaginoplasties or clitorectomies because of the serious psychological consequences they would have suffered if surgery had not been done. But the surgeries *had* been performed—and they were reporting longstanding psychological distress. They were certain that they would rather have had the "abnormal" genitals they [had] had than the "mutilated" genitals they were given. They were hostile and often vengeful towards the professionals who had been responsible for their care and sometimes, by transference, towards me. They were furious that they had been lied to.[33]

Given the lack of long-term follow-up studies it is unclear whether a majority of intersexuals wind up feeling this way, but even if only a small number do we must ask whether the practice of deception and "stonewalling" is essentially unethical.

Why would a physician ever withhold medical and personal historical information from an intersexed patient? Because she or he believes that the truth is too horrible or too complicated for the patient to handle. In a 1988 commentary in the *Hastings Center Report*, Brendan Minogue and Robert Tarszewski argued, for example, that a physician could justifiably withhold information from a sixteen-year-old AIS patient and/or her parents if he believed that the patient and/or family was likely to be incapable of handling the fact that she has testes and an XY chromosomal complement.[34] Indeed, this reasoning appears typical among clinicians treating intersexuality; many continue to believe that talking truthfully with intersexuals and their families will undo all the "positive" effects of the technological efforts aimed at covering up doubts. Thus despite intersexuals' and ethicists' published, repeated objections to deception, in 1995 a medical student was given a cash prize in medical ethics by the Canadian Medical Association for an article specifically advocating deceiving AIS patients (including adults) about the biological facts of their conditions. The prize-winner argued that "physicians who withhold information from AIS patients are not actually lying; they are only deceiving" because they *selectively withhold* facts about patients' bodies.[35]

But what this reasoning fails to appreciate is that hiding the facts of the condition will not necessarily prevent a patient and family from thinking about it. Indeed, the failure on the part of the doctor and family to talk honestly about the condition is likely only to add to feelings of shame and confusion. One woman with AIS in Britain writes, "Mine was a dark secret kept from all outside the medical profession (family included), but this [should] not [be] an option because it both increases the feelings of freakishness and reinforces the isolation."[36] Similarly, Martha Coventry, a woman who had her "enlarged" clitoris removed by surgeons when she was six, insists that "to be lied to as a child about your own body, to have your life as a sexual being so ignored that you are not even given the decency of an answer to your questions, is to have your heart and soul relentlessly undermined.[37]

Lying to a patient about his or her biological condition can also lead to a patient unintentionally taking unnecessary risks. As a young woman, Sherri Groveman, who has AIS, was told by her doctor that she had "twisted ovaries" and that they had to be removed; in fact, her testes were removed. At the age of twenty, "alone and scared in the stacks of a [medical] library," she discovered the truth of her condition. Then "the pieces finally fit together. But what fell apart was my relationship with both my family and physicians. It was not learning about chromosomes or testes that caused enduring trauma, it was discovering that I had been told lies. I avoided all medical care for the next 18 years. I have severe osteoporosis as a result of

a lack of medical attention. This is what lies produce."[38]

Similarly, as B. Diane Kemp—"a social worker with more than 35 years' experience and a woman who has borne androgen insensitivity syndrome for 63 years"—notes, "secrecy as a method of handling troubling information is primitive, degrading, and often ineffective. Even when a secret is kept, its existence carries an aura of unease that most people can sense.... Secrets crippled my life."[39]

Clearly, the notion that deception or selective truth-telling will protect the child, the family, or even the adult intersexual is extraordinarily paternalistic and naive, and, while perhaps well-intentioned, it goes against the dominant trend in medical ethics as those ethics guidelines are applied to other, similar situations. In what other realms are patients regularly not told the medical names for their conditions, even when they ask? As for the idea that physicians should not tell patients what they probably "can't handle," would a physician be justified in using this reasoning to avoid telling a patient she has cancer or AIDS?

In their commentary in the *Hastings Center Report* Sherman Elias and George Annas pointed out that a physician who starts playing with the facts of a patient's condition may well find himself forced to lie or admit prior deception. "Practically," Elias and Annas wrote, "it is unrealistic to believe that [the AIS patient] will not ultimately learn the details of her having testicular syndrome. From the onset it will be difficult to maintain the charade."[40] They also note that without being told the name and details of her condition any consent the AIS patient gives will not truly be "informed." As an attorney Groveman too argues "that informed consent laws mandate that the patient know the truth before physicians remove her testes or reconstruct her vagina."[41]

INFORMED CONSENT AND RISK ASSUMPTION

It is not at all clear if all or even most of the intersex surgeries done today involve what would legally and ethically constitute informed consent. It appears that few intersexuals or their parents are educated, before they give consent, about the anatomically strict psychosocial model employed. The model probably ought to be described to parents as essentially unproven insofar as the theory remains unconfirmed by broad-based, long-term follow-up studies, and is directly challenged by cases like the John/Joan case as well as by ever-mounting "anecdotal" reports from former patients who, disenfranchised and labeled "lost to follow-up" by clinicians, have turned to the popular press and to public protest in order to be heard. Of course, as long as intersex patients are not consistently told the truth of their conditions, there is some question about whether satisfaction can be assessed with integrity in long-term studies.

At a finer level, many of the latest particular cosmetic surgeries being used on intersexed babies and children today remain basically unproven as well, and need to be described as such in consent agreements. For example, a team of surgeons from the Children's Medical Center and George Washington University Medical School has reported that in their preferred form of clitoral "recession" (done to make "big" clitorises look "right"), "the cosmetic effect is excellent" but "late studies with assessment of sexual gratification, orgasm, and general psychological adjustment are unavailable..., and remain in question."[42] In fact the procedure may result in problems like stenosis, increased risk of infections, loss of feeling, and psychological trauma. (These risks characterize all genital surgeries.)

This lack of long-term follow-up is the case not only for clitoral surgeries; David Thomas, a pediatric urologist who practices at St. James's University Hospital and Infirmary in Leeds, England, recently noted the same problem with regard to early vaginal reconstructions: "So many of these patients are lost to follow-up. If we do this surgery in infancy and childhood, we have an obligation to follow these children up, to assess what we're doing."[43] There is a serious ethical problem here: risky surgeries are being performed as standard care and are not being adequately followed-up.[44]

The growing community of open adult intersexuals understandably question whether anyone should have either her ability to enjoy sex or her physical health risked without personal consent just because she has a clitoris, penis, or vagina that falls outside the standard deviation. Even if we *did* have statistics that showed that particular procedures "worked" a majority of the time we would have to face the fact that part of the time they would not work, and we need to ask whether that risk ought to be assumed on behalf of another person.

BEYOND "MONSTER ETHICS"

In a 1987 article on the ethics of killing one conjoined twin to save the other, George Annas suggested (but did not advocate) that one way to justify such a procedure would be to take "the monster approach." This approach would hold that conjoined twins are so grotesque, so pathetic, any medical procedure aimed at normalizing them would be morally justified.[45] Unfortunately, the present treatment of intersexuality in the U.S. seems to be deeply informed by the monster approach; ethical guidelines that would be applied in nearly any other medical situation are, in cases of intersexuality, ignored. Patients are lied to; risky procedures are performed without follow-up; consent is not fully informed; autonomy and health are risked because of unproven (and even disproven) fears that atypical anatomy will lead to psychological disaster. Why? Perhaps because sexual anatomy is not treated like the rest of human anatomy, or perhaps because we simply assume that any procedure which "normalizes" an "abnormal" child is merciful. Whatever the reason, the medical treatment of intersexuality and other metabolically benign, cosmetically unusual anatomies needs deep and immediate attention.

We can readily use the tools of narrative ethics to gain insight into practices surrounding intersexuality. There are now available many autobiographies of adult intersexuals.[46] Like that of John/Joan, whether or not they are characteristic of long-term outcomes these autobiographies raise serious questions about the dominant treatment protocols.

Narrative ethics also suggests that we use our imaginations to think through the story of the intersexual, to ask ourselves, if we were born intersexed, what treatment we would wish to have received. Curious about what adult non-intersexuals would have chosen for themselves, Suzanne Kessler polled a group of college students regarding their feelings on the matter. The women were asked, "Suppose you had been born with a larger than normal clitoris and it would remain larger than normal as you grew to adulthood. Assuming that the physicians recommended surgically reducing your clitoris, under what circumstances would you have wanted your parents to give them permission to do it?" In response,

> About a fourth of the women indicated they would not have wanted a clitoral reduction under *any* circumstance. About half would have wanted their clitoris reduced *only* if the larger than normal clitoris caused health problems. Size, for them, was not a factor. The remaining forth of the sample *could* imagine wanting their clitoris reduced if it were larger than normal, but *only* if having the surgery would not have resulted in a reduction in pleasurable sensitivity.[47]

Meanwhile, in this study, "the men were asked to imagine being born with a smaller than normal penis and told that physicians recommended phallic reduction and a female gender assignment." In response,

> All but one man indicated they would not have wanted surgery under any circumstance. The remaining man indicated that if his penis were 1 cm. or less *and he were going to be sterile*, he would have wanted his parents to give the doctors permission to operate and make him a female.[48]

Kessler is cautious to note that we need more information to assess this data fully, but it does begin to suggest that given the choice most people would reject genital cosmetic surgery for themselves.

As an historian, I also think we need to consider the historical and cultural bases for genital conformity practices, and realize that most people in the U.S. demonstrate little tolerance for practices in other cultures that might well be considered similar. I am, of course, talking about the recent passage of federal legislation prohibiting physicians from performing "circumcision" on the genitalia of girls under the age of eighteen, *whether or not the girls consent or personally request the procedure*. African female genital "cutting" typically involves, in part, excision of the clitoral tissue so that most or all clitoral sensation will be lost. While proponents of this traditional female genital "cutting" have insisted this practice is an important cultural tradition—analogous to male circumcision culturally—advocates of the U.S. law insist it is barbaric and violates human rights. Specifically, in the federal legislation passed in October 1996 Congress declared that: "Except as provided in subsection (b), whoever knowingly circumcises, excises, or infibulates the whole or any part of the labia majora or labia minora or clitoris of another person who has not attained the age of 18 years shall be fined under this title or imprisoned not more than 5 years, or both."[49]

Subsection "b" specifies that: "A surgical operation is not a violation of this section if the operation is (1) necessary to the health of the person on whom it is performed, and is performed by a person licensed in the place of its performance as a medical practitioner; or (2) performed on a person in labor or who has just given birth and is performed for medical purposes connected with that labor or birth."

Surgeons treating intersexuality presumably would argue that the procedures they perform on the genitals of girls (which clearly include excision of parts of the clitoris) are indeed "necessary to the health of the person on whom it is performed." While it is easy to condemn the African practice of female genital mutilation as a barbaric custom that violates human rights, we should recognize that in the United States medicine's prevailing response to intersexuality is largely about genital conformity and the "proper" roles of the sexes. Just as we find it necessary to protect the rights and well-being of African girls, we must now consider the hard questions of the rights and well-being of children born intersexed in the United States.

As this [article] was in process, the attention paid by the popular media and by physicians to the problems with the dominant clinical protocols increased dramatically, and many more physicians and ethicists have recently come forward to question those protocols. Diamond and Sigmundson have helpfully proposed tentative new "guidelines for dealing with persons with ambiguous genitalia."[50]

As new guidelines are further developed, it will be critical to take seriously two tasks. First, as I have argued above, intersexuals must not be subjected to different ethical standards from other people simply because they are intersexed. Second, the experiences and advice of adult intersexuals must be solicited and taken into consideration. It is incorrect to claim, as I have heard several clinicians do, that the complaints of adult intersexuals are irrelevant because they were subjected to "old, unperfected" surgeries. Clinicians have too often retreated to the mistaken belief that improved treatment technologies (for example, better surgical techniques) will eliminate ethical dilemmas surrounding intersex treatment. There is far more at issue than scar tissue and loss of sensation from unperfected surgeries.

Acknowledgements

The author wishes to thank Aron Sousa, Cheryl Chase, Michael Fisher, Elizabeth Gretz, Daniel Federman, the members of the Enhancement Technologies and Human Identity Working Group, and Howard Brody, Libby Bogdan-Lovis, and other associates of the Center for Ethics and Humanities in the Life Sciences at Michigan State University for their comments on this work.

Notes

1. Milton Diamond and H. Keith Sigmundson, "Sex Reassignment at Birth: Long-Term Review and Clinical Implications," *Archives of Pediatrics and Adolescent Medicine* 15 (1997): 298–304.
2. Ibid., 298.
3. Ibid., 300.
4. For a more in-depth biography, see John Colapinto, "The True Story of John/Joan," *Rolling Stone,* 11 December 1997, pp. 55ff.
5. Diamond and Sigmundson, "Sex Reassignment," p. 303.
6. I discuss this at length in Dreger, *Hermaphrodites and the Medical Invention of Sex* (Cambridge, Mass.: Harvard University Press, 1998); see especially prologue and chap. 1.
7. See Ethel Sloane, *Biology of Women*, 3d ed. (Albany: Delmar Publishers, 1993), p. 168. According to Denis Grady, a study of over 6,500 women athletes competing in seven different international sports competitions showed an incidence of intersexuality of one in 500 women, but unfortunately Grady does not provide a reference to the published data from that study (Denise Grady, "Sex Test," *Discover,* June 1992, pp. 78–82). That sampled population should not simply be taken as representative of the whole population, but this number is certainly higher than most people would expect.
8. Anne Fausto-Sterling, *Body Building: How Biologists Construct Sexuality* (New York: Basic Books, forthcoming 1999), chap. 2; Fausto-Sterling, "How Dimorphic Are We?" *American Journal of Human Genetics* (forthcoming); and personal communication. The highest modern-day estimate for frequency of sexually ambiguous births comes from John Money, who has posited that as many as 4 percent of live births today are of "intersexed" individuals (cited in Anne Fausto-Sterling, "The Five Sexes," *The Sciences* 33 [1993]: 20–25). Money's categories tend to be exceptionally broad and poorly defined, and not representative of what most

medical professionals today would consider to be "intersexuality."

9. Dreger, *Hermaphrodites,* chaps. 1–5; for a summary of the scene in Britain in the late-nineteenth century, see Dreger, "Doubtful Sex: The Fate of the Hermaphrodite in Victorian Medicine," *Victorian Studies* 38 (1995): 335–69.

10. Stuart R. Kupfer, Charmain A. Quigley, and Frank S. French, "Male Pseudohermaphroditism," *Seminars in Perinatology* 16 (1992): 319–31, at 325.

11. For summaries and critiques of Money's work on intersexuality, see especially: Cheryl Chase, "Affronting Reason," in *Looking Queer: Image and Identity in Lesbian, Bisexual Gay and Transgendered Communities,* ed. D. Atkins (Binghamton, N.Y.: Haworth, 1998); "Hermaphrodites with Attitude: Mapping the Emergence of Intersex Political Activism," GLQ 4, no. 2 (1998): 189–211; Anne Fausto-Sterling, "How to Build a Man," in *Science and Homosexualities,* ed. Vernon A. Rosario (New York: Routledge, 1997), pp. 219–25; and Ellen Hyun-Ju Lee, "Producing Sex: An Interdisciplinary Perspective on Sex Assignment Decisions for Intersexuals" (Senior Thesis, Brown University, 1994).

12. American Academy of Pediatrics (Section on Urology), "Timing of Elective Surgery on the Genitalia of Male Children with Particular Reference to the Risks, Benefits, and Psychological Effects of Surgery and Anesthesia," *Pediatrics* 97, no. 4 (1996): 590–94.

13. For example, see Patricia K. Donahoe, "The Diagnosis and Treatment of Infants with Intersex Abnormalities," *Pediatric Clinics of North America* 34 (1987): 1333–48.

14. Suzanne J. Kessler, "The Medical Construction of Gender: Case Management of Intersexed Infants," *Signs* 16 (1990): 3–26; compare the advice given by Cynthia H. Meyers-Seifer and Nancy J. Charest, "Diagnosis and Management of Patients with Ambiguous Genitalia," *Seminars in Perinatology* 16 (1992): 33239.

15. Lee, "Producing Sex," p. 45.

16. Melissa Hendricks, "Is It a Boy or a Girl?" *John Hopkins Magazine* (November, 1993): 10–16, p. 10.

17. Barbara C. McGillivray, "The Newborn with Ambiguous Genitalia," *Seminars in Perinatology* 16 (1991): 365–68, p. 366.

18. Kurt Newman, Judson Randolph, and Kathryn Anderson, "The Surgical Management of Infants and Children with Ambiguous Genitalia," *Annals of Surgery* 215 (1992): 644–53, pp. 651 and 647.

19. Meyers-Seifer and Charest, "Diagnosis and Management," p. 337. See also Kupfer, Quigley, and French, "Male Pseudohermaphroditism," p. 328; Rajkumar Shah, Morton M. Woolley, and Gertrude Costin, "Testicular Feminization: The Androgen Insensitivity Syndrome," *Journal of Pediatric Surgery* 27 (1992): 757–60, p. 757.

20. Justine Schober, personal communication; for data on this, see Justine M. Reilly and C.R.J. Woodhouse, "Small Penis and the Male Sexual Role," *Journal of Urology* 142 (1989): 569–71.

21. Robin J.O. Catlin, Appleton & Lange, *Review for the USMILE Step 2* (East Norwalk, Connecticut: Appleton & Lange, 1993), p. 49.

22. See the comments of John P. Gearhart in M. M. Bailez, John P. Gearhart, Claude Migeon, and John Rock, "Vaginal Reconstruction After Initial Construction of the External Genitalia in Girls with Salt-Wasting Adrenal Hyperplasia," *Journal of Urology* 148 (1992): 680–84, p. 684.

23. Kupfer, Quigley, and French, "Male Pseudohermaphroditism," p. 328.

24. Lee, "Producing Sex," p. 27.

25. See Donahoe, "The Diagnosis and Treatment of Infants with Intersex Abnormalities."

26. Reilly and Woodhouse, "Small Penis," p. 569.

27. Ibid., 571.

28. Ibid., 571.

29. Patricia K. Donahoe, David M. Powell, and Mary M. Lee, "Clinical Management of Intersex Abnormalities," *Current Problems in Surgery* 28 (1991): 515–79, p. 540.

30. Diamond and Sigmundson, "Sex Reassignment," pp. 300–301.

31. Cheryl Chase, personal communication.

32. Quoted in Justine M. Schober, "Long-Term Outcome of Feminizing Genitoplasty for Intersex," *Pediatric Surgery and Urology: Long Term Outcomes,* ed. Pierre D. E. Mouriquand (Philadelphia: William B. Saunders, forthcoming).

33. H. M. Malin, personal communication of 1 January 1997 to Justine M. Schober, quoted in Schober, "Long-Term Outcome."

34. Brendan P. Minogue and Robert Taraszewski, "The Whole Truth and Nothing But the Truth?" (Case Study), *Hastings Center Report* 18, no. 5 (1988): 34–35.

35. Anita Natarajan, "Medical Ethics and Truth Telling in the Case of Androgen Insensitivity Syndrome," *Canadian Medical Association Journal* 154 (1996): 568–70. (For responses to Natarajan's

recomendations by AIS women and a partner of an AIS woman, see *Canadian Medical Association Journal* 154 [1996]: 1829–33.)

36. Anonymous, "Be Open and Honest with Sufferers," *British Medical Journal* 308 (1994): 1041–42.

37. Martha Coventry, "Finding the Words," *Chrysalis: The Journal of Transgressive Gender Identities* 2 (1997): 27–30.

38. Sherri A. Groveman, "Letter to the Editor," *Canadian Medical Association Journal* 154 (1996): 1829, 1832.

39. B. Diane Kemp, "Letter to the Editor," *Canadian Medical Association Journal* 154 (1996): 1829.

40. Sherman Elias and George J. Annas, "The Whole Truth and Nothing But the Truth?" (Case Study), *Hastings Center Report* 18, no. 5 (1988): 35–36, p. 35.

41. Groveman, "Letter to the Editor," p. 1829.

42. Newman, Randolph, and Anderson, "Surgical Management," p. 651.

43. "Is Early Vaginal Reconstruction Wrong for Some Intersex Girls?" *Urology Times* (February 1997): 10–12.

44. Intersexuals are understandably tired of hearing that "long-term follow-up data is needed" while the surgeries continued to occur. On this, see especially the guest commentary by David Sandberg, "A Call for Clinical Research," *Hermaphrodites with Attitude* (Fall/Winter 1995–1996): 8–9, and the many responses of intersexuals in the same issue.

45. George J. Annas, "Siamese Twins: Killing One to Save the Other" (At Law), *Hastings Center Report* 17, no. 2 (1987): 2729.

46. See, for example, M. Morgan Holmes, "Medical Politics and Cultural Imperatives: Intersex Identities beyond Pathology and Erasure" (M.A. Thesis, York University, 1994); Chase, "Hermaphrodites with Attitude"; Geoffrey Cowley, "Gender Limbo," *Newsweek,* 19 May 1997, pp. 64–66; Natalie Angier, "New Debate Over Surgery on Genitals," *New York Times,* 13 May 1997; "Special Issue: Intersexuality," *Chrysalis: The Journal of Transgressire Gender Identities* 2 (1997) Intersexual autobiographies are also from peer support groups, including the Intersex Society of North America. For information about support groups see the special issue of *Chrysalis,* vol. 2, 1997.

47. Suzanne J. Kessler, "Meanings of Genital Variability," *Chrysalis: The Journal of Transgressive Gender Identities* 2 (1997): 33–37.

48. Ibid., 36.

49. *Omnibus Consolidated Appropriations Bill,* H.R. 3610, EL. 104–208.

50. Milton Diamond and Keith Sigmundson, "Management of Intersexuality: Guidelines for Dealing with Persons with Ambiguous Genitalia," *Archives of Pediatric and Adolescent Medicine* 151 (1997): 1046–50.

EPILOGUE

Alice Domurat Dreger

The editors of this volume have kindly chosen to reprint my 1998 article on the medical treatment of people born with atypical sex. A lot has changed since 1998—mostly for the better—so this epilogue is necessary to bring the reader up to date. Why not just create a new article? Three reasons: (1) today the medical care system for atypical sex is so in flux that it would be difficult to accurately capture the current variety of practices without that representation potentially becoming quickly out of date; (2) the ethical critiques I put forth in 1998 are still worth reviewing, even though some practices have changed; (3) the 1998 article when taken in

conjunction with this 2011 epilogue may provide the reader with a sense that medical practice *can change for the better* through the efforts of patient advocates (including clinicians) who are attuned to evidence and ethics.[1]

Public knowledge of sex variation has radically expanded since 1998. This matters to those interested in the medical treatment of intersex because the public's increased knowledge has changed how clinicians think. The success of the gay, lesbian, bisexual, and transgender rights movements has also changed how the public and clinicians think about atypical sex. In the early 1990s, many clinicians believed intersex

---

Epilogue reprinted by permission of the author.

to be taboo, and so they acted from places of shame and secrecy. Today clinicians find that parents and affected individuals often come with some background knowledge of intersex, often knowledge influenced by the rights movements of sexual minorities. As a consequence, intersex seems today to be generally treated with less shame, secrecy, homophobia, and transphobia.

The expansion of public understanding since 1998 has occurred largely through media attention to specific stories of intersex, including via television programs featuring leaders of the intersex rights movement such as Max Beck, Howard Devore, and Bo Laurent (also known as Cheryl Chase). In 2000, John Colapinto's excellent book, *As Nature Made Him*, told the full story of David Reimer, the man identified at the start of my 1998 article by Money's pseudonyms for him ("John/Joan").[2] Tragically, in 2004, Reimer committed suicide, an outcome that added to the public sense that Reimer had been abused by a problematic medical system based on shame, outdated sex norms, and lies. In 2002, Jeffrey Eugenides' novel *Middlesex* told the life story of a person with the intersex condition 5–alpha reductase deficiency, including an encounter with a John Money-like clinician.[3] *Middlesex* sold over three million copies and even landed on Oprah's Book Club, and curiously, it seemed to lead many doctors to rethink the treatment of intersex, in spite of being a fictional tale.

In 2009, international attention landed (unwittingly) on Caster Semenya, a young South African runner whose sex was called into question at the international games in Berlin. For the first time in response to a sex-test case in sports, an enormous—and enormously-open—international public dialogue occurred, with many commentators outraged at the way Semenya had been treated by sports officials and doctors. Her case has forced the International Olympic Committee and the International Association of Athletics Federations (as well as smaller sports bodies) to revise their policies.[4] The general theme among public commentators has focused on the rights of sexually atypical athletes to be treated as fully respected human beings. This represents real progress.

Clinicians today are much more likely to tell parents and affected individuals the full details of the intersex conditions with which they're dealing. Today when I visit with support groups, I meet teenagers who know their diagnoses and their full medical histories, and I meet parents who talk openly around their young children about their children's diagnoses and medical histories. This is a most radical and welcome development. Some clinicians actively refer patients and their families to the diagnosis-specific support groups, but many still do not. They typically tell me that they worry about what misinformation and "bad attitudes" their patients will pick up at the support groups, even though there are many high quality support groups like the Androgen Insensitivity Syndrome Support Group and the Hypospadias and Epispadias Association.

Probably the most visible change in medical practice since 1998 has been a shift in the nomenclature from "intersex" and words based on the root "hermaphrodite" (e.g., "male pseudohermaphrodite") to "disorders of sex development" (DSD).[5] I was one of the people who pushed for this change because: many clinicians refused to recognize conditions like hypospadias and ambiguous genitalia resulting from CAH as "intersex," so, while using the term "intersex," we could not get them to see the common problems and much-needed common solutions; many parents were frightened by the term "intersex," and so rushed to try to make it go away via surgery; the term "intersex" had become so politicized as to be wrapped up with adult queer rights in a way that muddied questions of care for sexually atypical children; many transgender (but not conventionally intersex) activists had started to adopt "intersex" for themselves, changing what "intersex" meant.[6]

The term "disorders of sex development" was officially adopted in 2006 by a consensus meeting in Chicago of the major North American and European pediatric endocrinology societies. DSD refers to "congenital conditions in which development of chromosomal, gonadal, or anatomic sex is atypical."[7] My colleagues and I also used the term "DSD" for the two handbooks

I coordinated and edited in 2005, one a set of clinical guidelines for pediatric care of DSD, the other a handbook for parents. These handbooks represented the first (and remain the only) consensus statements involving all three stakeholder groups, namely affected adults, parents of affected individuals, and specialist clinicians.[8]

The "Chicago consensus" of the pediatric endocrinology groups represented a great leap forward in terms of particular practices. For example, the consensus document states that "psychosocial care provided by mental health staff with expertise in DSD should be an integral part of management to promote positive adaptation." The consensus acknowledges the dangers of genital surgeries and states that, for clitoroplasties at least, "emphasis is on functional outcome rather than a strictly cosmetic appearance." The consensus also considers the data showing that testicular cancer is less common in cases of complete AIS than previously believed and suggests that watchful waiting (instead of removal with HRT) may be a reasonable option for women with complete AIS whose testes show no cancer. This is a sign that clinicians are becoming more long-term-data-driven and less phobic about sex atypical (but healthy) organs being left alone in patients. Specialists have also moved away from sex-changing baby males with small penises ("micropenis"). They also have moved away from recommending vaginoplasties in very young children, both because early vaginoplasties so often fail and require major revision at puberty, and because they require vaginal dilations which may traumatize children and the parents obligated to carry out dilations on their toddlers.

Unpublished survey data from DSD specialist David Sandberg of the University of Michigan suggest that clinicians' ideas about DSD care have shifted more than their practices, but a shift in attitude often precedes a shift in behavior, so this is hopeful. I find most exciting, in the DSD clinical literature, the move away from dialogues unreasonably focused on the nature-nurture debate of gender and sexual orientation towards dialogues more reasonably focused on reducing shame, secrecy, and medical trauma.[9] There is also substantially more discussion of what informed consent and a shared decision-making approach (where parents have real say) would really look like in these cases.[10] Since the closing of the Intersex Society of North America (ISNA) in 2008, the two organizations most actively in the lead in organizing clinical reform are Accord Alliance (focusing on implementing progressive team care for DSD) and Advocates for Informed Choice (focusing on using legal tools to defend the rights of people with atypical sex and their parents' rights).

I wish I could report that the "monster approach" to children with sex anomalies has become history, but we still see signs that this population (and their mothers) remains at risk for being treated extraordinarily in terms of their rights. For example, several colleagues and I have recently thrown light on what appears to have amounted to years of unconsented, risky, and badly managed medical experimentation on hundreds of pregnant women in an effort to prevent their daughters from being born with ambiguous genitalia.[11] We have also raised concerns about "clitoral sensory testing" performed on girls aged six and up who had been subjected to reduction clitoroplasties for cosmetic reasons before they are old enough to assent or consent to the surgery. This testing has included a surgeon touching conscious girls' genitals with Q-tips and "medical vibratory devices" and asking the girls how well they can feel him touching.[12] It is hard to imagine any other population of girls being subjected to such practices. Most disturbingly, some commentators on these recent stories have tried to argue that these extraordinary treatments should not trouble us because girls with ambiguous genitalia are simply not normal. Such attitudes suggest we still have a way to go.

Notes

1. Alice D. Dreger and April M. Herndon, "Progress and Politics in the Intersex Rights Movement: Feminist Theory in Action," *GLQ: A Journal of Lesbian and Gay Studies*, 2009, 15(2): 199–224.
2. John Colapinto, *As Nature Made Him: The Boy Who Was Raised as a Girl* (New York: Harper Collins, 2000).

3. Jeffrey Eugenides, *Middlesex: A Novel* (New York: Farrar, Straus and Giroux, 2002).

4. Alice Dreger, "Sex Typing for Sport," *Hastings Center Report*, 2010, 40(2): 22–24.

5. Alice Dreger, Cheryl Chase, Aron Sousa, Joel Frader, and Philip Gruppuso, "Changing the Nomenclature/Taxonomy for Intersex: A Scientific and Clinical Rationale," *Journal of Pediatric Endocrinology and Metabolism*, 2005, 18: 729–733.

6. Alice Dreger, "Why 'Disorders of Sex Development'? (On Language and Life)," at http://alicedreger.com/dsd.html.

7. Peter Lee et al., "Consensus Statement on Management of Intersex Disorders," *Pediatrics*, 2006, 118: e488–e500. Available at http://www.pediatrics.org/cgi/content/full/118/2/e488.

8. Consortium on the Management of Disorders of Sex Development in Childhood, *Clinical Guidelines* and *Handbook for Parents*, 2005, available at http://dsdguidelines.org.

9. Richard S. Hurwitz, "Long-term outcomes in male patients with sex development disorders—how are we doing and how can we improve?" *Journal of Urology*, 2010, 184(3): 831–832.

10. Katrina Karkazis, Anne Tamar-Mattis, and Alexander A. Kon, "Genital surgery for disorders of sex development: implementing a shared decision-making approach," *Journal of Pediatric Endocrinology and Metabolism*, 2010, 23(8): 789–805.

11. Catherine Elton, "A Prenatal Treatment Raises Questions of Medical Ethics," *Time*, June 18, 2010, at http://www.time.com/time/health/article/0,8599,1996453,00.html.

12. Alice Dreger and Ellen K. Feder, "Bad Vibrations," *Bioethics Forum*, June 16, 2010, at http://www.thehastingscenter.org/Bioethicsforum/Post.aspx?id=4730&blogid=140.

Human Cloning: Three Mistakes and an Alternative

Françoise Baylis

I. HUMAN CLONING: THREE MISTAKES AND AN ALTERNATIVE[1]

Human cloning by somatic cell nuclear transfer is arguably the most exciting and at the same time foreboding technological–biological development of our times. Specifically, the prospect of cloning humans using nuclear transfer technology challenges our understanding of ourselves (i.e., what it is to be human), and our place in the world. When we reproduce by sexual intercourse we do not reproduce ourselves, what we reproduce or perpetuate is our own kind. Significantly, our kind is one that reproduces by recombining genes. In marked contrast, with nuclear substitution there is no recombination of the genes. We do not reproduce our kind, rather we reproduce, or more precisely, replicate ourselves.[2] Thus,

the cloning of humans theoretically makes possible an important departure from species-typical functioning—one deserving of critical attention.

The term "cloning" properly applies to any procedure that produces a genetic replica of a cell or organism. In the literature on cloning humans, the term frequently refers to two distinct technologies used to create whole beings: embryo splitting (also referred to as twinning and blastomere separation) and somatic cell nuclear transfer. In late 1993, Jerry Hall and colleagues at George Washington University reported their success with cloning human polyploid embryos. The technique they developed involved blastomere separation at the two-cell to eight-cell stage, and transfer to an artificial zona pellucida for continued growth into separate but identical embryos (Hall et al.,

Baylis, F. (2002). "Human cloning: Three mistakes and an alternative." *Journal of Medicine and Philosophy* 27(3): pp. 319–337. 53

1993). Seventeen chromosomally abnormal human embryos were divided, and 48 developing embryos were obtained. A few years later, in February 1997, Ian Wilmut and colleagues at the Roslin Institute announced the existence of Dolly, the cloned sheep (Wilmut, Schnieke, McWhir, Kind, & Campbell, 1997). The nucleus of a cell from a six-year-old sheep was removed, transferred to an unfertilized enucleated egg, and encouraged to develop. Two hundred and twenty-seven embryos were reconstructed; Dolly was the only success. With the birth of Dolly (the first mammalian clone), the idea that humans might eventually be cloned by somatic cell nuclear transfer seized the public imagination and renewed the debate on the ethics of cloning people. Since then several other species have been cloned from adult somatic cells including mice, cows, the rhesus monkey and transgenic pigs (Kato et al., 1998; Onishi et al., 2000; PPL, 2000; Wakayama et al., 1998; Wells, Misica, & Territ, 1999; Wolf, Meng, Ouhibi, & Zelinski-Wooten, 1999). As regards the cloning of humans, in 1999 there was an unconfirmed report of human cloning from somatic cells by South Korean scientists (Watts & Morris, 1999). Then, in November 2001, Advanced Cell Technology (ACT) reported that it had cloned human embryos as a possible future source of stem cells for regenerative medicine (Cibelli et al., 2001).

Prior to the birth announcement of Dolly, and subsequent scientific and technological developments involving non-human animals, a number of countries had laws banning human cloning (Bonnicksen, 1995). As the prospect of human cloning appeared to draw nearer, however, additional committee reports, policy documents and legislation were issued specifically condemning human *reproductive*[3] cloning, where cloning technology is used to create whole beings. For example, in 1997, the Fiftieth World Health Assembly adopted the following resolution: "cloning for the replication of human individuals is ethically unacceptable and contrary to human dignity and integrity" (WHO,

1997). In the same year, the US National Bioethics Advisory Commission (NBAC) concluded that "it is morally unacceptable…to attempt to create a child using somatic cell nuclear transfer cloning," (NBAC, 1997, p. 106) and President Clinton enacted the NBAC recommendation to extend the moratorium on the use of federal funding for such research for five years. Under President Bush, the US House of Representatives passed a bill in July 2001 that would make it a federal crime to clone humans either to produce children or to create embryos for research purposes (the US Senate has yet to vote on the bill). Meanwhile, in the UK, it is legal to clone human embryos for research purposes (Human Fertilisation, 2001), but the use of cloning for human reproduction is prohibited. And, closer to home, the Canadian government is poised to introduce legislation in 2002 that would prohibit the cloning of humans for either research or reproductive purposes (Health Canada, 2001).

For some, these policy statements and legislative prohibitions are an important first step in precluding the further development of human cloning to replicate individuals. For others, these initiatives are at most useful temporizing maneuvers to preclude the trivial and misguided uses of cloning technology. Proponents of this latter view believe that the cloning of whole beings is inevitable. The underlying reasoning is as follows: (1) cloning humans represents an irresistible scientific and technological challenge which means that some research group(s) somewhere will develop the technology, and this effort will be defended on the grounds of freedom of scientific inquiry; (2) the commitment, in some jurisdictions, to free enterprise and personal choice, coupled with the burgeoning support for the compassionate use of cloning technology to assist certain infertile couples, means that the technology (once developed and shown to be reasonably safe and effective) will be "for sale"; and (3) once the technology is for sale, there will be eager customers.

The likely development and possible future use of cloning technology to create individuals raises important ethical questions about the common good and the integrity of the human species. These questions require timely and careful reflection. As Hans Jonas wrote more than twenty-five years ago: "Since no less than the very nature and image of man [sic] are at issue, prudence becomes itself our first ethical duty, and hypothetical reasoning our first responsibility" (Jonas, 1974, p. 141). In this spirit, the reader's attention is drawn to some of the more pervasive and egregious mistakes with the current debate on the ethics of cloning humans using nuclear transfer technology.

II. A FIRST MISTAKE

A first mistake with the public debate on the ethics of cloning humans is our apparent comfort with a discourse that lulls us into complacency about a technology that represents a fundamental challenge to our understanding of ourselves and the species to which we belong. Consider, for example, the following summary caricatures of potentially complex arguments against the cloning of humans as unnatural, as "playing God," as contrary to human dignity.

A. Cloning Humans is Unnatural

According to some, cloning humans is "contrary to nature". While the splitting of human embryos does occur in nature, spaced twinning (using both embryo splitting and freezing), and somatic cell nuclear transfer do not. Further, while asexual reproduction does occur in nature, it is unnatural for the species Homo Sapiens which practices sexual reproduction.

This argument against cloning humans presumes an understanding of nature as a primordial structure that is independent of, and authoritative with respect to, all other possible structures (for example, social structures). There are two common responses to this argument. One response posits a specific understanding of "human nature" that encompasses the desire for knowledge and the capacity for self-transformation. In this view, our nature includes mastering ourselves and choosing our own destiny (i.e., making plans for our own nature). Another response side-steps the debate about the scope and meaning of human nature and asks somewhat facetiously: "So what? So are all sorts of other interventions that we happily accept."

B. Cloning Humans is "Playing God"

Warnings against "playing God" have been interpreted in multiple ways. What is common to these interpretations "is the idea that there is a natural order or structure, perhaps divinely ordained, and that proposals to exceed the limits which this natural order defines should be rejected out of hand—or at least considered very carefully" (Grey, 1998). In its religious applications, the phrase "playing God" alludes to God's omniscience and omnipotence and serves to identify acts or decisions outside the realm of legitimate human activity. Some of the religious interpretations of the phrase "playing God" are helpfully summarized in the NBAC report, *Cloning Human Beings*:

> Human beings should not probe the fundamental secrets or mysteries of life, which belong to God. Human beings lack the authority to make certain decisions about the beginning or ending of life. Such decisions are reserved to divine sovereignty. Human beings are fallible and also tend to evaluate actions according to their narrow, partial, and frequently self-interested perspectives. Human beings do not have the knowledge, especially knowledge of outcomes of actions attributed to divine omniscience. Human beings do not have the power to control the outcomes of actions or processes that is a mark of divine omnipotence. (NBAC, 1997, pp. 42–43)

In response, some argue that God expects us to use our reason, imagination, and freedom to improve our quality of life. In this view, human beings are created co-creators and human action is an expression of divine will (Hefner, 1998). An alternative response to the "playing God" argument against cloning is that in a pluralistic society, discussions about the ethics of cloning humans should not be constrained by a particular conception of God as "the creator" (Silver, 1998, p. 172). More generally, others suggest that accusations of "playing God" sometimes operate as rhetorical devices that ultimately obfuscate rather than clarify discussion (Grey, 1998).

C. Cloning Humans is Contrary to Human Dignity

This admonition against cloning humans rests, in part, on the Kantian view that persons should be treated as ends in themselves (Kahn, 1997). In this view, cloning humans is morally wrong because typically clones are created exclusively as a means for benefitting another. For example, clones may be created solely to satisfy an interest in having a biologically related child, to replace a dying or deceased loved one or to serve as an organ or tissue donor.

In response, some insist that this argument against cloning is flawed insofar as it ignores the fact that typically there are multiple motives and reasons for procreating (whether by cloning or sexual relations), and that clones would never be created exclusively as a means to another's end. Others grant that some clones likely will be treated *as mere means,* but they argue that this problem is not unique to cloning since persons who conceive "in the usual way" sometimes also act instrumentally as, for example, when persons reproduce to save a failing marriage, to prove their virility, to continue their genetic line, or to have someone to care for them in their old age. Still others insist that it is a matter for debate whether human embryos fall within the scope of the Kantian categorical imperative (given their contested moral status) and, more generally, they argue that Kant's principle is sufficiently vague and open to selective interpretation as not to be very helpful (Harris, 1997).

These three arguments against cloning humans are "familiar" in that they rehearse old arguments against novel technologies. To be precise, versions of these arguments have been elaborated previously, for example, against the introduction of the contraceptive pill, the development of organ transplantation and the use of life-extending technologies. The pattern that has emerged is one of initial condemnation, followed by ambivalence, questioning and limited use, followed in turn by a change in public perceptions, advocacy and *finally* widespread acceptance. For those who are mindful of this pattern, there is a sense of *deja-vu* with the debate about cloning humans, and there is the expectation that both the debate and practice will evolve in a similar manner.

Another cluster of familiar arguments against cloning humans focus on the possible/probable harmful consequences of the technology for society and for the individuals thus created. These arguments are worn because although the objections raised are unique to cloning technology, they do little more than reiterate concerns identified years ago when the prospect of cloning humans was pure science fiction. Consider, for example, the claim that cloning technology will be used purposely to create inferior beings to do boring and menial work (think, for example, of the "Deltas" of *Brave New World).* Or, consider the claim that cloning technology will be abused by power-hungry authoritative regimes to more effectively oppress others (think, for example, of *The Boys from Brazil).* As well, there is the claim that human cloning violates the clone's right to a unique genetic identity, and the clone's right to an open future—that is, a future with a reasonable range of opportunities (Brock, 1997).

Typically, responses to these sorts of arguments begin with a basic lesson on the science of cloning in an effort to correct mistaken views about the science and about genetic determinism. For example, it is explained that individuals cloned by nuclear transfer technology are not really identical to one another, though they may be very similar. This is because genes are not constant, they mutate. As well, there can be important differences in gene expression. Added to this is the fact that a fraction (0.05%) of the human genome comes from mitochondrial genes contributed by the egg so that with cloning by somatic cell nuclear transfer, the clonant and the clone cannot be genetically identical unless they have the same maternal lineage. At the same time, it is also explained that identity is shaped by environmental as well as genetic factors: "genes do not *determine* in tight detail how a creature turns out…[they] merely propose possibilities. It is the environment that shapes the final outcome" (Wilmut, Campbell, & Tudge, 2000, pp. 302–303). For example, with cloning by somatic nuclear cell transfer, the clonant and the clone will have developed in different uterine environments. As well, they will be born years apart and thus be subject to different environmental choices and influences.

In addition to this introductory lesson, there are the usual responses to the specific concerns about societal harm. The most common of these express significant confidence in our ability to ensure that cloning technology will not be abused, but rather will be developed and practiced under controlled conditions (i.e., within appropriate professional, regulatory and legislative constraints). And as for the concerns about potential harm to individuals, it is noted that conventional identical twins are natural clones and they are not psychologically harmed by their lack of genetic uniqueness. This claim is morally relevant since genomic clones would be more different from each other than conventional identical twins. Further, it is argued that the concern about parents coercing their clones' development and subverting their independence by structuring the scope of their experiences and opportunities is not a unique feature of human cloning. This is also a risk for conventionally conceived children whose parents' hopes for their children quickly become expectations.

In my view, all of the arguments against cloning humans identified above and the typical rejoinders are not particularly interesting or challenging. Consistent with this view is Daniel Callahan's recent conclusion, based on his review of the cloning debate from the early 1970s to the present, that "[n]o arguments have been advanced this time that were not anticipated and discussed in the 1970s" (Callahan, 1998,

p. 141). Interestingly, on this basis, Callahan credits bioethicists writing in the early 1970s—in particular, Paul Ramsey, Hans Jonas and Leon Kass—with remarkable prescience. But isn't this hubris on the part of bioethics? Shouldn't the fact that no new arguments have been introduced in the post-Dolly era be cause for concern, not congratulations? Others suggest that our imagination has stagnated even longer—that the issues currently addressed in the debate about cloning humans are no different from those that concerned Aldous Huxley in the 1930s when he originally published *Brave New World,* his fictional account of a cloned "utopia". How is it that greater knowledge of the science and a better understanding of the technological possibilities has not introduced new ethical questions or concerns, has not sparked the moral imagination? Are we to believe those who insist that "there are no new ethical issues in relation to the current hysteria over cloning" (Wolpert, 1999, p. 282)?

III. A SECOND MISTAKE

A second mistake with the current debate on the ethics of cloning humans—a mistake informed, in part, by a fear of eugenics—is that much of the discussion remains at the level of the personal, as though the *raison d'etre* of the technology were to address individual needs and wants. This perspective is clearly evident in discussions about the motives for pursuing human cloning (Robertson, 1998).

It has been suggested, for example, that some couples may want to use cloning technology because it is the only way to have a child that is biologically related to each of the partners. This might include: infertile couples where both have no gametes (where the male partner could provide the somatic cell and the female partner could provide the enucleated oocyte); women undergoing *in vitro* fertilization (IVF) with too few oocytes who might benefit from embryo splitting; and lesbian couples (where one partner could provide the somatic cell and the other could provide the enucleated oocyte) (Baird, 1999). Others possibly interested in human cloning are couples at high risk of having a child with a serious genetic disease. Cloning could also be used to satisfy a wish to re-create a deceased loved one; the usual example given is of parents who want to re-create a dying or deceased child. There may also be those who would use cloning technology to get a compatible organ or tissue donor for themselves or their offspring. Finally, there may be individuals who for reasons of "curiosity, vanity, the wish for personal power, or an undoubtedly misguided desire for immortality" (Wilmut et al., 2000, p. 306) want a genetic replica of themselves.

One consequence of the unrelenting focus on the personal is the perception of human cloning as a bi-generational issue. Human clones are described as "spaced twins," "later-born identical twins," "'delayed' genetic twins," and the "ultimate single-parent child." As well, the dominant image for human cloning is one of mass production with multiple images of the identical phenotype—"xeroxed human beings" and "carbon-copied humans"—not the traditional pedigree chart or family tree with missing or unusual linkages. Cloning is thus portrayed as horizontal multiplication, not as vertical, multi-generational replication.

With attention focused on the present and the next generation, priority is given to concerns about possible medical and psychological harms to future children and fundamental questions about what it means to be human are set aside. Notably, this dominant perspective is highly compatible with contemporary silence on the possible uses of human cloning to pursue public health or broader societal goals.

When the possibility of cloning humans was discussed in the 1960s, there was considerable speculation about the potential societal benefits of human cloning. One suggestion was to clone individuals with a high pain threshold or resistance to radiation (Haldane, 1963, pp. 353, 355). Another suggestion was to clone individuals skilled at certain jobs, for example, soldiers (Fletcher, 1971, p. 779). Today, the examples have changed and the focus is on cloning specific persons of extraordinary talent such as Beethoven or Einstein. As well, there is particular attention to the potential societal harms of human cloning resulting from the replication of persons with undesirable traits—the most common example being Hitler. In response to such fanciful claims, scientists have been successful in labeling most speculation about the eugenic applications of human cloning as "stupid talk" that obscures the real scientific issues (Butler & Wadman, 1997). To avoid the charge of "stupid talk" serious academics dutifully focus on the "more immediate and realistic possibilities" and abdicate their responsibility to engage in hypothetical reasoning.

IV. A THIRD MISTAKE

A third mistake with the current debate on the ethics of cloning humans is that it wrongly focuses much of the discussion on reproductive issues and reproductive freedom. Physicians and researchers, for example, justify human cloning as an aid for infertile couples and an aid in pre-implantation diagnosis. They also frequently note that cloning technology promotes procreative autonomy.

Among those who view cloning as a form of assisted conception are those who believe that the principle of reproductive freedom entrenches the right to reproduce by any means chosen. Dan Brock, for example, maintains that the right to reproductive freedom presumptively includes the right to select the means of reproduction that best serve one's interests and needs, including human cloning (Brock, 1997). Some even go so far as to argue that, in the United States at least, this is a constitutionally protected right. John Robertson, for example, maintains that "[t]he right of married and arguably even unmarried persons to procreate is a fundamental constitutional right that cannot be restricted unless clearly necessary to protect compelling state interests" (Robertson, 1994, p. 13). In his view, cloning appears to fall within this fundamental freedom. At the other extreme are those who insist that human cloning is intrinsically wrong. George Annas, for example, counters that reproductive rights are not absolute and that cloning by somatic cell nuclear transfer is sufficiently different from other means of reproduction as not to be considered constitutionally protected (Annas, 1997). The Vatican insists that "human beings have a right to be 'born in a human way, and not in a laboratory'" (Butler & Wadman, 1997, p. 8).

Between these extremes are those who maintain that cloning humans should be prohibited for the time being because of potential medical and psychological harms to future clones (including harms arising from possible commodification). Only when human cloning is shown to be reasonably safe and effective might it become available to further reproductive goals, subject to appropriate constraints aimed at preventing possible abuses.[4] For example, a distinction might be drawn between frivolous reasons for cloning such as vanity, and "legitimate" socio-medical reasons for cloning such as allowing persons with otherwise untreatable infertility to have a biologically related child.

The cloning of humans, however, ought not to be construed narrowly as a reproductive technology. While it is certainly the case that cloning technology likely will be provided by those who currently work in, or are affiliated with, IVF clinics, it is a serious mistake to believe that cloning is just another means of assisted reproduction. As George Annas writes, cloning "represents a difference in kind, not in degree in the way that humans continue the species" (Annas, 1997, p. 80). With reproduction by means of sexual intercourse, each offspring (except for identical twins, triplets, or rarely even quadruplets) has a unique genetic make-up that is a combination of genes from his or her biological parents. Assisted reproductive technologies preserve this feature of human reproduction. In marked contrast, human cloning by somatic cell nuclear transfer not only separates reproduction from sexual relations, it also separates reproduction from recombination, as there is no reshuffling of the genes. Unlike current assisted reproductive technologies, therefore, this type of human cloning transgresses species norms. The ethics of transgressing species norms, though widely discussed in the literature on xenotransplantation, is not central to discussions about human cloning; instead, autonomy (procreative liberty), utility and safety appear to be the predominant concerns.

Attempts to map the cloning debate onto the debate about reproductive freedom is not surprising since the domain of reproductive ethics is reasonably familiar territory. There is, for instance, much material in the bioethics literature on autonomy and reproductive choice on the one hand, and the sanctity of human life and the concept of family on the other. In comparison, there is little on transgenerational justice that spans more than one or two generations, and still less on the notion of species integrity that is not about the creation of transgenic animals—these issues merit careful consideration.

V. AN ALTERNATIVE

The way in which any discourse is framed informs (if not determines) the issues identified, the questions asked, the interpretations offered and the range of responses advocated. The common view of cloning technology as a reproductive technology thus explains the current interest in rights (both reproductive rights and property rights), personal autonomy, informed consent, family privacy, safety and potential harms to children. According to the NBAC, for example, "The unique and distinctive ethical issues raised by the use of somatic cell nuclear transfer to create children relate to, for example, serious safety concerns, individuality, family integrity, and treating children as objects" (NBAC, 1997, pp. 3–4). To be sure, these are important issues. There are, however, other equally important issues that are not identified, much less debated, with the current analytical framework. To correct this, an alternative framework is recommended where human cloning is also viewed as an individual and a species enhancement technology—a mechanism for environmental and biological improvements on a scale never before possible.

Humans have always sought to enhance their own and their children's physical, intellectual, emotional and moral capacities with a view to improving health and increasing the prospects for happiness and "success". Common contemporary enhancements include: vaccines to enhance the immune response to specific diseases; good nutrition to enhance physical development; sound education to enhance intellectual, social and other abilities; music lessons to enhance manual dexterity and mathematical ability; dance lessons and gymnastics to enhance balance and posture; sports training (and/or steroids) to enhance athletic ability, build muscle mass and strength; and cosmetic surgery to enhance physical appearance. With adults the use of these enhancements is generally a matter of personal choice. With children, some of these enhancements are legally and morally required (e.g., vaccinations and basic education), others are optional (e.g., music lessons and cosmetic surgery). Elective enhancements are generally used at the discretion of parents, with or without consultation with the child, and based on their assessment of their child's abilities and interests. Significantly, parents may choose enhancements that will expand the range of opportunities for their child, or they may choose enhancements that will considerably narrow the range of opportunities because of a very limited focus on select talents that are not widely adaptable.

With the cloning of whole beings, parental efforts at enhancing children's capacities will intensify because of the available knowledge regarding the child's genetic structure. The cloning of humans thus will not simply be about having children but about having a unique opportunity to improve on a desired specimen (e.g., a clone of oneself or a loved one) by investing in enhanced genes and/or enhanced environments in order to increase/accentuate desired traits and/or to modify/eliminate negative traits. Consider the following scenario. A talented concert violinist chooses to clone herself using her egg (enucleated oocyte), her nucleus (somatic cell) and her uterus to achieve near perfect cloning. Like all parents, she wants her child to have a

"better" life. This motivates her to embark on a unique enhancement project made possible by her decision to reproduce asexually. She does not want her daughter to suffer the disappointments she has known and is thus intent on enhancing her child's talent for creating (her understanding of) beautiful music. With germline gene transfer, the violinist hopes to improve her clone's dexterity, hearing and memory. To be sure, attempts at genetically enhancing these traits will be difficult (if not ultimately impossible) because many genes affect these abilities and each of these genes may affect multiple body systems. Nonetheless, the violinist is willing to experiment. Also, persuaded that a little melancholy (sweet sorrow) will add a creative edge to her clone's music, she agrees to altering the genes responsible for the production of serotonin. When her child is a toddler, the environmental enhancement begins in earnest.

The violinist teaches her clone special exercises to improve the genetically improved dexterity and memory. As well, there is the drug regimen to alter the serotonin levels, the Stradivarius and the Juilliard School music lessons that her own parents could not afford to give her until she reached her mid-teens. In these ways the violinist hopes that her child—a genetic replica of herself—will have a better future.

As illustrated above, with cloning by somatic cell nuclear transfer the parent (i.e., clonant) has intimate knowledge of the child's (i.e., clone's) future possibilities because of their shared genotype. This unique foreknowledge necessarily influences (possibly skews) the enhancements chosen, and this is not because of misguided views about genetic determinism. Our genes do not determine who we are, but they clearly do suggest certain possibilities and set certain boundaries. Foreknowledge of these possibilities and boundaries, which becomes possible with cloning technology, will influence the genetic, surgical, pharmaceutical and other medical enhancements that will be pursued in order to improve the clone's form. In turn, these biological enhancements may influence behaviour. For example, a physical change can alter/improve an individual's psychological and social dispositions. As well, this unique foreknowledge will influence the choice of social, cultural, ecological, physical and other environments to which the clone will be exposed in an effort to further improve performance. In this way, human cloning technology to produce a genetic replica of a person whose potential is known makes possible a unique and complex kind of biological and environmental enhancement.

To be sure, any cloning experiment ultimately may fail to achieve its objective. For example, the violinist's clone may become a disgruntled clerk at an airport car rental. Nonetheless, the point remains. Cloning (at least of those who have lived a reasonable life span) is not simply about reproduction. Rather, it is very much about "getting it right" (avoiding the errors of a previous generation), on the basis of unique advance knowledge about which genetic and environmental factors might benefit from enhancement.

If we now move the discussion from the means of enhancement to the goals of enhancement, an important difference emerges between the goals of *intentional individual enhancement* and the goals of *intentional species enhancement.* With the intentional biological and environmental enhancement of individual human beings, the goals are typically to promote health, happiness, and "success". In turn, these will be the *de facto* goals of inadvertent species enhancement—a phenomenon that will occur over time, as enhancements made at the individual level are passed on to subsequent generations (with or without further alterations), and as the environment of which these individuals are an integral part continues to evolve. In marked contrast, with *intentional species enhancement,* where changes are not merely the inadvertent cumulative long-term side-effect of idiosyncratic changes at the individual level, more communal goals can be pursued such as the survival of the species, the elimination of misery and an improvement in the quality of life.

For example, in the not-too-distant future, if pollution and overpopulation were to cause our environment to deteriorate so significantly that our survival on the planet were threatened, the cloning of humans might be an important element of a survival strategy for the species. Individuals with certain biological traits conducive to survival in this emerging inhospitable environment could be cloned (and possibly genetically enhanced) while at the same time efforts were made to stabilize the deteriorating environment. In this way, it would be possible to enhance the species in a single generation and thereby increase the probability of survival.

From the perspective of some, however, a more immediate threat to our survival and the cause of considerable misery is "our limited capacity for altruism, and for the imaginative sympathy it depends on" (Glover, 1984, p. 181). Jonathan Glover suggests, for example, that although war may appear to be the result of particular economic, social and political arrangements, our failure to eliminate war suggests that psychological changes may be required in addition to political and social reforms. In this view, species enhancement using both genetic and environmental methods may be necessary to overcome certain emotional and imaginative limitations. This might involve direct genetic intervention to ensure that genes we value, such as those that contribute to our capacity for altruism and human sympathy, survive through cloning and are genetically and environmentally enhanced.

Finally, a less dramatic reason for pursuing biological species enhancement would be to improve our quality of life perhaps by enhancing our intellectual capacities. We can, for example, imagine a time in the remote future when we will have exhausted our capacity to understand our world: "Just as calculus is too much for a dog's brain to grasp, so some parts of physics might turn out to be too difficult for us as we are" (Glover, 1984, p. 180). At that time, "[b]ecause our growing understanding of the world is so central a part of why it is good to be human," we may want to select from among us a number of good specimens for replication and genetic enhancement in order that we might transcend our intellectual limitations (Glover, 1984, p. 180). Before any such hypothetical need should arise, however, we can perhaps more easily imagine a world in which the increasing abilities of machines are fast outpacing those of humans. In response to this threat, humans might want to genetically enhance their cognitive skills by cloning good specimens to be genetically engineered in order to acquire new and increasingly sophisticated judgment, decision-making, and adaptation skills.

In addition to the obvious genetic planning that cloning technology makes possible for the species, it is important to stress the interesting possibilities for environmental species enhancement. The cloning of humans provides us with a unique opportunity to study the nature/nurture question on a grand scale. For the first time, it would be possible to hold constant one element of this dyad and, in so doing, to learn how best to cultivate/nurture desirable traits. Leaving aside, for the sake of argument, questions of research ethics, the same "gene bundles" could be exposed to different social, environmental and generational influences so that we might better understand human development and evolution. In an ideal world, this knowledge could then be used to improve our quality of life—to modify our political and economic systems, to alter our educational programs and to introduce social changes that would nurture the traits we value for ourselves and subsequent generations.

In closing, the benefit of regarding the cloning of humans as an enhancement technology is twofold. The first benefit is that this perspective will shed a new light on questions that are already the subject of intense debate. Among these questions: What are the moral costs of human cloning? What obligations do we have to subsequent generations who will be subject to an unprecedented measure of control from preceding generations? How are these obligations to be weighed against obligations to those who are living? What about issues of social justice? While many live in poverty and lack basic health care, can we responsibly devote energy and resources to the project of cloning humans? Is human cloning necessary? If so, necessary for what? Is human cloning progressive? If so,

progressive towards what end? Is it efficient? If so, effecting what? Is it good for the species, for the individual clonant, for the individual clone, or is it good for its own sake? Answers to these questions will differ significantly depending upon the framework for analysis—whether one considers cloning to be a reproductive and/or an enhancement technology.

The second benefit of considering the cloning of humans as an enhancement technology is that this perspective will bring into sharp focus a range of novel questions that merit thoughtful reflection. For example: With the cloning of humans are we bound to embrace "volitional evolution" whereby we intentionally intervene in the shaping of human purpose? Would volitional evolution result in a domestication of the species? What is the value of diversity? What is the value of homogeneity? What social norms regarding race, gender and appearance might (inadvertently or intentionally) be entrenched with cloning technology? While undeniably offensive in its eugenic implications, in the long term, would homogenization of the species be a cure for such social and political ills as racism, sexism, classism, homophobia and so on, or would any initiative of this kind only serve to exacerbate existing prejudices?

As well, another cluster of questions might stem from an understanding of human cloning as the modern equivalent to reincarnation. This perspective might refashion our understanding of such concepts as "a life span" and "a life plan". For example, given the belief that reincarnation is a mechanism that allows individuals to improve upon themselves over time, in our modern production-oriented society would there develop an expectation that persons should avail themselves of cloning technology for the express purpose of improving upon the prior incarnation? What would be the end-point? Would it be culturally informed or socially stipulated? What would be the social, political and moral responses to this new eugenics?

When the cloning of humans is considered solely as a reproductive technology, the questions listed above garner hardly any serious attention. Instead we concentrate on questions about possible harms to children and personal choice: "Is a clone any worse off than a 'normal' but unwanted child? Is Steve, who wants to clone himself, any more egotistical than Saul, who wants to conceive naturally, though his children will have a 25 percent chance of getting Tay-Sachs disease? And if cloning should be outlawed because it may undermine family values, should we outlaw divorce as well?" (Bilger, 1997, p. 19). In marked contrast, when the cloning of humans is considered an individual or species enhancement technology, broader societal and species-type questions outside the protected realm of personal and reproductive autonomy are "front and center".

Thus, it is salient to understand that the current debate on the ethics of cloning humans with its predominant focus on autonomy (individuals' rights, desires and choices) is profoundly unsatisfactory and lacking in imagination. This debate is sustained and remains sustainable, however, because it occurs in a social context sympathetic to the claim that "the principles of personal liberty and personal fortune are the primary determinants of what individuals are allowed and able to do" (Silver, 1997, p. 9). As a result, the debate about cloning humans stagnates at the level of the personal; it never really moves beyond the framework of private relationships and reproductive choice. Thus, profound value questions are set aside and potentially dramatic societal and species consequences arising from the use of cloning technology are inappropriately downplayed or exaggerated. Only in recognizing the individual and species enhancement dimensions of cloning technology can we begin to recognize the broader issues and grapple with the threat/opportunity that cloning humans represents. For all of us.

Notes

1. The research for this paper was supported by grants from the Social Sciences and Humanities Research Council of Canada and from Dalhousie University. This is a revised version of the *Dr. John P. Maclean Memorial Lecture, Department of Internal Medicine, University of Manitoba,* Winnipeg, Manitoba, April 1999, that was also presented at the Second Annual *International Bioethics Retreat,* Florence, Italy, October 1999.

2. I owe the distinction between "reproducing our kind" and "reproducing ourselves" to Ford Doolittle, Dalhousie University.

3. In the literature a distinction is drawn between *reproductive* cloning, where the aim is to reproduce whole beings, and *therapeutic* cloning, where the aim is to reproduce cell lines for the treatment of disease or disability.

4. The Report of the National Bioethics Advisory Commission would appear to fall in this general category. See National Bioethics Advisory Commission (1997). The Executive Summary (1997) of this report is reprinted in the *Hastings Center Report,* 27(3), 7–9.

References

Annas, G.J. (1997). Human cloning. *ABA Journal,* 83, 80–81.

Baird, P.A. (1999). Cloning of animals and humans: What should the policy response be? *Perspectives in Biology and Medicine,* 42(2), 179–194.

Bilger, B. (1997, September/October). Cell block. *The Sciences,* 17–19.

Bonnicksen, A.L. (1995). Ethical and policy issues in human embryos twinning. *Cambridge Quarterly of Healthcare Ethics,* 4(3), 268–284.

Brock, D. (1997). Cloning human beings: An assessment of the ethical issues pro and con. In: National Bioethics Advisory Commission. *Cloning human beings: Report and recommendations of the National Bioethics Advisory Commission, Volume II Commissioned Papers.* Rockville, Maryland.

Butler, D., & Wadman, M. (1997). Calls for cloning ban sell science short. *Nature,* 386, 8.

Callahan, D. (1998). Cloning: Then and now. *Cambridge Quarterly of Healthcare Ethics,* 7(2), 141–144.

Cibelli, J.B., Kiessling, A.A., Cunniff, K., Richards, C., Lanza, R.P., & West, M. (2001). Somatic cell nuclear transfer in humans: Pronuclear and early embryonic development. *E-biomed: The Journal of Regenerative Medicine,* 2, 25–31.

Fletcher, J. (1971). Ethical aspects of genetic controls. *New England Journal of Medicine,* 285, 776–783.

Glover, J. (1984). *What sort of people should there be?* Great Britain: Richard Clay (The Chaucer Press) Ltd.

Grey, W. (1998). Playing God. *Encyclopedia of applied ethics* (Vol. 3). USA: Academic Press.

Haldane, J.B.S. (1963). Biological possibilities for the human species in the next ten thousand years. In: G.E.D. Wolstenhome (Ed.), *Man and his future* (pp. 337–361). London: Churchill.

Hall, J.L., Engel, D., Gindoff, P.R., Motto, G.L., & Stillman, R.I. (1993). Experimental cloning of human polyploid embryos using an artificial zona pellucida. *The American Fertility Society, Co jointly With the Canadian Fertility and Andrology Society. Program Supplement* [Abstract of the Scientific and Oral Poster Sessions, Abstract 0-001S1].

Harris, J. (1997). 'Goodbye Dolly?' The ethics of human cloning. *Journal of Medical Ethics, 23,* 353–360.

Health Canada. (2001). *Draft Legislation on Assisted Human Reproduction.* http://www.hc-sc.gc.ca/English/reproduction/legislation.pdf.

Hefner, P. (1998). Cloning as quintessential human act. In: M. Ruse (Ed.), *Philosophy of biology* (pp. 352–256). Amherst, New York: Prometheus Books.

Human Fertilisation and Embryology (Research Purposes) Regulations. (2001). Statutory Instrument 2001 No. 188. http://www.legislation.hmso.gov.uk/si/si2001/20010188.htm.

Jonas, H. (1974). Biological engineering—a preview. In: H. Jonas (Ed.), *Philosophical essays: From ancient creed to technological man* (pp. 141–167). Englewood Cliffs, NJ: Prentice Hall.

Kahn, A. (1997). Clone mammals…clone man. *Nature, 386,* 119.

Kato, Y., Tani, T., Sotomaru, Y., Kurokawa, K., Kato, J., Doguchi, H., Yasue, H., & Tsunoda, Y. (1998). Eight calves cloned from somatic cells of a single adult. *Science, 282,* 2095–2098.

National Bioethics Advisory Commission (NBAC). (1997). *Cloning human beings: Report and recommendations of the National Bioethics Advisory Commission.* Rockville, MD: National Bioethics Advisory Commission.

Onishi, A., Iwamoto, M., Akita, T., Mikawa, S., Takeda, K., Awata, T., Hanada, H., & Perry, A.C.F. (2000). Pig cloning by microinjection of fetal fibroblast nuclei. *Science, 289,* 1188–1190.

PPL Therapeutics plc. (2000). *PPL produces world's first cloned pigs.* Press release March 5, http://www.ppl-therapeutics.com.

Robertson, J. (1994). The question of human cloning. *Hastings Center Report, 24*(2), 6–14.

Robertson, J. (1998). Human cloning and the challenge of regulation. *New England Journal of Medicine,* 339(2), 119–122.

Silver, L.M. (1997). *Remaking Eden: Cloning and beyond in a brave new world.* New York: Avon Books.

Silver, L.M. (1998). Cloning, ethics, and religion. *Cambridge Quarterly of Healthcare Ethics,* 7(2), 168–172.

Wakayama, T., Perry, A.C., Zuccotti, M., Johnson, K.R., & Yanagimachi, R. (1998). Full-term development of mice from enucleated oocytes injected with cumulus cell nuclei. *Nature, 394,* 369–374.

Watts, J., & Morris, K. (1999). Human cloning trial met with outrage and scepticism. *The Lancet, 353,* 43.

Wells, D.N., Misica, P.M., & Territ, H.R. (1999). Production of cloned calves following nuclear transfer with cultured adult mural granulosa cells. *Biology of Reproduction, 60,* 996–1005.

Wilmut, I., Schnieke, A.E., McWhir, J., Kind, A.J., & Campbell, K.H.S. (1997). Viable offspring derived from fetal and adult mammalian cells. *Nature, 385,* 810–812.

Wilmut, I., Campbell, K., & Tudge, C. (2000) *The second creation: The age of biological control by the scientists that cloned Dolly.* London, England: Headline.

Wolf, D.P., Meng, L., Ouhibi, N., & Zelinski-Wooten, M. (1999). Nuclear transfer in the rhesus monkey: Practical and basic implications. *Biology of Reproduction, 60,* 199–204.

Wolpert, L. (1999). Is science dangerous? *Nature, 398,* 281–282.

World Health Organization. (1997, May 14). *Cloning in human reproduction.* Fiftieth World Health Assembly. WHA50.37 Supplementary agenda item. Geneva.

The Inevitability of Genetic Enhancement Technologies

Françoise Baylis and Jason Scott Robert

INTRODUCTION

For some, the development and use of any technology to enhance human capacities and traits is laudable—likely to improve the human condition.[1] For others, the development and use of all but a narrow set of environmental enhancements (such as education) is deeply problematic.[2] Between these extremes are those who are not so much concerned with the technical means of enhancement—that is, whether the alterations are sought by environmental, surgical, pharmacological or genetic means—but rather who are worried about the nature of the alterations sought—that is, whether the enhancement technology will be used (alone or in combination) to make physical, intellectual, psychological or moral alterations to the self.[3] In the category of *physical enhancements* there might be a range of alterations aimed at improving size, increasing muscle mass, reducing sleep dependence, increasing endurance, decelerating aging, altering skin colour, or changing gender. *Intellectual enhancements* might include alterations aimed at improving memory and cognitive ability, promoting multidimensional thinking, and increasing imagination. *Psychological enhancements* might include efforts to improve sociability, reduce shyness, and instil confidence. And, *moral enhancements* could seek to control violent behaviour, encourage kindness, and promote the capacity for sympathy. Some of these types of enhancements are considered worthy of pursuit, while others are thought to be of questionable value.

Moreover, for some individuals the worry is not with the technical means of enhancement or with the human characteristics to be enhanced, but rather with the underlying motivation(s). In very general terms, enhancements may be sought for a variety of reasons: to be in fashion; to improve performance; to gain a competitive advantage; to secure and exercise power; to promote and protect health and well-being; to increase the lifespan; to assuage or even overcome existential angst; or to meet the demands of justice.[4] And, depending upon the underlying motivation, the resulting alterations may be conservative (i.e., used to normalize the self), liberal (i.e., used to liberate the self), or radical (i.e., used to fashion a self that effectively challenges others' conception of oneself).[5] From the perspective of some theorists, not all of these reasons for seeking to enhance human capacities and traits are equally meritorious.

With this rough taxonomy of means, objects, and motivations in mind, we turn our attention to genetic enhancement technologies in particular. For our purposes, a *genetic enhancement technology* is any technology that directly alters the expression of genes that are already present in humans, or that involves the addition of genes that have not previously appeared within the human population (including plant, animal, or custom-designed genes), for the purpose of human physical, intellectual, psychological, or moral improvement. This includes somatic cell nuclear transfer (SCNT) technology, somatic and germ line gene transfer technology, cosmetic gene insertion, cosmetic stem cell transfer, and the creation of human-to-human and animal-to-human chimeras, as well as animal-to-human hybrids.

Baylis, F. & Robert, J.S. (2004) "The Inevitability of Genetic Enhancement Technologies." *Bioethics* 18(1): pp. 1–26.

We contend that attempts to develop and use such technologies are inevitable. While the argument offered here might be developed and applied more broadly to encompass additional or even all new forms of (bio)technology, we restrict our attention, and so the scope of our claim, to genetic enhancement technologies as defined above.

To be sure, not all of the envisioned genetic enhancements will come to pass. The complexities of organismal development[6] are such that some of the genetic tinkering imagined and promoted by enhancement enthusiasts will prove to be impossible.[7] This fact is irrelevant to our argument, however. What matters to our argument is that *despite* the likely failure of particular genetic enhancements, there are some among us who will *inevitably attempt* to engineer the human genome[8] for the purpose of improving *Homo sapiens*. And, to our surprise (and perhaps our disgust or delight) some will succeed.

… We explore various reasons for the inevitability of genetic enhancement technologies, and conclude that accepting the inevitability of genetic enhancement will spur us to profitably redirect ethical energy to the all-important tasks of ensuring that the process of attempting genetic enhancement is morally acceptable, and that successfully developed genetic enhancements are used in a socially responsible manner. In this way we hope to guard against a defeatist interpretation of our inevitability claim, while simultaneously opening moral space for a more productive dialogue.[9]

ESCHEWING BOUNDARIES: SUPPORT FOR GENETIC ENHANCEMENT TECHNOLOGIES

Some insist that the pursuit of all enhancement technologies is not just ethically permissible, but also a moral imperative for humans,[10] and that specific objections to the development and use of genetic enhancement technologies are wrongheaded. Among the proponents of this view are those who maintain that humans are sorely imperfect, and so humans should do whatever

can be done to augment human traits and capacities. In many respects, however, this suggestion is less an argument than a manifesto.[11] What we take to be the standard argument in support of genetic enhancement technologies must be reconstructed; abstracted, it runs as follows: (1) *Enhancing* human capacities and traits is a worthy ideal, as evidenced by the general social commitment to education, medicine, and welfare; (2) *genetically* enhancing human capacities and traits—for example, somatic cell nuclear transfer (i.e., cloning) for the purpose of replicating and improving upon a desired specimen,[12] and cosmetic stem cell transfer to supplement the functioning of normal genes—represents but one end of a continuum of enhancement technologies to pursue the goal of enhancing human capacities and traits; (3) if the *goal* of genetic enhancement is the same as the (laudable) goal of generic enhancement, then the *means* of enhancement do not matter morally; (4) the goal of genetic enhancement is in fact the same as the goal of generic enhancement, and so is itself laudable; therefore, (5) genetic enhancement technologies should be developed and their use promoted and supported.

While the first premise seems unassailable, and the conclusion does indeed follow from the premises taken together, premises (2–4) deserve further scrutiny. The second and fourth premises are the subject of many of the objections outlined below. The third premise is the subject of the final objection surveyed.

ESPOUSING LIMITS: OBJECTIONS TO GENETIC ENHANCEMENT TECHNOLOGIES

Current objections to genetic enhancement technologies are many and varied. Though some of the arguments to be discussed below have been treated in considerably more detail by others,[13] it will become evident that sketching them here is necessary to our programmatic endeavour to change the subject and tenor of ethical debates about genetic enhancements. In our view, the objections to genetic enhancement technologies cluster around the following themes: (i) the technologies are intrinsically wrong; (ii) whether the technologies are effective or not, there likely will be negative biological consequences; (iii) if the technologies are effective and their use is widespread, this will result in harmful social consequences; and (iv) the means of achieving laudable ends are not all equally morally meritorious. Below, we briefly elaborate on each of these concerns...[14]

1. *Transgression of divine laws.* There are two major thrusts to the argument against genetic enhancement technologies as 'playing God.' The first focuses on God's omniscience. The claim is that the requisite knowledge and capacities to plan for the physical, intellectual, psychological and moral well-being of distant future generations is beyond the grasp of humans. On this view, volitional evolution—the intentional genetic shaping of human purpose—should remain beyond human reach. It is sheer hubris for anyone to attempt to directly manipulate the human genetic structure, for only God can know (and accordingly plan for) the future of the species. The second major thrust of the argument against 'playing God' focuses on God's omnipotence. The claim is that the planned (hoped for) use of genetic enhancement technologies aimed at creating or modifying life is an unwarranted, unwise and profoundly immoral attempt to usurp God's power.[15]

2. *Transgression of natural laws.* According to some, the use of genetic enhancement technologies is unnatural for at least two reasons: it is contrary to the natural course of events; and it is contrary to human nature. The putatively unnatural features of genetic enhancement technologies are objectionable from the perspective of those who believe that the natural order has intrinsic value, independently of human valuers. On this view, nature deserves respect; this respect sets limits on human intervention; and these limits preclude the use of genetic enhancement technolo-

gies. Despite a wide range of opinion on the nature of human nature,[16] and against the historically prevalent view that humans are by nature meant to master nature,[17] the second, related objection is that as humans are part of nature, rather than separate from nature, the essence of humans is to nurture and protect the natural world, not to dominate it through, for instance, genetic engineering.

3. *Introduction of an unacceptable risk of harm.* There is considerable speculation about the possible negative biological consequences of the introduction and use of genetic enhancement technologies. The possibility of error, and the potential for serious correlative physical, psychological and other harms to individuals, are typical objections to enhancement technologies especially during their early research phases. These objections are particularly significant in the case of genetic enhancement technologies where: (i) any error may be irreversible; (ii) the underlying risk of harm is unknown and unknowable; and (iii) the direct consequences of any error will be borne by many in addition to the individual who may be enhanced, particularly if the error is perpetuated into future generations.

4. *Introduction of a threat to genetic diversity.* It is said that genetic enhancement technologies will have a deleterious impact on the genetic variability characteristic of the human gene pool. Though it is widely recognized that there is no real prospect of eliminating genetic diversity altogether,[18] some argue that even small changes could lead to serious harm.[19] One possible reason for concern is that scientists know so little about gene function in organismal development, and not much more about development above the level of the genes....

5. *Introduction of a threat to our common genetic heritage.* The United Nations Educational, Scientific, and Cultural Organization adopted a *Universal Declaration on the Human Genome and Human Rights* in 1997. In Article 1 of that document,

UNESCO declared that "the human genome underlies the fundamental unity of all members of the human family, as well as the recognition of the inherent dignity and diversity of each of its members."[20] If the human genome represents humanity's common heritage....then this heritage may be seriously threatened by genetic enhancements. Some believe that there is the distinct possibility that with the genetic enhancement of successive generations—by altering the expression of genes that are already present or adding new genes that have not previously appeared in humans—a segment of society will engineer itself out of the species *Homo sapiens*. Already those who worry about the possibility of radical transformation jest about the creation of a new species—*Homo Glaxo Wellcomus*.[21]

6. *Paradoxical counterproductivity.* In liberal democratic societies, at least, decisions about the use of genetic enhancement technologies are thought to be a private matter. This view is mistaken, however, insofar as there would be enormous social ramifications to the millions of individual decisions to use genetic enhancement technologies. Consider, for example, the potentially devastating social impact of a genetic technology to alter the aging process and extend life. If it were possible to genetically optimise human biology to be resistant to disease and the ravages of old age, and the middle classes in economically advanced industrialised countries availed themselves of this technology for themselves and their children, enormous social problems would result from ever-increasing population density,[22] not to mention ever-increasing healthcare spending for a population that is (by global standards and at least for now) very healthy.[23] This is an instance of what Ivan Illich refers to as 'paradoxical counterproductivity,' the process by which an institution or technology, in its normal course of operation, paradoxically subverts the very purpose it was intended to serve.[24]...[A] genetically enhanced human

species, by threatening to overwhelm existing social institutions and practices, may become, paradoxically, disabled.[25] Consider, for example, the elective use of genetic enhancement technologies to increase height with the aim of securing competitive advantage. Particular social and economic advantages may be accessible only to tall people; but there are of course height limits beyond which being tall would in fact be disadvantageous. As Dan Brock notes, "to be nine feet tall would on balance be harmful in nearly any human society because our social world is constructed for persons whose height rarely reaches beyond seven feet. One would literally become, in a physical respect, unfit for human company."[26] Now, if everyone were to be nine feet tall, the expected competitive advantage would dissipate; and if instead the social world were to be reconstituted so as to accommodate those who are nine feet tall (if not everyone were), then the competitive advantage would be a result of social, rather than genetic, enhancement.

7. *A misuse of social resources.* Considerable time, money and talent typically are required for the development of new technologies. When these technologies respond to a widespread need (or even the needs of a very deserving few), and there is the political will to ensure their just distribution, one may legitimately conclude that financial and human resources have been invested wisely. This is not the case, however, when the new technologies address the perceived needs of an affluent minority and serve to entrench existing power relations. In these instances, there are likely huge opportunity costs as other needed social and health objectives are not pursued.[27]

8. *A widening of the gap between the 'haves' and the 'have-nots'.* The first genetic enhancements available, and quite possibly the only ones, will likely be physical and intellectual enhancements. These enhancements will initially be very expensive and

only the rich (and powerful) will be able to gain access. As with other advanced technologies (such as computers and electronics), however, in time the cost of these enhancements should decrease. Even so, in all likelihood the technologies will still only be available to the middle classes, and only in some countries. A potential problem with this is that the widespread use of these technologies by those who can afford them will accentuate both the vagaries of the natural lottery as well as socio-economic differences.[28] The idea that humans are all created equal is a useful political fiction helping to establish solidarity amongst humans and to undergird social commitment to a principle of equality of opportunity, namely that despite the differences between individuals, each individual should have the opportunity to strive for success (however defined). Mehlman notes that, "in the worst case scenario, unequal access to genetic enhancement will divide society into the enhanced and the un-enhanced."[29] He argues that this split would critically threaten the basis of the principle of equality of opportunity by freezing prospects of upward social mobility. Shenk, citing Thomas Jefferson's observation that "the mass of mankind has not been born with saddles on their backs, nor a favored few booted and spurred, ready to ride them," worries that we simply cannot be confident in either the truth or the rhetorical power of those words in future.[30] More globally, Silver notes that:

> ...the social advantage that wealthy societies currently maintain could be converted into a genetic advantage. And the already wide gap between wealthy and poor nations could widen further and further with each generation until all common heritage is gone. A severed humanity could very well be the ultimate legacy of unfettered global capitalism.[31]

The claim, then, is that use of genetic enhancement technologies will increase the gap between the haves and have-nots, unmask the myth of social equality, and result in significant social disruptions both within and between societies.

9. *Promotion of social conformity and homogeneity.* While genetic enhancement technologies are commonly thought to be liberating, they can be very constraining. Experience shows that enhancement technologies are often used to reinforce inappropriate social roles, prejudices and stereotypes as people seek to advantage themselves or their children relative to others. Consider, for example, cosmetic surgery for women to achieve their ideal(ised) shape, for individuals of Japanese descent to 'Westernize' their eyes, and for individuals of Jewish heritage to alter their 'Jewish' noses. These sorts of physical enhancements promote a harmful conception of normality and hide the fact that such norms are socially and culturally constructed. This problem can only be exacerbated with genetically based physical and intellectual enhancements.[32]

10. *Undermining free choice.* Many are familiar with the aphorism 'more is not always better.' In this context, the point is that 'more options' does not mean necessarily 'more choice.' While the use of genetic enhancement technologies can be described as empowering, as when rational individuals autonomously choose to avail themselves of the technologies,[33] the fact remains that choice is always constrained by context. If the context includes the widespread use of a particular enhancement technology, personal freedom may be seriously threatened as people feel obliged to avail themselves of the technology. For example, if a significant minority of people freely choose to genetically alter their children's ability to produce growth hormone and the average height shifts upward, it will be extremely difficult, if not impossible, for parents to freely choose not to provide their child with this genetic

enhancement. There will be strong social pressure to conform, as there already is in the case of prenatal diagnosis;[34] concerning genetic enhancements, parents may well feel the need to conform just to compete.[35]

11. *The means matter morally.* While some would suggest that enhancement technologies from education to germ-line engineering exist on a continuum and are of a piece in promoting a single goal—the laudable augmentation of human capacities and traits—it is not clear that the end justifies the use of any and all possible means. Consider that particular means may be valuable in themselves (because edifying, or taxing, or demanding persistence)—independently of the overarching end—and not merely instrumentally (as means to that pre-specified end, no matter how valuable). The idea is that the experience of accomplishment (the means by which accomplishment is achieved) could itself be valuable, and not just the accomplishment (the end) alone: value is not exclusively consequential. Moreover, different means target different variables, and alternative means may well have different opportunity costs and collateral consequences—some of which will have a moral dimension—independently of shared ends. The objection is, thus, that it is inappropriate to pretend that genetic enhancement technologies are just 'more of the same' and so are therefore ethically unproblematic.[36]

TO STEER, BUT NOT TO STOP

Not all of the ethical objections described above will be persuasive for everyone, and some will persuade no one…. In our view, however, the concerns raised about the negative social consequences can be developed most persuasively, as can the worry about paradoxical counter-productivity and the notion that means matter morally….

These objections, [properly elaborated and] taken together, would seem to provide ample good reason to forsake the development and use of genetic enhancement technologies. There is no evidence as yet, however, that these arguments in particular, or any other arguments, *however well developed*, will suffice to stop the refinement and use of genetic enhancement technologies. As it happens, contemporary Western democracies have no experience with permanently halting the development and use of any enhancement technology on ethical grounds.

The typical response to the development and use of enhancement technologies involves a complex mix of outright 'condemnation' and what might be described as 'passive-aggressive resignation.' Policy statements and legislative or regulatory prohibitions are introduced with full knowledge (and acceptance) of the fact that these 'barriers' will not be entirely effective. The overarching pragmatic goal is not to stop the development and use of a specific technology, but rather to slow and possibly to steer basic and applied research. Examples in this category include the use of performance enhancement drugs, the use of psychedelic drugs and the current effort to clone a human being.

… In each of these instances, prohibitions have been, and continue to be, introduced with the putative goal of stopping the deleterious activity, knowing that in practice, the prohibitions are at most containment initiatives or speed bumps.

We fully anticipate that a similar pattern of response will prevail with the development and use of human genetic enhancement technologies. If so, we can further anticipate the following progression: "initial condemnation, followed by ambivalence, questioning and limited use, followed in turn by a change in public perceptions, advocacy and widespread acceptance."[37] Examples of enhancement technologies where the progression from 'condemnation' to 'widespread acceptance' are evident include cosmetic surgery, organ transplantation and gender reassignment. Though initially criticised, these alterations to the self are now either commonplace or well on their way to being so considered.

In anticipation of this sequela, we are driven to ask: why do arguments underscoring probable, unsavoury and unethical consequences have such a limited prospect of stopping the development and use of enhancement technologies, the potential for benefit notwithstanding? More precisely, *why is the development and use of genetic enhancement technologies inevitable?* As will become evident in what follows, by 'inevitability' we do not mean to invoke either a technological imperative or a slippery slope, but rather something more akin to "resilient to (moral) argument and resultant from particular conceptions of contemporary humanity."[38]

THE INEVITABILITY THESIS

According to some, genetic enhancement technologies are inevitable—and welcome—because they promise to secure health, success, wealth and happiness, especially for the presently disadvantaged.... [D]espite its popularity, this hypothesis surely strains one's credulity. Ours is not a kind, caring, compassionate world, but rather a capitalist, heedlessly liberal, curiosity-driven, competition-infused world in which some are intent on controlling the human evolutionary story.

Genetic enhancement technologies are inevitable because so many of us are crass capitalists, eager to embrace biocapitalism.[39] In economically advanced industrialised countries, ours is a corporate world where there is a shared commitment to capitalism, privatisation and a market-driven global economy. In this world, marked by globalisation, free markets and consumer choice, there is no enhancement technology that is too dangerous, or too transgressive, for it not to be pursued. Unrestrained consumerism is good and if this results in a free-market eugenic meritocracy, so be it.

In this worldview, only commercial viability (marketability and profitability) matters. If a genetic enhancement technology can be developed and sold (at a profit), it will be made and marketed (and not necessarily in that order). Particular nation-states can try to prohibit the development of the technology, but ultimately are unlikely to be successful. One reason, explored by Gardner, is that once any nation-state endorses human genetic enhancement as

a way to gain an industrial-commercial edge, other nation-states will be forced to follow suit.[40] A second reason concerns not nation-states but multinational corporations. The state's authority and power have been seriously eroded by globalisation. Multinationals are widely recognised as more powerful than elected governments and thus, not surprisingly, their commercial interests prevail.[41] Whether at the level of nation-states or multinational industries, ethical concerns are easily swept aside when there is (serious) money to be made.

This mercantile account of the modern world is critically incomplete, however—not least because very many of us aim to transcend crass capitalism. So, eagerness to embrace biocapitalism cannot completely explain the inevitability of genetic enhancement technologies.

Genetic enhancement technologies are inevitable because heedless liberalism is rampant. Leon Kass observes that prohibitionists are struggling "against the general liberal prejudice that it is wrong to stop people doing something."[42] Jeffrey Kahn similarly notes the (perhaps uniquely) American reticence to prohibit certain types of research and development because of the prevailing attitude that "capitalistic acts between consenting adults are none of its business."[43] Within states, the liberal reduction of the ethical complexities of genetic enhancement technologies to the sacred paradigm of individual free choice virtually guarantees the inevitability of the technologies; meanwhile, more globally, the liberal reluctance to move beyond this paradigm engenders a more general attitude of cultural relativism whereby there is neither the imperative nor the opportunity to deem some activities as just plain wrong.

Such a political diagnosis of the modern world is also seriously incomplete, however—not least because it invokes an unfair caricature of liberalism and fails to appreciate the complexities of political life both nationally and globally. So heedless liberalism is also unable to completely account for the inevitability of genetic enhancement technologies.[44]

Genetic enhancement technologies are inevitable because humans are naturally inquisitive (and tinkering) beings. Ours is a curiosity-driven, knowledge-based world that is fascinated with technology and in which the guiding mantra is 'if it can be done, it will be done, and so we should do it first.' In this world, the quest for knowledge for knowledge's sake is an all-consuming passion; understanding ourselves, unravelling the mystery of our existence, is our Holy Grail. Add to this our love of technology, and the inevitability of embracing genetic enhancement technology becomes evident. With research on genetic manipulation there is the prospect "to improve our understanding of the most complex and compelling phenomenon ever observed— the life process. We cannot be expected to deny ourselves this knowledge."[45] Nor can we be expected to restrain ourselves from harnessing and applying this knowledge.

A key feature of this worldview is the belief that scientific knowledge is value-free and yet immensely valuable…. In this view, while knowledge can be used to pursue less than praiseworthy technological interventions, this is not sufficient reason to halt the quest for scientific knowledge and understanding. If there are concerns about the misuse of knowledge in the development of a particular technology, then these should appropriately be directed to the eventual application of the technology, not hinder the search for purest scientific knowledge.

Again, some would argue that this view of the world is seriously flawed, not least because scientific knowledge, like all knowledge, is value-laden.[46] Moreover, the distinction between (basic) scientific knowledge and (applied) technology does not withstand critical scrutiny. While some would want to restrict or forbid genetic engineering in humans, it must be remembered 'that it would be difficult to separate…knowledge of molecular genetics from the know-how that manipulates the chromosome.'[47]

This account of the inevitability of genetic enhancement technologies is therefore also incomplete, as the pursuit of knowledge is bound up with social and political (and economic) factors.

A worldview according to which knowledge is neutral and can be sought for its own sake, is impoverished and so cannot completely explain the inevitability of genetic enhancement technologies.

Genetic enhancement technologies are inevitable because humans are competitive beings, always looking for new and challenging opportunities to maximize personal, social and economic advantage. Competition is (and has been) a valued human activity not only in itself but also instrumentally—competition promotes the drive to succeed and thus fosters improvement. In work, in sport, in reproduction, (and in other contexts as well), competition is both encouraged and rewarded. Humans have, throughout the ages, repeatedly shown themselves to be competitive beings driven to succeed (and/or to exceed), and willing to use most any means available to achieve the desired end.

In this view, there can be no doubt that genetic enhancement technologies will be among the means used to secure competitive or positional advantage. To be sure, this use of genetic enhancement technologies may be unfair (as when the genetic enhancements are available only to a small elite) or it may be self-defeating (as when the genetic enhancements are universally available and electively used by all so that no relative advantage is gained).[48] No matter. The point remains that genetic enhancement technologies will be used (by some or all) in attempts to gain a competitive advantage either by strengthening a particular capacity needed to pursue a specific life goal (increased height for the aspiring basketball player, or increased dexterity for the budding pianist), or by strengthening a range of capacities likely to increase one's ability to effectively pursue and master a range of options.

This worldview is flawed, however, in its narrow account of the human drive to compete and succeed. As Dan Brock astutely notes, and as we make clear above regarding means mattering morally, "sometimes a valued human activity is defined in part by the means it employs, not just by the ends at which it aims."[49] While competition is a valued human activity, this is, in large measure, because of the way it engages our physical, intellectual and other capacities. For many of us it is not only about winning, but also about how the game is played. In large part this explains the ban on the use of performance enhancement drugs in Olympic competition. On this view, achieving success in the workplace or elsewhere by means of genetic enhancement would hardly be worth the candle. As such, our competitive spirit alone cannot account for the inevitability of genetic enhancement technologies.

In sum, a common flaw with each of these characterisations of the modern world—characterisations of worldviews—is that they are one-dimensional: based either in simplistic economic, political, scientific, or sociological terms. The inevitability of genetic enhancement technologies demands a more encompassing, multi-dimensional diagnosis.

Genetic enhancement technologies are inevitable because the future is ours for the shaping. Ours is a dynamic world in which change is a constant, characterised historically by a variety of cultural revolutions (in language development, agriculture, political organization, physical technologies and, now, biotechnologies) each of which has significantly shaped the human species.[50] Given the economic, political, scientific and sociological realities sketched above, some firmly believe that the time has come for humans to shape our own destiny and to direct the course of evolution. Genetic enhancement technologies are seen as our most powerful tool for this purpose.

In previous times, humans saw themselves as beings created in the image of a divine God, later as products of natural selection and more recently as bundles of selfish genes shaped by selection.[51] Now some see humans as self-transforming beings capable of, and intent on, refashioning ourselves in our own image of what we should be.[52] In this worldview there are and should be no restrictions—financial, moral, epistemic, biological—on what is possible.

This worldview would appear to rest on a particular understanding of human purpose. Following Maslow,[53] what distinguishes humans is the drive toward self-actualization—the desire to realize human potentialities. For generations, increasing percentages of the population in many countries have not had to strive to meet lower-order physiological and safety needs. A direct consequence of this is that some humans have been able to direct their energies to the pursuit of higher order needs, the ultimate goal being to satisfy their desire to realise themselves to the fullest. These individuals have tested their physical, intellectual, emotional and moral limits seeking to learn, for example, what are the limits of the human body? What are the limits of the human mind? What are the limits to human suffering? What are the limits to human evil? These limits have been tested in sport, in business, in play, in war and in love—not with the hope of actually identifying any limits, but rather with the evolutionary goal of transcending all possible limits.

As needed, some among these few have avidly pursued physical, intellectual, psychological and moral enhancements. Now the option of pursuing these enhancements using genetic technologies is on the horizon and keenly awaited....

Here we offer an *avant garde* sketch of human nature. Humans are indeed imperfect creatures, but imperfection is not a necessary condition for humanness. Humans are not merely inquisitive or competitive; rather, we posit that the essential characteristics of humanness are *perfectibility* and the biosocial drive to pursue perfection. These essential characteristics are neither merely naturally present nor culturally driven, but rather biosocially overdetermined. We are on the cusp of what may prove to be our final evolutionary stage.

CONCLUSION

To summarise, there are good reasons to believe that attempts to develop and use genetic enhancement technologies are fraught with moral peril. Nevertheless, in our view, their development and use are inevitable, not simply because of capitalist forces (though these are by no means inconsequential), or because of heedless liberalism (which surely plays a role), or because of a natural desire for knowledge (which is also a significant consideration), or because of a natural or fostered desire to outperform (which, too, is partly explanatory), but also because this is our destiny chosen by those among us who are intent on achieving self-actualisation by controlling the human evolutionary story.

In closing, we maintain that accepting the inevitability of genetic enhancement technologies is an important and necessary step forward in the ethical debate about the development and use of such technologies. We need to change the lens through which we perceive, and therefore approach, the prospect of enhancing humans genetically. In recognizing the futility of trying to stop these technologies, we can usefully direct our energies to a systematic analysis of the appropriate scope of their use. The goal of such a project would be to influence how the technologies will be developed, and the individual, social, cultural, political, economic, ecological and evolutionary ends the technologies should serve. It is to these tasks that bioethical attention must now fully turn.

Acknowledgements

The research for this paper was supported by grants from the Social Sciences and Humanities Research Council of Canada, Dalhousie University, and the Canadian Institutes of Health Research (to FB), and from the Canadian Institutes of Health Research and Associated Medical Services, Inc. (to JSR). We are grateful to John MacMillan and other members of the Strategic Research Network on Enhancement Technologies and Human Identity, as well as several anonymous referees, for detailed comments on a draft; we are also grateful to members of the Department of Bioethics at Dalhousie University, and to participants at the Fifth World Congress (2000) of the *International Association of Bioethics*, London, UK, and the 2001 meeting of the *Society for Social Studies of Science*, Cambridge MA, for lively discussion of early versions of this article.

Notes

1. See, for instance: B. Stableford. 1984. *Future Man.* New York. Crown; and A Sandberg. (n.d.). Genetic Modifications. Available online at: *http://www. aleph.se/Trans/Individual/Body/ genes.html* (accessed 7 February, 2002).

2. For instance: L.J. Kass. 1985. *Toward a More Natural Science: Biology and Human Affairs.* New York. Free Press; and L.J. Kass. The Wisdom of Repugnance. *New Republic* 1997; 216: 17–27.

3. L. Walters & J.G. Palmer. 1997. *The Ethics of Human Gene Therapy.* New York. Oxford University Press.

4. Generally, see: E. Parens, ed. 1999. *Enhancing Human Traits: Ethical and Social Implications.* Washington. Georgetown University Press. For considerations of justice specifically, see, for instance: N. Holtug, Does Justice Require Genetic Enhancements? *Journal of Medical Ethics* 1999; 25: 137–143; and A. Buchanan, D.W. Brock, N. Daniels & D. Wikler. 2000. *From Chance to Choice: Genetics and Justice.* New York. Cambridge University Press.

5. A.D. Dreger, personal communication.

6. J.S. Robert. Interpreting the Homeobox: Metaphors of Gene Action and Activation in Evolution and Development. *Evolution & Development* 2001; 3: 287–295.

7. J.W. Gordon. Genetic Enhancement in Humans. *Science* 1999; 283: 2023–2024.

8. A caveat about *the* human genome: at the genetic level, humans differ from each other by 1/10 of 1%, but it is not the case that there is some "one" genome shared by all humans that is 99.9% identical. There is no single human genome representative of all humans, for genetic variation is the norm. See: A.L. Tauber & S. Sarkar. The Human Genome Project: Has Blind Reductionism Gone Too Far? *Perspectives in Biology and Medicine* 1992; 35: 220–235, at 228; see also E.A. Lloyd. 1994. Normality and Variation: The Human Genome Project and the Ideal Human Type. In *Are Genes Us? The Social Consequences of the New Genetics.* C.F. Cranor, ed. New Brunswick, N.J. Rutgers University Press: 99–112; and J.S. Robert. Illich, Education, and the Human Genome Project: Reflections on Paradoxical Counterproductivity. *Bulletin of Science, Technology, and Society* 1998; 18: 228–239, at 229–230.

9. In a broad discussion of genetic engineering, Heta Häyry has warned against a particular kind of defeatist pessimism, one that we avoid here.

That attitude 'cynically assumes that nothing can be done,' and that 'the total prohibition of gene-splicing activities is the only way to save humankind from the slippery slope to which mad scientists and big corporations are leading us.' Such pessimism may be self-fulfilling, in the sense that 'ordinary citizens' may decide not even to bother attempting to influence the development and use of genetic engineering technologies. Our inevitability claim, as will become evident below, is a different sort of claim altogether; it does not rest on slippery-slope foundations, and its objective is rather to spur attention to the question of how best to mediate the consequences of the development of genetic enhancement technologies. See H Häyry. 1994. How to Assess the Consequences of Genetic Engineering? In *Ethics and Biotechnology*. A. Dyson & J. Harris, eds. New York. Routledge: 144–156, at 152. See also note 38, below.

10. Sandberg, *op. cit.* note 1.

11. Stableford, *op. cit.* note 1; see also hints in this direction offered by Joseph Rosen in: L. Slater. Dr. Daedalus: A Radical Plastic Surgeon Wants to Give You Wings. *Harper's Magazine* 2001; July:57–67.

12. F. Baylis. Human Cloning: Three Mistakes and an Alternative. *Journal of Medicine and Philosophy* 2002; 27: 319–337.

13. See, for instance: J. Glover. 1984. *What Sort of People Should There Be? Genetic Engineering, Brain Control and Their Impact on Our Future World*. New York. Penguin Books; J. Harris. 1992. *Wonderwoman and Superman: The Ethics of Human Biotechnology*. Oxford. Oxford University Press; D. Heyd. 1992. *Genethics: Moral Issues in the Creation of People*. Berkeley. University of California Press; J. Wood-Harper. 1994. Manipulation of the Germ Line: Towards Elimination of Major Infectious Diseases? In *Ethics and Biotechnology, op. cit.* note 9, pp. 121–143; P. Kitcher. 1996. *The Lives to Come: The Genetic Revolution and Human Possibilities*. New York. Simon & Schuster; Walters and Palmer, *op. cit.* note 3, especially Chapter 4; and M-W. Ho. 1999. *Genetic Engineering: Dream or Nightmare?* 2nd edition. New York. Continuum.

14. Nils Holtug has noted that intuitive worries about human gene therapy are generally of the slippery slope variety and, moreover, he has argued that such slippery slope arguments can generally be overcome in the context of human gene therapy. We have thus striven to avoid explicit slippery slope objections to genetic enhancement technologies (though some of the objections may be reconstructed in slippery slope terms). See N. Holtug. Human Gene Therapy: Down the Slippery Slope? *Bioethics* 1993; 7: 402–419. See also note 38, below.

15. P. Ramsey. 1970. *Fabricated Man: The Ethics of Genetic Control*. New Haven. Yale University Press; N. Messer. Human Cloning and Genetic Manipulation: Some Theological and Ethical Issues. *Studies in Christian Ethics* 1999; 12:1–16.

16. R. Trigg. 1988. *Ideas of Human Nature: An Historical Introduction*. Oxford. Basil Blackwell.

17. As documented in: C. Merchant. 1989. *The Death of Nature: Women, Ecology, and the Scientific Revolution*. New York. Harper and Row.

18. G.E. Pence. 1998. *Who's Afraid of Human Cloning?* Lanham, MD. Rowman and Littlefield: 129–131.

19. D.T. Suzuki & P. Knudtson. 1990. *Genethics: The Ethics of Engineering Life*. Revised edition. Toronto. Stoddart.

20. UNESCO. 11 November, 1997. *Universal Declaration on the Human Genome and Human Rights*. 29th Session of the General Conference. Paris. Available online at: *http://unesdoc.unesco. org/images/0010/001096/109687eb.pdf* (accessed 7 February 2002); see also C. Byk. A Map to a New Treasure Island: The Human Genome and the Concept of Common Heritage. *Journal of Medicine and Philosophy* 1998; 23: 234–246.

21. Anonymous. Editorial: The Big Test. *New Republic* 2001; 223. Of course, it is worth emphasising again that there is no such thing in nature as *the* human genome, given the predominance of genetic variability; moreover, there is no such thing in nature as the *human* genome, given that humans share significant DNA sequences with virtually all extant and extinct creatures from apes to amoebae.

22. J. Harris. Intimations of Immortality. *Science* 2000; 288: 59.

23. D. Callahan. 1999. *False Hopes: Overcoming the Obstacles to a Sustainable, Affordable Medicine*. New Brunswick, NJ. Rutgers University Press.

24. Robert. *op. cit.* note 8, p. 229; see also: I. Illich. 1978. *Toward a History of Needs*. Berkeley. Heyday: 35, 117; and I. Illich. Disabling Professions, I.K. Illich, I.K. Zolal, J. McKnight, J. Caplan, H. Shaiken, eds. 1977. *Disabling Professions*. New York. Marion Boyars: 11–39, at pp. 28–31.

25. On 'detrimental enhancements,' see: D. Shickle. Are 'Genetic Enhancements' Really Enhancements? *Cambridge Quarterly of Healthcare Ethics* 2000; 9: 342–352, at 344–345.

26. D.W. Brock. 1998. Enhancements of Human Function: Some Distinctions for Policymakers. In *Enhancing Human Traits, op. cit.* note 4, pp. 48–69, at 59.

27. See, for instance: A. Lippman. Led (Astray) by Genetic Maps: The Cartography of the Human Genome and Health Care. *Social Science and Medicine* 1992; 35: 1469–76.

28. M.H. Shapiro. The Impact of Genetic Enhancement on Equality. *Wake Forest Law Review* 1999; 34: 561–637; L.M. Silver. 1997. *Remaking Eden: Cloning and Beyond in a Brave New World.* New York. Avon Books.

29. M.J. Mehlman. How Will We Regulate Genetic Enhancement? *Wake Forest Law Review* 1999; 34: 671–714, at 687.

30. D. Shenk. Biocapitalism: What Price the Genetic Revolution? *Harper's* 1997; December: 37–45, at 45.

31. L.M. Silver. 9 November, 1999. Reprogenetics: How Do a Scientist's Own Ethical Deliberations Enter into the Process? Paper presented at the conference *Humans and Genetic Engineering in the New Millenium—How Are We Going to Get 'Genethics' Just in Time?* Available online at: *http://www.etiskraad.dk/publikationer/genethics/ren.htm#kap02* (accessed 7 February 2002).

32. See, for instance: S. Bordo. 1998. *Braveheart, Babe,* and the Contemporary Body. In *Enhancing Human Traits: Ethical and Social Implications, op. cit.* note 4, pp. 189–221; M.O. Little. 1998. Cosmetic Surgery, Suspect Norms, and the Ethics of Complicity. In *Enhancing Human Traits, op. cit.* note 4, pp. 162–176.

33. K. Davis. 1995. *Reshaping the Female Body: The Dilemma of Cosmetic Surgery.* New York. Routledge.

34. B. Duden. 1993. *Disembodying Women: Perspectives on Pregnancy and the Unborn.* Translation by Lee Hoinacki. Cambridge. Harvard University Press; see also: Robert, *op. cit.* note 4; and J.S. Robert. Moral Truthfulness in Genetic Counseling. *Business and Professional Ethics Journal* 1998; 17: 73–93.

35. W. Gardner. Can Human Genetic Enhancement Be Prohibited? *Journal of Medicine and Philosophy* 1995; 20: 65–84.

36. Brock, *op. cit.* note 26; see also R. Cole-Turner. 1998. Do Means Matter? In *Enhancing Human Traits op. cit.* note 4, pp. 151–161; E. Parens. Is Better Always Good? The Enhancement Project. *Hastings Center Report* 1998; 28: S1–S15; S. Goering. Gene Therapies and the Pursuit of a Better Human. *Cambridge Quarterly of Healthcare Ethics* 2000; 9: 330–341; and Shickle, *op. cit.* note 25.

37. Baylis, *op. cit.* note 12.

38. An anonymous reviewer suggested that we expand on our notion of inevitability, especially to distinguish it from other arguments for inevitability. There is, for instance, a large literature on slippery slope arguments for inevitability, ably summarised in Holtug *op. cit.* note 14. Holtug follows W. van der Burg (The Slippery Slope Argument. *Ethics* 1999; 102: 42–65) in distinguishing between logical and empirical versions of the slippery slope argument. Some commentators would, of course, respond to our question ('why is the development and use of genetic enhancement technologies inevitable?') by invoking an argument to the effect that no line (or no principled line) can be drawn to prevent particular enhancements once genetic enhancement technologies have been developed (a logical slippery slope argument), or to the effect that the mere possibility of developing a technology leads to the development of that technology, and further that the mere existence of a technology leads to its inevitable use (and, possibly, abuse) (the technological imperative—an empirical slippery slope argument). It should be evident that our notion of inevitability is not of the slippery slope variety— in fact, we are not certain that there is anything at the bottom of the slope toward which to slip! Rather, we interpret inevitability in the sense of political immunity to moral criticism, on the basis of common views of the nature of humans and/ in the contemporary world. This is, of course, an empirical claim; we hope to be shown to be wrong (and if we are wrong, then, ironically, our aim will have been accomplished). But it is not a pessimistic claim in the sense objected to by Häyry; and it is not a slippery slope claim in any of the senses addressed by Holtug.

39. As cited in Shenk, *op. cit.* note 30, p. 41.

40. Gardner, *op. cit.* note 37.

41. See, for instance, R. Sandbrook. Neoliberalism's False Promise. *Literary Review of Canada* 2000; 8.8: 20–24.

42. As cited in Anonymous. The Politics of Genes: America's Next Ethical War. *Economist* 2001; 14 April: 21–24, at 21.

43. Ibid. p. 22.

44. We make this claim with some hesitation, inasmuch as Buchanan et al., in *From Chance to Choice (op. cit.* note 4), offer a sophisticated defense of

liberalism generative of the result that genetic enhancements should in principle be permissible (subject to the satisfaction of particular requirements of justice).

45. Gordon, *op. cit.* note 7, p. 2024.
46. See, for instance: H. Longino. 1990. *Science as Social Knowledge.* Princeton. Princeton University Press; L. Code. 1991. *What Can She Know? Feminist Theory and the Construction of Knowledge.* Ithaca. Cornell University Press; and R. Campbell. 1998. *Illusions of Paradox: A Feminist Epistemology Naturalized.* Lanham, MD. Rowman & Littlefield.

47. B. Allen. Forbidding Knowledge. *Monist* 1996; 79: 294–310, at 307–308.
48. Brock, *op. cit.* note 26, p. 60.
49. Ibid. p. 58.
50. J. Lederberg. 1963. Biological Future of Man. In *Man and His Future.* G.E.W. Wolstenholme, ed. Toronto. Little, Brown and Company: 263–273, at 269.
51. R. Dawkins. 1976. *The Selfish Gene.* Oxford. Oxford University Press.
52. Stableford, *op. cit.* note 1; Sandberg, *op. cit.* note 1; and Slater, *op. cit.* note 11.
53. A.H. Maslow. 1954. *Motivation and Personality.* New York. Harper.

Smart Drugs for Cognitive Enhancement: Ethical and Pragmatic Considerations in the Era of Cosmetic Neurology

Vince Cakic

In ancient Greece, it is said that students would entwine rosemary sprigs into their hair in the belief that it would improve their memory.[1] Although the desire to enhance one's cognitive abilities has not abated since then, modern advances in psychopharmacology now offer the possibility of one day realising this ancient dream. Cognitive enhancing drugs, smart drugs or ''nootropics'' (from the Greek roots noo-, mind and -tropo, turn, change), not only represent important pharmacotherapies for neurocognitive disorders such as dementia, attention deficit disorder and schizophrenia, but might also augment the minds of the healthy.[2] The possibility of purchasing ''smartness in a bottle'' is likely to have broad appeal to students with normal or above average cognitive functioning to begin with.

Need to finish that 5000–word paper on contemporary Russian literature by the morning?

Then pop the psychostimulants modafinil (Provigil) or methylphenidate (Ritalin). Or, for the old fashioned, there is still always caffeine or amphetamine (Dexedrine). Need to memorise all of the steps in the Krebs cycle? Fear not, for the likes of brahmi, piracetam (Nootropil), donepezil (Aricept) and galantamine (Reminyl) are your trusty companions! Overcome by a lack of motivation? Perhaps selegiline (Deprenyl) is for you.

As the latest incarnation of ''cosmetic neurology''—the off-label and non-prescription use of drugs in the healthy for the purposes of enhancement rather than treatment[3]—nootropics have captured the imagination of popular media as a sign of the brave new world in which we now live.[4–8] A world where we must be bigger, better and faster, where to err is all too human, and to realise one's highest potential demands that one be unfettered by their own biological limitations.

As the post-war baby boomer generation ages, there will be an increase in demand for and development of drugs that treat neurocognitive disturbances such as Alzheimer's disease, and it is likely that nootropics for the purposes of cosmetic neurology will be derived from this therapeutic market.[9] Although they currently offer modest improvements in cognitive performance at best, it is thought that future nootropics will encompass a wide array of drugs that enhance memory, attention, alertness, motivation, executive function, creativity or the need for sleep. Refer to Lanni et al[10] and de Jongh et al[11] for a review of current nootropics and future drug targets.

As evidenced by the literature,[3,12–14] the increasing use of nootropics and other forms of cosmetic neurology have been presaged for some time. However, although several authors[15–18] have considered the issue of ''academic doping'', none have examined the main ethical issues to any large extent. This is despite the widespread non-medical use of psychostimulants such as methylphenidate across universities for the purposes of enhancing concentration.[19] It seems apparent that cognitive enhancing drugs would be highly attractive to high school and university students, and the largest non-therapeutic market for future nootropics could very well be this demographic. As a corollary, the ethical and pragmatic issues that will emerge from the use of nootropics by students warrants earnest consideration.

In the absence of any existing ethical framework with which to view this issue, it may be relevant to examine the one paradigmatic human endeavour that has already wrested with the problem of performance-enhancing drugs for several decades: competitive sport.[14,20] This article will briefly consider four critical themes regarding the use of drugs in sport as they apply to nootropics in academia: (1) the argument that they are a form of cheating because they offer an unfair advantage; (2) the problem of indirect coercion; (3) the argument that they are dangerous; and that (4) regardless of the ethical implications of their use, prohibition is likely to

fail. Although this is by no means an exhaustive treatise on the matter, it is hoped that this article will provoke greater discussion of the issue than is presently the case.

PERFORMANCE-ENHANCING DRUGS CREATE AN UNEVEN PLAYING FIELD

One of the most frequently invoked arguments against the use of performance-enhancing drugs in sport is that they confer an unfair advantage to those who use them.[21–23] If the difference between winning and losing were determined not on the running track but in the chemical laboratory, it would result in an ''uneven playing field'' because athletes would not be competing on equal grounds. It is often concluded, therefore, that doping in sports is a form of cheating, because it provides doping athletes an unfair advantage over their clean competitors.[22,23]

The contention that a student's use of nootropics would produce an uneven playing field is a peculiar one. One implicit assumption of this argument appears to be the belief that without the use of nootropics, an even playing field either exists or is entirely possible. However noble an aspiration this may seem, it assumes the validity of the level playing field concept without reconciling itself with the reality of widespread biological and environmental inequalities that already exist.[12,24]

Unsurprisingly, cognitive ability is a significant predictor of academic performance[25] and twin studies indicate that IQ has a heritability of approximately 50%.[26] That is, a sizeable proportion of one's academic successes are due to the genes with which one has been naturally endowed. Moreover, resources that influence academic performance are also unevenly distributed across social classes. Home computer access,[27] private tuition[28] and even better childhood nutrition[29] are all examples of environmental factors that contribute to improved academic performance, factors that are less readily available to individuals from lower socioeconomic backgrounds.

It is clear, then, that some students have a distinct genetic or environmental advantage over others from the [outset]. Academic performance is not merely the product of hard work, discipline and other laudable personal attributes, but, it would seem, is a competition partly won by the genes and socioeconomic background of one's parents. It follows, therefore, that prohibiting nootropics would not even the playing field, because there never was an even playing field to begin with.

To be sure, nootropics would probably make an already uneven playing field more unfair, and one that is likely only to favour the wealthy who can afford to purchase them.[2,17] Not only do the rich get richer, but in the future it seems that they might also get smarter. However, using unequal distribution to justify the prohibition of nootropics is akin to prohibiting private tuition, which also increases academic performance while exacerbating educational inequalities between social classes. If socioeconomic inequalities in education are readily tolerated by society, then it would be hypocritical to apply this criterion selectively to nootropics and not to other performance-enhancing strategies.[3,12]

It is interesting to consider under what conditions society might have an obligation to ensure universal access to nootropics should highly effective compounds emerge.[14,18] If nootropics represented the most cost-effective means of enhancing academic performance, social programmes might seek to make them accessible to the underprivileged. Moreover, it is entirely possible that some nootropics would primarily benefit those in whom cognitive deficits are present, with little, no, or perhaps even deleterious effects upon the healthy.[11,12] This appears to be the case with modafinil, in which the greatest improvements in cognitive performance are seen in those with lower IQs.[30] Nootropics might therefore free underperforming students from their "neurological handicaps"—rather than creating an uneven playing field, nootropics could help to level it, increasing standards in academic performance in the process.

EVERYBODY ELSE IS TAKING THEM

Some athletes are motivated to use performance-enhancing drugs because they believe their competitors are doing so.[20,22,31] Although it is difficult to determine the prevalence of drug use in sports, anecdotal reports suggest up to 95% of elite athletes have taken them[31] and the general opinion of athletes is that few successful Olympians do not dope.[32] Therefore, in order to compensate for what might be considered an unfair advantage against them, an athlete who would otherwise not be compelled to dope may decide that this is the only avenue through which they can remain competitive against those who do.[20,31]

One concern surrounding the widespread use of nootropics is that it may indirectly coerce other students into taking them in order to keep up with their peers.[2,12,33] For example, if the majority of students were to use modafinil and their doing so vastly improved their academic performance, then the remaining non-users would feel a certain amount of pressure to follow suit in order to remain competitive. The Red Queen Principle applies here, in which an individual must continue developing in order to maintain their fitness relative to others with whom they are competing.[3] Ergo, a student must make use of every possible advantage afforded to them, eg, nootropics, as failing to do so might result in a relative loss of academic performance.

It would appear that for a student to be indirectly coerced into using nootropics, several criteria must be fulfilled. First, nootropics would need to confer substantial improvements in performance such that not taking them would place one at a distinct academic disadvantage against those who do. In addition, a sufficiently high proportion of the student's peers must use nootropics in order to edify the perception that "everybody else is taking them". Moreover, it is likely that the most successful students would need to use nootropics, so as to perpetuate the presumption that it is either impossible or prohibitively difficult for a drug-free student to attain high grades.

In the absence of empirical data, one can only speculate if any of these factors presently hold true in academia. For example, caffeine is a widely used nootropic that can reduce fatigue and promote alertness and vigilance,[34] but it is unlikely that its use is necessary for academic success and that many feel coerced into consuming it. However, some speculate that indirect coercion may already be felt by students who attend schools with high rates of methylphenidate use.[12,35]

McCabe et al[19] report that in the USA the non-medical use of methylphenidate and amphetamine in the previous year is as high as 25% in some college campuses. The most commonly cited reason for using these stimulants is to enhance concentration (58%) and increase alertness (43%), indicating that they are being used for their performance-enhancing properties.[11] Others have reported similar findings.[36,37] Interestingly, that the prevalence of methylphenidate is over two times greater at colleges with more competitive admission criteria[19] hints at indirect coercion, but this remains to be evaluated explicitly.

Although indirect coercion would imaginably be an unpleasant experience in those who feel it, the expectation that one restrain their actions for fear that it may evoke feelings of coercion in others is not a particularly cogent reason for prohibiting these actions. Students who are not employed are more likely to perform better academically than those who are.[38] As a consequence, nootropics would be no more coercive than the pressure that one should not work to support oneself financially in order to remain academically competitive. Placing constraints on people's actions so as to protect others from feelings of coercion is arguably no less an attack on personal freedom.

However, difficulties in this reasoning arise when considering indirect coercion with respect to dangerous or toxic nootropics. Should individuals be protected from the pressure of taking potentially dangerous drugs such as methylphenidate in order to succeed academically? What if the nootropic were innocuous? Would this relegate indirect coercion to a moot point? It seems reasonable to argue that few would raise the same level of concern about indirect coercion regarding caffeine use as they would towards methylphenidate. It is apparent then, that the issue of indirect coercion to use performance enhancers hinges upon the safety profile of the drug in question and that this may be a major determinant of future policy towards nootropics use.

PERFORMANCE-ENHANCING DRUGS ARE DANGEROUS

According to the World Anti-Doping Agency (WADA) one criterion for prohibiting a drug in sport is whether or not it poses an actual or potential risk to an athlete's health.[39] Chronic use of anabolic steroids, for instance, may produce hepatic disease and cardiovascular complications resulting in death.[40] Although the dangers of drugs are often overstated, these dangers seemingly justify their prohibition because legalisation may be perceived as tacit endorsement of their use. Indeed, the safety profile of a performance-enhancing drug appears to be a large determinant of whether or not it is prohibited. Caffeine, for example, reliably increases performance in a range of sports including swimming, cycling and running at doses allowed by WADA.[41] Yet despite being a form of ''cheating'' in the same vein as anabolic steroids, caffeine's use in sport is permitted because it is relatively harmless.[22]

Similar considerations have been made with regard to nootropics.[2] For nootropic psychostimulants such as methylphenidate, the dangers are real and relatively well known. Aside from its abuse potential, methylphenidate may aggravate mental illness, produce sleep disturbances and is associated with cerebrovascular complications.[42] Therefore, inadequacies of prohibition notwithstanding, restricting methylphenidate's use would be justified in the eyes of many.

In contrast, common nootropics such as caffeine and brahmi have an extensive history of use and are generally well tolerated.[41,43] For the majority of nootropics, however, there are few data on the effects of long-term use of these drugs on humans. Although many display minimal adverse effects and in some cases appear to be neuroprotective, eg, modafinil,[44] it remains to be seen whether nootropics represent a pharmacological "free lunch" or if the enhancement of some cognitive functions can only be realised at the expense of others.[10,12] For example, transgenic mice with increased expression of the NR2B protein subunit of the *N*-methyl-D-aspartate receptor display improved learning and memory functioning.[45] However, they also possess a greater ability to recall aversive events;[46] enhancing memory might not only increase the ability to recall exam material, but also negative and traumatic experiences that might otherwise be forgotten. Happiness, as they say in the classics, is good health and a bad memory, and augmenting the latter may have untoward effects upon general mental well-being.

It is clear that there are risks inherent in the use of any drug, and given that the use of nootropics by the healthy would be for the purposes of enhancement rather than treatment, some clinicians would deem any risk unacceptable.[2,3] On the other hand, the general libertarian perspective argues that provided that the individual is cognisant of the potential side effects, they are free to make their own decision to take nootropics.[3] If we take this perspective to its logical and extreme conclusion, however, is this no different to allowing the use of any nootropic, no matter how dangerous, eg, methamphetamine, provided that individuals are aware of the dangers in doing so? It would appear that both extremes are untenable—on one hand people should have a right to decide whether or not the risks of nootropics are acceptable, but civil liberties must also be balanced by the need to safeguard the public good.[47]

DRUG USE WOULD BE IMPOSSIBLE TO CONTROL

The widespread access to and use of performance-enhancing drugs in sport despite their prohibition suggests that current anti-doping measures are inadequate.[22] The competitive advantages derived from their use, the low likelihood of drug testing and the relatively minor punishment for getting caught make them attractive to many athletes.[48] As a consequence, Foddy and Savulescu[22] contend that any attempt to prohibit performance-enhancing drugs is condemned to failure. This is not influenced by ethical considerations concerning such use, but rather the belief that any attempt at prohibition is not pragmatic and possibly more harmful than regulation.[21,22,24,49] Let us consider a future scenario in which highly effective nootropics are developed: would the prohibition of these drugs for academic gain even be possible?

As in the case of controlled substances such as methylphenidate and amphetamine, the high rates of non-medical use and the ease with which they can still be obtained[36] demonstrate the inability of prohibition to control their illicit supply effectively. As nootropics would probably have legitimate therapeutic applications in the treatment of neurocognitive disorders such as dementia,[50] diversion from legitimate sources—as is the case with the aforementioned—would be highly likely.

Considerations of supply notwithstanding, just how the prohibition of nootropics in academic contexts could be enforced remains unclear. One conjures to mind the scenario of students taken to one side, cup in hand, and asked to provide a urine sample to test officials.[15] Scandal would erupt and rumours abound when the magna cum laude is stripped of his title for testing positive for modafinil—a drug that gave him near-superhuman levels of mental endurance. As laughable as it may seem, it is possible that scenarios such as this could very well come to fruition in the future. However, given that the benefits of nootropics can also be derived from periods of study at any time leading up to examinations, this would also require drug testing during non-exam periods.[14] If the current situation in competitive sport is anything to go by, any attempt to prohibit the use of nootropics will probably be difficult or inordinately expensive to police effectively.

CONCLUSIONS

In any highly competitive environment it is inevitable that people will seek to gain advantages over their competitors. This is no more apparent than in competitive sport, in which pharmacologically based performance enhancers are prohibited yet widely used. Therefore, with the development of highly effective nootropics in the future, it is likely that their use by healthy students will become more widespread. With this come a number of ethical dilemmas that warrant deeper consideration. Is there something intrinsically wrong about enhancing our minds pharmacologically? What is it about swallowing a pill to improve our cognitive abilities that offends our sensibilities, when we will happily drink a cup of coffee to increase our alertness? Should the use of nootropics by students be prohibited, and if so, on what grounds? Finally, would it even be possible to enforce the prohibition of drugs in academia?

In this article I have briefly touched upon these issues by examining some themes that have arisen from the drugs in sport debate. Ostensibly, academia is not as competitive as sport, in which the mantra ''nobody remembers second place'' governs the latter. However, high school and university are the primary competitive spheres of many people's lives, and ones that have significant bearing upon their lives in terms of both career opportunities and future earning capacity. The pressure to succeed academically is very real and in a climate in which high-stakes public examinations have increased demand for private tuition,[51] it is likely that all avenues for performance enhancement will be exhausted. Whether this culminates in the widespread use of performance-enhancing drugs to the level seen in sports remains unclear, and will probably be influenced by the competitiveness of the scholastic setting, eg, university or school entrance exams versus end of semester final exams.

By examining the main considerations from the drugs in sport debate, we may draw from almost 50 years of discussion regarding the use of performance-enhancing drugs. Those who forget history are doomed to repeat it, and it is apparent that the failures and inconsistencies inherent in anti-doping policy in sport will be mirrored in academia unless a reasonable and realistic approach to the issue of nootropics is adopted. Taking caffeine as an exemplar nootropic whose use is both safe and culturally endorsed, it is likely that drug safety will be an important factor in determining the acceptability of nootropics use within academia. If this is to be the case, then there is a greater need to examine the safety and efficacy of putative nootropics in the healthy rather than only in clinical populations. However, the widespread non-medical use of methylphenidate[36] suggests that students will use nootropics regardless of their safety or legality. Perhaps the most that can be hoped for is to have a better understanding of the dangers of nootropics so that students will take this into consideration when deciding whether or not to use them.

Acknowledgements

The author would like to thank Janin Bredehoeft, Jacob Potkonyak and Alex Marshall for suggestions on earlier drafts.

Notes

1. Le Strange R. *A history of herbal plants.* London: Angus and Robertson, 1977.
2. Chatterjee A. The promise and predicament of cosmetic neurology. *J Med Ethics* 2006;32:110–13.
3. Chatterjee A. Cosmetic neurology: the controversy over enhancing movement, mentation, and mood. *Neurology* 2004;63:968–74.
4. Szalavitz M. Popping smart pills: the case for cognitive enhancement. *Time* 6 January 2009. http://www.time.com/time/health/article/0,8599,1869435,00.html (accessed Jul 2009).
5. Fallik D. Improve my mind, please. *Philadelphia Inquirer* 2005 March:D1.
6. Douglas K, George A, Holmes B, et al. 11 Steps to a better brain. *New Scientist* 28 May 2005. http://www.newscientist.com/article/mg18625011.900–11–steps-to-a-better- brain.html (accessed Jul 2009).
7. Kher U. Can you find concentration in a bottle? *Time* 8 January 2006. http://www. time.com/time/magazine/article/0,9171,1147202,00.html (accessed Jul 2009).

8. Lawton G. Get ready for 24–hour living. *New Scientist* 18 February 2006. http:// www.newscientist.com/article/mg18925391.300–get ready-for-24hour-living.html (accessed Jul 2009).

9. Dekkers W, Rikkert MO. Memory enhancing drugs and Alzheimer's disease: enhancing the self or preventing the loss of it? *Med Health Care Philos* 2007;10:141– 51.

10. Lanni C, Lenzken SC, Pascale A, et al. Cognition enhancers between treating and doping the mind. *Pharmacol Res* 2008;57:196–213.

11. de Jongh R, Bolt I, Schermer M, et al. Botox for the brain: enhancement of cognition, mood and pro-social behavior and blunting of unwanted memories. *Neurosci Biobehav Rev* 2008;32: 760–76.

12. Farah MJ. Emerging ethical issues in neuroscience. *Nat Neurosci* 2002;5:1123–9.

13. Rose SPR. 'Smart drugs': do they work? Are they ethical? Will they be legal? *Nat Rev Neurosci* 2002;3:975–9.

14. Whitehouse PJ, Juengst E, Mehlman M, et al. Enhancing cognition in the intellectually intact. *Hastings Cent Rep* 1997;27:14–22.

15. `Turner DC, Sahakian BJ. The cognition-enhanced classroom. In: Zonneveld L, Dijstelbloem H, Ringoir D, eds. *Reshaping the human condition: exploring human enhancement.* The Hague: Rathenau Institute, 2008:107–13.

16. Sheridan K, Zinchenko E, Gardner H. Neuroethics in education. In: Illes J, ed. *Neuroethics in the 21st century: defining the issues in theory, practice, and policy.* New York: Oxford University Press, 2005:265–75.

17. Levy N. The presumption against direct manipulation. In: Levy N, ed. *Neuroethics: challenges for the 21st century.* Cambridge: Cambridge University Press, 2007:88–135.

18. Schermer M. On the argument that enhancement is ''cheating''. *J Med Ethics* 2008;34:85–8.

19. McCabe SE, Knight JR, Teter CJ, et al. Non-medical use of prescription stimulants among US college students: prevalence and correlates from a national survey. *Addiction* 2005;99:96–106.

20. Murray TH. The coercive power of drugs in sports. *Hastings Cent Rep* 1983;13:24– 30.

21. Smith ACT, Stewart B. Drug policy in sport: hidden assumptions and inherent contradictions. *Drug Alcohol Rev* 2008;27:123–9.

22. Foddy B, Savulescu J. Ethics of performance enhancement in sport: drugs and gene doping. In: Ashcroft RE, Dawson A, Draper H, McMillan JR, eds. *Principles in health care ethics.* New York: John Wiley and Sons, 2007:511–19.

23. Loland S. *Fair play in sport: a moral norm system.* London: Routledge, 2002.

24. Kayser B, Mauron A, Miah A. Current anti-doping policy: a critical appraisal. *BMC Med Ethics* 2007;8:1–10.

25. Rohde TE, Thompson LA. Predicting academic achievement with cognitive ability. *Intelligence* 2007;35:83–92.

26. Devlin B, Daniels M, Roeder K. The heritability of IQ. *Nature* 2001;388:468–70.

27. Attewell P, Battle J. Home computers and school performance. *Inf Soc* 1999;15:1–10.

28. Bloom BS. The 2 sigma problem: the search for methods of group instruction as effective as one-to-one tutoring. *Educ Res* 1984;13:4 16.

29. Glewwe P, Jacoby HG, King EM. Early childhood nutrition and academic achievement: a longitudinal analysis. *J Public Econ* 2001;81:345–68.

30. Randall DC, Shneerson JM, File SE. Cognitive effects of modafinil in student volunteers may depend on IQ. *Pharmacol Biochem Behav* 2005;82:133–9.

31. Morgan WJ. Fair is fair, or is it?: a moral consideration of the doping wars in American sport. *Sport Soc* 2006;9:177–98.

32. Rabinowicz V. Athletes and drugs: a separate pace? *Psychol Today* 1992;25:52–3.

33. Degrazia D. Prozac, enhancement, and self-creation. *Hastings Cent Rep* 2000;30:34–40.

34. Brice C, Smith A. The effects of caffeine on simulated driving, subjective alertness and sustained attention. *Hum Psychopharmacol Clin Exp* 2001;16:523–31.

35. Diller LH. The run on Ritalin: attention deficit disorder and stimulant treatment in the 1990s. *Hastings Cent Rep* 1996;26:12–18.

36. Graff Low K, Gendaszek AE. Illicit use of psycho-stimulants among college students: a preliminary study. *Psychol Health Med* 2002;7:283–7.

37. Teter CJ, McCabe SE, LaGrange K, et al. Illicit use of specific prescription stimulants among college students: prevalence, motives, and routes of administration. *Pharmacotherapy* 2006;26: 1501–10.

38. McKenzie K, Schweitzer R. Who succeeds at university? Factors predicting academic performance in first year Australian university students. *Higher Educ Res Dev* 2001;20:21–33.

39. World Anti-Doping Agency. *World-anti-doping code.* Montreal, Canada: World Anti-Doping Agency, 2003.

40. Thiblin I, Petersson A. Pharmacoepidemiology of anabolic androgenic steroids: a review. *Fund Clin Pharmacol* 2004;19:27–44.

41. Burke LM. Caffeine and sports performance. *Appl Physiol Nutr Metab* 2008;33:1319–34.

42. Leonard BE, McCartan D, White J, et al. Methylphenidate: a review of its neuropharmacological, neuropsychological and adverse clinical effects. *Hum Psychopharmacol Clin Exp* 2004;19:151–80.

43. Russo A, Borrelli F. Bacopa monniera, a reputed nootropic plant: an overview. *Phytomedicine* 2005;12:305–17.

44. Jenner P, Zeng B-Y, Smith LA, et al. Antiparkinsonian and neuroprotective effects of modafinil in the MPTP-treated common marmoset. *Exp Brain Res* 2000;133:178–88.

45. Tang Y-P, Wang H, Feng R, et al. Differential effects of enrichment on learning and memory function in NR2B transgenic mice. *Neuropharmacology* 2001;41: 779–90.

46. Tang Y, Shimizu E, Tsien JZ. Do 'smart' mice feel more pain, or are they just better learners? *Nat Neurosci* 2001;4:453.

47. Warren OJ, Leff DR, Athanasiou T, et al. The neurocognitive enhancement of surgeons: an ethical perspective. *J Surg Res* 2009;152:167–72.

48. Haugen KK. The performance-enhancing drug game. *J Sports Econ* 2004;5:67–86.

49. Savulescu J, Foddy B, Clayton M. Why we should allow performance enhancing drugs in sport. *Br J Sports Med* 2004;38:666–70.

50. Cheshire WP. Drugs for enhancing cognition and their ethical implications: a hot new cup of tea. *Expert Rev Neurother* 2006;6:263–6.

51. Kenny DT, Faunce G. Effects of academic coaching on elementary and secondary school students. *J Educ Res* 2004;98:115–26.

Medical Innovation versus Stem Cell Tourism

Olle Lindvall and Insoo Hyun

Stem cell tourism is a worrying new form of medical travel driven by hope and pretense. Clinics around the world are offering unproven stem cell-based therapies to desperate patients for an array of intractable medical conditions. Such stem cell clinics have come under attack by scientists, clinicians, and bioethicists on grounds that they exploit seriously ill patients and threaten legitimate progress in the stem cell field.[1] These concerns have found support in two recent publications. An analysis by Lau et al.[2] of online advertisements for stem cell therapies reveals that many clinics worldwide overpromise the benefits of their purported treatments and grossly downplay or ignore their attendant risks. And none backs up their claims with credible preclinical studies or other published scientific evidence. This is not simply another case of buyer beware; at stake is the potential for serious harm to vulnerable patients, many of whom may be too young to opt out of the proffered treatment. As a case in point,

Amariglio et al.[3] report of a child who developed tumors in his brain and spinal cord after being treated with a series of poorly defined fetal stem cell transplants administered at a stem cell clinic. One might conclude from these examples that stem cell tourism—as the travel metaphor suggests—is teeming with medical tourist traps selling inauthentic representations of real medical treatment to unsuspecting consumers. The solution, many would argue, is for scientists to work with regulatory bodies to tighten regulations in offending locales and better educate patients.

These are sensible responses, but we must proceed carefully. The difficulty lies in being able to distinguish clearly between objectionable stem cell tourism and legitimate attempts at medically innovative stem cell-based interventions. This is crucial for two reasons: First, failure to draw such a distinction makes it difficult to sanction against objectionable stem cell tourism and may hinder the development of ethically and scientifically responsible avenues for innovative stem cell-based care for patients with few or no acceptable alternatives. We must discourage objectionable stem cell tourism without eliminating the possibility of responsible medical innovation.

Second, the general issue of medical travel is complex, and demonizing all stem cell tourism runs the risk of giving short shrift to patients' legitimate ethical motivations for such travel. Patients are not to blame, since medical travel may represent for them their last grasp at hope. Indeed, medical travel occurs in other areas of medicine, often involving highly innovative interventions at great cost to seriously ill patients, as happens today in cardiac centers of excellence all over the United States. Likewise, medical travel now and in the future may include "proven stem cell therapies," i.e., stem cell-based treatments that have been established in the clinic and accepted by the scientific and clinical community. Such treatments, e.g., hematopoietic stem cell transplantation for leukemia, may not be available to patients in their own country. In due course, other proven treatments may be banned for political or religious reasons because of their use of human embryonic stem cells. Patients should remain free to travel to clinics offering established stem cell-based therapies. Thus, we must be able to distinguish between acceptable medical travel for innovative or proven therapies and problematic stem cell tourism.

The key question, therefore, is what are the hallmarks of an innovative stem cell-based medical intervention? To answer this question, we have to clarify the central difference between research, as carried out in a clinical trial process, and medical innovation. As explained in the seminal U.S. research ethics document, the Belmont Report, research aims at scientifically generalizable results (not patient care), whereas the goal of medical innovation is the benefit of the individual patient.[4-6] Because of these disparate aims, the regulatory requirements for clinical research do not serve as a proper surrogate for the ethical standards appropriate for attempts at medically innovative therapies.[7] In short, the ethics of medical innovation is the ethics of patient care, not research. The research ethics paradigm views innovative treatment as a departure from standard treatment and overlooks clinical situations in which the currently accepted treatments are ineffective or burdensome.[7]

From many patients' point of view, consenting to medically innovative care may be preferable to enrolling in a clinical trial, especially where patient care is decidedly not the purpose of the trial—expanding knowledge is. Patients with precious little time might not care much about expanding knowledge; what they care about is getting better and surviving. Demonizing stem cell tourism will never squelch this vital instinct. Acceptable channels must be made available to seriously ill patients.

There are additional reasons why we must reserve space for stem cell-based medical innovations. One may not be able to rely solely on the clinical trials process—moving from Phase I, through Phase II, to Phase III trials to demonstrate safety, efficacy, and possible advantages compared to available treatments—to advance the field. We believe medically innovative care could be a powerful route, in combination with the clinical trials process, for developing proven therapies if conducted with rigorous oversight and scientific integrity. There exists an enormous array of possible stem cell-based interventions, depending, e.g., on cell type, homologous or nonhomologous use, site of delivery, autologous or allogeneic transplantation, and disease indication. The result of this plurality is that some stem cell-based interventions may be more akin to a drug intervention amenable to a multistage clinical trials approach, whereas others may align more along a surgical or transplantation paradigm, for which a clinical trials approach may be practically quite difficult to use, at least initially. In the last 40 years, only 10 to 20% of all surgical techniques were developed through a clinical trials process. Some specialties, such as cardiac transplant and laparoscopic surgery, developed entirely without clinical trials.[8] Responsible medical innovation could be an important avenue for the development of stem cell-based therapies that follow a surgical paradigm or otherwise do not fit neatly into the square peg of the clinical trials process. Other approaches may evolve through the "off-label" use of approved stem cell-based interventions outside of a clinical trial, as has happened with many medical innovations in the past.

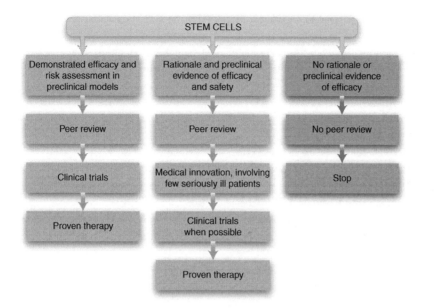

Fig.1: Different steps in alternative processes for developing new stem cell-based therapies.

In either of these cases, tough standards must be set forth to protect patients.

Developing a stem cell-based therapy via medical innovation alone is, however, not optimal. The clinical trials process enables one to compare the results of a procedure with the long-term outcome of alternative interventions, which is particularly relevant for stem cell-based therapies. These are in most cases meant to be replacement or regenerative therapies, for which long-term survival, lasting efficacy, and lack of serious side-effects are essential. The stem cell-based therapies must also be clinically competitive. Compared to available treatments, stem cell-based therapies have to offer more pronounced clinical improvement, fewer side effects, and/or lower costs.

Given the importance of both clinical trials and medical innovation, how should we proceed? The *Guidelines for the Clinical Translation of Stem Cells,*[9] drafted by the International Society for Stem Cell Research (ISSCR), emphasize the clinical trials process in the absolute majority of translational stem cell studies (Fig. 1, left track). The principles include consistent starting materials, tests in animal models, review of protocols, and informed consent from patients.

Similarly, the ISSCR Guidelines offer standards for stem cell-based medical innovation. Currently, almost all stem cell-based approaches— aside from hematopoietic stem cell transplantation for blood disorders—are "unproven." But there are important differences. The "magic cure by stem cells" approach (Fig. 1, right track), for which there is no scientific rationale or preclinical evidence of efficacy and safety, must be condemned in all circumstances. If there are no chances of improvement, the "therapy" is both unethical and scientifically and clinically unacceptable. Stem cell-based medical innovation (Fig. 1, middle track) encompasses approaches where there is a scientific rationale and for which efficacy without serious side effects has been demonstrated in animal models but the approach has not yet been established clinically. This may be due to poor availability of cells, limiting the number of patients who can be transplanted, or to rapid scientific development with a need of further optimization before formal clinical trials should be started. This category should be acceptable outside formal clinical trials in few seriously ill patients who lack good therapeutic options. Although this proposal may seem radical to some, this is not a unique approach to medical advancement. As others have argued, efforts must often be made to advance a procedure to the point at which a formal research protocol can be developed.[7,10] These initial efforts may include clarifying the types of patients who might benefit from the proposed intervention and standardizing the procedures.[7]

We emphasize, however, that stem cell-based medical innovations should be subject to a combined scientific and ethical review and proper patient protections.[9] Again, this is not a new concept. In surgery, where medical innovation is both widespread and necessary for improving patient care, medical professional societies have previously wrestled with similar questions. As a result of this vital dialogue, The Society of University Surgeons recently issued ethical guidelines for surgical innovation.[10] According to these guidelines, surgical innovators ought to submit a proposal to a local surgical innovations committee, which, like an ethical research board, would provide appropriate oversight, but within the context of patient care.[10,11] An analogous process for stem cell-based innovations has to be sensitive to the complexities of stem cell science. There should be a written plan that includes a scientific rationale, available evidence of efficacy and safety from preclinical studies in animal models as well as from applications of this intervention for other indications in humans, full characteristics of the cells to be delivered, and description of mode of cell delivery and of clinical follow-up. This plan should be approved through a review process performed by experts, and there should then be a rigorous voluntary informed consent. Transparency of this review process and institutional accountability are also desirable and crucial for continued public support of the stem cell field. Following the experience with the medically innovative procedure, the physician-scientists should, whenever possible, initiate a clinical trials process. Due to the complexity of stem cell-based approaches and their strong foundation on basic research, medical innovations should only be applied by clinicians who are experts in the field and with close links to stem cell laboratories. Our recommenda-

tion here echoes the concept of "field strength" advanced by some writing in the liver transplantation field—namely, that the team performing the innovative procedure should have proven successes in relevantly similar procedures.[12]

Given the current state of our knowledge about stem cells and their actions, patients should continue to be counseled against medical travel for unproven stem cell-based therapies at this time. In the near future, however, there will be a need to articulate further the acceptable conditions under which "unproven" stem cell therapies for specific diseases may be attempted, as medical innovation, in patients outside of clinical trials. In a world already flattened by the Internet and easy travel, this task will become increasingly difficult, especially as authoritative preclinical stem cell studies and legitimate clinical trials begin to offer promising results to the public. Thus, the public's interest in stem cell tourism is likely to increase as stem cell science advances toward the clinic. There is much work ahead for the international community of researchers, clinicians, patient advocates, and regulators.

Notes

1. I. Hyun et al., *Cell Stem Cell* 3, 607 (2008).
2. D. Lau et al., *Cell Stem Cell* 3, 591 (2008).
3. N. Amariglio et al., *PLoS Med.* 6, e1000029 (2009).
4. The Belmont Report; available at http://ohsr.od.nih.gov/guidelines/belmont.html.
5. C. E. Margo, *J. Med. Ethics* 27, 40 (2001).
6. H. Morreim, *Am. J. Bioeth.* 5, 42 (2005).
7. G. J. Agich, *J. Med. Ethics* 27, 295 (2001).
8. D. M. Cosgrove, *Cleve. Clin. J. Med.* 75, S6 (2008).
9. International Society for Stem Cell Research (ISSCR), *Guidelines for the Clinical Translation of Stem Cells*; available at www.isscr.org.
10. W. L. Biffl et al., *J. Am. Coll. Surg.* 206, 1204 (2008).
11. A. M. Reitsma, J. D. Moreno, Eds., *Ethical Guidelines for Innovative Surgery* (University Publishing Group, Hagerstown, MD, 2006).
12. D. C. Cronin, J. M. Millis, M. Siegler, *N. Engl. J. Med.* 344, 1633 (2001).
13. We are grateful to E. Borgelt for research assistance on this paper.

Useful Resources

APOGEE-Net/CanGèneTest

"APOGEE-Net/CanGèneTest is an international research and knowledge network studying health care and health policy challenges in genetic services, including genetic laboratory services. Its general objective is to streamline the technology transfer of clinically useful and cost/effective genetic innovations towards the health care system and support the development of evidence-informed health policies."

BioEdge.org: Bioethics News from Around the World

BioEdge is a weekly electronic newsletter about cutting-edge bioethical issues

Bioethics Blogs

Arthurdobrin's Weblog http://arthurdobrin.wordpress.com/
Bioethics blog http://blog.bioethics.net/
Bioethics discussion blog http://bioethicsdiscussion.blogspot.com/
Bioethics forum http://www.thehastingscenter.org/bioethicsforum/
Biopolitical Times http://www.biopoliticaltimes.org/
Clinical bioethics blog http://www.clinicalbioethics.com/
Ethics, technology, and society http://jasonmillar.ca/ethicstechnologyandsociety/
Global bioethics blog http://globalbioethics.blogspot.com/
Lost in translation http://lostintranslationethics.blogspot.com/
Neuroethics and law blog http://kolber.typepad.com/
Patients, medicine, science and trust http://johnhoey.blogspot.com/
Udo Schuklenk's Ethx blog http://ethxblog.blogspot.com/
Women's bioethics blog http://womensbioethics.blogspot.com/

Body Integrity Identity Disorder (BIID) Info

This website aims to provide accurate and complete information about Body Integrity Identity Disorder (BIID)—"a relatively unknown and misunderstood condition which leads people to need an impairment of some sort. The most often sought impairments are: amputation, paraplegia, blindness, deafness."

Bionews.org

A Web-based biotechnology resource.

Canada's Biotechnology Strategy (CBS)

"The Canadian Biotechnology Strategy (CBS) is Canada's plan for the emerging field of biotechnology that supports and compliments the regulatory and research activities of various federal departments and agencies."

Center for Genetics and Society (CGS)

"The U.S. Center for Genetics and Society is a non-profit information and public affairs organization working to encourage responsible uses and effective societal governance of the new human genetic and reproductive technologies."

European Commission: Research and Innovation—Science in Society: Governance and Ethics of New and Emerging Technologies

"As science advances, new guiding principles and rules are necessary to ensure that fundamental rights and values are preserved. The Science in Society (SIS) Programme has a role to play in making sure dialogue that frames decision-making on the governance and ethics of new and emerging technologies is rigorous, comprehensive, and transparent."

GE³LS, Genome Canada

"GE³LS stands for genomics and its related ethical, economic, environmental, legal and social aspects. GE³LS research complements genomics research by addressing questions that lie at the interface between science and society."

International Neuroethics Society

This is an "interdisciplinary group of scholars, scientists, clinicians and other professionals who share an interest in the social, legal, ethical and policy implications of advances in neuroscience." The society aims "to promote the development and responsible application of neuroscience through interdisciplinary and international research, education, outreach and public engagement for the benefit of people of all nations, ethnicities, and cultures."

International Society for Stem Cell Research (ISSCR)

"ISSCR is an independent, nonprofit organization established in 2002 to promote and foster the exchange and dissemination of information and ideas relating to stem cells, to encourage the general field of research involving stem cells, and to promote professional and public education in all areas of stem cell research and application."

Intersex Society of North America (ISNA)

"ISNA was founded in 1993 in an effort to advocate for patients and families who felt they had been harmed by their experiences with the health care system." This organization closed in 2008, but the website remains a useful resource.

National Institutes of Health (NIH), Stem Cell Information

This NIH website aims to collate information and updates about stem cell research from the scientific community.

READINGS

Allhoff, F. (2007). On the autonomy and justification of nanoethics. *Nanoethics*, 1(3), 185–210.

Benatar, D. (Ed.). (2006). *Cutting to the core: Exploring the ethics of contested surgeries*. Lanham, MD: Rowman & Littlefield Publishing.

Cotton, M. (2010). Discourse, upstream public engagement and the governance of human life extension research. *Poiesis Praxis, 7,* 135–150.

Elliott, C. (2003) *Better than well: American medicine meets the American dream.* New York: W. W. Norton.

Elliott, C. (2000). A new way to be mad: Amputations sought by healthy people. *The Atlantic Monthly,* 2866, 73–84.

Glannon, W. (2011). *Brain, body and mind: Neuroethics with a human face.* New York, NY: Oxford University Press.

Glannon, W. (2006). *Bioethics and the brain.* New York, NY: Oxford University Press.

Harris, J. (2007). *Enhancing evolution: The ethical case for making better people.* Princeton, NJ: Princeton University Press.

Jasanoff, S. (2007). *Designs on nature: Science and democracy in Europe and the United States.* Princeton, NJ: Princeton UP.

Kaplan, D. M. (2004). *Readings in the philosophy of technology.* Lanham, MD: Rowman & Littlefield.

Kimmelman, J. (2009). *Gene transfer and the ethics of first-in-human research: Lost in translation.* New York, NY: Cambridge University Press.

Levy, N. (2005). Amputees by choice: Body integrity identity disorder and the ethics of amputation. *Journal of Applied Philosophy*, 22(1), 75–86.

Levy, N. (2007). *Neuroethics: Challenges for the 21st century.* Cambridge, MA: Cambridge University Press.

Nordmann, A. (2007). If and then: A critique of speculative NanoEthics. *Nanoethics*, 1(1), 31–46.

Rose, N. (2004). Becoming neurochemical selves. In N. Stehr (Ed.), *Biotechnology, commerce and Civil Society* (pp. 89–128). New York, NY: Transaction Press.

Twine, R. (2010). *Animals as biotechnology: Ethics, sustainability and critical animal studies.* London, UK & Washington, DC: Earthscan Publications.